AF780947

Surgery of the Hip Joint

Second Edition

Volume II

Surgery of the Hip Joint

Second Edition

Volume II

Edited by Raymond G. Tronzo

With contributions by Jeffrey J. Eckardt, Michael Gitelis, Steven Gitelis, Kim Hammerberg, Michael N. Jolley, Paul A. Lotke, Dana C. Mears, Joseph H. Moll, Douglas J. Pritchard, Harry E. Rubash, Eduardo A. Salvati, Richard F. Santore, Mitchell B. Sheinkop, David R. Steinberg, Marvin E. Steinberg, Raymond G. Tronzo, B. G. Weber, and Philip D. Wilson Jr.

With 287 halftone illustrations in 506 parts and 157 line illustrations

Springer-Verlag
New York Berlin Heidelberg
London Paris Tokyo

Raymond G. Tronzo, M.D.
Palm Beach Joint Replacement Center
1114 North Olive Avenue
West Palm Beach, Florida 33401
USA

Library of Congress Cataloging-in-Publication Data
(Revised for vol. 2)
Surgery of the hip joint.
Includes bibliographies and index.
1. Hip joint—Surgery. I. Tronzo, Raymond G.
[DNLM: 1. Hip joint—Surgery. WE 860 S961]
RD549.S87 1984 617.581 84–1450

Surgery of the Hip Joint was originally published in 1973, © Lea & Febiger.

© 1987 by Springer-Verlag New York Inc.

Softcover reprint of the hardcover 2nd edition 1987

All rights reserved. This work may not be translated or copied in whole or in part without the written permission of the publisher (Springer-Verlag, 175 Fifth Avenue, New York, New York 10010, USA), except for brief excerpts in connection with reviews or scholarly analysis. Use in connection with any form of information storage and retrieval, electronic adaptation, computer software, or by similar or dissimilar methodology now known or hereafter developed is forbidden.
The use of general descriptive names, trade names, trademarks, etc. in this publication, even if the former are not especially identified, is not to be taken as a sign that such names, as understood by the Trade Marks and Merchandise Marks Act, may accordingly be used freely by anyone.
While the advice and information in this book are believed to be true and accurate at the date of going to press, neither the authors nor the editors nor the publisher can accept any legal responsibility for any errors or omissions that may be made. The publisher makes no warranty, express or implied, with respect to the material contained herein.

Typeset by Arcata/Kingsport, Kingsport, Tennessee.

9 8 7 6 5 4 3 2 1

ISBN-13: 978-1-4613-8630-8 e-ISBN-13: 978-1-4613-8628-5
DOI: 10.1007/978-1-4613-8628-5

This book is dedicated to those teachers who showed us how; to those students at all levels who challenged us to learn more; and to those patients whose comfort brought us our rewards.

Preface

The first edition of *Surgery of the Hip Joint* has had certain measures of success. Its cover won the Outstanding Award for art at a publishers trade show. A year later it was translated into Spanish for exposure to the vast world of the Spanish speaking peoples. As I traveled through Europe, it was repeatedly a pleasant surprise to have the book recognized as an authoritative reference. This was a great tribute to the experts whose diligent efforts made it all possible. Apparently the book has stood the test of time to judge from the many inquiries and constructive comments made toward urging us on to write a second edition.

It was not an easy task to gather another cadre of authorities to update our knowledge of the hip joint. People who have earned respected positions in their field are unavoidably burdened with a busy schedule, so a chapter in this text must be appreciated as coming from someone devoted to giving up some of his precious time for the sake of sharing his knowledge with peers and students.

As we struggled along, it became obvious that the book would require more than one volume because outdated concepts had to be scrapped if an up-to-date text were to be offered. Time passed so rapidly that total hip arthroplasties would not become stabilized because of a never-ending parade of implant designs with increasing bioengineering considerations. More recently the bone-cement interface has become a major source of failure which has ushered in a new era of biological bonding of the implant. Consequently, three divisions of the book have evolved. Volume I covers basics plus children's diseases of the hip; Volume II is devoted to adult hip problems and all of their surgical management with the notable exception of total hip arthroplasties, which will be explored comprehensively at a later date.

The main focus of the current book has remained the same: a comprehensive treatise on the surgical treatment of conditions of the hip joint. "There are many ways of skinning a cat" is most applicable to orthopedic surgery. Each author has been charged with giving an overview of the options and then presenting the reader with the reasons for his personal surgical approach to the problem at hand. Although this book has been used in the courtroom as a reference to support various positions, the views as stated represent only one man's opinion. They are not the last word on what is right and what is wrong.

Finally, two axioms are humbly offered. Oftentimes we as surgeons become obsessed with the mechanics of a single implant while losing sight of the principles of the operation. We, therefore, must be masters of the operation, not slaves to any device. Furthermore, we must realize that the success of any given operation will depend on whether the skill of our hands matches the quickness of our minds.

Preface to the First Edition

Whereas hand surgery must be shared with hand surgeons, foot surgery with podiatrists, fractures with general surgeons, and spine surgery with neurosurgeons, hip surgery is clearly becoming the exclusive domain of orthopedic surgeons. With the drama surrounding total hip arthroplasties, new careers are being carved out for the hip surgeon. Hip clinics are sprouting up and hip fellowships are being offered for super-subspecialty training. Indeed, hip centers are being built; although Mr. Charnley currently has the only bona fide hip center, at Wrightington, England, more will surely be established elsewhere.

Certainly the hip joint deserves all this attention. It is not only the largest joint in the body but is the site of major diseases in patients of all ages from infancy to senility. It has become the crossroads in orthopedics where clinician and basic researcher meet. Biomaterials and biomechanics were just emerging areas until their meteoric growth resulting from the complex search for the ideal artificial hip joint.

Much is being learned from the intense research surrounding the hip joint. Few problems have as yet been solved, but the future holds promises for many breakthroughs. There are signs, too, of a more aggressive surgical attack against crippling deformities. Orthopedists are increasingly inventive about new surgical procedures and are willing to treat lesions early in the evolution of the disease. With careful planning, it is hoped that this new approach will bring about happy solutions to problems rather than create new ones.

Interestingly enough, there are few books devoted to the vital hip region. Most that have been published were focused on a specific area. The need for a comprehensive text is unchallenged.

The challenge of being realistically comprehensive, up to date and authoritative has been formidable. It could not have been done alone, for no individual alive is knowledgeable enough to be a single author. What has been gathered together here, then, is a group of surgeons who come closest to being "the experts" in given areas because of their devoted interest. Overlapping has been kept to a minimum, and each author was asked to be generally comprehensive only in the sense of presenting meaningful material to the reader. The final mode of treatment was to be individualized; no one was to defend a middle ground but was urged to provide a personalized view of what he believed to be successful.

Finally, the theme of the book, as its title, was to be *Surgery of the Hip Joint,* with little emphasis on the theoretical or medical aspects of hip diseases. A notable exception to this is the chapter on soft-tissue lesions, which was included only as a means of keeping the surgical conditions in their proper perspective.

It is hoped that the book's audience will be orthopedic surgeons, both young and old, who need a global reference for the surgical management of hip disorders.

Contents

Contributors

Jeffrey J. Eckardt, M.D.
Associate Professor, Division of Orthopedic Surgery, UCLA Medical Center, Los Angeles, California, U.S.A.

Michael Gitelis, M.D.
Instructor, Orthopedic Surgery, Rush Medical College, Rush–Presbyterian–St. Lukes Medical Center, Chicago, Illinois, U.S.A.

Steven Gitelis, M.D.
Assistant Professor, Orthopedic Surgery, Rush Medical College, Rush–Presbyterian–St. Lukes Medical Center, Chicago, Illinois, U.S.A.

Kim Hammerberg, M.D.
Assistant Professor/Attending Surgeon, Orthopedic Surgery, Rush Medical College, Rush–Presbyterian–St. Lukes Medical Center, Chicago, Illinois, U.S.A.

Michael N. Jolley, M.D.
Attending Physician, Medical Center at Princeton, Princeton, New Jersey, U.S.A.

Paul A. Lotke, M.D.
Professor, Orthopedic Surgery, Chief of the Implant Surgery, Hospital of the University of Pennsylvania, University of Pennsylvania School of Medicine, Philadelphia, Pennsylvania, U.S.A.

Dana C. Mears, M.D., PH.D.
Associate Professor, Department of Orthopedic Surgery, University of Pittsburgh, Pittsburgh, Pennsylvania, U.S.A.

Joseph H. Moll, M.D.
Orthopedic Surgeon, 931 East Ocean Boulevard, Stuart, Florida, U.S.A.

Douglas J. Pritchard, M.D.
Consultant, Department of Orthopedics, Mayo Clinic and Mayo Foundation; Professor of Orthopedic Surgery, Mayo Medical School, Rochester, Minnesota, U.S.A.

Harry E. Rubash, M.D.
Assistant Professor, Department of Orthopedic Surgery, University of Pittsburgh, Pittsburgh, Pennsylvania, U.S.A.

Eduardo A. Salvati, M.D.
Chief of Hip Clinic, The Hospital for Special Surgery; Clinical Professor of Surgery, Orthopedics, Cornell University Medical College; Attending Orthopedic Surgeon, The Hospital for Special Surgery and The New York Hospital, New York, New York, U.S.A.

Richard F. Santore, M.D.
Professor of Surgery, University of California Medical School; Chief, Arthritis Program Rehabilitative Hospital, San Diego, Donald Sharp Memorial Hospital, San Diego, California, U.S.A.

Mitchell B. Sheinkop, M.D.
Associate Professor, Orthopedic Surgery, Rush Medical College, Rush–Presbyterian–St. Lukes Medical Center, Chicago, Illinois, U.S.A.

David R. Steinberg, M.D.
Assistant Instructor, Department of Orthopedic Surgery, Hospital of the University of Pennsylvania, University of Pennsylvania School of Medicine, Philadelphia, Pennsylvania, U.S.A.

Marvin E. Steinberg, M.D.
Professor and Vice Chairman, Department of Orthopedic Surgery, Hospital of the University of Pennsylvania, University of Pennsylvania School of Medicine, Philadelphia, Pennsylvania, U.S.A.

Raymond G. Tronzo, M.D.
Clinical Professor of Orthopedic Surgery, Section of Joint Replacement Surgery University of Miami Medical School, Miami; (in private practice) Palm Beach Joint Replacement Center, West Palm Beach, Florida, U.S.A.

B. G. Weber, M.D.
Professor, Chefarzt Clinic for Orthopedic Surgery, Kantonsspital, St. Gallen, Switzerland.

Philip D. Wilson Jr., M.D.
Surgeon-in-Chief, The Hospital for Special Surgery; Professor of Surgery, Orthopedics, Cornell University Medical College, New York, New York, U.S.A.

CHAPTER 1

Avascular Necrosis of the Femoral Head

MARVIN E. STEINBERG

Avascular or aseptic necrosis of bone was probably first described in 1738 by Alexander Munro.[68] In 1794 James Russell published a text on necrosis of bone,[84] and between 1829 and 1842 Jean Cruveilhier, the noted French anatomist, recorded gross deformation of the femoral head as a late complication of trauma, presumably as a result of vascular damage.[26,57,64,67] Kragelund in 1886 and Konig in 1888 published more comprehensive reports on this subject.[26,57] Freund, however, is generally credited with the first detailed description of bilateral idiopathic aseptic necrosis of the femoral heads.[34,47] The more recent works by Phemister and his associates have become classics on the etiology, pathogenesis, and treatment of this condition.[58,79-81]

Avascular necrosis of the femoral head is not a specific disease. It is the common end-result of a number of conditions, all of which presumably lead to impairment of the blood supply to the femoral head. The diagnosis is usually based on a characteristic x-ray picture and is supported by clinical and laboratory findings.

This condition has assumed a place of major importance among disorders of the hip. In 1962 Mankin and Brower reported five cases of bilateral idiopathic aseptic necrosis of the hip and stated that only 22 additional cases could be found in the English literature.[70] Since then many more idiopathic cases have been reported, and it has been recognized that this is not an uncommon disorder. Unfortunately, avascular necrosis afflicts young individuals and is frequently bilateral. It thus presents the orthopedist with a major dilemma concerning treatment. Certain measures which might have been advised only a few years ago are no longer generally recommended; others have become available, however, and newer methods of treatment are currently being evaluated. There is often disagreement over the indications for and the effectiveness of a specific procedure. The series are often too small and the follow-up too short to allow definitive conclusions. We are therefore somewhat in a state of flux concerning the treatment of avascular necrosis at the present time. This chapter can thus best serve the reader by providing an understanding of the basic etiology and pathogenesis, as well as the general principles of management, rather than limiting itself to a didactic review of the more popular operative procedures.

The material herein is based not only on a comprehensive review of the literature but also on a detailed study of more than 400 cases of avascular necrosis seen during the past 20 years. In several of these the femoral heads were available for radiological and histological examination. A number of personal communications with authorities in this field are included so as to provide current information which is not yet available in the literature.

Etiology

A variety of etiological factors may contribute to avascular necrosis of the femoral head. The disorders most frequently encountered in association with this condition are listed in Table 1–1. The phenomenon common to most if not all of these disorders is a mechanical interruption of the blood supply. We therefore prefer the terms avascular

TABLE 1–1 Conditions Associated with Avascular Necrosis of the Femoral Head

- Fracture of the femoral neck
- Traumatic dislocation of the hip
- Trauma to the hip without fracture or dislocation
- Legg-Calve-Perthes' disease
- Excessive alcohol intake
- Chronic liver disease
- Systemic steroid administration
- Renal transplantation
- Lupus erythematosus and other collagen-vascular disorders
- Caisson disease or decompression sickness
- Exposure to high altitude
- Sickle cell disease and sickle cell variants
- Miscellaneous hemoglobinopathies and coagulopathies
- Pancreatitis
- Hyperlipidemias
- Burns
- Pregnancy
- Gout
- Gaucher's disease
- Fabry's disease
- Arteriosclerosis and other vascular-occlusive disorders
- Radiation
- Slipped capital femoral epiphysis
- Reconstructive hip surgery (including cup arthroplasty, surface replacement arthroplasty, cuneiform osteotomy of the femoral neck, and synovectomy)
- Hip manipulation (including treatment of CDH and use of traction in the correction of slipped epiphysis)
- Idiopathic

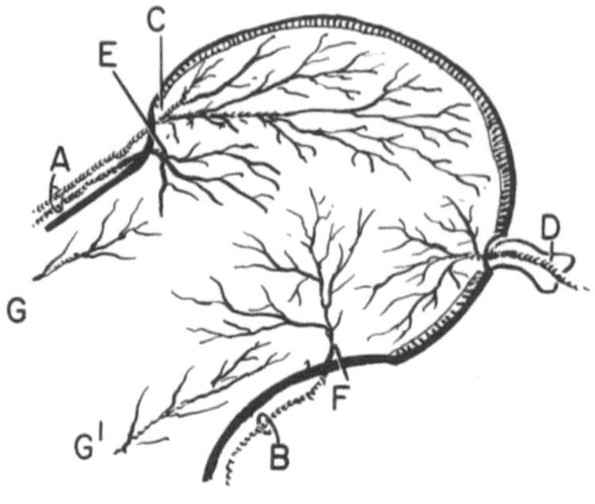

FIG. 1–1 Blood supply to the femoral head. *A*, Superior retinacular vessels. *B*, inferior retinacular vessels. *C*, lateral epiphyseal artery. *D*, medial epiphyseal artery. *E*, superior metaphyseal artery. *F*, inferior metaphyseal artery. *G* and *G'*, intramedullary vessels from the neck.

and ischemic necrosis rather than the more general terms aseptic necrosis and osteonecrosis.

The circulation to the femoral head has been described by a number of investigators,[16,18,23,89,102] most notable among these being Trueta and Harrison,[103] and is depicted in Fig. 1–1. The medial femoral circumflex artery gives rise to the superior (A) and inferior (B) retinacular vessels. These in turn give off superior metaphyseal (E) and lateral epiphyseal (C), and inferior metaphyseal (F), vessels, respectively. The obturator artery, through its acetabular branch, supplies the artery of the ligamentum teres, which ends as the medial eiphyseal artery (D). Vessels which travel upward from the femoral shaft and trochanteric region assume a subcortical position and terminate within the proximal portion of the neck (G and G'). Although anastomoses occur, these vessels possess a certain autonomy. The lateral epiphyseal artery, for example, supplies the superior lateral two-thirds of the head. The medial epiphyseal artery supplies the remaining one-third. In the neck the inferior metaphyseal vessels are the most important.

Fracture of the Femoral Neck

By far the largest group of cases of avascular necrosis of the femoral head are those seen in conjunction with trauma to the region of the hip, usually transcervical fracture or complete dislocation.[10,15,46,53] As can be seen from Fig. 1–1, significantly displaced femoral neck fractures can and usually do interrupt a major part of the blood supply to the head, leaving only the medial epiphyseal and rarely the inferior metaphyseal vessels intact. Claffey found that the superior retinacular vessels were usually torn if the neck was displaced upward by one-half the diameter of the head. When reviewing x-ray films of 178 neck fractures, he found that in 24 the fracture line crossed the course of the lateral epiphyseal arteries in the subcapital region. Of these, all 24 had clinical and x-ray evidence of avascular necrosis. In an additional 20 cases where the fracture line questionably involved the path of these arteries, avascular necrosis developed in 10.[20]

Between 65 and 85% of the heads examined during the first few weeks following transcervical fracture show areas of avascular necrosis on histological examination. Some degree of revascularization occurs, and thus the clinical evidence of avascular necrosis is lower than those figures imply. Boyd and George, excluding basilar and impacted fractures, found that 34% of transcervical fractures showed x-ray evidence of avascular necrosis within 3 years, and 14% did not unite.[11] They noted that avascular necrosis was twice as common in the nonunited fractures as in the united ones, and Bonfiglio and Voke reported it to be four to five times as common.[10] Catto, after an extensive review of the literature, concluded that approximately one-third of severely displaced femoral neck fractures failed to unite. Of those which did unite, 28% developed evidence of avascular necrosis manifested by gross collapse of the upper weight-bearing surface of the head.[15,16]

It is difficult to compile accurate statistical data on avascular necrosis, as the incidence varies considerably with the means of evaluation, the diagnostic criteria, the type of fracture, and the method of treatment. The following generalizations can be made, however. The incidence of avascular necrosis is increased in fractures which are grossly displaced, occur in the middle or high cervical region, are allowed to remain unreduced for prolonged periods, and undergo forceful manipulation or inadequate reduction and fixation. Delayed union or nonunion predisposes toward avascular necrosis, and conversely the incidence of delayed union or nonunion is increased in cases showing avascular necrosis.[9,52,53,54,85,86]

Trauma to the Hip Without Fracture

Avascular necrosis of the femoral head is also seen following trauma to the hip without fracture. In a series of 125 cases reported by Hastings and Macnab, 78% followed neck fractures, 6% followed dislocations, and 2% were related to trauma without fracture or dislocation.[47] In children the incidence of avascular necrosis following hip dislocation is 4 to 10%. This complication appears to be directly related to a delay in effecting reduction and to a lesser extent to the degree of initial trauma.[25,43] Iatrogenic trauma must also be considered in this discussion. It can include prolonged or forceful hip manipulation, as in the treatment of congenital hip dysplasia or slipped epiphysis, arthroplasties and synovectomies with dislocation and excision of the capsule and ligamentum teres, and cuneiform osteotomy for correction of slipped epiphysis or coxa vara. In these cases, as in fractures, the cause of avascular necrosis is direct mechanical disruption of the circulation.[53,68]

Legg-Calve-Perthes' Disease

Legg-Calve-Perthes' disease is covered thoroughly in Volume 1, Chapter 11 and therefore is not discussed in detail here. Although the etiology has not been definitely established, it is presumably related in some way to altered blood supply to the femoral head. This condition is unique in that it affects only children in the 4- to 12-year-old group and follows a more or less defined clinical course. Wide variations are noted in age of onset, degree of involvement, duration of disease process, and end-result. Spontaneous healing occurs over a period of 1 to 4 years, leaving patients with varying degrees of anatomical disturbance of the hip joint. In general, the smaller the area of head involvement and the shorter the healing period, the better is the end-result.[54,82]

Sickle Cell Anemia and Miscellaneous Hemoglobinopathies

Sickle cell anemia and other hemoglobinopathies account for a small but interesting group of patients with avascular necrosis of the femoral head. This lesion has been seen in at least five varieties of sickle cell disease, including classic sickle cell anemia (SS), sickle cell trait (AS), sickle cell hemoglobin C disease (SC), sickle cell thalassemia (S-thal), and hereditary persistence of fetal hemoglobin with sickle hemoglobin (SF). Of these, hip involvement is most commonly seen in those with SC disease, reports varying between 20 and 68%, whereas in patients with SS disease the incidence has been cited as 0 to 12%, presumably because of the decreased life expectancy. Accurate statistics for the other variants are not available.

The appearance of lesions in bone may be similar in all these conditions. There is diffuse or localized osteoporosis due to erythroid hyperplasia as well as the more dramatic picture of localized sclerosis or avascular necrosis due to thrombosis and infarction. Virtually any area of bone may be affected by these changes. In the femoral head different degrees of involvement have been noted, including well-localized changes resembling the so-called osteochondritis dissecans, more extensive involvement similar to that seen in Legg-Calve-Perthes' disease, and severe deformity in advanced cases. Although Legg-Perthes' disease is uncommon in Blacks, it does occur and the final diagnosis should therefore not be made without hemoglobin electrophoresis. Infarction of the humeral head has been noted in almost one-half of the patients with femoral head involvement (M. E. Steinberg, J. Rudick, and D. R. Steinberg, *unpublished data*).

Bone changes in these conditions, as well as in other hemoglobinopathies, are presumed to be the direct results of mechanical interruption to the blood supply of a region. In the case of the sickle cell variants, this occurs when systemic factors lead to sickling of red blood cells with a resultant increase in relative blood viscosity, stasis, and thrombosis of smaller vessels.[18,19,53,54,57,85]

Decompression Sickness or Dysbaric Osteonecrosis

Decompression sickness, or caisson disease, is a symptom complex involving virtually every organ of the body; it is caused by the rapid release of air bubbles from within the tissues as a result of too-rapid decompression, as well as by other factors. Although this situation occurs most commonly upon return to atmospheric pressure after prolonged exposure to hyperbaric conditions, as with caisson workers, deep-sea divers, and scuba divers, it has also been described in high-altitude fliers who go rapidly from atmospheric pressure to hypobaric conditions, thus producing a similar situation.[72] Most of the oxygen and carbon dioxide can be transported via the bloodstream to the lungs where it is expelled. Nitrogen bubbles, however, are not removed so readily and tend to accumulate within the tissues and in smaller blood vessels. Because nitrogen is approximately five times as soluble in fat as in water, this accumulation is most pronounced in those tissues richest in fat, e.g., the fatty marrow of the long bones. Confined as they are within a rigid structure, these nitrogen bubbles are able to build up a sufficient pressure to cause external compression of intramedullary vessels in addition to forming intraarterial gas emboli. The result may be local infarction of bone. The first such case was reported in 1888 by Twynam.[72]

The true incidence of bone infarction due to decompression is difficult to determine, as the reports of different series vary widely. Radiological evidence does not appear until months or even years after the circulatory insult, and clinical symptoms are often lacking unless there is involvement of an articular surface. Multiple small areas of infarction presumably occur quite frequently and defy diagnosis. In general, the incidence seems highest in those subjected most frequently to episodes of too-rapid decompression. Sites of most frequent involvement are the proximal and distal femur, proximal humerus, and proximal tibia.[1,17,53,54,57–59,72]

Alcoholism

Although the incidence of alcoholism in the general U.S. population approximates 4% "excessive" alcohol intake has been reported in 14 to 74% of patients with nontraumatic avascular necrosis of the femoral head. A high incidence of pancreatitis, liver disorder, and unrecognized trauma is also noted in these patients. The mechanism for the production of avascular necrosis, however, has not been definitely established.

Excessive alcohol intake itself, as well as liver disease, lead to significant hyperlipemia and to a variety of alterations in blood coagulability. Thus sludging, thrombosis, hemorrhage, or fat embolization could ultimately be responsible for circulatory occlusion and avascular necrosis. It has also been postulated that the sclerotic lesions within the bone represent areas of calcified fat necrosis caused by release of pancreatic enzymes, although this seems unlikely.[7,46,51,57,70,95]

Renal Transplantation

Avascular necrosis of bone is a recognized complication following renal transplantation. Initially it was reported in as many as 40% of these patients; however, more recent data suggest that the incidence has dropped to between 10 and 15%, and perhaps lower. Patients undergoing renal transplantation have generally been on chronic dialysis and have varying degrees of osteodystrophy related perhaps to both the dialysis and the renal insufficiency. Following surgery they are maintained on high doses of corticosteroids and immunosuppressive agents. Thus several factors are present which might predispose to avascular necrosis. Although most investigators have reported that steroid administration is the most probable cause, Kenzora and Glimcher concluded that the presence of the underlying renal bone disease was possibly just as important.[60]

In our own prospective series of 72 renal transplant patients, we found that despite advanced stages of renal osteodystrophy virtually none of the patients developed avascular necrosis in the absence of steroid administration. Conversely, this condition was found in 13% of those patients receiving corticosteroids.[89]

We therefore concluded that of the various etiological factors present in the transplantation patient steroid administration is probably the most important. The gratifying decline in the incidence of avascular necrosis after transplantation may be due to both a decrease in the steroid used and better medical management of these patients in general.[14,23,44,60,89]

Systemic Steroid Administration

In virtually every significant series of cases of nontraumatic avascular necrosis of the femoral head, a large proportion of patients is noted to have received steroid therapy. The incidence of steroid administration ranges from 18 to 57%. Usually patients have received relatively high doses of corticosteroids for prolonged periods, but we have encountered cases in which a moderate dose of steroid given for only 10 to 14 days apparently resulted in aseptic necrosis. Although in some cases steroid administration was presumably started after the hip involvement was present, and in a small number it was given in response to hip pain, in most instances steroid administration antedated the onset of hip disease. In most of these cases some other significant disease process was also present. Thus the question can be raised as to whether the primary systemic disorder or the steroid administration itself was responsible for the vascular changes in the femoral head. The conditions most frequently encountered include rheumatoid arthritis, renal transplantation, various dermatological conditions, asthma and other allergic disorders, the nephrotic syndrome, lupus erythematosus, and head or spinal cord trauma. Some authors have claimed that these diseases in themselves can lead to avascular necrosis and are quick to cite the occasional case of lupus erythematosus in which avascular necrosis developed without a history of steroid therapy.[83,88] In our opinion, association with such a wide variety of conditions cannot be ascribed to mere coincidence, and it must be noted that in most of these disorders there is no history of avascular necrosis in the absence of corticosteroid therapy.

Although the pathogenesis of steroid-induced avascular necrosis is unproved, several explanations have been put forth. Steroid-induced vasculitis, compression fractures of osteoporotic bone, and increased use and traumatization of a joint rendered less painful after steroid therapy are hypotheses which we find less acceptable. Of greater importance are the known hyperlipemic effects of corticosteroids, the increase of blood viscosity with sludging, and the increased incidence of fatty liver. Experimentally, intraarterial lipid injections have been shown to cause fat emboli in the small vessels of bone. In a limited number of clinical specimens investigators have noted the presence of fat emboli. Accordingly, it is our belief that many systemic conditions, e.g., lupus erythematosus and renal transplantation, previously considered as separate entities in the etiology of avascular necrosis, should be included under the general category of steroid-induced avascular necrosis.[22,23,26,32,33,44,47,54,55,57,60,66,83,103,105]

Miscellaneous Conditions

Other conditions have been mentioned occasionally in connection with avascular necrosis. These include gout,[49] Gaucher's disease,[7,30,57,70] arteriosclerosis,[51,57] Fabry's disease,[7] pelvic irradiation,[35,36] burns, and hyperlipidemias. The number of cases studied in any one category is too small to afford a direct discussion of pathogenesis. In virtually all of these situations a clear mechanism exists which could cause vascular impairment through changes in vessel walls, external occlusion, or embolization by clumped blood cells or fat droplets.[45,46,57] Arlet, Ficat, and Hungerford have postulated that an increase in the marrow pressure of the femoral head and neck may be the cause of the avascular necrosis, although they do not explain the reason for this increased pressure in all instances.[29,50,51] We therefore prefer to consider this increased pressure as part of the pathogenesis in most cases rather than as a separate etiological factor.

"Idiopathic" Avascular Necrosis

Bilateral idiopathic avascular necrosis in the adult was first reported by Freund in 1926.[34,47] Later, Chandler gave thorough consideration to this condition and described it as "coronary disease" of the hips. It is thus not surprising that the eponym

"Chandler's disease" came into being.[70] As with most idiopathic conditions, the cases which can be included here have diminished steadily with advancing knowledge. We must now delete from this group those patients in whom alcoholism, steroid administration, Cushing's disease, and hematological disorders, for example, have been noted. It seems that we might reasonably expect fewer reports of idiopathic avascular necrosis in future years.[45,46,52,53,57]

Pathogenesis

Except in the case of fresh fracture of the femoral neck, we rarely have the opportunity to examine a whole human femoral head during the early stages of avascular necrosis. The pathological changes found shortly after the vascular insult have therefore been determined primarily from cases involving trauma and from work with experimental animals.[62] These data have been supplemented by examination of core biopsies removed during early femoral head decompression as reported by Arlet, Ficat, and Hungerford.[24,50,51] Sophisticated angiographic studies by Theron have confirmed vascular occlusion during the early phase in humans.[101] Clinical and radiological abnormalities do not appear until months or years after circulatory impairment, but histological and metabolic changes occur within hours.

Although the extent of the involvement and the rate and degree of repair vary considerably, depending in part on the specific etiological factors involved, the basic pathological changes follow a similar pattern. The superior-lateral area of the head, which is most involved, not only has the most isolated blood supply but also receives the maximum stress during weight-bearing. Both of these factors contribute to the pathological changes seen. Early in the course of this disorder a significant increase may occur in the intraosseous pressure of the femoral head and neck. Although the reason for this increased pressure has not been established, it is presumed to play a role in the pathogenesis by further impairing the local circulation, as discussed.[29,50,51]

Early Stage

The earliest changes have been reported in studies of femoral heads excised within the first few days or weeks following fresh fractures. Notable among these are the works by Phemister,[79,80] Sherman and Phemister[87] and Catto.[15,16] Similar changes were noted by Kenzora et al. in experimental studies involving rabbits.[62]

The degree of involvement depends initially on the size of the area deprived of circulation, the completeness of this deprivation, and its duration. Experimental and clinical observations led to the conclusion that cells totally deprived of a blood supply for 12 hours are no longer viable; however, the first histological evidence of cell death may not be present until 48 hours later and consists of cellur dissolution and liquefaction in the marrow. The only indicator of death of bony trabeculae is the disappearance of osteocytes from within their lacunae, which does not begin to occur until 2 weeks and may not be complete until 3 to 4 weeks from the time of the vascular insult. Early in the course of this disorder no changes in articular cartilage are seen, as basic nourishment is derived from the synovial fluid.[6]

During the first few weeks a vigorous attempt at repair is often noted. An ingrowth of vascular fibrous tissue takes place from areas with intact circulation, most notably from the region supplied by the vessels of the ligamentum teres and to a lesser extent by the inferior metaphyseal arteries. A similar process occurs at the fracture site itself and is most advanced in cases with anatomical replacement and rigid fixation of the fracture fragments. Removal and replacement of necrotic marrow debris take place, new bone is laid down on dead trabeculae, and later dead bone is partially resorbed. Several investigators have reported that in virtually all femoral neck fractures some degree of avascular necrosis is present initially, often with involvement of a very large portion of the head. Because only a relatively small percent of these heads go on to the clinical and x-ray picture of established avascular necrosis, it must be presumed that a large degree of repair can and does occur in most instances.[1,6,9,15,39,42,53,87,95]

Later Stages

In a number of cases healing is not complete. The advancing front of vascular fibrous tissue seems to outstrip its blood supply and turns into a dense avascular barrier which blocks further repair. In these cases the classic findings of avascular necrosis eventually develop, as described below.

Gross Picture The articular cartilage is usually well preserved until late. Often, however, it is undermined, particularly in the anterior-superior quadrant, the main weight-bearing region of the head. This is brought about because of collapse of the underlying bone. In this area the cartilage has a somewhat wrinkled surface and can easily be pushed inward with the pressure of a finger. It may remain intact or exhibit an irregular slit or fissure in its surface, at times creating a large movable flap (see Fig. 1–16C, below). Usually a thin layer of dense cortical bone remains attached to the undersurface of the cartilage and is in turn separated from the deeper compressed trabeculae by a few millimeters. This accounts for the subchondral radiolucent line seen occasionally on x-ray films. In the most advanced cases gross fragmentation of the head occurs, and superimposed degenerative arthritis involving both the head and the acetabulum is noted.

Microscopic Picture Figure 1–2 is a representation of the classic findings in the advanced stage of avascular necrosis. Figure 1–3 is a low-power photomicrograph of a cross-section through the anterior-superior quadrant of the head which shows these changes. Five distinct zones can be identified.

Zone A represents the articular cartilage which exhibits varying degrees of abnormality in different areas of the same head. Some regions appear al-

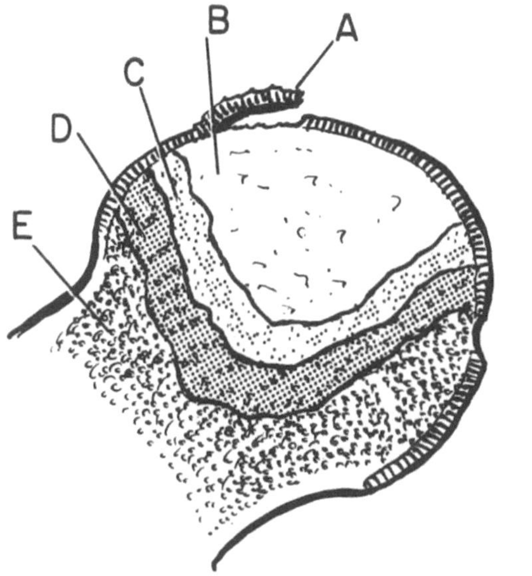

FIG. 1–2 Cross-section of the femoral head showing an advanced degree of avascular necrosis. *A*, articular cartilage. *B*, necrotic bone and marrow elements. *C*, fibrous tissue. *D*, hypertrophic new bone. *E*, normal trabeculae of the femoral neck.

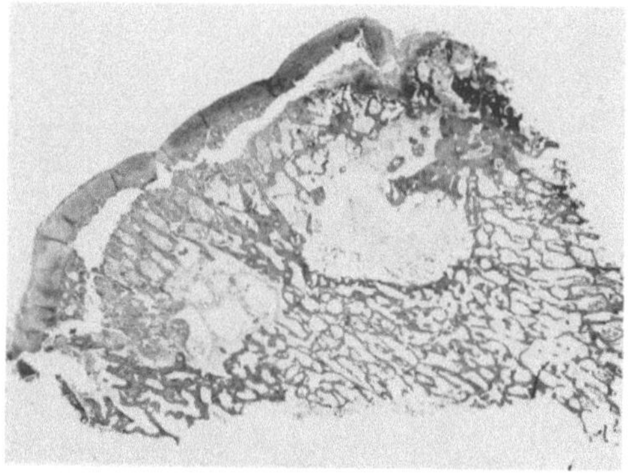

FIG. 1–3 Low-power photomicrograph of cross-section through the anterior-superior quadrant of the femoral head showing an advanced degree of avascular necrosis

most normal with only slight alteration in cellular detail and a smooth surface (Fig. 1–4A). Other regions may be totally lacking in viable cells and may show gross surface irregularity and fibrillation (Fig. 1–4B). The fact that an area of cartilage is completely undermined and lifted as a free flap from the underlying trabeculae does not necessarily mean that it loses its viability, as the primary nutrition of the cartilage is from the synovial fluid. Usually a thin layer of cortical bone remains adherent to the undersurface of articular cartilage. This bone, unlike its adjacent cartilage, is nonviable (Fig. 1–5).

Zone B represents the central area of the infarct, which has not been involved in any reparative processes. It is usually located in the anterior-superior quadrant of the head, the major weight-bearing area. Trabeculae are dead, as evidenced by the absence of osteocytes within the lacunae. Marrow elements have been replaced by acellular necrotic debris, which in areas has undergone calcification (Fig. 1–6). Occasionally, large pseudocysts filled with necrotic debris or avascular fibrillar material are present (Fig. 1–7). Toward the margins of this zone ingrowth of viable elements may be noted (Fig. 1–8). In some regions fibro-osseous metaplasia and new bone formation can be seen (Fig. 1–9), whereas in others nests of cartilage cells are found in conjunction with endochondral bone formation (Fig. 1–10).

Zone C represents the irregular border of fibrous tissue which often acts to wall off the necrotic bone from the adjacent viable bone and which has already been noted in Fig. 1–8. In some areas it is dense and avascular, whereas in others it is loosely arranged and adequately supplied with

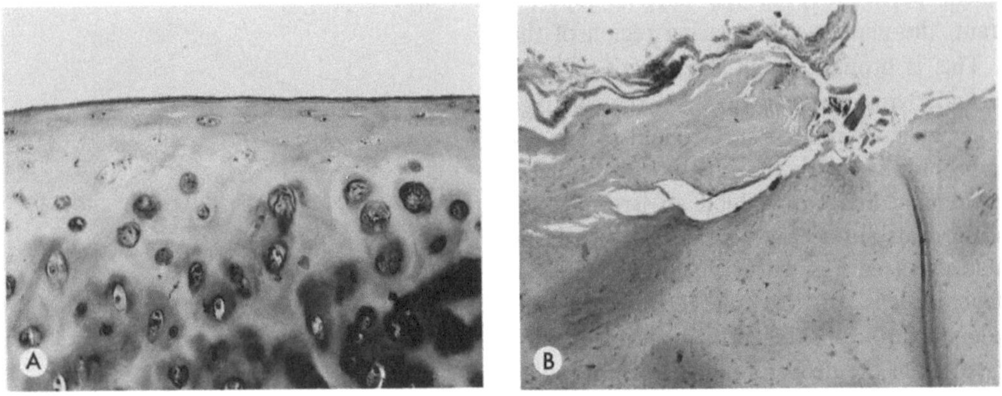

FIG. 1–4 Articular surface of the head shown in Fig. 1–3 **A** Area of intact cartilage (×42). **B** Area of dead and fibrillated cartilage (×21).

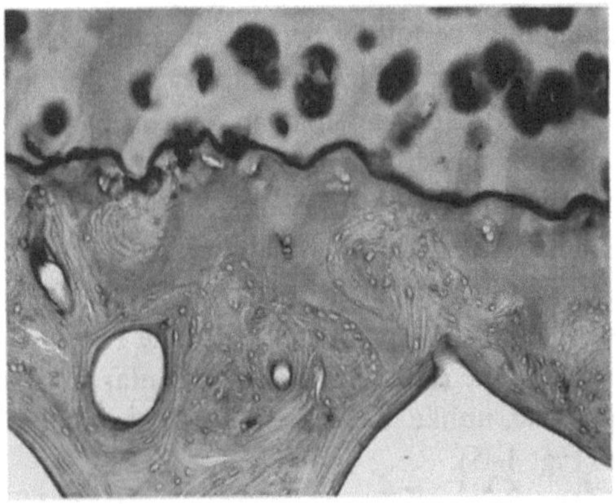

FIG. 1–5 Dead subchondral bone lying just deep to the section shown in Fig. 1–4*A* (×42).

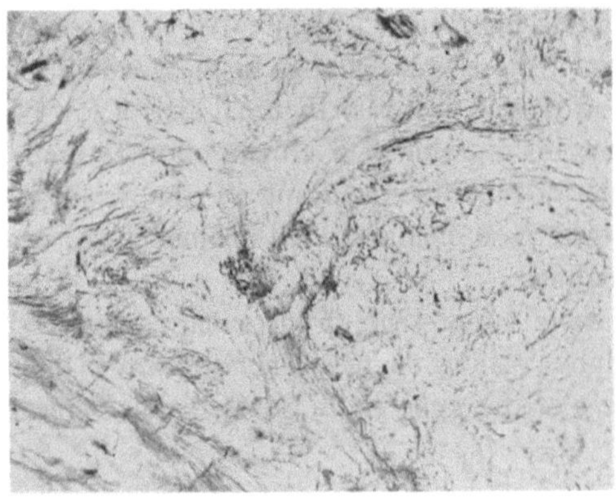

FIG. 1–7 Loose fibrillar material at the center of a large "cyst" seen in Fig. 1–3 (×21).

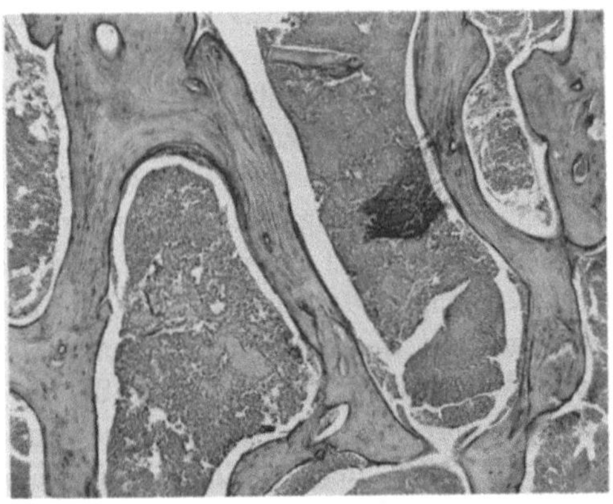

FIG. 1–6 Necrotic bone and marrow elements at the center of the avascular region (×21).

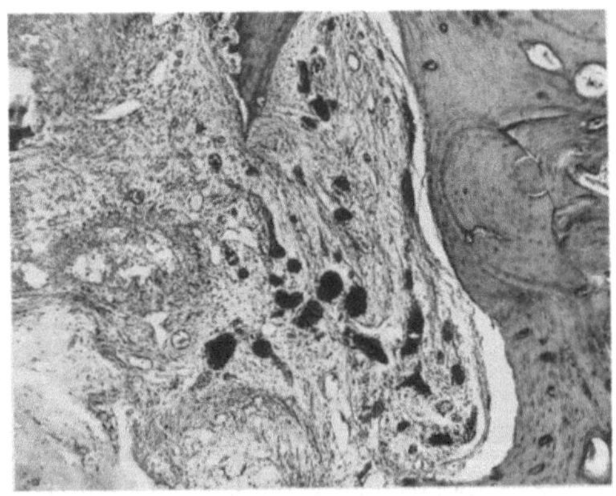

FIG. 1–8 Junction between the necrotic trabeculae and the zone of cellular fibrous tissue (×21).

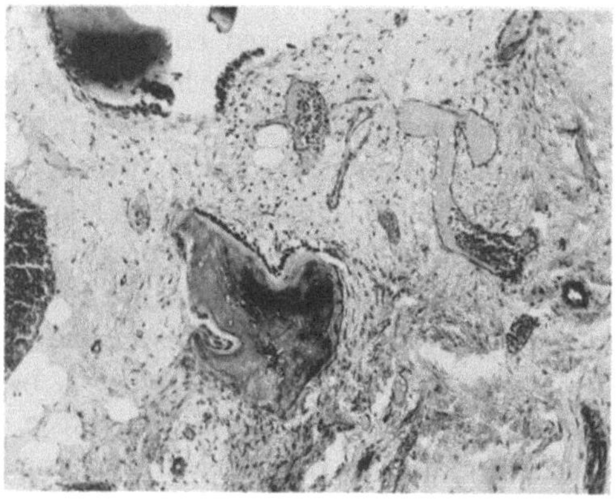

FIG. 1–9 New bone formation within fibrous tissue (×42).

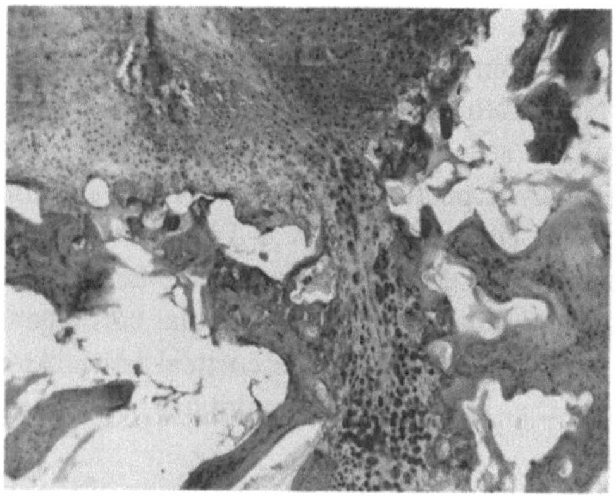

FIG. 1–10 Cartilage formation at the margin of the necrotic zone (×21).

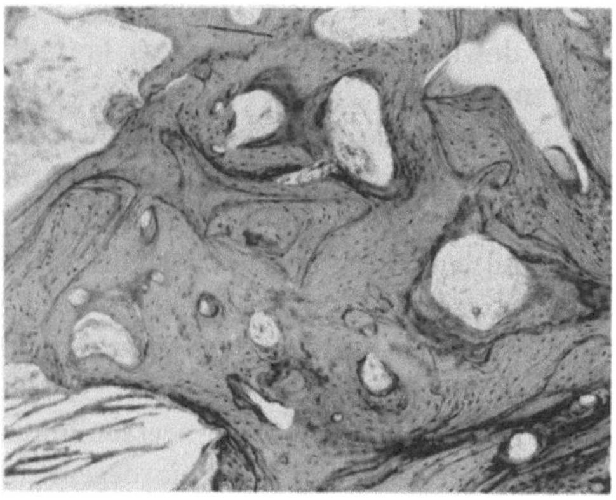

FIG. 1–11 Area of dense bone consisting in new bone formation directly on dead trabeculae (×21).

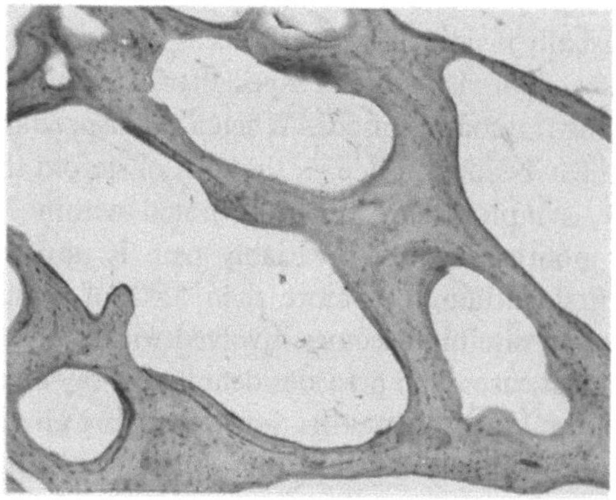

FIG. 1–12 Return to normal trabeculae of the viable inferior portion of the head (×21).

blood vessels. In some regions no true fibrous zones can be noted, and viable and nonviable trabeculae merge.

Zone D represents the hypertrophic trabeculae which are largely responsible for the sclerotic areas noted on x-ray films. These thickened trabeculae may be composed of dead bone, living bone, or more often a mixture of live bone laid down on the preexisting framework of dead trabeculae (Fig. 1–11).

Zone E represents the normal trabeculae of the femoral neck. The trabeculae are considerably more slender than those in zone D and contain abundant marrow-filled interstices (Fig. 1–12).

In most cases the synovium exhibits some degree of nonspecific synovitis. The acetabulum may remain grossly normal, even with moderately advanced disease of the femoral head. On histological examination, however, surface irregularities and chondrocyte injury may be seen. Eventually gross acetabular changes do occur, and the typical picture of degenerative arthritis develops.

Clinical Characteristics

Although avascular necrosis occurs in conjunction with and as a result of many disorders, a general clinical pattern can be noted. The picture to be described applies primarily to those cases unrelated to local trauma.

Approximately 70% of cases are diagnosed in men, with the peak incidence occurring between the ages of 30 and 50 years. The onset of symptoms is usually insidious; however, occasionally an acute onset of pain is reported, especially following some minor traumatic episode. When a predisposing insult can be identified, e.g., the start of steroid therapy, symptoms are generally noted within 3 to 18 months. Almost invariably pain is unilateral at first, although in more than 55% of patients the opposite hip becomes involved within 2 years. In most cases pain precedes definitive x-ray abnormalities by 2 to 6 months; however, x-ray changes are occasionally noted prior to the onset of pain. Adequate x-ray studies, often including laminograms or computed tomography (CT) scans and bone scans when necessary, are essential for early diagnosis. Magnetic resonance imaging (MRI) has been shown to be perhaps the best method for early diagnosis of this condition.[97] In the high-risk patient, especially one in whom the opposite hip is already involved, unexplained hip pain should alert the examiner to the possibility of avascular necrosis, even though routine x-ray studies are within normal limits.

Early in the course of the disease the range of motion is well preserved. This is in contrast to degenerative arthritis, where considerable loss of motion usually develops before pain is reported. Eventually, however, decreased motion and a limp develop. The course then becomes one of gradual deterioration as progressive degenerative changes take place.[39-42,62,69,95]

Radiological Changes

Correlation between the x-ray picture and the actual viability of the femoral head may be poor initially. Although tissue death begins within 12 hours after the circulatory insult, radiographic changes are not seen before 2 months and usually appear much later. The diagnostic accuracy of the x-ray study improves with the passage of time. For example, following high femoral neck fracture with displacement, x-ray examination leads to the diagnosis of avascular necrosis in 25% of cases by 1 year, 38% of cases by 2 years, and 56% of cases examined 3 to 7 years after trauma (Fig. 1–13).

The earliest sign is usually an increase in the density of the superior lateral area of the femoral head. This is in part relative and in part actual. Disuse of the involved extremity leads to osteoporosis of adjacent vascularized bone in the neck and acetabulum. That area of the head which lacks circulation is unable to undergo this same osteoporotic response with bone resorption. More important, however, is the actual increase in bone mass in those regions of the head undergoing a process of repair. Here thickened trabeculae are noted and are often composed of new living bone laid down on the framework of dead trabeculae (Fig. 1–11). Calcification of interstitial debris also adds a certain measure to the radiopacity. Occasionally, however, diffuse osteopenia is the first radiographic abnormality noted. In the later stages of the disease gross segmental collapse leads to increased density of the mechanically compressed bone. Areas of radiolucency also develop within the head and are usually composed of granulation or fibrous tissue which accompany the process of resorption or repair. Pseudocyst formation is frequently seen (Fig. 1–14).

Not infrequently a radiolucent line, or "crescent sign," is seen beneath the subchondral bone of the superior portion of the head on the anteroposterior or lateral film (Figs. 1–14B and 1–15). This occurs when dead cancellous bone begins to collapse and separate from the articular cartilage with its attached plate of dense cortical bone. At this stage the head usually maintains its spherical shape.

With the passage of time, flattening of the superior weight-bearing surface almost inevitably occurs as the supporting trabeculae continue to collapse. The crescent, if present earlier, gradually becomes obliterated, although a crescent sign occasionally follows rather than precedes gross collapse. The area of primary involvement stands out as a blunted wedge of sclerotic bone with its apex directed downward. Scattered areas of radiolucency remain.

Because avascular necrosis affects the bone of the femoral head rather than the articular cartilage or the acetabulum, the joint line remains well preserved until late in the course of the disease (Fig. 1–16). The irregularity of the collapsed head ultimately leads to cartilage damage and to joint line narrowing, as seen on x-ray films. Secondary changes begin to occur in the acetabulum with the appearance of sclerosis, cystic degeneration, and osteophyte formation. Eventually the picture becomes one of an end-stage degenerative hip (Fig. 1–17).[7,21,53,73,78]

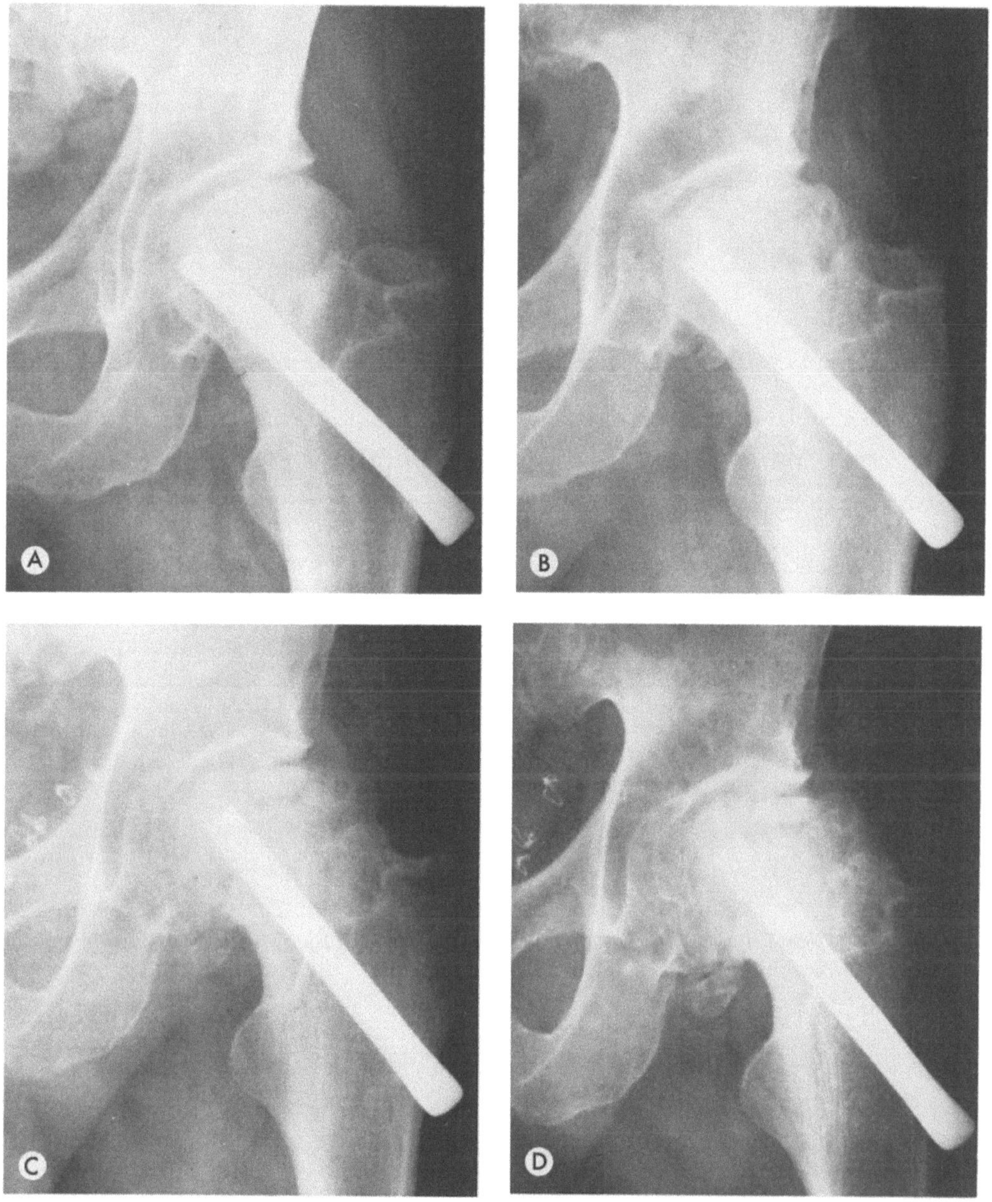

FIG. 1–13 Sequence of changes in the femoral head following high transcervical fracture with early nailing. **A** Two years after trauma. **B** Three years. **C** Five years. **D** Six years.

Although the femoral head is the site of most frequent involvement in nontraumatic avascular necrosis, occasionally other bones are affected as well. In our series this has occurred in approximately 15% of cases. The second most common area of involvement is the humeral head (Fig. 1–18).[22] Other areas may also be involved, such as the femoral condyles, dome of the talus, carpal bones, and proximal tibia. Rarely, involvement at these sites occurs before femoral head involvement.

There are clinical and radiological syndromes in which a similar picture is noted in certain areas without involvement of the femoral head. We are uncertain as to the relation between these syndromes and avascular necrosis of the femoral head in regard to etiology and pathogenesis.

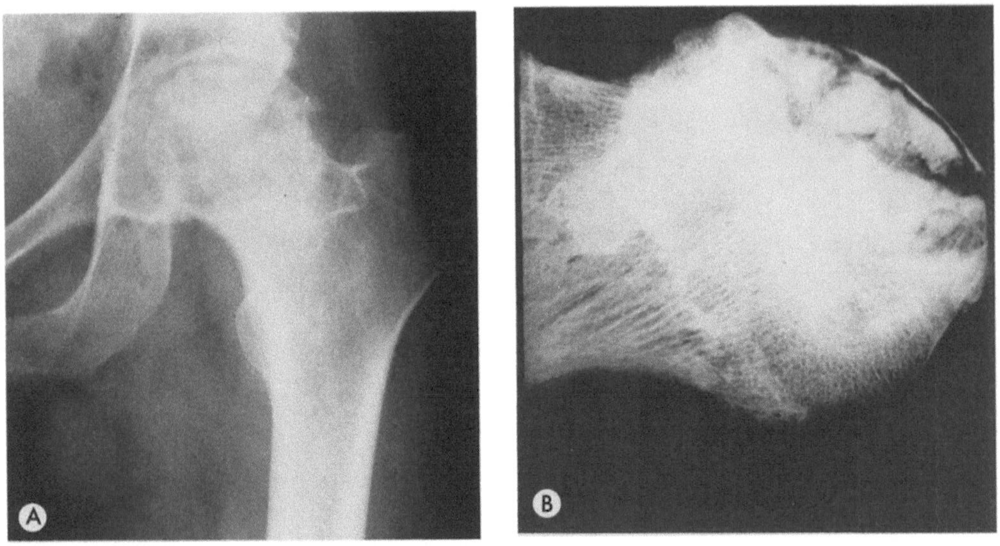

FIG. 1–14 Typical radiological changes in an advanced stage of avascular necrosis secondary to steroid administration. **A** Anteroposterior view of the hip. **B** Fine-grain x-ray film of the bisected femoral head.

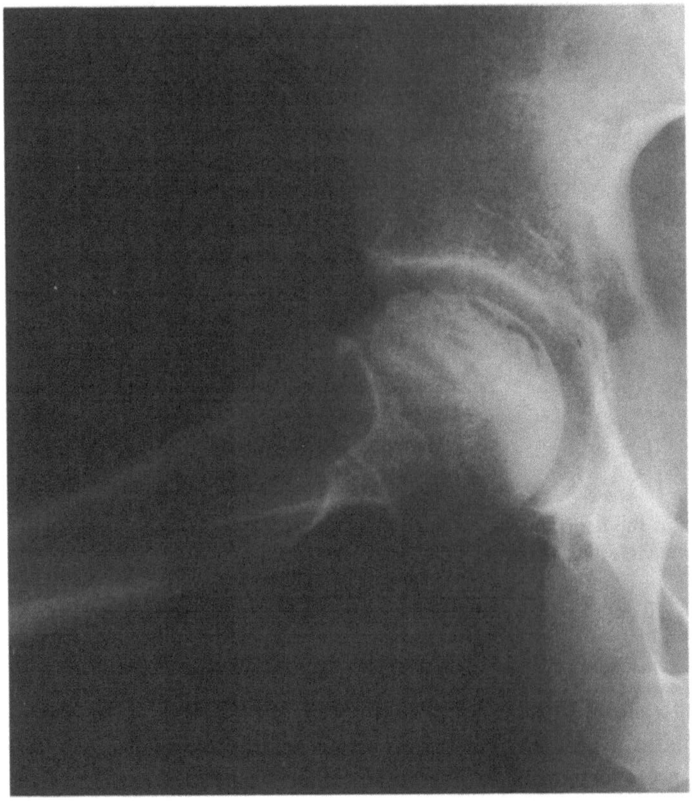

FIG. 1–15 Clear demonstration of the "crescent sign" in a lateral x-ray film.

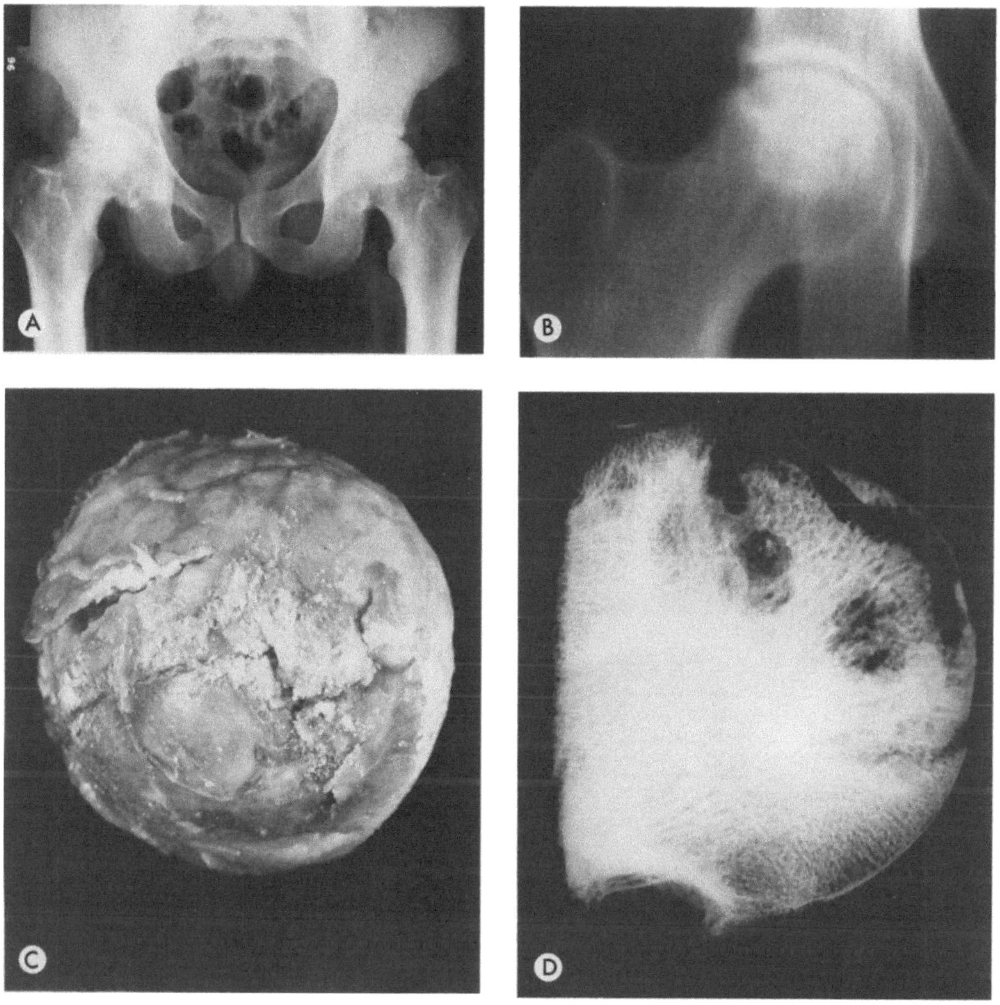

FIG. 1–16 Bilateral femoral head necrosis in a chronic alcoholic. Articular cartilage with the attached subchondral plate remains relatively intact, although the underlying cancellous bone has collapsed. **A** Anteroposterior view of the pelvis. **B** Laminogram of the right hip. **C** Gross photograph of the right femoral head following excision. **D** Fine-grain x-ray film of the anterior half of the femoral head and neck.

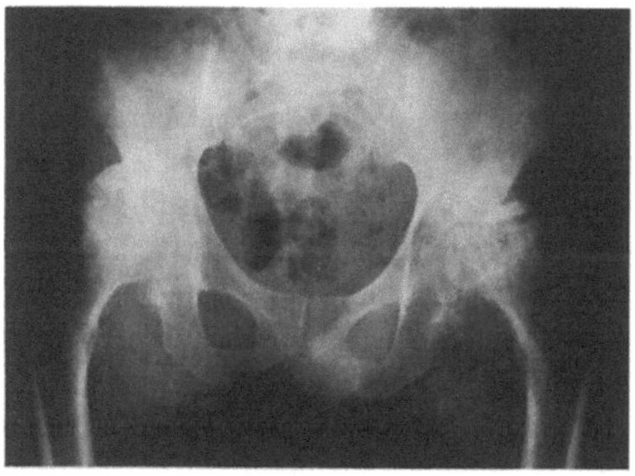

FIG. 1–17 Advanced stage of degenerative arthritis following bilateral avascular necrosis in a chronic alcoholic with pancreatitis.

Special Techniques

As mentioned earlier, there is a delay of a few to several months between the onset of avascular necrosis and the appearance of radiological changes. Because an early diagnosis is important clinically, special imaging techniques should be used when ordinary films do not confirm the suspected clinical diagnosis. Laminograms in both the anteroposterior and lateral planes are occasionally helpful (Fig. 1–16B). Bone scans using technetium-99M diphosphonate are important for early diagnosis as they generally indicate areas of avascular necrosis before such abnormalities show up

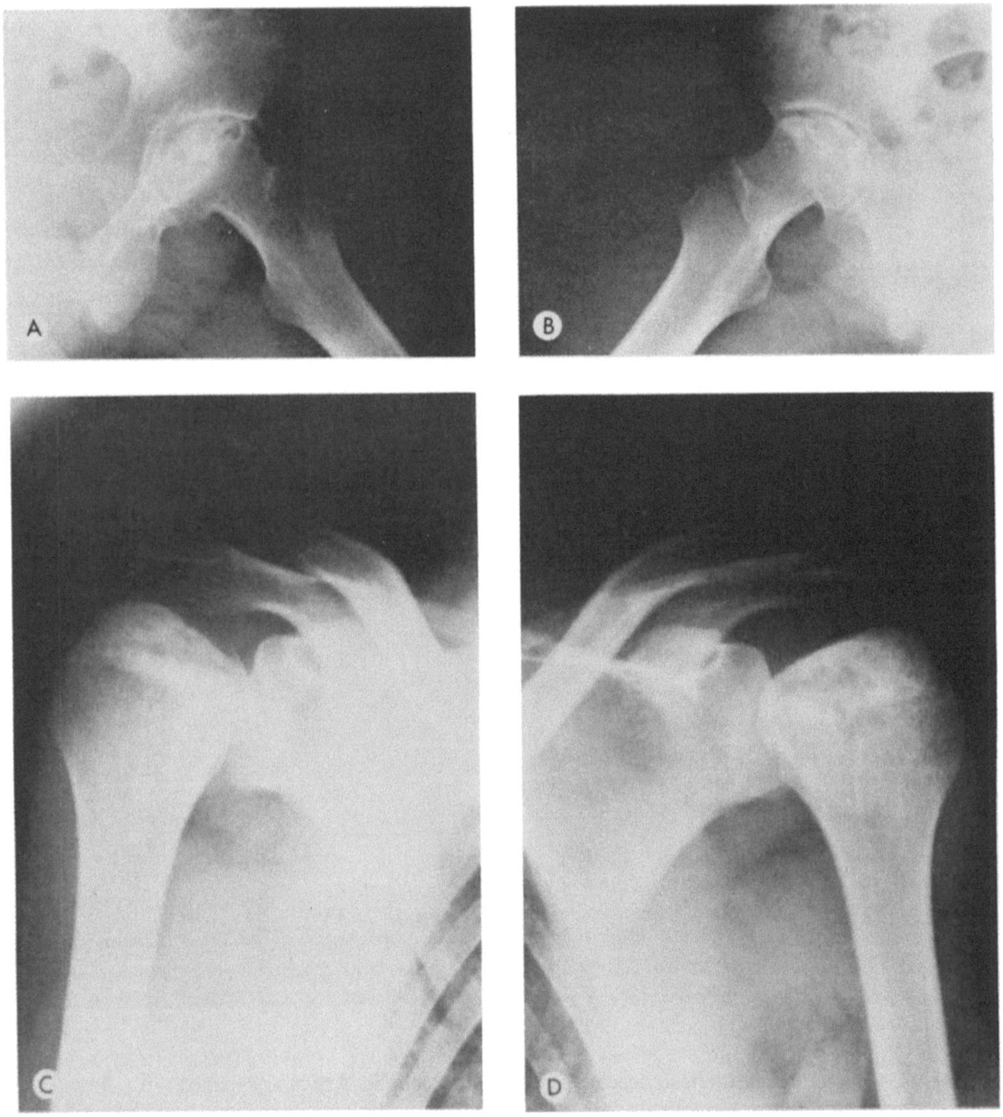

FIG. 1–18 Avascular necrosis of the femoral and humeral heads bilaterally in a patient subjected to prolonged corticosteroid treatment for the nephrotic syndrome. **A** Lateral view of the right hip. **B** Lateral view of the left hip. **C** and **D** Anteroposterior views of the shoulders.

on routine x-ray films (Fig. 1–19). This is due to a local increase in isotope uptake in conjunction with the attempted processes of repair. In some cases decreased uptake may be seen over the avascular segment in place of or in addition to the surrounding area of increased uptake. Although very sensitive, the bone scan is not selective and does not distinguish avascular necrosis from a number of other conditions. Ideally this technique leads to a diagnosis in the asymptomatic hip; however, in our series the scan generally became positive only after the onset of pain.[2,18,24]

Computed tomography (CT) has proved useful in detecting the lesion once structural changes have occurred in the bone. This technique may eventually replace conventional laminography Fig. 1–20). Specialized angiographic techniques may prove useful for the early diagnosis of avascular necrosis, but further experience is needed in this area.[102]

Magnetic resonance imaging is a technique which is proving valuable for the diagnosis of a number of musculoskeletal disorders. It is capable of detecting avascular necrosis before changes appear on plain x-ray films (Fig. 1–21). It combines the advantages of CT and radionuclide imaging

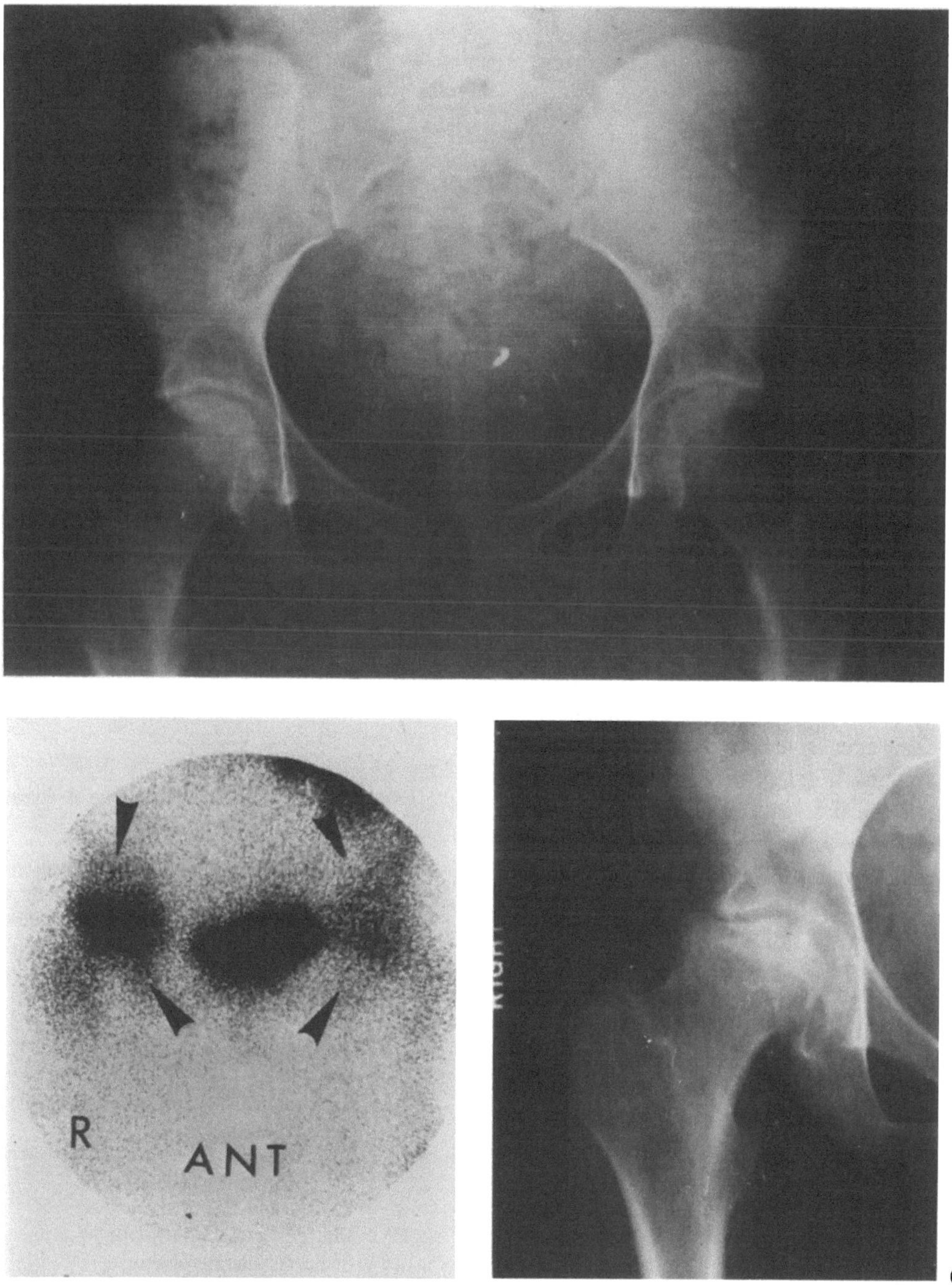

A B C

FIG. 1–19 A 19-year-old woman developed right hip pain 4 months after renal transplantation. **A** Initial x-ray films were read as "within normal limits." **B** A bone scan done at the same time was "positive," and a tentative diagnosis of avascular necrosis was made. *Arrows* = femoral head. **C** Films 3 months later showed gross collapse of the femoral head.

(bone scan) without exposing the patient to ionizing radiation. Studies have indicated that it is perhaps the best method for early diagnosis of this condition.[97]

Arlet, Ficat, and Hungerford believed that intraosseous pressure measurements and venography are sensitive methods for early diagnosis.[20,50,51] It is uncertain how well they can differentiate between avascular necrosis and other conditions involving the femoral head. A major drawback is that this is an invasive technique and may require anesthesia.

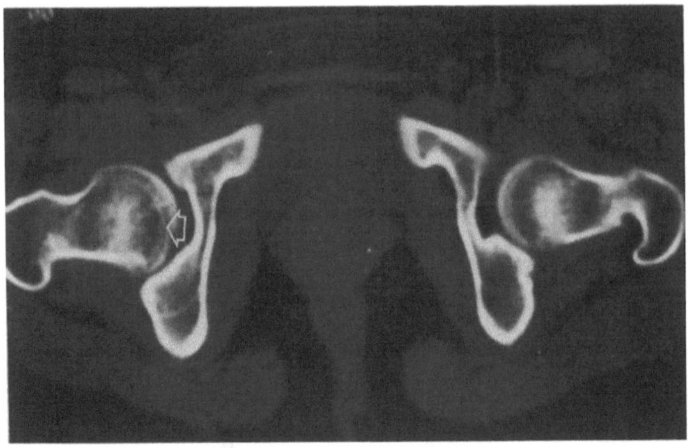

FIG. 1–20 The CT shows an extensive area of necrosis in the femoral head posteriorly.

Stages of Involvement

Evaluating the degree or stage of involvement of the femoral head is important in determining the prognosis and the optimal method of treatment. Although a number of grading systems have been devised, we have found the system described below to give us the most precise and comprehensive results without sacrificing relative simplicity (Table 1–2). It offers some important advantages over older systems. First, it provides two stages into which the earliest cases can be placed prior to the appearance of radiologic abnormalities. This is especially important as our goal is to diagnose and treat this condition as early as possible. With increasing use of radionuclide scans, MRI, and other diagnostic modalities mentioned, more cases will be diagnosed in the preradiologic stage. Second, unlike other systems, it allows us to quantitate the degree of involvement in addition to categorizing the nature of the pathological changes. For strictly clinical purposes this can be simply estimated as mild, moderate, or severe. When more precise quantitation is required, the degree of in-

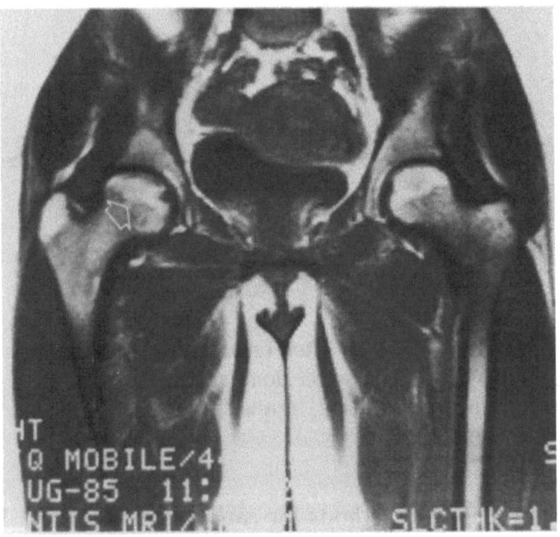

FIG. 1–21 The MRI is more sensitive in delineating the necrosis area and is more accurate in picking up the earliest lesions.

TABLE 1–2 Radiological Staging of Avascular Necrosis of the Femoral Head

Stage	Criteria
0	Normal x-ray film, normal bone scan
I	Normal x-ray film, abnormal bone scan
II	Sclerosis and/or cyst formation in femoral head
	A. Mild (<20%)
	B. Moderate (20–40%)
	C. Severe (>40%)
III	Subchondral collapse (crescent sign) without flattening
	A. Mild (<15%)
	B. Moderate (15–30%)
	C. Severe (>30%)
IV	Flattening of head *without* joint narrowing or acetabular involvement
	A. Mild (<15% of surface and <2 mm depression)
	B. Moderate (15–30% of surface *or* 2–4 mm depression)
	C. Severe (>30% of surface or >4 mm depression)
V	Flattening of head *with* joint narrowing and/or acetabular involvement
	A. Mild; B. Moderate; C. Severe (determined as above plus estimate of acetabular involvement)
VI	Advanced degenerative changes

volvement can be measured objectively by the use of point counting, concentric circles, and planimetry. This systems allows us to determine quite accurately the progression or resolution of the condition, evaluate the effectiveness of various treatment modalities, establish a prognosis, and decide on the best method of treatment.[93]

Treatment

In order to determine the best treatment for avascular necrosis, several factors must be considered: stage or degree of involvement, etiology, amount of pain and disability, duration of symptoms, age and health of the patient, social and economic situation, and whether the condition is unilateral or bilateral.

In children with avascular necrosis, e.g., in Legg-Calve-Perthes' disease, the potential for healing is far greater than in the adult, and the treatment therefore differs considerably. This is discussed in detail in Volume 1, Chapter 11.

In the adult perhaps the most significant factor is the amount of bone which has become devitalized. If the area is small, and especially if it is not adjacent to the weight-bearing surface, it may remain asymptomatic and go undiagnosed. Such "silent" infarcts are probably more common than we recognize. These areas may remain avascular and asymptomatic, or they may be replaced with living bone. In virtually all intracapsular fractures some degree of avascular necrosis is present; but if it is not extensive and if the fracture is treated appropriately, the avascular area eventually heals. In such circumstances no specific treatment is required for the avascular necrosis itself.

The best treatment for any disease is prevention. This applies equally to avascular necrosis of the femoral head. With increasing awareness of the causes of this condition, we should be able to increase our effectiveness in preventing it. In those intracapsular fractures in which the femoral head can be saved, early and optimum reduction and fixation decrease the incidence of avascular necrosis. In the badly displaced fractures in which the blood supply has almost certainly been interrupted, primary prosthetic replacement is often the best treatment. In various medical conditions requiring steroid treatment, the dose should be kept as low as possible and another agent used when equally effective. In renal disorders, in addition to keeping the steroid dose low, optimal management of the renal failure itself and improved dialysis techniques are important in decreasing the incidence of avascular necrosis. Measures are available to decrease the incidence of dysbaric osteonecrosis in divers and caisson workers, and these should be employed.[56] Similarly, it is important that optimal management be instituted in the case of sickle cell disease and that care be exercised in the use of irradiation to the pelvis and hip region.

In most clinical cases of avascular necrosis of the femoral head, a significant percentage of the weight-bearing area is involved. If left untreated, virtually all eventually collapse and develop significant pain and disability.[29,63,90,94] It is therefore important to diagnose this condition as early as possible and to proceed quickly with the appropriate treatment, even though the measures currently available are not completely effective. We must maintain a high index of suspicion in the patient who is particularly susceptible to this condition, such as the individual on long-term steroids or the heavy drinker. This is especially true if the opposite hip is already involved, as the incidence of bilaterality is more than 55%.

If x-ray studies are not diagnostic, a bone scan and perhaps MRI studies should be obtained. In selected instances intraosseous pressure measurements, as advocated by Arlet, Ficat, and Hungerford,[29,50,51] and angiography, as described by Theron,[101] are also to be considered, although these techniques are not in general use at the present time. Ideally, diagnosis is made before symptoms develop; however, in practice the majority of cases are initially diagnosed after the onset of pain.

The specific therapeutic measures to be considered are listed in Table 1–3. Each of these is discussed in some detail initially, and we then attempt to indicate which measures are most applicable to each stage of the disorder. The basic determination which must be made is whether the goal is symptomatic management, preservation of the femoral head, or joint reconstruction.[3,28,31,42,50,63,65,71,76,90,94,95]

Symptomatic Management

During the earliest stages of the disorder symptomatic measures alone have generally been used. Limited weight-bearing has often been instituted

TABLE 1–3 Treatment of Avascular Necrosis of the Femoral Head

Symptomatic management
Observation, analgesics
Limited weight-bearing
Preservation of the femoral head
Drilling or "core decompression"
Grafting
Cancellous bone
Cortical bone
Muscle-pedicle bone graft
Bone graft with microvascular anastomosis
Osteochondral allograft
Osteotomy
Angulation
Rotation (Sugioka)
Electrical stimulation
Joint reconstruction
Cup arthroplasty
Standard
"Adjusted cup"
Femoral head replacement
Single component
Multicomponent
Surface replacement arthroplasty
Total hip replacement
Miscellaneous
Fusion
Girdlestone pseudarthrosis

in the hope that it will prevent or at least retard collapse of the femoral head. Although this approach may be successful when the area of involvement is minimal, it is unsuccessful in the majority of cases we are called on to treat. In our series, 92% of cases progressed with no indication that limited weight-bearing retarded this progression. It therefore seems that prescribing a cane or crutches, except for pain relief, is an unnecessary restriction.[29,63,90,94]

Symptomatic management is indicated when the diagnosis is not yet established, when measures designed to preserve the femoral head cannot yet be instituted for one reason or another, or when the condition has progressed beyond the point where the joint can be preserved but has not yet reached the stage where reconstruction is required.

Preservation of the Femoral Head

Preservation of the femoral head, although often not achievable, must always be our goal. If collapse can be prevented, secondary degenerative changes in the articular cartilage and in the acetabulum will not occur.

Drilling and "Core Decompression"

Drilling has long been advocated as a means of restoring circulation to the avascular segment by forming a pathway for the ingrowth of new vessels. These vessels in turn enable the necrotic bone to be resorbed and new bone to be formed. Arlet, Ficat, and Hungerford have advocated early "core decompression" to decrease the intramedullary pressure which they have found elevated in most cases of avascular necrosis. Instead of simply drilling the head, they remove one or more cylindrical cores of bone, going from just below the greater trochanter and extending well into the necrotic segment. These cores are examined histologically to confirm the diagnosis. In their opinion the primary value of the procedure is to decompress the head and neck, thereby eliminating what they believe is a significant link in the chain of events leading to necrosis of bone. Weight-bearing is restricted for at approximately 3 months. Using this approach, they achieved favorable results and in many cases prevented femoral head collapse, particularly if the procedure was employed early (D. S. Hungerford, *personal communication*).[29,50,51] Results reported by other investigators have been less successful, however (J. E. Kenzora and M. J. Glimcher, *personal communication*).[94]

Grafting

The use of bone graft was first popularized by Phemister[81] and later modified by Bonfiglio and associates.[8,10] The hip is approached laterally, and one or more channels are created with a drill or a coring device from just below the greater trochanter, through the necrotic segment, and to or through the articular cartilage. These investigators advocated the use of cortical-cancellous bone struts from the tibia to provide mechanical support for the articular surface, thereby preventing collapse during the healing process. If an unstable nonunion is also present, the fixation may be supplemented by threaded pins. They reported satisfactory results in more than 70% of cases. Although best in early cases (without collapse), Bonfiglio (*personal communication*) has also used it after collapse has begun and believes it retards progression.[28,71,90,94]

When avascular necrosis is not complicated by nonunion of the neck, the hip may be approached anteriorly. A window is made in the neck, and the necrotic area is curetted widely and packed with cancellous bone graft. Although this provides more direct visualization of the affected area and allows more complete removal, it necessitates violation of the joint with the possibility of increased morbidity. The results of this technique have been disappointing according to Sugioka. (*personal communication*).

In 1978 Meyers reported his experience with a muscle-pedicle bone graft inserted into a posterior window at the femoral head–neck junction after curettage of the necrotic area and packing with cancellous bone. Of 23 cases followed 1 to 4 years, all eight which were operated on before femoral head collapse obtained good results, whereas 9 of 15 operated on after collapse obtained poor results.[75,76]

These experiences led him to a second approach. In five patients followed 6 months to 2 years, areas of gross collapse were excised, filled with cancellous bone, and then resurfaced with fresh cadaver osteochondral grafts. Of these, three obtained excellent early results, and two had good results.[75] Other authors have reported mixed results with similar techniques. At the present time this approach must be considered experimental because of the technical problems involved, the small number of cases done, and the short follow-up.

In general, grafting procedures have not worked uniformly well, and many competent hip surgeons have been unable to achieve the degree of success reported in the literature (J. E. Kenzora and M. J. Glimcher, *personal communication*).[94] This may be due to the need for more careful patient selection and meticulous attention to the details of surgical technique. Grafting should be limited to patients without collapse for best results, although the indications may be extended somewhat under special circumstances.

We have modified the grafting technique by using a graft made from a core of normal cancellous bone removed from the trochanter and distal neck, taking care to remove the avascular segment. Sufficient bone is available to fill the cored-out defect in the head without the need for a surgical approach to a separate site. The core is reversed and placed loosely into the head and neck (Fig. 1–22). We believe that the defect can be filled with living bone more rapidly and more completely if a graft is available, in contrast to leaving a large defect completely devoid of bone. Decompression of the head and neck as well as access to vascular ingrowth are also provided by this technique, as these factors may be important elements in the process of repair. The cancellous bone is incorporated more readily than a cortical strut and does not require that a tibial defect be created, a situation which has occasionally resulted in tibial fracture. Our results with this technique, although occasionally excellent, have been quite variable and rather unpredictable.[92] However, this is our preferred approach at the present time for treatment of femoral heads prior to collapse of the articular surface. In most cases it affords significant relief of pain and will usually retard, if not completely halt, progression.

With the development of microvascular surgery, attempts have been made to insert living bone grafts into the necrotic segment of the femoral

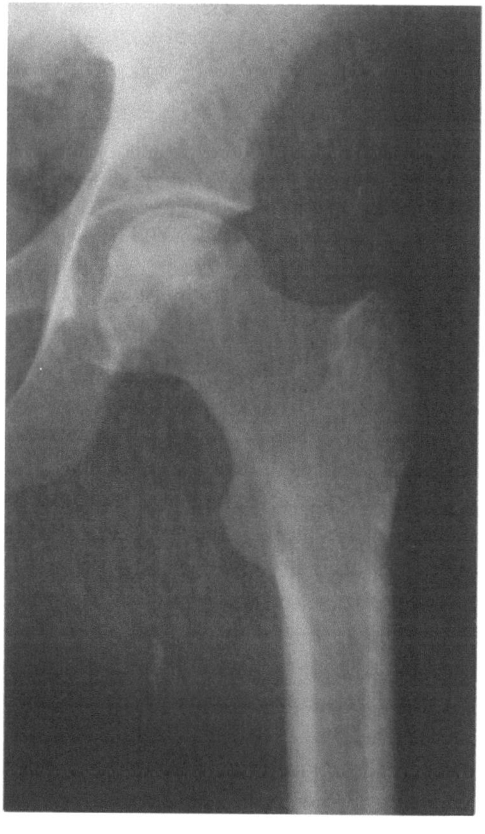

FIG. 1–22 A femoral head which has undergone core decompression and grafting with cancellous bone.

head using a microvascular anastomosis. Urbaniak has employed this technique in approximately 30 cases with promising initial results (*personal communication*).

Gantz and Buchler[37] reported promising results with revascularization techniques using the Hori procedure (implanting a distally ligated arteriovenous pedicle), arteriovenous fistula loop, or vascularized bone grafts. They combined one or the other of these micrografting procedures with a flexion/varus/trochanteric realignment osteotomy. Gilbert and colleagues[38] reported their early experience with a microvascular transfer of the fibula. It remains experimental; their conclusion: "There is no one method yet to treat osteonecrosis of the femoral head."

Osteotomy

Merle d'Aubigné et al. reported on 56 varus or flexion/extension osteotomies performed prior to 1963. In 47 the initial results were considered good and very good.[76] In 1974 they reported a combined total of 92 osteotomies which were followed between 1 and 13 years. Forty percent of these were considered failures, and eventually all showed progressive or degenerative changes.[65] They concluded that if the necrotic area is small and can be completely removed from weight-bearing by the osteotomy satisfactory results might be obtained. However, if it is large, other procedures should be considered. Wagner[104] has reported good results with a valgus/flexion osteotomy when the total necrosis angle was 200 degrees or less (measured as the angle between the two borders of the lesion in the AP x-ray). He would flex them from 30–60 degrees with an average of 45 degrees and valgization of not more than 15 to 20 degrees. He noted poorer results with a varus/flexion osteotomy probably because the necrotic segment was left in a weight bearing position and because there was residual abductor insufficiency due to elevation of the greater trochanter. He "viewed selected use of a valgus/flexion osteotomy as a valuable method for treating ischemic necrosis of the femoral head of limited extent in those patient who are typically younger and not good candidates for a replacement arthroplasty." Millis[77] at the same seminar voiced similar enthusiasm. Ten cases were treated. They were young, active people with osteonecrotic lesions which could be shifted out of weight bearing stresses as much as possible. When the lesion was primarily anterolateral, the technique of Wagner (valgus/flexion osteotomy) was used. When it was more central so that at least 50% of it could be not be delivered from the acetabulum, a varus or varus/extension osteotomy was performed in an attempt at containing the area inside of the acetabulum as far away from stress as possible (see Chapter 10). They were all Stage II, III, and IV. They had a three-year follow-up with all patients experiencing complete relief of pain and no signs of any progression of their collapse. He recommended such biplane osteotomies in such selected patients. One must caution, however, that the upper end must not be left too distorted by an aggressive osteotomy, otherwise a revision to a total hip replacement will be difficult resulting in less than satisfactory function.

Sugioka in 1973 reported a new type of rotational osteotomy by which the femoral head and neck could be rotated 60° or more on the long axis of the neck. Using this technique even large areas of necrosis could be relieved of weight-bearing and replaced with healthy bone (Figs. 1–23 and 1–24). This procedure has now been performed on more than 300 patients with the maximum follow-up more than 10 years. Results have been gratifying, with prevention of collapse and preservation of joint surfaces in most cases. Although it has been most successful in early cases, it has also been effective in cases with marked collapse of the head, so long as the acetabulum remained grossly normal (Y. Sugioka, *personal communication*).[99,100,101] This procedure is one of the few which may allow preservation of the femoral head even after significant collapse has occurred. It is technically very demanding, however, and most other surgeons have been unable to duplicate Sugioka's dramatic results in the relatively few cases that have been attempted.

Electrical Stimulation

Electrical stimulation of established nonunions has given dramatic results, with 80 to 85% going on to solid bony union.[5,15] Histologically, certain areas in the femoral head afflicted with avascular necrosis bear a close resemblance to the tissue found at the site of a nonunion. This has prompted the use of electrical stimulation as a treatment for the early stages of avascular necrosis.

Bassett et al. and Eftekhar et al. have reported encouraging preliminary results using pulsed elec-

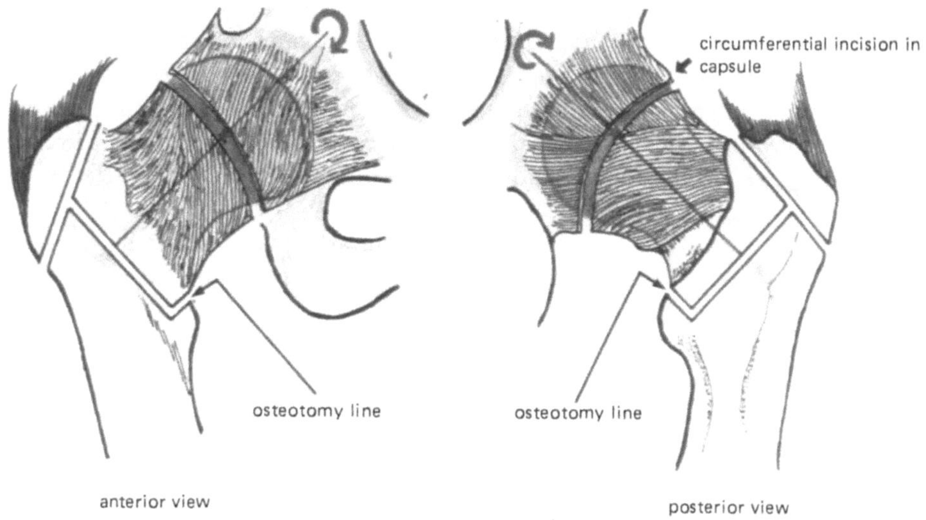

FIG. 1–23 Transtrochanteric anterior rotational osteotomy of Sugioka. More than 60° of rotation is possible, allowing healthy bone and cartilage to replace the collapsed segment in the weight-bearing area. (Courtesy of Dr. Y. Sugioka.)

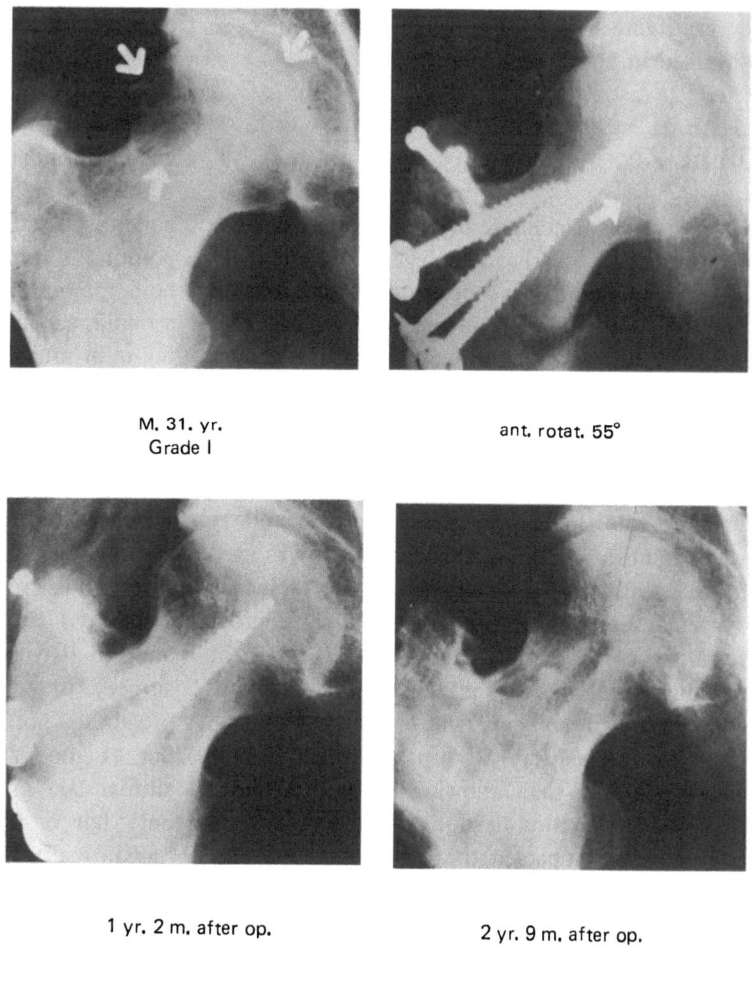

FIG. 1–24 X-ray appearance 2 years 9 months after Sugioka rotational osteotomy. Collapse has not occurred. (Courtesy of Dr. Y. Sugioka.)

tromagnetic fields without surgery. In the majority of cases clinical improvement was noted, and radiographic progression was retarded or reversed.[5,27] To date, the number of cases has been too small and the follow-up too short for definitive conclusions to be drawn. A multicenter study is currently in progress which should provide a conclusive evaluation of this method over the next few years (C. A. L. Bassett, *personal communication*). We are now evaluating the role of direct current stimulation as an adjunct to decompression and bone grafting. This method has been used on 65 hips with the longest follow-up to date being 4 years. Results have been considerably better than in patients treated nonoperatively with limited weight-bearing; but so far there has been no evidence that supplementation with direct current has improved on the results obtained with decompression and grafting alone.[91,92] We are presently evaluating the effects of capacitive coupling, a newer method of electrical stimulation.

At the present time the role of electrical stimulation in the treatment of avascular necrosis must be considered still experimental. It would indeed be gratifying if it yielded results similar to those obtained in nonunions.

Joint Reconstruction

Once significant collapse of the femoral head has occurred, particularly after degenerative changes in the acetabulum have been noted, attempts to preserve the femoral head are generally of little avail. At this point reconstructive measures should be considered.

Cup Arthroplasty

Prior to total hip replacement, cup arthroplasty was a mainstay of hip reconstruction. It was used for the treatment of a variety of disorders including avascular necrosis. Results were not satisfactory for a number of reasons, including collapse of the necrotic head beneath the cup. In 1974 Kerboul et al. described their experience with the "adjusted cup" arthroplasty in 80 hips followed 1 to 6 years.[63] Rather than allowing the cup to move freely on the femoral head, as in the standard approach, they impacted the cup firmly onto the reamed head so as to protect it and to discourage motion. The acetabular cartilage was preserved and was not reamed. They reported good results in 66% of cases in regard to both function and relief of pain, fair results in 16%, and failure in 13%. They concluded that the procedure was useful in cases without excessive involvement, but that total hip replacement was preferred in advanced cases.

Cup arthoplasty, either by the standard technique or as reported by Kerboul et al., is not often used in the United States for the treatment of avascular necrosis because of the unpredictable results. However, the basic concept of covering the femoral head with a fixed metallic cup has been incorporated in the surface replacement arthroplasty to be discussed.

Femoral Head Replacement

Because the primary pathology is present initially in the head rather than the acetabulum, it seems reasonable to replace the head alone with a prosthetic component and preserve the acetabulum if it is not involved. This approach has been used extensively in the past and is still in use. A variety of prostheses are available, including single-component devices such as the Austin Moore device (Fig. 1–25), and the Thompson device; and multicomponent or bipolar devices such as the Bateman and the Giliberty. These may be used with or without cement. Although the early results are generally satisfactory, long-term results are disappointing. Problems have been encountered with both femoral loosening and deterioration of the articular cartilage of the acetabulum, often resulting in protrusio acetabuli. Kerboul et al. reported that of 46 cases following 3 to 10 years, results were excellent in 3, good in 16, fair in 12, and poor in 15.[3,63] In our own series of 36 endoprostheses in patients under age 50, most of which were inserted for avascular necrosis, results were not as good as with total hip replacement in a similar age group. The overall incidence of revision was 47%. The 5-year revision rate was 38%, and the 10-year rate was 56%. Mean time from surgery to revision was 5.4 years. In those prostheses not revised, the functional result was not as good as in total hip arthroplasties in a similar age group, with 42% of patients rated only fair or poor.[96] Even a normal acetabulum has difficulty withstanding the pressures imposed by a rigid metal ball, and in most cases of advanced femoral head collapse the acetabular carti-

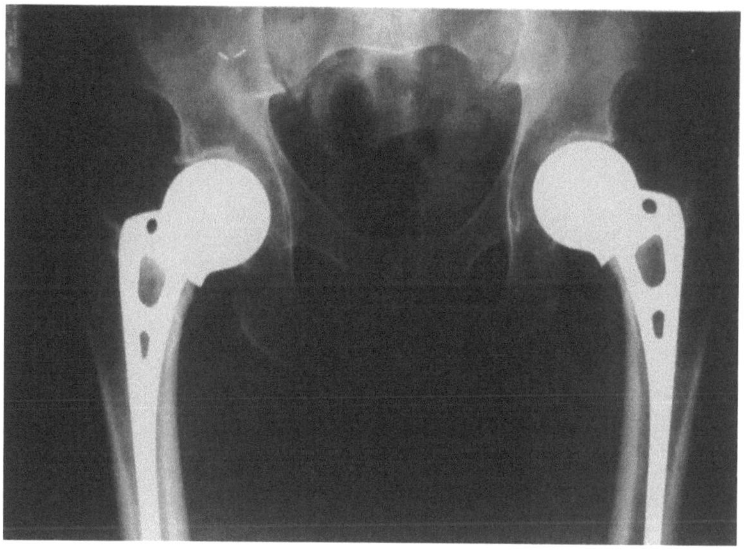

FIG. 1–25 Bilateral femoral head replacement with Austin Moore prostheses. This was a satisfactory clinical result despite the joint line narrowing.

lage is no longer biologically normal despite the x-ray appearance. Opinions vary as to whether the multicomponent devices spare the acetabulum better than the single-component prostheses. The real advantage may be less than the theoretical one, as abnormal pressure rather than friction is most likely the major problem, and this is caused equally by both types of device. If the medullary canal is large and firm fixation cannot be achieved without cement, the prosthesis should be cemented into place. Where a tight fit can be obtained without cement, however, there is no general agreement as to whether cement should or should not be used.

Thus the role of and the optimum technique for femoral head replacement have not been clearly determined. The procedure remains a therapeutic alternative and is favored by many. Others, however, prefer total hip replacement once significant collapse of the femoral head has occurred.

Surface Replacement

This procedure has engendered a great deal of interest, as it has, at least on a theoretical basis, certain definite advantages over conventional total hip replacement. Paramount, of course, is preservation of the femoral head and neck and the ability to perform subsequent procedures quite adequately should they become necessary. It is important to have good bone stock in the femoral head on which to seat the femoral component. Otherwise it is feared that collapse of the head and loosening of the femoral cap will take place (Fig. 1–26). Amstutz et al.,[3] among others, has reported surface replacement in a number of patients with avascular necrosis and has obtained good results. The results reported by others have not been so encouraging, and many believe that avascular necrosis is a relative contraindication to the performance of a surface replacement arthroplasty. All agree that if the procedure is to be done the prosthesis must be seated on structurally sound and primarily viable bone. Thus it can be performed in certain cases of avascular necrosis where involvement of the head is not very extensive. One should be prepared, however, to proceed with conventional total hip arthroplasty or femoral head replacement if at the time of surgery it is found that the involvement of the femoral head is extensive.

Unfortunately, there have been a number of reports indicating a high failure rate for surface replacement arthroplasty. The initial enthusiasm has waned considerably, and it has been all but abandoned at many centers. This procedure should be done only by those experienced in hip surgery and should be approached with caution as it is still in a stage of evaluation and development.

Total Hip Replacement

Total hip replacement arthroplasty is perhaps the most frequent reconstructive procedure used in the management of avascular necrosis. It has withstood the test of time, and it virtually guarantees

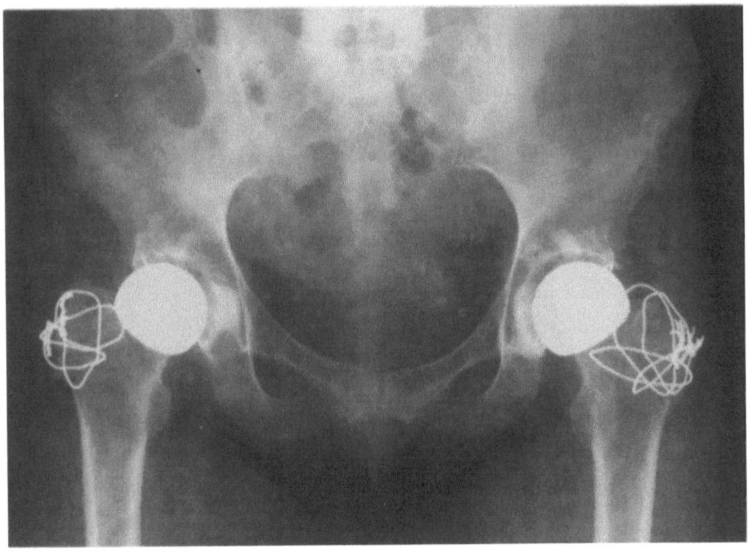

FIG. 1–26 Good clinical result in a patient 4 years after bilateral surface replacement arthroplasty for avascular necrosis secondary to steroid administration.

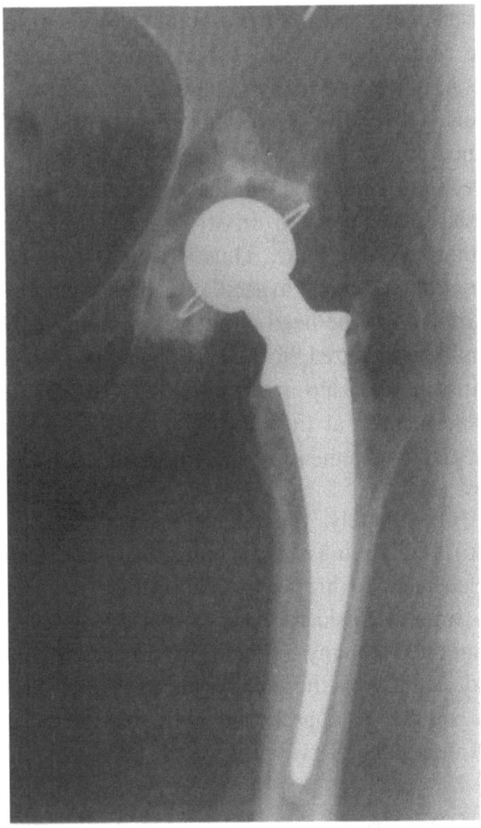

FIG. 1–27 Muller total hip replacement with an excellent clinical result 5 years after surgery for avascular necrosis following a renal transplant.

a high percentage of success. It is the preferred approach when there is involvement of the acetabulum as well as of the femoral head (Fig. 1–27).[28,90,96] Although some surgeons prefer simple femoral head replacement when the acetabulum appears to be grossly normal, we believe that the relatively high failure rate of femoral endoprostheses after 5 years justifies a primary total hip replacement even in these cases. This procedure should not, however, be undertaken lightly in the young individual. Studies have shown a 15 to 20% 5-year failure rate of cemented total hip replacements in individuals younger than 40. This figure may become even higher if the individual is heavy or physically active. Interest has been growing in the role of noncemented total hips, particularly for the young patient. If this procedure withstands the test of time, it may prove to be the treatment of choice for avascular necrosis of the femoral head.

Miscellaneous Procedures

Hip Fusion

Hip fusion, although a procedure to be considered, is rarely indicated for avascular necrosis. Most patients prefer to have a movable rather than a fused hip. If a fusion is to be done, the high incidence of bilaterality must be fully considered. It is contraindicated if there is evidence of involvement of the opposite hip. In those cases in which fusion has been attempted, the failure rate has been high because of the avascularity of the femoral head.

Girdlestone Pseudarthrosis

Girdlestone pseudarthrosis should be reserved for special circumstances in which other procedures are not applicable. Thus it might be considered in the case of a painful hip in which sepsis has been superimposed on avascular necrosis. It is also useful as a salvage procedure for the failed total hip replacement, particularly when sepsis is present and occasionally without sepsis when there is no longer sufficient bone stock available to perform a revision of the total hip.

If this procedure is performed properly so as to leave smooth, parallel surfaces to articulate with each other, and if a sufficient period of traction and nonweight-bearing is pursued, the results are often quite satisfactory. Good motion and pain relief should be achieved. The hip will not be stable, and the patient should anticipate using a cane to minimize the abductor lurch which is generally present. The Girdlestone can of course be converted to a total hip replacement at a later date; but if performed properly with adequate resection of the acetabular margins as well as the femoral neck, this may be technically difficult.

Treatment by Degree of Involvement

Having reviewed in some detail the specific advantages and disadvantages of various approaches to the treatment of the avascular head, we conclude and summarize this section with a brief description of which approaches, in our opinion, are most indicated for the various stages of involvement of the hip, as listed in Table 1–2.

Prior to Collapse: Stages 0 through II

In the earliest stages, prior to any collapse of the femoral head, prophylactic measures should be considered to retard the progression of the disorder and hopefully prevent collapse. Under certain circumstances observation and conservative management are indicated, but in our experience this almost inevitably leads to progression; therefore we believe that a more aggressive approach should be taken if possible. Among these we include drilling or core decompression and grafting. The rotational osteotomy of Sugioka has yielded good results in his hands but is a technically difficult procedure and should probably be reserved for cases in which there are no other good alternatives. Electrical stimulation at this stage is still experimental though promising. We personally favor grafting the femoral head through the lateral approach, as described, using cancellous bone, which also provides for decompression and a channel for vascular ingrowth. The use of a viable graft with a microvascular anastomosis should also be considered. If results after longer follow up are as good as the preliminary results, it might become the procedure of choice. It is technically demanding, however, and should be attempted only by those skilled in this technique.

Subchondral Collapse: Stages III through IVA

So long as there is no flattening, and perhaps even with minimal flattening of the articular surface, attempts to preserve the femoral head are justified. In such cases we take the same approach as outlined above, recognizing, however, that the end-results will generally be less satisfactory.

Flattening of the Head Without Acetabular Involvement: Stages IVB and IVC

Once definite collapse of the articular surface has occurred, measures to preserve the femoral head generally fail. Grafting may retard the rate of collapse but does not provide a completely satisfactory result. Only the rotational osteotomy of Sugioka has been successful in preserving the femoral head, and this procedure might be considered at this stage. As mentioned, however, it is technically quite demanding, and few surgeons have been able to equal the results reported by Sugioka. If pain and disability are mild to moderate, conservative measures should be continued. However, if symptoms warrant, joint reconstruction at this stage is indicated. Although some prefer to replace only the femoral head with either a single or multicomponent device, we believe that long-term results are better with replacement of both the femoral head and the acetabulum. Surface replacement arthroplasty is now used infrequently, and for the majority of patients total hip replacement is the procedure of choice. Care must be exercised during the postoperative period to minimize stress on the components so as to give maximum useful life to this device in the young and active patient. Cemented components are still the standard, but time may prove the noncemented total hip best in the young patient.

Degenerative Changes Involving the Acetabulum: Stages V and VI

Once the acetabulum has become involved, attempts to preserve the femoral head or to use a femoral endoprosthesis alone usually give poor results. At this stage, if conservative management is no longer sufficient to relieve pain and disability, total hip replacement is usually indicated. Under special circumstances, other procedures, discussed earlier, may be considered.

Acknowledgments

We wish to thank Drs. Raymond G. Tronzo, John L. Sbarbaro Jr., James Koh, Gerald D. Hayken, David R. Steinberg, and other members of the Department of Orthopedic Surgery at the University of Pennsylvania School of Medicine for the clinical material on which a large portion of this chapter was based. Dr. Yoichi Sugioka, Professor and Chairman of the Department of Orthopedic Surgery of Kyushu University deserves special thanks for sharing with us his clinical material and providing us with detailed information concerning his rotational osteotomy.

References

1. Aegerter, E., Kirkpatrick, J. A., Jr.: *Orthopedic Diseases,* 3rd ed. Philadelphia, Saunders, 1968.
2. Alavi, A., McCloskey, J. R., and Steinberg, M. E.: Early detection of avascular necrosis of the femoral head by ^{99m}technetium diphosphonate bone scan: a preliminary report. Clin. Orthop., 127:137, 1977.
3. Amstutz, H. C., Christie, J., Mensch, J. S.: Treatment of osteonecrosis of the hip. In: *The Hip: Proceedings of the Third Open Scientific Meeting of the Hip Society.* St. Louis, Mosby, 1975, pp. 19–34.
4. Bassett, C. A. L., Mitchell, S. N., Gaston S. R.: Treatment of ununited tibial diaphyseal fractures with pulsing electromagnetic fields. J. Bone Joint Surg., 63A:511, 1981.
5. Bassett, C. A. L., Schink-Ascani, M. M., Lewes, S. N.: Treatment of femoral head osteonecrosis with pulsed electromagnetic fields (PEMFs). In: *Bone Circulation* (Arlet, J., Ficat, R. P., and Hungerford, D. A., eds.) Baltimore, Williams & Wilkins, 1983, pp. 343–354.
6. Bobechko, W. P., Harris, W. R.: The radiographic density of avascular bone. J. Bone Joint Surg., 42B:626, 1960.
7. Boettcher, W. G., Bonfiglio, M., Hamilton, H. H., et al.: Non-traumatic necrosis of the femoral head. I. Relation of altered hemeostasis to etiology. J. Bone Joint Surg., 52A:312, 1970.
8. Boettcher, W. G., Bonfiglio, M., Smith K.: Non-traumatic necrosis of the femoral head. II. Experiences in treatment. J. Bone Joint Surg., 52A:322, 1970.
9. Bohr, H., Larsen, E. H.: On necrosis of the femoral head after fracture of the neck of the femur. J. Bone Joint Surg., 47B:330, 1965.
10. Bonfiglio, M., Voke, E. M.: Aseptic necrosis of the femoral head and nonunion of the femoral neck. J. Bone Joint Surg., 50A:48, 1968.
11. Boyd, H. B., George, I. L.: Complications of fractures of the neck of the femur. J. Bone Joint Surg., 29B:13, 1947.
12. Brighton, C. T., Black, J., Friendenberg, Z. B., et al.: A multicenter study of the treatment of nonunion with constant direct current. J. Bone Joint Surg., 62A:2, 1981.
13. Brodetti, A.: The blood supply of the femoral neck and head in relation to the damaging effects of nails and screws. J. Bone Joint Surg., 42B:794, 1960.
14. Burton, D. S., Mochizuki, R. M., Halpern, A. A.: Total hip arthroplasty in the cardiac transplant patient. Clin. Orthop., 130:186, 1978.
15. Catto, M.: A histological study of avascular necrosis of the femoral head after transcervical fracture. J. Bone Joint Surg., 47B:749, 1965.
16. Catto, M.: The histological appearances of late segmental collapse of the femoral head after transcervical fracture. J. Bone Joint Surg., 47B:777, 1965.
17. Chryssanthou, C. P.: Dysbaric osteonecrosis: etiological and pathogenetic concepts. Clin. Orthop., 130:94, 1978.
18. Chung, S. M. K., Alavi, A., Russell, M. O.: Management of osteonecrosis in sickle-cell anemia and its genetic variants. Clin. Orthop., 130:158, 1978.

19. Chung, S. M. K., Ralston, E. L.: Necrosis of the femoral head associated with sickle-cell anemia and its genetic variants. J. Bone Joint Surg., 51A:33, 1969.
20. Claffey, T. J.: Avascular necrosis of the femoral head. J. Bone Joint Surg., 42B:802, 1960.
21. Coleman, S. S., Compere, C. L.: Femoral neck fractures: pathogenesis of avascular necrosis, nonunion, and late degenerative changes. Clin. Orthop., 20:247, 1961.
22. Cruess, R. L.: Experience with steroid-induced avascular necrosis of the shoulder and etiologic considerations regarding osteonecrosis of the hip. Clin. Orthop., 130:86, 1978.
23. Cruess, R. L., Blennerhassett, J., MacDonald, F. R., et al.: Aseptic necrosis following renal transplantation. J. Bone Joint Surg., 50A:1577, 1968.
24. D'Ambrosia, R. D., Shoji, H., Riggins, R. S., et al.: Scintigraphy in the diagnosis of osteonecrosis. Clin. Orthop., 130:139, 1978.
25. Donaldson, W. E., Jr., Rodriquez, E. E., Skovron, M., Gartland, J. J.: Traumatic dislocation of the hip joint in children. J. Bone Joint Surg., 50A:79, 1968.
26. Dubois, E. L., Cozen, L.: Avascular (aseptic) bone necrosis associated with systemic lupus erythematosus. JAMA, 174:108, 1960.
27. Eftekhar, S. A., Schink-Ascani, M. M., Mitchell, S. N., et al.: Osteonecrosis of the femoral head treated by pulsed electromagnetic fields (PEMFs): a preliminary report. In *The Hip* (Hungerford, D. S., ed.) St. Louis, Mosby, 1983, pp. 306–330.
28. Enneking, W. F.: The choice of surgical procedures in idiopathic aseptic necrosis. In: *The Hip: Proceedings of the Seventh Open Scientific Meeting of the Hip Society.* St. Louis, Mosby, 1979, pp. 218–237.
29. Ficat, R. P., Arlet, J.: *Ischemia and Necrosis of Bone* (Hungerford, D. S., ed.) Baltimore, Williams & Wilkins, 1980.
30. Finby, N., Begg, C. F.: Correlation conferences in radiology and pathology: aseptic necrosis of hip. New York J. Med., 68:796, 1968.
31. Fischer, S. J.: Non-traumatic avascular necrosis: a review of its causes, diagnosis, and treatment. Orthop. Rev., 2:113, 1979.
32. Fisher, D. E.: The role of fat embolism in the etiology of corticosteroid-induced avascular necrosis: clinical and experimental results. Clin. Orthop., 130:68, 1978.
33. Fisher, D. E., Bickel, W. H., Holley, K. E.: Histologic demonstration of fat emboli in aseptic necrosis associated with hypercortisonism. Mayo Clin. Proc., 44:252, 1969.
34. Freund, E.: Bilateral aseptic necrosis of the femoral head. Ann. Surg., 104:100, 1936.
35. Fries, G.: Uberwachung der Huftgelenke nach Bestrahlung weiblicher Genitalkarzinome. Munch. Med. Wochenschr., 109:1499, 1967.
36. Fries, G.: Zur Rontgen-Diagnostik Osteoradionekrotischer Huftveranderugen nach Rontgen-Radiumbestrahlung weiblicher Genitalkarzinome. Strahlentherapie, 132:113, 1967.
37. Gantz, R., Buchler, U.: Overview of attempts to revitalize the dead head in aseptic necrosis of the femoral head–osteotomy and revascularization (Chapter 18). The Hip Society, 1983.
38. Gilbert, A., Judet, H., Judet, J., Agatti, A.: Microvascular transfer of the fibula for necrosis of the femoral head. Ortho. 9:885, June, 1986.
39. Glimcher, M. J., Kenzora, J. E.: The biology of osteonecrosis of the human femoral head and its clinical implications. I. Tissue biology. Clin. Orthop., 138:284, 1979.
40. Glimcher, M. J., Kenzora, J. E.: The biology of osteonecrosis of the human femoral head and its clinical implications. II. The pathological changes in the femoral head as an organ and in the hip joint. Clin. Orthop., 139:283, 1979.
41. Glimcher, M. J., Kenzora, J. E.: The biology of osteonecrosis of the human femoral head and its clinical implications. III. Discussion of the etiology and genesis of the pathological sequelae; comments on treatment. Clin. Orthop., 140:273, 1979.
42. Glimcher, M. J., Kenzora, J. E.: Osteonecrosis: The Pathobiology, Clinical Manifestations, Therapeutic Dilemmas. Instructional Coruse 103, American Academy of Orthopaedic Surgeons, Annual Meeting, Atlanta, 1980.
43. Haliburton, R. A., Brockenshire, F. A., Barber, J. R.: Avascular necrosis of the femoral capital epiphysis after traumatic dislocation of the hip in children. J. Bone Joint Surg., 43B:43, 1961.
44. Hall, M. C., Elmore, S. M., Bright, R. W., et al.: Skeletal complications in a series of human renal allografts. JAMA, 208:1825, 1969.
45. Hamilton, H. E., Bonfiglio, M., Sheets, R. F., Connor, W. E.: Relation of altered hemostasis to idiopathic aseptic necrosis of the femoral head. J. Clin. Invest., 44:1058, 1965.
46. Hastings, D. E., Macnab, I.: Spontaneous avascular necrosis of the femoral head. Can. J. Surg., 8:68, 1965.
47. Heimann, W. G., Frieberger, R. H.: Avascular necrosis of the femoral and humeral heads after high-dosage corticosteroid therapy. N. Engl. J. Med., 263:672, 1960.
48. Hulth, A.: Necrosis of the head of the femur. Acta Chir. Scand., 122:75, 1961.
49. Hunder, G. G., Worthington, J. W., Bickel, W. H.: Avascular necrosis of the femoral head in a patient with gout. JAMA, 203:101, 1968.
50. Hungerford, D. S.: Bone marrow pressure, venography, and core decompression in ischemic necro-

sis of the femoral head. In: *The Hip: Proceedings of the Seventh Open Scientific Meeting of the Hip Society.* St. Louis, Mosby, 1979, pp. 218–237.
51. Hungerford, D. S., Zizic, T. M.: Alcoholism associated ischemic necrosis of the femoral head: early diagnosis and treatment. Clin. Orthop., 130:144, 1978.
52. Jacobs, B.: Epidemiology of traumatic and nontraumatic osteonecrosis. Clin. Orthop., 130:51, 1978.
53. Jaffe, H. L.: Ischemic necrosis of bone. Med. Radiogr. Photogr., 45:58, 1969.
54. Johnson, L. C.: Histogenesis of avascular necrosis. In: Proceedings of a Conference on Aseptic Necrosis, sponsored by the National Institutes of Health, St. Louis, December 1964.
55. Johnson, R. L., Smyth, C. J., Holt, G. W., et al.: Steroid therapy and vascular lesions in rheumatoid arthritis. Arthritis Rheum., 2:224, 1959.
56. Jones, J. P., Jr., Behnke, A. R., Jr.: Prevention of dysbaric osteonecrosis in compressed-air workers. Clin. Orthop., 130:118, 1978.
57. Jones, J. P., Jr., Engleman, E. P.: Osseous avascular necrosis associated with systemic abnormalities. Arthritis Rheum., 9:728, 1936.
58. Kahlstrom, S. C., Burton, C. C., Phemister, D. B.: Aseptic necrosis of bone. Surg. Gynecol. Obstet., 68:129, 1939.
59. Kawashima, M., Torisu, T., Hayashi, K., Kitano, M.: Pathological review of osteonecrosis in divers. Clin. Orthop., 130:107, 1978.
60. Kenzora, J. E., Glimcher, M. J.: The role of renal bone disease in the production of transplant osteonecrosis. Orthopaedics, 4:305, 1981.
62. Kenzora, J. E., Steele, R. E., Yosipovitch, Z. H., Glimcher, M. J.: Experimental osteonecrosis of the femoral head in adult rabbits. Clin. Orthop., 130:8, 1978.
63. Kerboul, M., Thomine, J., Postel, M., Merle d'Aubigne, R.: The conservative surgical treatment of idiopathic aseptic necrosis of the femoral head. J. Bone Joint Surg., 56B:291, 1974.
64. Lampe, C. E.: Osteochondritis dissecans of the head of the femur. Acta Orthop. Scand., 26:33, 1957.
65. Leach, R. E., Lynch, J.: Management of idiopathic aseptic necrosis. In: *The Hip: Proceedings of the Fourth Open Scientific Meeting of the Hip Society.* St. Louis, Mosby, 1976, pp. 9–20.
66. Lee, K. D., Corcoran, S. F., Parsons, J. R.: Hyperlipidemia and idiopathic aseptic necrosis of the femoral head in adults. Orthopaedics, 3:651, 1980.
67. Lowe, H. G.: Avascular necrosis after slipping of the upper femoral epiphysis. J. Bone Joint Surg., 43B:688, 1961.
68. Luck, J. V.: *Bone and Joint Diseases.* Springfield, Charles C Thomas, 1950.
69. Malka, S.: Idiopathic aseptic necrosis of the head of the femur in adults. Surg. Gynecol. Obstet., 123:1057, 1966.
70. Mankin, H. J., Brower, T. D.: Bilateral idiopathic aseptic necrosis of the femur in adults: "Chandler's disease." J. Hosp. Joint Dis., 23:42, 1962.
71. Marcus, N. D., Enneking, W. F., Massam, R. A.: The silent hip in idiopathic aseptic necrosis—treatment by bone grafting. J. Bone Joint Surg., 55A:1351, 1975.
72. Markham, T. N.: Ann Arbor case reports: aseptic necrosis in a high-altitude flier. J. Occup. Med., 9:123, 1967.
73. Martel, W., Sitterley, B. H.: X-ray findings are numerous in osteonecrosis. Mod. Med., May 18, 1970.
74. Merle d'Aubigné, R., Postel, M., Mazabraud, A., et al.: Idiopathic necrosis of the femoral head in adults. J. Bone Joint Surg., 47B:612, 1965.
75. Meyers, M. H.: The treatment of osteonecrosis of the hip with fresh osteochondral allografts and with the muscle pedicle graft technique. Clin. Orthop., 130:202, 1978.
76. Meyers, M. H., Harvey, J. P., Jr., Moore, T. M.: Treatment of displaced subcapital and transcervical fractures of the femoral neck by muscle-pedicle-bone graft and internal fixation. J. Bone Joint Surg., 55A:257, 1973.
77. Millis, M. M.: Biplane intertrochanteric osteotomy for osteonecrosis. Presented at the Symposium on Osteotomy of the Hip and Knee, Boston, 1986.
78. Patterson, R. J., Bickel, W. J., Kahlin, D. C.: Idiopathic avascular necrosis of the head of the femur. J. Bone Joint Surg., 46A:267, 1964.
79. Phemister, D. B.: Changes in bones and joints resulting from interruption of circulation. I. General consideration and changes resulting from injury. Arch. Surg., 41:436, 1940.
80. Phemister, D. B.: Fractures of neck of femur, dislocations of hip, and obscure vascular disturbances producing aseptic necrosis of head of femur. Surg. Gynecol. Obstet., 59:415, 1934.
81. Phemister, D. B.: Treatment of the necrotic head of the femur in adults. J. Bone Joint Surg., 31A:55, 1949.
82. Ralston, E. L.: Legg-Calve-Perthes disease—factors in healing. J. Bone Joint Surg., 43A:249, 1961.
83. Ruderman, M., McCarty, D. J., Jr.: Aseptic necrosis in systemic lupus erythematosus: report of a case involving six joints. Arthritis Rheum., 7:709, 1964.
84. Russell, J.: An essay on necrosis. Section I. General remarks and description of appearances. Clin. Orthop., 130:5, 1978.

85. Sennara, H., Gorry, F.: Orthopedic aspects of sickle cell anemia and allied hemoglobinopathies. Clin. Orthop., 130:154, 1978.
86. Sevitt, S.: Avascular necrosis and revascularization of the femoral head after intracapsular fractures. J. Bone Joint Surg., 46B:270, 1964.
87. Sherman, M. S., Phemister, D. B.: The pathology of ununited fractures of the neck of the femur. J. Bone Joint Surg., 29A:19, 1947.
88. Siemsen, J. K., Brook, J., Meister, L.: Lupus erythematosus and avascular bone necrosis: a clinical study of three cases and review of the literature. Arthritis Rheum., 5:492, 1962.
89. Spence, R. K., Alavi, A., Barker, C. F., et al.: Osteonecrosis in the renal transplant recipient—a prospective study. In: *Bone Circulation* (Arlet, J., Ficat, R. P., and Hungerford, D. S., eds.) Baltimore, Williams & Wilkins, 1984, pp. 246–249.
90. Springfield, D. S., Enneking, W. J.: Surgery for aseptic necrosis of the femoral head. Clin. Orthop., 130:175, 1978.
91. Steinberg, M. E., Brighton, C. T., Hayken, G. D., et al.: Early results in the treatment of avascular necrosis of the femoral head with electrical stimulation. Orthop. Clin. North Am., 15:1, 1984.
92. Steinberg, M. E., Brighton, C. T., Steinberg, D. R., et al.: Treatment of avascular necrosis of the femoral head by a combination of bone grafting, decompression, and electrical stimulation. Clin. Orthop., 186:137, 1984.
93. Steinberg, M. E., Hayken, G. D., Steinberg, D. R.: A new method for evaluation and staging of avascular necrosis of the femoral head. In: *Bone Circulation* (Arlet, J., Ficat, R. P., and Hungerford, D. S., eds.) Baltimore, Williams & Wilkins, 1984, pp. 398–403.
94. Steinberg, M. E., Hayken, G. D., Steinberg, D. R.: The "conservative" management of avascular necrosis of the femoral head. In: *Bone Circulation* (Arlet, J., Ficat, R. P., and Hungerford, D. S., eds.) Baltimore, Williams & Wilkins, 1984, pp. 334–337.
95. Steinberg, M. E., Koh, J. K., Alavi, A., et al.: Non-traumatic avascular necrosis of the femoral head in adults. Orthop. Digest, March 1977, pp. 17–22.
96. Steinberg, M. E., Unger, A. S.: Femoral endoprosthetic replacement in younger patients. Presented to the American Academy of Orthopaedic Surgeons, 52nd Annual Meeting, Las Vegas, Nevada, 1985.
97. Steinberg, M. E., Chen, H. H., Thickman, D., et al.: Early diagnosis of avascular necrosis by nuclear magnetic resonance imaging. Presented to American Academy of Orthopaedic Surgeons, 52nd Annual Meeting, Las Vegas, Nevada, 1985.
98. Sugioka, Y.: Transtrochanteric anterior rotational osteotomy of the femoral head in the treatment of osteonecrosis affecting the hip: a new osteotomy operation. Clin. Orthop., 130:191, 1978.
99. Sugioka, Y.: Transtrochanteric rotational osteotomy in the treatment of idiopathic and steroid-induced femoral head necrosis, Perthes disease, slipped capital femoral epiphysis, and osteoarthritis of the hip. Clin. Orthop., 184:12, 1984.
100. Sugioka, Y., Katsuki, I., Hotokebuchi, T.: Transtrochanteric rotational osteotomy of the femoral head for the treatment of osteonecrosis. Clin. Orthop., 169:115, 1982.
101. Theron, J.: Superselective angiography of the hip. Radiology, 124:649, 1977.
102. Trueta, J., Harrison, M. H. M.: The normal vascular anatomy of the femoral head in adult man. J. Bone Joint Surg., 35B:442, 1953.
103. Velayos, E. E., Leidholt, J. D., Smyth, J. J., Priest, R.: Arthropathy associated with steroid therapy. Ann. Intern. Med., 64:759, 1966.
104. Wagner, H., and Bauer, W.: Five year follow-up of intertrochanteric osteotomy for ischemic necrosis of the femoral head. Presented at the Symposium on Osteotomy of the Hip and Knee, Boston, 1986.
105. Wang, G., Moga, D. B., Richemer, W. G., et al.: Cortisone-induced bone changes and its response to lipid clearing agents. Clin. Orthop., 130:81, 1978.

Chapter 2

Tumors

Douglas J. Pritchard

The region of the hip may be defined as that area which contains the proximal femur, the acetabulum, the adjacent innominate bone, and all of the surrounding soft tissues. A wide variety of benign and malignant bone and soft-tissue tumors occur in this region, including almost all of the primary bone tumors, many soft-tissue tumors, and many metastatic lesions.

The patient may complain of pain in the buttock, the groin, the lateral aspects of the thigh, or even the knee. Depending on the nature of the lesion, the pain is usually present even at rest, and it may be aggravated by weight-bearing. The patient also may complain of a local mass or of a swelling in the thigh or distal extremity. Infrequently, the patient presents with a pathological fracture of the hip.

A high index of suspicion is necessary in order to detect some of the more subtle tumors. For example, chondrosarcoma typically arises from the triradiate cartilage on the inner aspect of the acetabulum. In its early stages the lesion may be extremely difficult to visualize on a routine roentgenogram. With the advent of computed tomography (CT), some lesions can now be detected which in the past may have been overlooked. Other diagnostic modalities also are helpful on occasion. For example, the patient with persistent pain may have normal roentgenograms and a positive radionuclide bone scan. Arthrography of the hip joint is occasionally useful, particularly for the detection of synovial tumors. Plane tomograms sometimes are more useful than CT. For the patient with persistent pain in the region of the hip, any one or all of these diagnostic modalities may be necessary to reveal the tumor.

After the treatment of any tumor in the region of the hip, as with mesenchymal tumors in other locations, careful follow-up is necessary. Almost all mesenchymal tumors have the potential to recur locally, and of course malignant tumors have the potential to metastasize. The frequency of follow-up examinations depends on the nature of the particular lesion. For highly malignant tumors, such as osteosarcoma, follow-up examinations should be conducted at least every 3 months during the first 18 months after treatment. After that, the intervals between examinations may be lengthened to 6-month intervals. After several years they may again be lengthened, to yearly examinations. With each follow-up examination, the type of procedure employed depends on the biological potential of the lesion in question. Almost all the sarcomas have great potential for metastasis to the lung fields; therefore CT scans of the lung fields should be obtained at each follow-up visit. Some tumors, such as Ewing's sarcoma, tend to metastasize to bones; therefore technetium bone scans are useful for follow-up purposes. However, osteosarcoma has a minimal tendency to metastasize to bone unless there is intervening evidence of pulmonary metastasis, and therefore technetium bone scans are not routinely obtained for follow-up purposes.

For benign tumors, ideal follow-up again depends on the nature of the underlying lesion. For tumors such as giant cell tumors, which have a great tendency to recur, frequent follow-up is indicated. However, lesions such as osteochondroma, which rarely recurs, probably can safely be observed at 6-month intervals for the first 1.5 years and yearly thereafter for several more years. There can be no set rule for the frequency of follow-up examinations; each case must be individualized.

Benign Bone Tumors

Although any benign tumor may involve bones in the hip region, several lesions are particularly common. These are osteoid osteoma, giant cell tumors, and osteochondroma.

Osteoid Osteoma

In the Mayo Clinic experience reported by Dahlin,[3] 43 of 158 osteoid osteomas occurred in the proximal femur and 5 in the ilium. Patients with this tumor complain of pain, which is frequently relieved by salicylates. Sometimes the complaint is of referred pain, particularly in the knee. Physical examination may reveal considerable atrophy of the thigh muscles. Not uncommonly, a neurological cause for the symptoms is considered.

Even when the presence of an osteoid osteoma is suspected, it may be difficult to find evidence of a lesion on the roentgenogram. Classically, an area of sclerosis is seen with a central, small, lucent area usually referred to as a nidus (Fig. 2–1). However, sclerosis is not always present, and the nidus may not be apparent on routine roentgenograms. If the diagnosis is suspected and the roentgenograms are not helpful, a technetium-99 bone scan is obtained,[14] which should reveal an area of intense uptake. Once the area is localized, tomography may be helpful in visualizing the lesion. If there is no intense uptake on bone scan, the patient probably does not have an osteoid osteoma. The most difficult problem is localizing the tumor. It must be precisely localized before surgical intervention so that the operation can be planned to minimize the sacrifice of normal tissues.

Intraoperative roentgenograms are usually needed to localize the lesion further. The entire nidus should be reomoved, but the surrounding sclerotic bone need not be because it is reactive bone that will gradually remodel once the nidus is removed. Bone grafts may or may not be needed to fill the resulting defect, depending on the location of the tumor and the extent of the defect. A pathologist should confirm that the lesion has been removed. Cultures should probably be prepared in every case to check for Brodie's abscess, which may mimic an osteoid osteoma.

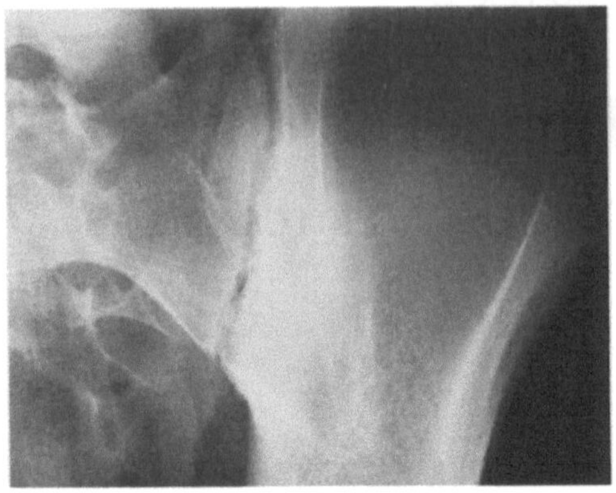

A

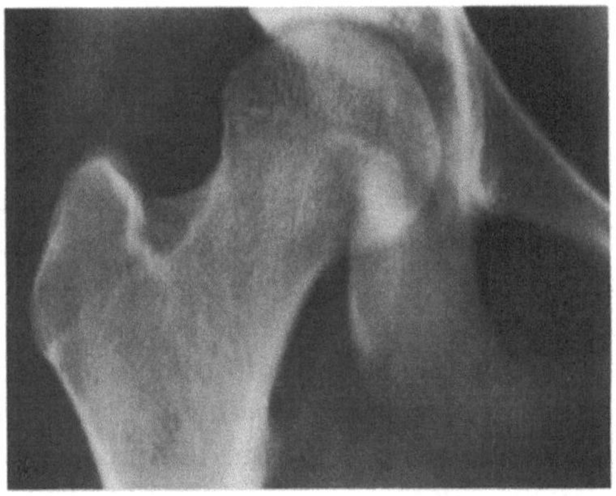

B

FIG. 2–1 Osteoid osteoma. **A** Of the ilium. **B** Involving the superior aspect of the base of the femoral neck in a 22-year-old man.

Giant Cell Tumor of Bone

In the Mayo Clinic experience, Dahlin[3] reported 23 benign giant cell tumors involving the hip region. Eighty-five percent of the benign giant cell tumors occurred in patients more than 19 years old, with females more often affected than males. Patients usually complain of pain and occasionally note swelling. Giant cell tumors tend to behave in a locally malignant manner and therefore must be completely removed if recurrence is to be avoided. However, because complete removal of a giant cell tumor in the hip region is a drastic measure, particularly for young adults, excision by curettage probably should be considered as a preliminary approach.[9] The radiographic classification of Campanacci[2] is helpful in deciding whether excision by curettage is likely to be successful. In this system, lesions that are entirely intraosseous and appear roentgenographically to be indolent are probably the most favorable lesions for excision by curettage. However, lesions that have broken through cortical bone and extend into the surrounding soft tissues and which appear roentgenographically to be aggressive probably will not be cured by curettage and will require more aggressive surgical resection.

If curettage is selected, the technique is very important. Probably most important is to make a "window" over the tumor large enough so that the entire cavity can be visualized. Once the tumor has been completely curetted, a dental burr can be used on the surface of the entire cavity and another 1 to 2 mm of bone tissue removed. Undiluted phenol is used to cauterize the tumor cavity. The phenol must be neutralized with alcohol and flushed with copious quantities of saline; great care must be taken to avoid spillage of the phenol onto the adjacent structures. Cryosurgery with liquid nitrogen also may be used to achieve the same purpose. Pulsating lavage (Water-Pik) may be utilized to thoroughly irrigate the tumor cavity as well as the entire wound. In the hip region, autogenous iliac bone grafts usually are needed to fill the resulting defect.

For the giant cell tumor of the proximal femur which is large or aggressive, primary resection of the proximal femur and replacement with a custom-type endoprosthesis may be needed. (See Special Surgical Considerations, below.) Various endoprosthetic prostheses in different sizes should be available so that the correct size can be inserted at surgery. If these are not available, a custom-designed device can be ordered, obviously necessitating a delay. In this case treatment is either delayed or surgery is performed in two stages: first the resection and later, when the prosthesis is available, the reconstruction. Because giant cell tumors occasionally grow rapidly, any delay in treatment requires careful observation, with frequent roentgenograms. If rapid growth becomes apparent, surgical intervention becomes mandatory.

Giant cell tumors tend to be implanted into the surrounding soft tissues. Therefore follow-up with periodic roentgenographic examinations may reveal soft-tissue implants; such lesions tend to have a characteristic roentgenographic appearance: a rim of sclerotic bone around the periphery of the tumor. Sometimes it is difficult to differentiate roentgenographically between soft-tissue implants and heterotopic bone.

When autogenous bone grafts are obtained from a remote incision, separate gowns, gloves, drapes, and instruments should be utilized. This precaution minimizes the risk of tumor implantation at the donor site.

Radiation therapy for giant cell tumor probably should be avoided unless the tumor is unresectable. In the past, a number of giant cell tumors were treated by radiation therapy, and some became malignant. Most lesions in the hip region can be treated surgically.

Osteochondroma

Osteochondroma is the most common primary bone tumor; however, most patients with such lesions probably never undergo operation. Of 579 surgically removed lesions reported by Dahlin,[3] 53 occurred in the hip region and 29 in the ilium. Most of the lesions are solitary, but some patients have multiple osteochondromas. The latter condition appears to be familial. When multiple tumors are present, each lesion has the gross and microscopic appearnace of a solitary lesion. However, patients with multiple lesions are at much greater risk for the development of subsequent malignant transformation of one or more osteochondromas. Although the true incidence of such malignant transformation has not been accurately determined, it probably is somewhat greater than 10% for multiple tumors and less than 1% for solitary osteochondromas.

Generally, most of these lesions are asymptomatic and are found incidentally when roentgenograms are obtained for other purposes. This is particularly true for lesions in the hip region because much soft tissue overlies the hip and the mass may not be detected by the patient or the physician. When a lesion impinges on surrounding structures, pain or other disability may result. Occasionally, pain is due to fracture at the base of the lesion.

The roentgenographic appearance is usually characteristic: a pedunculated, mushroom-shaped mass projecting from the surface of the bone. The stalk may be either narrow or broadly based (sessile). The lesion commonly arises at the site of tendon insertion and hence tends to project away from the joint and toward the pull of the tendon.

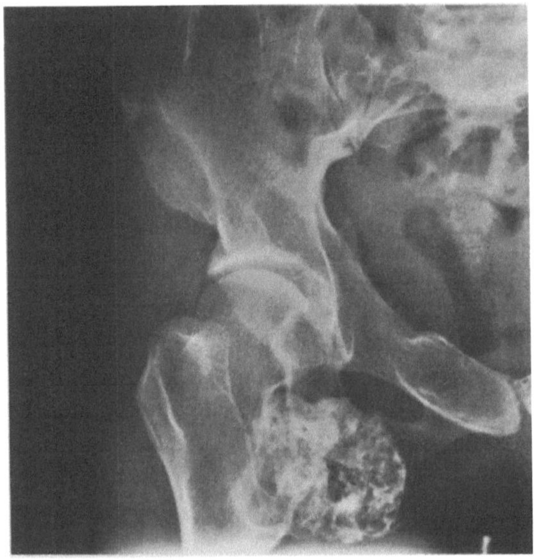

FIG. 2–2 Large osteochondroma arising from the base of the femoral neck.

An osteochondroma that arises from the femoral neck tends to be broad-based and may encircle the femoral neck (Fig. 2–2). The cartilage cap of the lesion has a less-dense roentgenographic appearance than usual. When the lesion is large and there is considerable calcification and irregularity of the cap, malignant transformation should be suspected (Fig. 2–3).

The normal cortex of the involved bone extends into the base of the tumor stalk. This feature may be helpful in differentiating osteochondroma from parosteal osteosarcoma, which on occasion has a somewhat similar roentgenographic appearance.

Surgical treatment is indicated when the lesion is either producing symptoms or is so large that malignant transformation is a consideration. In this regard, the size and, specifically, the thickness of the cartilage cap are directly related to the potential for malignancy; the thicker the cap, the more likely it is that malignant cells will be found. Sometimes roentgenograms do not reveal the size of the cartilage cap, and clinical examination suggests that the lesion is larger than it appears to be on the roentgenogram.

When an osteochondroma is excised, the stalk needs only to be osteotomized in line with the normal underlying bone; underlying medullary bone tissue need not be removed. This approach makes recurrence of an isolated osteochondroma unlikely.

The cartilage cap should be examined histologically. At least one section should be taken at a right angle to the surface of the lesion so that the true thickness of the cartilage cap can be determined. The chondrocytes of the cartilage cap usually are arranged in clusters and have a benign appearance. Malignant transformation of an osteo-

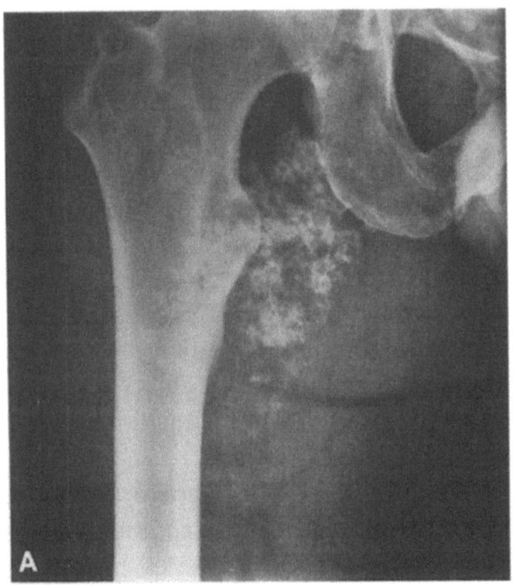

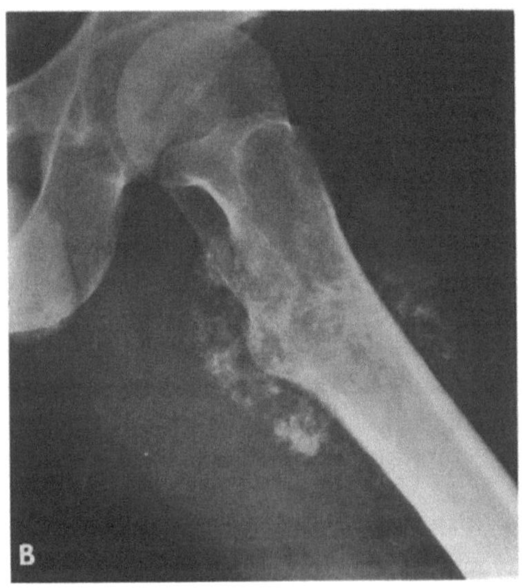

FIG. 2–3 **A** Anteroposterior view of a large osteochondroma which appears to be arising from the region of the lesser trochanter. The margins of the lesion are indistinct. **B** Lateral view of the same lesion. The tumor had areas of chondrosarcoma on its surface.

chondroma is usually to a chondrosarcoma; hence the chondrocytes need to be carefully examined.[6] A cartilage cap that is more than 1 cm thick is particularly worrisome.

Malignant Bone Tumors

Chondrosarcoma

The region of the hip is a common site for chondrosarcoma. In Dahlin's series[3] of 470 chondrosarcomas, 58 tumors arose in the proximal portion of the femur. An additional 128 chondrosarcomas arose in the pelvis adjacent to the hip. As with most bone tumors, males are more commonly affected than females. Chondrosarcoma tends to arise in older persons, although those of any age may be afflicted.

A chondrosarcoma in the hip region is difficult to detect until it has been present for a long time. Patients may complain of referred pain in a site remote from the hip. Most patients with chondrosarcoma complain of pain, which is usually present at rest but may be aggravated by weight-bearing. The patient may complain for several years before the true nature of the problem is identified.

Most chondrosarcomas appear to arise de novo and are called *primary chondrosarcomas;* however, some lesions arise in preexisting benign tumors, such as an osteochondroma or an enchondroma in a patient with multiple enchondromas. Such lesions are referred to as *secondary chondrosarcomas.* My colleagues and I have not seen a chondrosarcoma arise in a documented preexisting solitary enchondroma (Figs. 2–4 and 2–5).

The roentgenographic features of chondrosarcoma are often characteristic and helpful in the

A
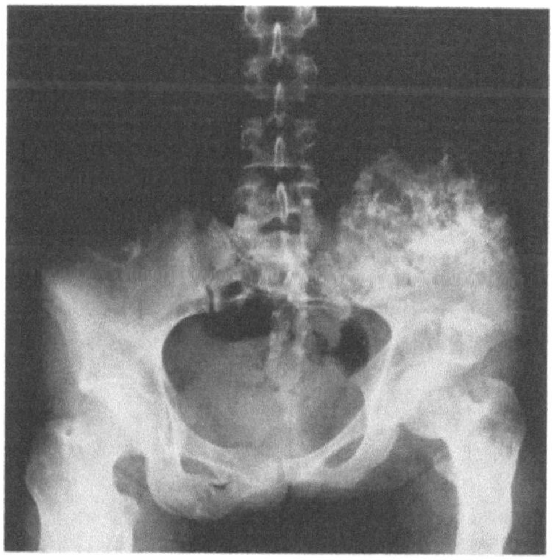

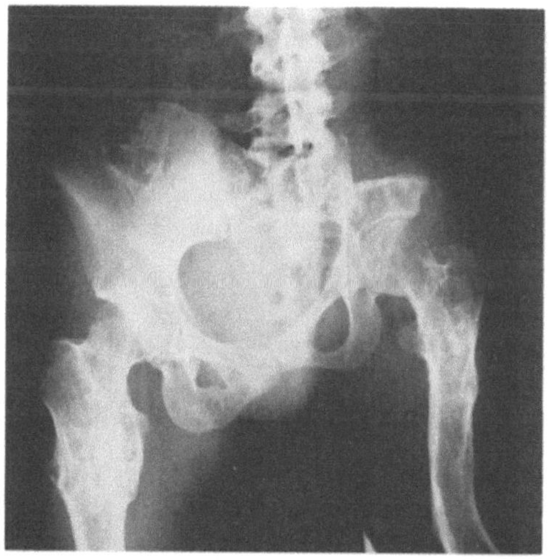
B

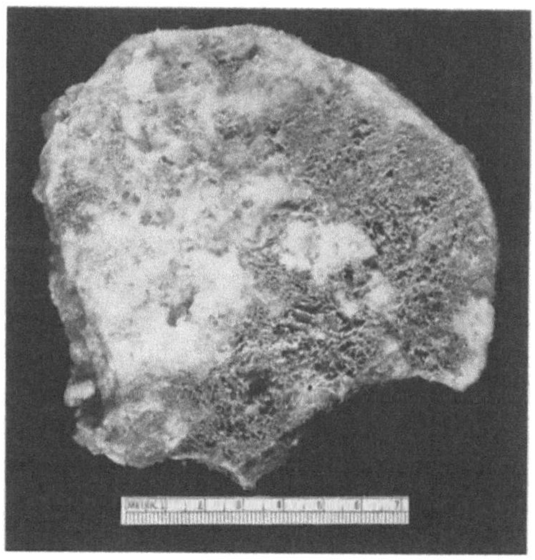
C

FIG. 2–4 Secondary chondrosarcoma in a 24-year-old woman with multiple osteocartilaginous exostoses. **A** The patient had recent enlargement of the left iliac crest. Note the mottled calcification and scalloped periphery. **B** At 2 years after excision her hip function is normal, with some pain on stress. The migrated inferior ilium has stabilized to the sacrum with fibrous union; there are 2 inches of shortening but no evidence of recurrence. **C** Gross appearance of the removed ilium containing the tumor. Peripheral borders showed no malignancy. The pathological diagnosis was grade 2 chondrosarcoma.

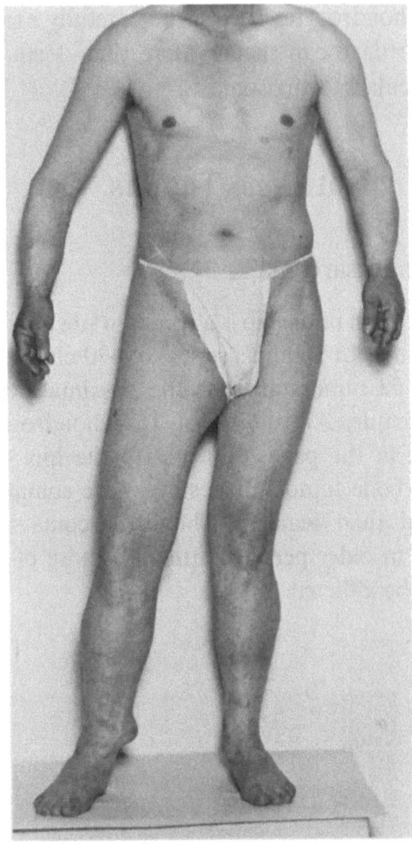

A

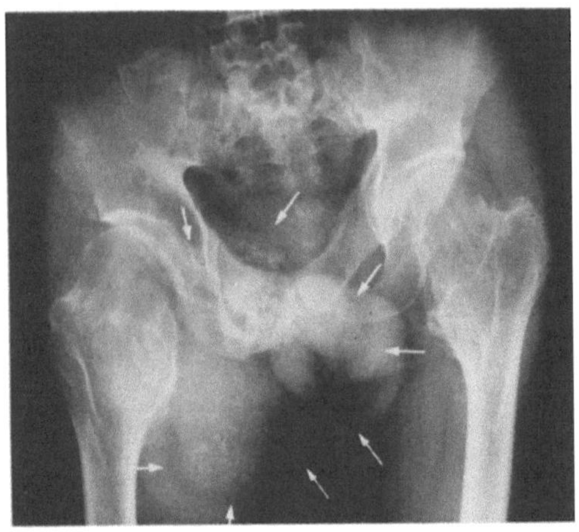

B

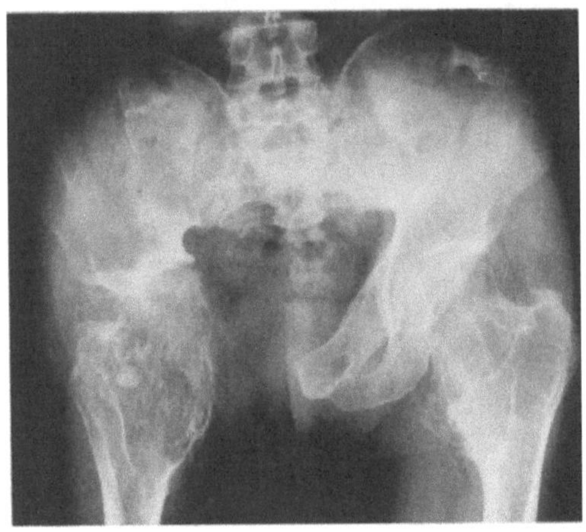

C

FIG. 2–5 Secondary chondrosarcoma in a 40-year-old man with multiple osteocartilaginous exostoses. **A** There is slight dwarfing as well as prominences and deformities about the major joints. The tumor in the right groin was growing and painful, and was disturbing the normal gait. **B** *Arrows* define the soft-tissue extent of the large chondrosarcoma (grade 1) arising from the right ischium. Note the characteristic increase in mottling and calcification, indicating a probable malignant nature. **C** Appearance of the pelvis 2 years after local removal. Despite the absence of ischium, including a large portion of the acetabulum, the patient has a stable hip with good function and works on his feet 10 to 12 hours daily.

diagnosis. For lesions that arise in the intertrochanteric region, there may be a fusiform expansion of the bone associated with thickening of the cortex. If the lesion arises in the medullary cavity, there is usually characteristic scalloping of the endosteal surface of the cortex. Characteristic stippling, or calcification, within the lesion is also a helpful clue. When the lesion extends outside the bone, there may be a large mass of calcific material. Lesions that arise on the inner wall of the acetabulum may be difficult to detect on the roentgenogram, particularly if the lesion is predominantly lytic. Some lesions have the typical appearance of a benign enchondroma, except that some scalloping of the cortical bone is present. These lesions usually are low-grade chondrosarcomas (Fig. 2–6).

Histopathological analysis of the lesion is par-

FIG. 2–6 Typical low-grade chondrosarcoma showing expansion of bone and scalloping of the endosteal cortical surface.

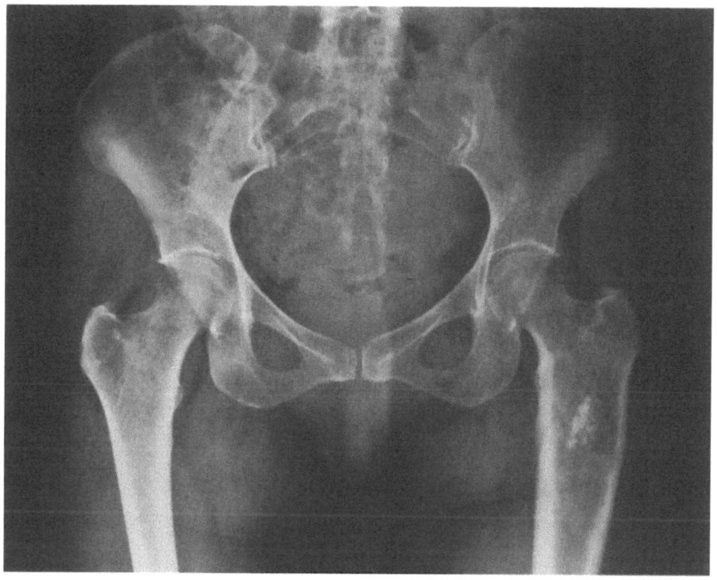

ticularly important because even the most experienced bone pathologists may have difficulty differentiating a benign cartilage tumor from a low-grade chondrosarcoma. Grading of this tumor is also important.[11] High-grade chondrosarcomas require ablative surgery, just as other high-grade sarcomas do. However, the borderline or very low-grade lesions do not require such radical treatment. Low-grade lesions grow slowly, but they tend to recur if not completely excised. Any statement about prognosis for this condition must take into account the necessity for prolonged follow-up because recurrences may not manifest until many years after the original treatment. In fact, statistically, the chance of recurrence is as great during the twentieth year as during the first year after surgery. This lesion also has the potential to metastasize; even very low-grade chondrosarcomas occasionally do so.

Chondrosarcoma is probably one of the most difficult of the primary bone tumors for the orthopedic surgeon to treat. Treatment planning depends on the findings of the pathologist and the radiologist. If the tumor has the roentgenographic appearance of a very low-grade lesion and if other circumstances are favorable, something less than total resection of the lesion might be considered. For example, if the lesion is in the trochanteric area of the proximal femur and has the roentgenographic appearance of an enchondroma but is worrisome because of some scalloping, a hemicylindrical resection of the affected area might be done. The remaining tumor might then be excised with a curet, the cavity cauterized, and bone grafts applied. If the pathologist confirms that the lesion is a borderline, very low-grade (grade ½) lesion, this treatment is probably satisfactory, although the patient must be followed for many years to rule out the possibility of local recurrence. However, if the pathologist finds that the tumor is higher grade, a more radical procedure is necessary. If a high-grade lesion is suspected, a generous biopsy specimen should be taken at the outset and results of the final pathology report known before proceeding with the definitive surgery.

If the lesion is entirely intraosseous or has only minimal cortical breakthrough, and if histologically the lesion is not too wildly malignant, resection of the proximal end of the femur might be considered. The hip can be reconstructed using a cutom-type total hip prosthesis (Fig. 2–7).

For lesions of the acetabulum and adjacent pelvis, local resections may be done if they can be accomplished without entering the tumor and without spilling tumor into the surrounding soft tissues. Chondrosarcoma tends to be implanted into soft tissues, and so care must be taken to avoid seeding the tumor.

If the acetabulum itself is involved with the tumor, hemipelvectomy may be required; however, if the lesion is small, resection may be considered. For example, the acetabulum and the adjacent femoral head and neck may be resected and reconstruction done by attempting arthrodesis of the

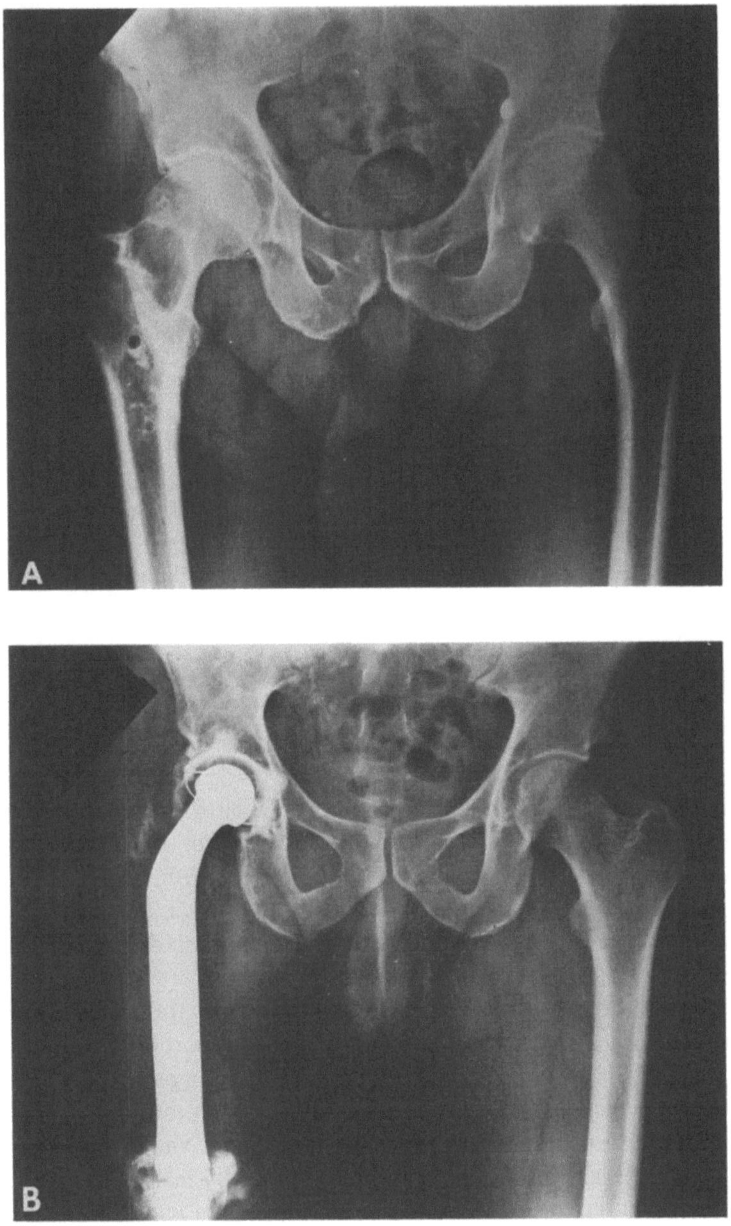

FIG. 2–7 **A** Atypical chondrosarcoma involving the proximal femur. The lesion was resected, and a custom-type total hip arthroplasty was utilized to reconstruct the hip. **B** Appearance of reconstruction with a custom-type prosthesis.

proximal femur to either the remaining ilium or the pubic bone. Although such procedures may be suitable for some small, low grade chondrosarcomas, most chondrosarcomas are high grade and are of considerable size before they are discovered. Such large lesions require radical treatment, and this usually necessitates hemipelvectomy.

An entity referred to as dedifferentiated chondrosarcoma accounts for about 10% of all chondrosarcomas.[4] Histologically, this lesion contains easily recognizable areas of ordinary chondrosarcoma, but it also may contain areas of high-grade fibrosarcoma, osteosarcoma, or malignant fibrous histiocytoma. The clinical behavior of the tumor is predicted by the more malignant dedifferentiated area. Hence the patient with dedifferentiated chondrosarcoma usually requires radical amputation surgery.

Osteosarcoma

Osteosarcoma is the most common primary sarcoma of bone, accounting for about 20% of all bone sarcomas. In Dahlin's series of 962 cases,[3]

47 were in the upper femur and hip region and 81 were in the adjacent pelvis. Osteogenic sarcoma occurs most often in patients who are in their second and third decades, with males more commonly affected than females. As with most of the tumors in the hip region, pain or a mass (or both) is the most frequent presenting symptom. Osteosarcoma rarely presents with a pathological fracture in the hip joint.

The roentgenographic appearance of osteosarcoma in the hip region is not likely to be characteristic. The lesion probably will show evidence of cortical destruction with evidence of a soft-tissue mass, which may be calcified or ossified, and there may be considerable adjacent reactive sclerosis. Some osteosarcomas present as almost exclusively lytic lesions, though they usually have an obviously aggressive appearance with indistinct margins at the periphery of the lesion.

The older patient may have evidence of Paget's disease in the same area as the destructive lesion. The incidence of malignant transformation of Paget's disease is unknown, but it is probably small. Nevertheless, malignant transformation of Paget's disease should be suspected whenever there is a change in the roentgenographic appearance of the lesion in an older adult or when there is a change in symptoms. In addition, the serum alkaline phosphatase level may be elevated at the time of malignant transformation. However, this finding in itself does not necessarily imply that malignant transformation has taken place.

In addition, the presence of osteogenic sarcoma should be suspected in the older adult if the patient has had radiation therapy either for carcinoma of the pelvic organs or for any preexisting condition in the same general region. Postirradiation sarcoma can arise even many years after the initial radiation treatment.

An open biopsy specimen should be obtained to establish the diagnosis of osteosarcoma. An adequate amount of representative tissue must be available so the pathologist can make an accurate diagnosis. However, great care must be taken when placing a biopsy incision, as subsequent ablative surgery is required in the vast majority of patients. The biopsy site must be placed in such a way that it can be removed together with the tumor specimen at the time of definitive surgery. As with other locations, transverse incisions in the hip region should be avoided because they make the subsequent definitive surgery much more difficult and, on occasion, even make it necessary to perform a hemipelvectomy when some lesser procedure might otherwise be indicated.

The treatment of osteosarcoma remains controversial. In 1967 Dahlin and Coventry[5] reported on 650 patients treated at the Mayo Clinic and established that 23.3% were alive at 5 years and 17.3% at 10 years. Lesions located in the hip region, however, were associated with a somewhat worse prognosis. Since 1967, survival of patients with osteosarcoma has improved considerably. The reasons for this improvement remain obscure. In the Mayo Clinic experience, this improvement in survival has been independent of any adjunctive treatment.[16] Many other investigators have utilized various forms of adjunctive treatment, however, including numerous combination chemotherapy regimens. The latter investigators tend to believe that the improvement in prognosis is related to the adjunctive treatment utilized.

There is much confusion at the present time as to whether adjunctive chemotherapy is necessary for all patients. It also remains unsettled as to whether the limb-salvage procedures are preferable to amputation surgery, particularly for tumors in the hip region. For a very small lesion that is entirely intraosseous and involves the proximal portion of the femur, it is very tempting to resect the proximal femur together with a wide cuff of surrounding normal muscles. The hip can then be reconstructed with a custom-type total hip implant (Fig. 2–8). This concept is particularly tempting if one believes that preoperative chemotherapy allows less ablative surgery to be done. To date, however, the exact value of such an approach has not been definitely established. In the hip region, amputation surgery is needed to achieve adequate margins, at least in most patients. Techniques for resection and reconstruction, however, are now available, and if some of the more promising current chemotherapy programs prove to be useful, more patients may undergo limb-salvage procedures.

Fibrosarcoma and Malignant Fibrous Histiocytoma

The clinical and roentgenographic findings associated with fibrosarcomas and malignant fibrous histiocytomas are similar to those of osteogenic sarcoma. The treatment is essentially identical for all these entities; at the present time it is not known

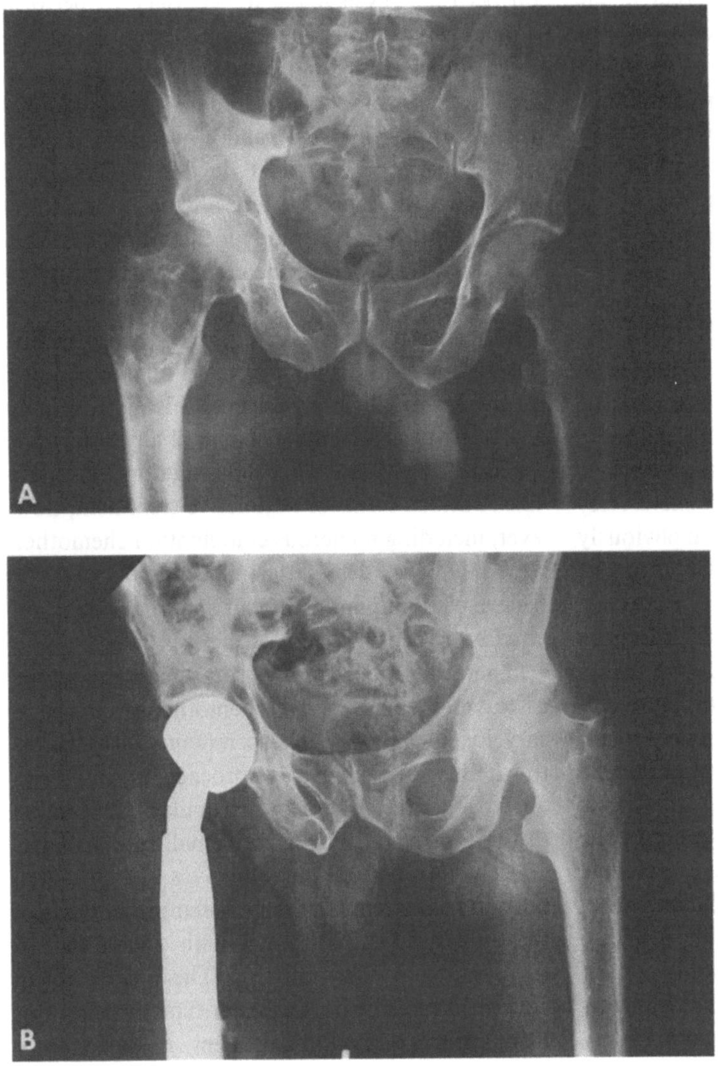

FIG. 2–8 **A** Unusual-appearing osteosarcoma in a 49-year-old man. **B** The lesion was resected and the hip reconstructed with a Bateman-type prosthesis. The patient subsequently developed metastatic disease.

if these conditions have different prognoses. They must be differentiated if one is to know whether there are any important differences among them.

Ewing's Sarcoma

Ewing's sarcoma of bone is much less common than osteogenic sarcoma, accounting for about 5% of all bone sarcomas. Approximately 25% of Ewing's sarcomas occur in the hip region. Mature adults rarely have Ewing's sarcoma, with most of the lesions occurring in patients less than 20 years old. In addition to having pain and swelling, patients with Ewing's sarcoma may complain of intermittent low-grade fever. Mild anemia or leukocytosis (or both) may be noted. Occasionally, patients with Ewing's sarcoma present with pathological fractures. The roentgenographic appearance is not characteristic. The so-called onionskin layering of reactive periosteal tissue is not commonly seen in the hip region. Usually, there is an indistinct area of cortical bone destruction with evidence of an adjacent soft-tissue mass.

In the past, no more than about 10% of patients with Ewing's sarcoma survived longer than 5 years. It was recognized that the primary lesion is sensitive to irradiation. With the use of radiation therapy to control the primary tumor and chemotherapy to eliminate micrometastases and control systemic disease, survival has improved considerably. With patients surviving longer, it has become apparent that local control of the primary lesion with radiation therapy is not always achieved. Indeed, recent information indicates that

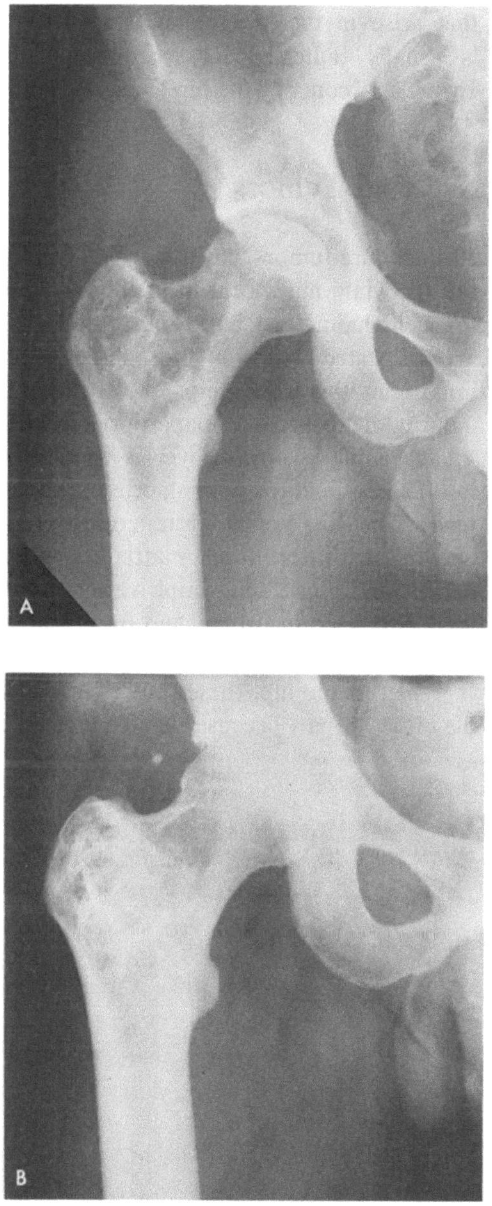

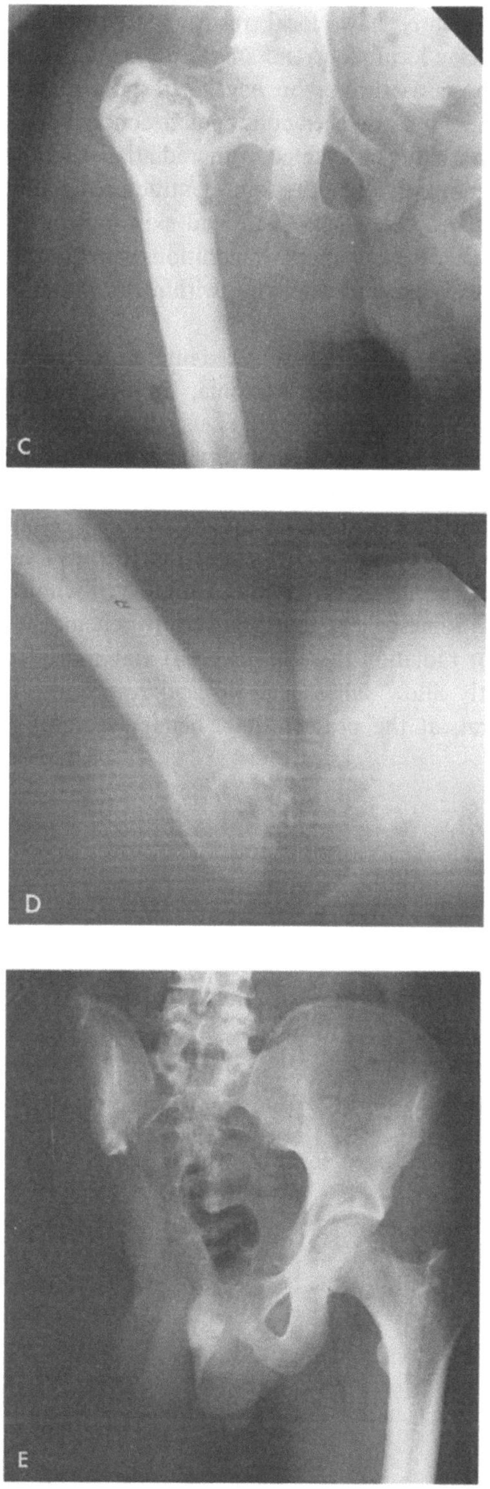

FIG. 2–9 Ewing's sarcoma in an 18-year-old man. **A** There was chiefly lytic involvement of trochanteric and femoral neck regions at the time of biopsy. Treatment was irradiation. **B** Two years later there was good response to the irradiation, with some sclerosis of the tumor. **C** and **D** Four years after radiation therapy, a pathological fracture occurred, and hindquarter amputation was then done. **E** The pelvis after amputation. The patient was alive and well 17 years after the initial diagnosis.

15 to 20% of patients who survive the initial period subsequently have local recurrences.[10] Patients who have local recurrences have the same general prognosis as those who have metastatic disease.

There has also been considerable concern about the morbidity associated with radiation therapy. This morbidity includes joint contractures, pathological fractures, soft-tissue and skin induration, and other local changes. In addition, patients with late osteosarcoma occurring within the radiation field also have been noted.[15]

Thus there has been renewed interest in surgical resection for Ewing's sarcoma; however, in the region of the hip joint it is usually difficult to achieve a wide excision of Ewing's sarcoma because most of the lesions have considerable extension into the soft tissues. Currently, various combinations of chemotherapy, radiation therapy, and surgery are being explored in a number of clinical trials. Some believe that preoperative chemotherapy or radiation therapy (or both) may more frequently allow subsequent surgical resections. In general, at the present time, hemipelvectomy is not advocated for patients with Ewing's sarcomas that arise in the hip region. Radiation therapy is usually indicated for treatment of primary Ewing's sarcoma of the hip (Figs. 2–9 and 2–10).

Synovial Tumors

Various rare tumors and tumor-like conditions of the synovium may occur in the region of articulations, including the bursae and tendon sheaths. When located within a joint, these lesions may imitate another condition, e.g., arthritis, and remain undiagnosed and inappropriately treated.

The actual synovial layer is usually one cell in thickness, and these lining cells are slightly flattened. The subsynovial tissues consist of a fibrous network with a collagen matrix, as well as fat, nerves, and blood and lymph vessels. This entire layer is termed *synovium,* and from it arise synovial tumors.

When in the hip, these tumors are difficult to diagnose, in part because they cannot be seen or

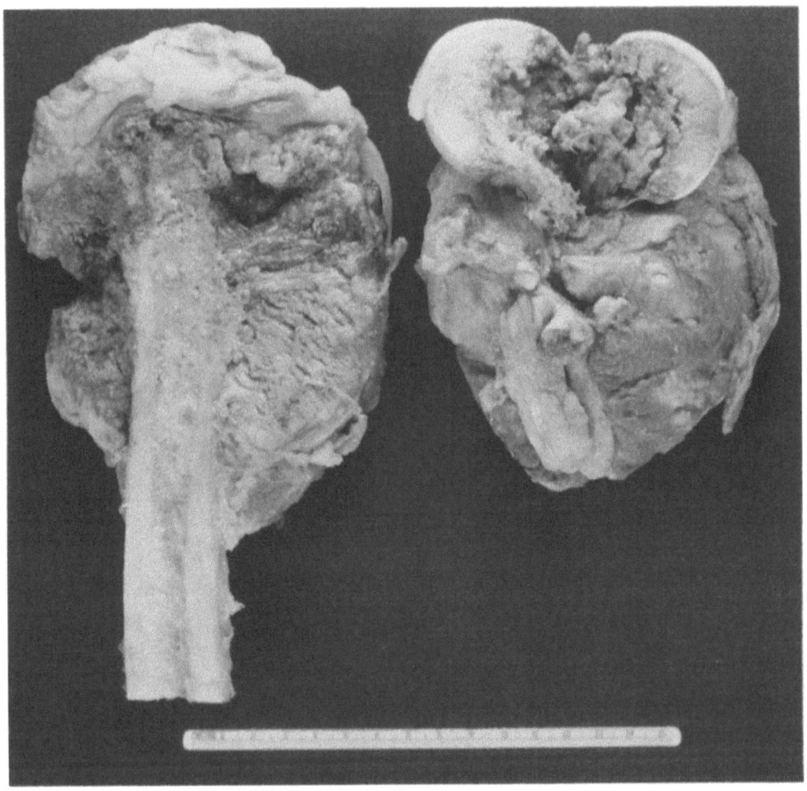

FIG. 2–10 Same case as in Fig. 2–9, showing extensive involvement, evident in the surgical specimen.

palpated as they may be in the knee (the more common location for synovial tumors). The examiner should be aware, however, that such tumors can exist in the hip. Synovial tumors, all benign, are classified as (1) pigmented villonodular synovitis, (2) xanthoma, (3) (osteo)chondromatosis, (4) hemangioma, (5) lipoma, and (6) plexiform neuroma, vascular myoma, myxoma, and perhaps some other rare tumors (Figs. 2–11 and 2–12).

Malignant tumors of the synovium are almost nonexistent. Synovial sarcoma occurs near a joint but very seldom in one; it is so named because of the appearance of the tumor cells, and it arises de novo from the mesenchyma of the somatic soft tissues rather than from preexistent synovial tissue.

The differential diagnosis of synovial tumors about the hip includes cysts of synovium, either rheumatoid or degenerative in origin, and adventitious or typical tumors of the bursae, particularly the greater trochanteric and the iliopectineal bursae.

Pigmented Villonodular Synovitis

Pigmented villonodular synovitis does not commonly involve the hip, but when it does it presents a fairly typical appearance and should be suspected when a single joint is involved. The condition—

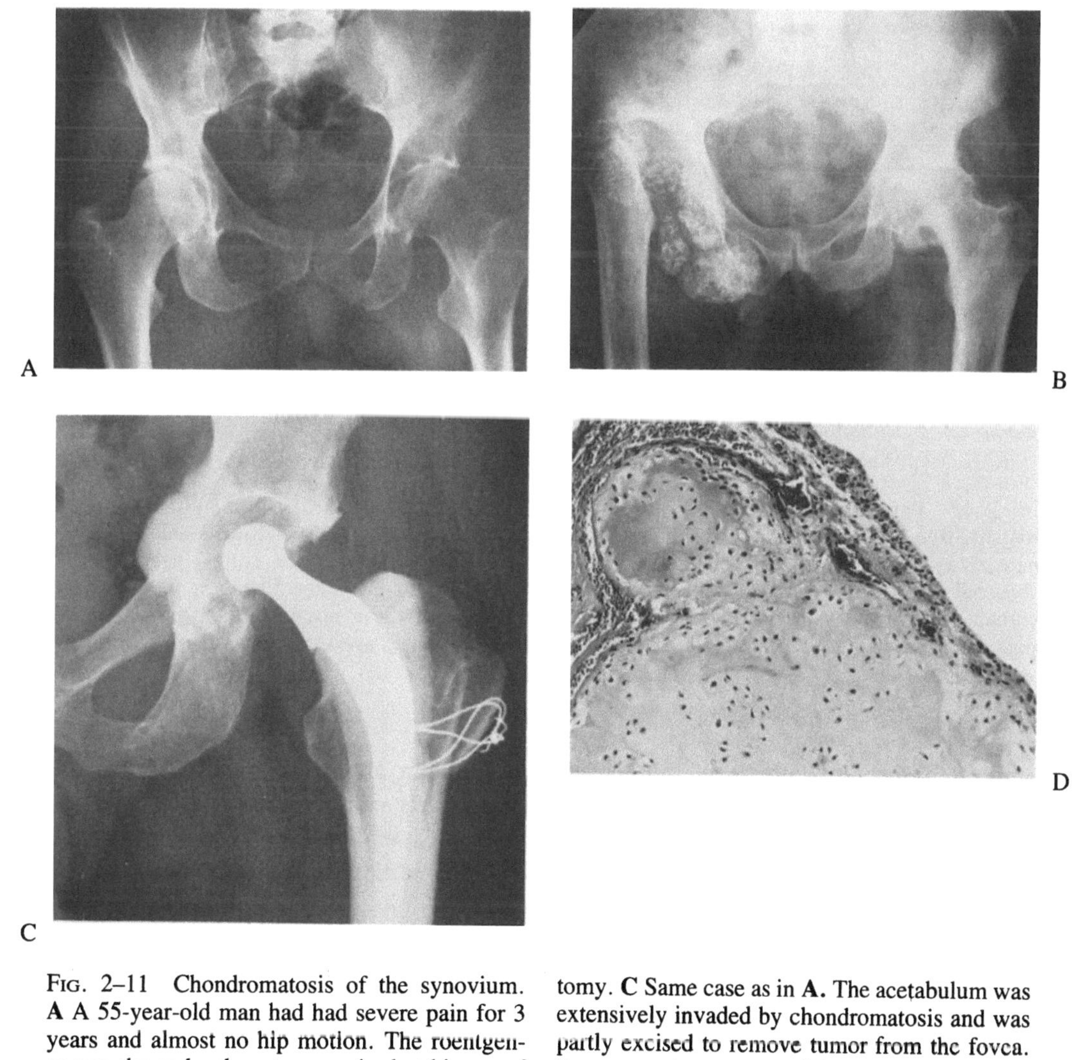

FIG. 2–11 Chondromatosis of the synovium. **A** A 55-year-old man had had severe pain for 3 years and almost no hip motion. The roentgenogram showed only osteoporosis, but biopsy of the synovium revealed multiple diffuse chondromatosis. **B** By contrast, there is marked, diffuse osteochondromatosis in this 62-year-old man which recurred after removal of the femoral head and neck and an attempt at complete synovectomy. **C** Same case as in **A**. The acetabulum was extensively invaded by chondromatosis and was partly excised to remove tumor from the fovea. Reconstruction was possible by total hip arthroplasty after complete synovectomy. This is the appearance 8 weeks after removal and total hip arthroplasty. **D** Same case as in **A** and **C**. Proliferated cartilaginous masses are seen below the synovial layer. (Hematoxylin and eosin, ×175.)

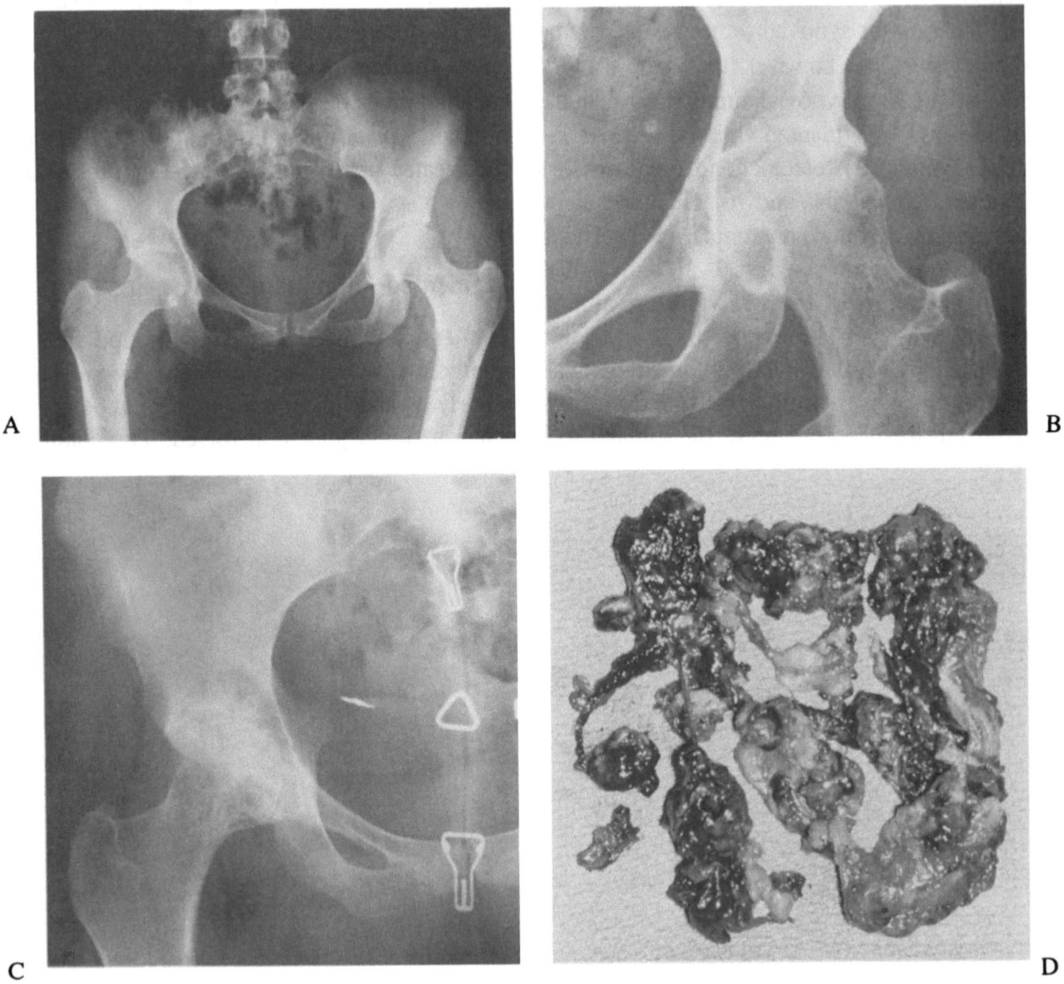

FIG. 2–12 Pigmented villonodular synovitis. **A** Involved right hip of a 32-year-old woman. Note the early changes, chiefly osteoporosis. **B** More advanced changes are seen in this 30-year-old woman, including cystic formation; the joint space is still fairly normal. **C** Note the far-advanced changes in this 19-year-old woman, with loss of joint space. This is difficult to differentiate roentgenographically from degenerative arthritis, but the age of the patient decreases the probability of the latter diagnosis. **D** Gross appearance of the synovium of the patient in **A**. The pigmented synovium is evident.

a pigmented, xanthic, inflammatory, tumor-like proliferation of stromal cells—initially was described by Jaffe and associates in 1941.[7]

Grossly, the synovium has an abundant, diffuse, reddish brown, shaggy-beard appearance. Sometimes the lesion is localized. The brown discoloration is due to intra-articular hemorrhage from a variety of causes. The diffuse villous and nodular microscopic transformation of the synovium results from proliferation of synovial lining and stromal cells that fill the interstices and infiltrate the subsynovial fat. These fibroid xanthic components are histiocytic, form multinucleated giant cells, and contain abundant lipoids and hemosiderin. There also is an accompanying inflammatory component of lymphocytes and some plasma cells.

The condition may affect persons of either sex and of almost any age, exclusive of childhood. Swelling is common about the knee but is not evident when the hip is involved. Pain may be present for months to many years.

Unilateral hip involvement, most commonly during the fourth or fifth decade of life, characterized by pain which is increased by activity and relieved by rest should make one suspect pigmented villonodular synovitis. A slight limp, limitation of hip motion, and other findings which suggest synovial involvement of the hip are present. There usually is no restriction of hip motion, except by pain. Laboratory findings are of no help, but the roentgenographic appearance is reasonably typical, at least when the lesion is in the advanced stages. Predominant findings are multiple cystic-like areas in the acetabulum and femoral head and occasionally in the femoral neck—wherever there is synovial attachment to bone but not necessarily at the points of maximal weight-bearing load, as in degenerative arthritis. These "cysts" consist of the tumor itself eroding into the subjacent bone and cartilage. Usually, there is no distortion of the contour of the femoral head compared with that seen in osteoarthritis, and seldom do osteoarthritic lippings or spurs form. However, the joint space may narrow as the disease progresses.

The most common differential diagnostic problem is degenerative arthritis, although rheumatoid arthritis, tuberculosis, and other granulomas also must be considered.

Surgical exploration is indicated when the condition is suspected. In most cases reported in the literature, the initial diagnosis was osteoarthritis when operation was done. The gross findings are so characteristic that as soon as the synovium is opened the correct diagnosis should be immediately suspected because the thick, exuberant, frond-like synovium with its characteristic color is evident. The diagnosis is confirmed by microscopic examination.

Synovectomy, with removal of all the synovium including that in the "cysts," is indicated. Although irradiation may be of some help, it probably should not be used because of its relatively poor curative value and its potential for causing later malignancy. Perhaps total hip arthroplasty will prove to be the most effective procedure, especially when involvement is extensive. We have had limited experience with hip arthroplasty for this condition.

Chondromatosis of the Synovium

Chondromatosis includes osteochondromatosis of the synovium, but occasionally there is no actual bone present in the discrete cartilaginous tumors. It is the same process as osteochondromatosis, and the same treatment is used. Chondromatosis is a benign, tumorous, multifocal, chondromatous or chondro-osseous meta-plastic proliferation involving the subsynovial connective tissue of joints, tendon sheaths, or bursae. In the experience at the Mayo Clinic, the hip was involved in 16% of the cases (the knee in almost 70%).[8] The process can involve any joint. The average age of the patients is about 40 years, and males are affected more often than females. Symptoms include pain and limited motion about the hip. Swelling in the synovium cannot be diagnosed as such by the patient or the examiner (as it can in the knee). Duration of symptoms may be long or relatively short before diagnosis is made. In the Mayo Clinic series, only two-thirds of the roentgenograms showed radiopaque masses. Diagnosis is difficult because the roentgenogram may not reveal ossific bodies even when they are present.

Whereas the disease is readily recognized in the knee—where the synovium can be palpated, there is less soft tissue obscuring the roentgenogram, and surgical diagnosis by arthrotomy is more readily done—recognition in the hip is another matter. Long-standing pain localized to one joint may be associated roentgenographically with only mild osteoporosis or with multiple, diffuse, calcified, osteocartilaginous bodies. If only slightly calcified, osteochondromatous bodies may be seen with special roentgenographic techniques to blur out soft-tissue shadows. If calcific deposits are present but few in number, oblique and lateral views sometimes show them because, if the osteochondromatous bodies have become loose and fall into the recesses of the joint, they do so inferiorly and medially in the normal synovial pocket in this region. These bodies are often best seen in a lateral view.

When the roentgenological diagnosis is indefinite and symptoms persist without any other obvious cause, diagnostic arthrotomy is indicated. This is a difficult problem because one wishes to do as little damage to the joint as possible during exploration. An anterior iliofemoral approach is sufficient. This approach exposes the anterior portion of the hip capsule, which then is carefully opened so as not to injure the articular cartilage of the head; the anterior and anteromedial aspects of the hip are inspected. This is an inadequate exposure for the entire hip joint; and if the diagnosis is still suspected but cannot be confirmed this way, the exposure must be extended into a classic Smith-Petersen approach. The hip joint must then be dislocated—something one wishes not to do because avascular necrosis may follow. If the dislocation is needed only for a short time, however, this sequela is unlikely. Because osteochondromatosis may be sharply localized and may not be a diffuse condition of the entire synovium, careful inspection of the entire synovial lining is important. Generally, diagnosis can be made by the gross appearance and confirmed by immediate histological examination using frozen section technique.

The treatment of osteochondromatosis consists in removing any loose osteochondromatous bodies and the involved synovium from which they arise. In general, complete synovectomy is necessary, and thus complete exposure of the hip joint is required.

The condition may recur because nests of synovium may be left behind. If this happens, a second arthrotomy is necessary. Damage to the hip by this procedure may be fairly extensive, and in certain instances a primary arthroplasty is advisable if the synovial chondromatosis is extensive.

Radiation therapy is to be condemned. Although irradiation may have some inhibiting effects on synovial growth, its potential for causing malignant change later is notorious.

Frequently, the long-standing synovial osteochondromatosis creates secondary osteoarthritis. If this occurs, it can be managed primarily by total hip replacement.

Other Synovial Tumors

Other synovial tumors of the hip are rare. Localized xanthomas are perhaps the most common of these, and whether they are primarily the cause of the problem or incidental to it is not known. Usually such lesions are found incidentally at operation for degenerative arthritis.

Benign and Malignant Soft-Tissue Tumors

A wide variety of soft-tissue somatic tumors are seen in the hip region. Several classifications of these tumors are available. That of Soule is presented because of its completeness (Table 2–1).

Lipoma is the most common benign soft-tissue tumor. It arises in the fat of the buttock and upper part of the thigh. Malignant fibrous histoicytoma, liposarcoma, synovioma, fibrosarcoma, and rhabdosarcoma are the most common malignant tumors of soft tissue about the hip.

TABLE 2–1 Classification of Somatic Soft-Tissue Tumors

- I. Fibromatous tumors
  - A. Benign tumor-like proliferations
    - 1. Hypertrophic scar
    - 2. Keloid
    - 3. Fibromatoses
      - a. Nodular fascial fibromatosis
        - (1) Plantar
        - (2) Palmar
        - (3) Penile (?)
      - b. Juvenile fibromatosis
        - (1) Fibromatosis colli (congenital torticollis)
        - (2) Diffuse muscular fibromatosis (?)
        - (3) Congenital generalized fibromatosis
        - (4) "Juvenile" aponeurotic fibroma
        - (5) Infantile dermal fibromatosis
        - (6) Aggressive infantile fibromatosis
        - (7) Fibrous hamartoma of infancy
      - c. Desmoid (aggressive fibromatosis, desmoid fibromatosis)
    - 4. Elastofibroma dorsi
  - B. Benign neoplasms
    - 1. Fibroma
    - 2. Dermatofibroma (?)
    - 3. Myxoma (fibromyxoma) (?)
  - C. Malignant neoplasms
    - 1. Fibrosarcoma
      - a. Adult type
      - b. Juvenile type (?)
    - 2. Myxosarcoma (?)
    - 3. Dermatofibrosarcoma protuberans (?)
- II. Xanthofibrohistiocytic tumors (tumors of histiocytes) (?)
  - A. Benign neoplasms
    - 1. Xanthoma
      - a. Histiocytoma
      - b. Nevoid xanthogranuloma (nevoid histiotiocytoma)
    - 2. Fibrous xanthoma
      - a. Giant cell tumor of tendon sheath
      - b. Villonodular synovitis
    - 3. Atypical fibrous xanthoma
      - a. Dermatofibroma
      - b. Sclerosing hemangioma
      - c. Reticulohistiocytic granuloma
      - d. Dermatofibrosarcoma protuberans
      - e. Xanthogranuloma
  - B. Malignant fibrous xanthoma (giant cell sarcoma); malignant histiocytoma
- III. Proliferative tumefactive lesions (pseudosarcomatous lesions)
  - A. Proliferative (nodular) fasciitis
  - B. Proliferative myositis
  - C. Myositis ossificans
  - D. Irradiation fibromatosis
- IV. Lipomatous tumors
  - A. Benign tumor-like proliferations
    - 1. Lipogranuloma
      - a. Traumatic fat necrosis

b. Injection granuloma (paraffinoma)
c. Sclerosing lipogranuloma
2. Symmetrical lipomatosis
B. Benign neoplasms
1. Lipoblastomatosis
2. Lipoblastoma (hibernoma)
3. Lipoma (numerous types)
a. Infiltrating (myolipoma)
b. Myelolipoma
C. Malignant liposarcoma
1. Myxoid
2. Lipogenic
3. Pleomorphic
V. Angiomatous tumors
A. Benign neoplasms
1. Hemangioma
a. Capillary
b. Cavernous
c. Mixed
d. Venous
2. Juvenile hemangioma (hemangioendothelioma)
3. Congenital hemangiomatosis
4. Congenital arteriovenous malformation
5. Lymphangioma
a. Capillary and cavernous
b. Cystic hygroma
6. Hemangioendothelioma
7. Glomus tumor
8. Hemangiopericytoma
B. Malignant neoplasms
1. Angiosarcoma
2. Lymphangiosarcoma and chronic lymphedema
3. Kaposi's sarcoma
4. Malignant hemangiopericytoma
VI. Neuromatous tumors
A. Nonneoplastic tumors
1. Traumatic neuroma
2. Sclerosing neuroma
B. Benign neoplasms
1. Neurilemmoma
2. Neurofibroma
3. Neurofibromatosis, multiple
4. Granular cell neurilemmoma (?)
C. Malignant neoplasms
1. Neurofibrosarcoma (malignant schwannoma)
2. Sarcoma associated with neurofibromatosis
3. Neuroepithelioma, malignant
VII. Myomatous tumors
A. Benign neoplasms
1. Leiomyoma
a. Vascular (angioneuromyoma)
b. Leiomyomatosis cutis
c. Leiomyoblastoma
2. Rhabdomyoma (glycogen tumor)
3. Granular cell myoblastoma (?)
B. Malignant neoplasms
1. Leiomyosarcoma
2. Malignant (organoid) granular cell myoblastoma (?)
3. Rhabdomyosarcoma
a. Pleomorphic (adult)
b. Embryonal (juvenile)
(1) Solid
(2) Alveolar
(3) Botryoid
VIII. Synovial tumors
A. Benign tumors
1. Ganglion cyst (myxoma) (?)
2. Popliteal cyst (synovial cyst) (?)
3. Villonodular synovitis (?)
4. Osteochondromatosis of bursae
5. Adventitious bursa
B. Malignant synovial sarcoma
IX. Miscellaneous mesenchymal tumors
A. Benign tumors
1. Calcinosis, generalized
2. Tumorous calcinosis
3. Myositis ossificans, progressive
4. Heterotopic bone or cartilage
5. Benign mixed mesenchymoma
6. Granular cell tumor (myoblastoma)
7. Chondroma or chondroid tumor
B. Malignant tumors
1. Malignant lymphoma (reticulum cell sarcoma)
2. Solitary plasmacytoma
3. Extraskeletal osteogenic sarcoma
4. Extraskeletal chondrosarcoma
5. Malignant mixed mesenchymoma
6. Clear cell sarcoma
7. Malignant granular cell tumor (myoblastoma)
X. Malignant mesenchymal sarcoma of indeterminate type (undifferentiated mesenchymal sarcoma; round-cell sarcoma, Ewing's type)

[From Coventry, M. B.: Tumors in and about the hip. In *Surgery of the Hip Joint.* (Tronzo, R. G., ed.) Philadelphia, Lea & Febiger, 1973, pp. 378–410.]

Soft-tissue tumors often may be diagnosed by visual and tactile means. Although some of them, buried deep in the tissues about the hip, defy recognition on palpation by the examiner, the patient may be aware of a swelling. A few of the tumors cast characteristic shadows on the roentgenogram.

Lipoma

The lipoma usually is classified as either infiltrating or encapsulated, and it may grow to a considerable size. The roentgenographic appearance is characteristic if the roentgenogram shows the tumor in profile: it is the only tumor that is less dense than the surrounding muscle. At excisional biopsy, care must be taken to remove all of the tumor and

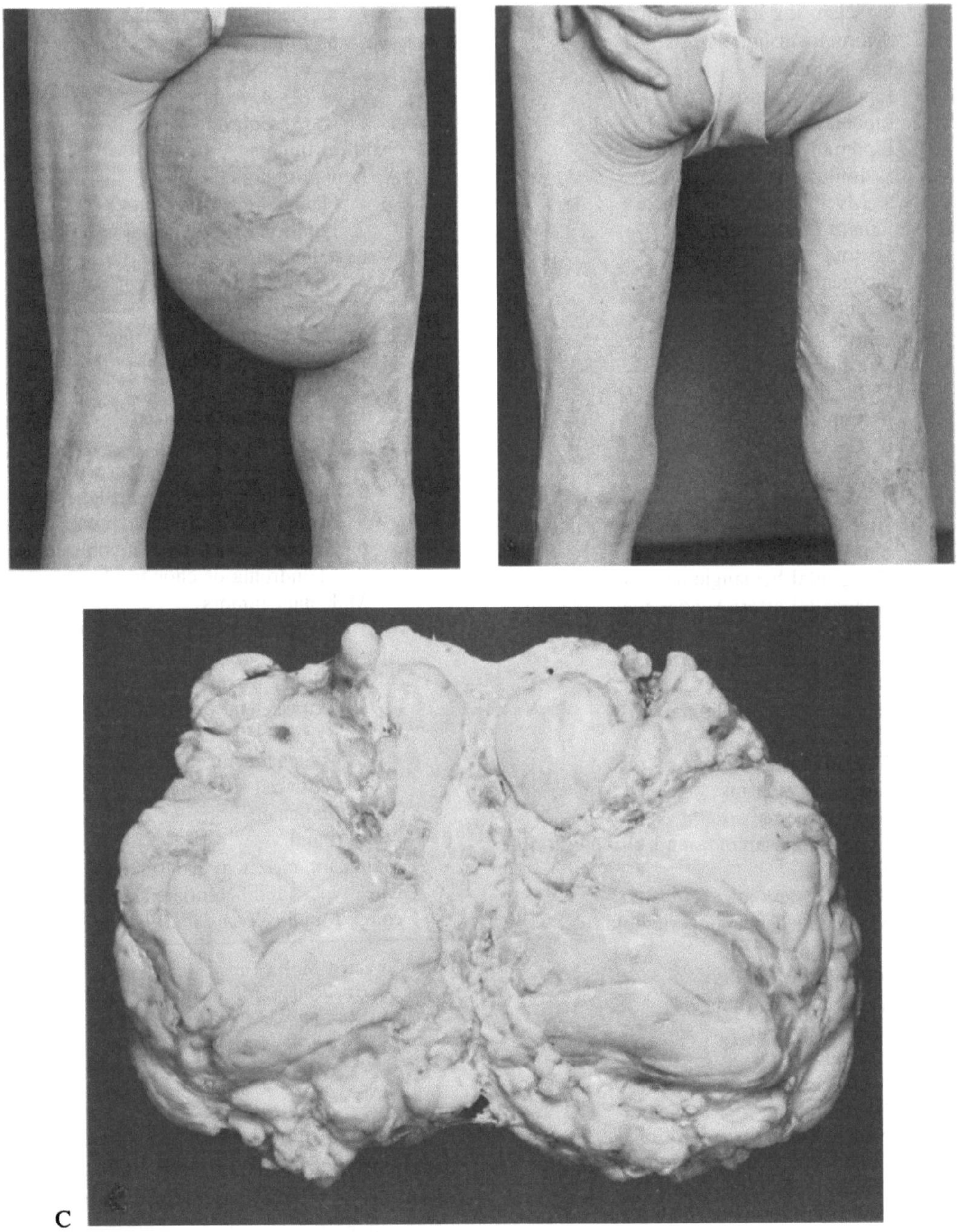

A B

C

FIG. 2–13 Lipoma in an 81-year-old man. **A** Appearance before removal of the lipoma. **B** Appearance after removal. **C** The removed tumor weighed 10 kg (22 lb).

not simply shell it out lest small bits of pedunculated tumor be left and continue to grow (Fig. 2–13).

Liposarcoma

The liposarcoma, a malignant counterpart of the lipoma, is commonly found about the hip. Of 169 liposarcomas in the lower extremity reported from the Mayo Clinic,[12] 123 were in the thigh (usually upper) and 13 in the buttock.

The diagnosis of liposarcoma, in contrast to that of lipoma, may be difficult, especially when the lesion is Broders' histological grade 1 or 2. Any lipoma that is growing should be suspected of being malignant. Furthermore, on palpation the liposarcoma is frequently firmer, and most liposarcomas do not have enough normal fat to be radiolucent, compared with the surrounding muscle. However, of 66 roentgenograms of patients with liposarcoma reviewed, 10 showed a combination of radiolucency and radiopacity.[12] Thus roentgenograms are not as diagnostic as they are for lipoma, but the combination of more-dense and less-dense tissue may be characteristic of liposarcoma.

Computed tomography is very helpful not only in defining the extent of the lesion but also in revealing relative densities: most soft-tissue sarcomas are not homogeneous. If the entire lesion is of one density, it is less likely to be malignant.

Before operation, the patient must be prepared to accept the fact that the "lipoma" may be malignant. Excisional biopsy is mandatory, and care is taken to remove all gross tumor. As was found in our review of these tumors, the grade 1 or 2 lesion could be removed locally if it was excised widely with a healthy margin of several centimeters. However, there is a significant chance of recurrence. Even at the second recurrence of the tumor, wide local removal is usually effective for the lower-grade tumors. If the tumor recurs a second time, more radical surgery, e.g., amputation, must be considered.

The higher-grade lesion (grades 3 and 4) probably should be treated by amputation primarily unless the tumor can be removed widely without sacrifice of limb function. This is difficult to do about the hip, and radical surgery such as hindquarter amputation frequently is necessary for cure. The 5-year survival rates in the Mayo Clinic

A
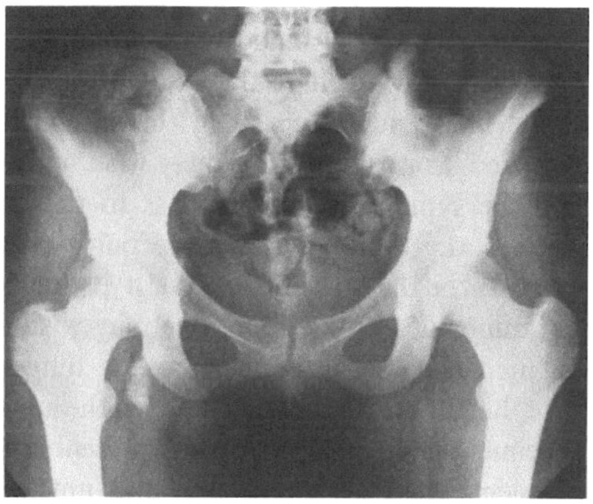

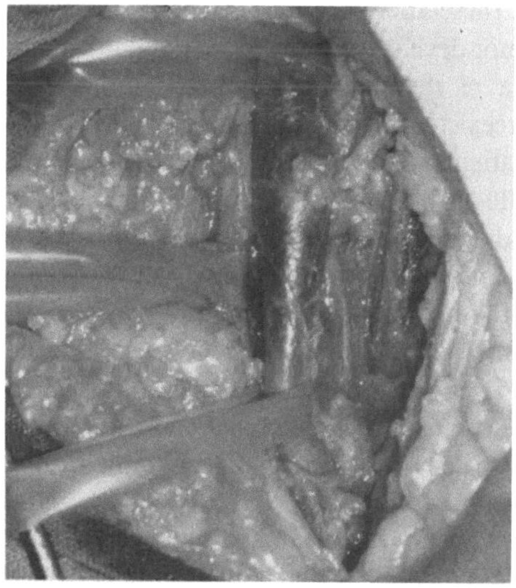
B

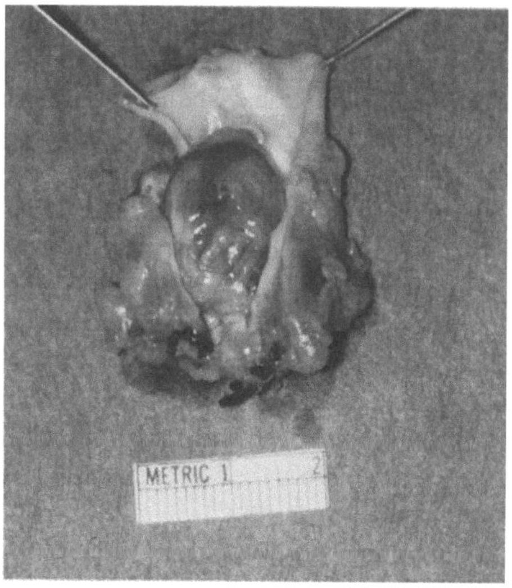

C

FIG. 2–14 Synovioma of the right hip region of a 17-year-old girl. **A** Note the calcification in the region of the iliopectineal bursa. **B** At operation a tumor was seen to be perforating the external iliac vein. Hindquarter amputation was done. **C** Inner aspect of the external iliac vein, with a synovioma growing into it. Despite this, the patient was alive 15 years after hindquarter amputation.

study were 60% for lipogenic lesions, 47.3% for myxoid lesions, and 33.3% for pleomorphic lesions.[12] According to the grade of differentiation, the rates were 75.0% for grade 1, 40.0% for grade 2, 37.3% for grade 3, and 31.8% for grade 4. The overall 5-year survival rate for all grades (166 cases) was 44.6%, and the 10-year survival rate was 22.8%.

Synovioma

Synovioma, or synovial sarcoma, usually arises in an extremity or a limb girdle; rarely, it occurs in the trunk or neck. In the Mayo Clinic experience, about 70% of the tumors involved the lower extremities, usually the thigh, followed in decreasing frequency by the knee, foot, hand, and leg.[17] Only 18% of the 185 Mayo Clinic patients had evidence of origin from anatomical synovium, and even in these the evidence was only suggestive. This tumor develops de novo from ubiquitous mesenchyma of the somatic soft tissue rather than from preexistent synovial tissue. The age range of the patients is considerable, but most are young or middle-aged adults.

The diagnosis is particularly difficult because the mass or swelling is often deep in the hip region. Pain is the dominant symptom and may occur 1 to 20 years before diagnosis, the average duration being 2.5 years. Careful roentgenographic evaluation often is of value; Cadman et al.[1] found evidence of calcification on roentgenograms in one-third of 57 cases.

The synovial sarcoma is a lobular, circumscribed, grayish tumor that shows zones of hemorrhage, necrosis, calcification, or cyst formation. Microscopically, it is characterized by bimorphic cells ranging from plump spindle cells to epithelium-like elements that line glandular spaces or clefts.

Synovial cell sarcoma tends to have a prolonged course, with multiple recurrences after local excision. Thus local excision generally is to be condemned. However, the confusion regarding diagnosis often leads to inadequate treatment. In the Mayo Clinic series[17] the overall 5-year survival rate was 38% and the 10-year rate 23%, with a median survival time of 39 months. However, for patients treated since 1960, the 5-year survival rate was 55% and the 10-year rate 38%.

As with all tumor surgery, close cooperation between the pathologist and the orthopedist is essential if the diagnosis is to be made at operation. Radical surgery is necessary, and in the area about the hip this generally means hindquarter amputation (Fig. 2–14).

Special Surgical Considerations

Each tumor, soft tissue or bony, should be judged individually. Several factors are considered, including the benign or malignant nature of the lesion, the possibility of local recurrence, the function of the hip, and the precise anatomical location of the lesion. Even such routine approaches as the anterior iliofemoral or the straight lateral approach must at times be modified, depending on the site and nature of the lesion. Most high-grade radioresistant malignant lesions, whether bony or soft tissue in origin, require hindquarter amputation when they occur in the hip region.

The technique of hindquarter amputation must be modified to exclude the tumor from the incisional lines and include it in the specimen to be removed. For example, one may wish to disarticulate the symphysis of even pass to the opposite pubis if the tumor involves the pubic region, or to go through the pubic ramus if it does not. If the tumor lies in the ilium, one may wish to pass far medially even into the sacrum at times, to ensure that all the tumor is included in the amputated specimen. Soft-tissue sarcomas present a similar problem when designing skin and muscle flaps. One must always include the biopsy site in the amputated specimen, even if biopsy is done by needle or small incision, because cells spilled along the biopsy tract may implant. A thorough knowledge of the anatomy in this area is obviously necessary.

The preoperative emotional preparation of the patient and his or her family is important. It should be emphasized that hindquarter amputation can produce cure in many patients and that satisfactory prostheses are available to allow reasonably good function, particularly for younger patients.

The surgical preparation of the patient includes the usual preoperative sedation and shaving of the buttocks, perineum, upper part of the thigh, and abdomen. Bowel preparation and enemas are usually given for 2 days preceding the surgical procedure. Placement of an indwelling urethral catheter is essential because it not only allows accurate monitoring of urine output during the procedure

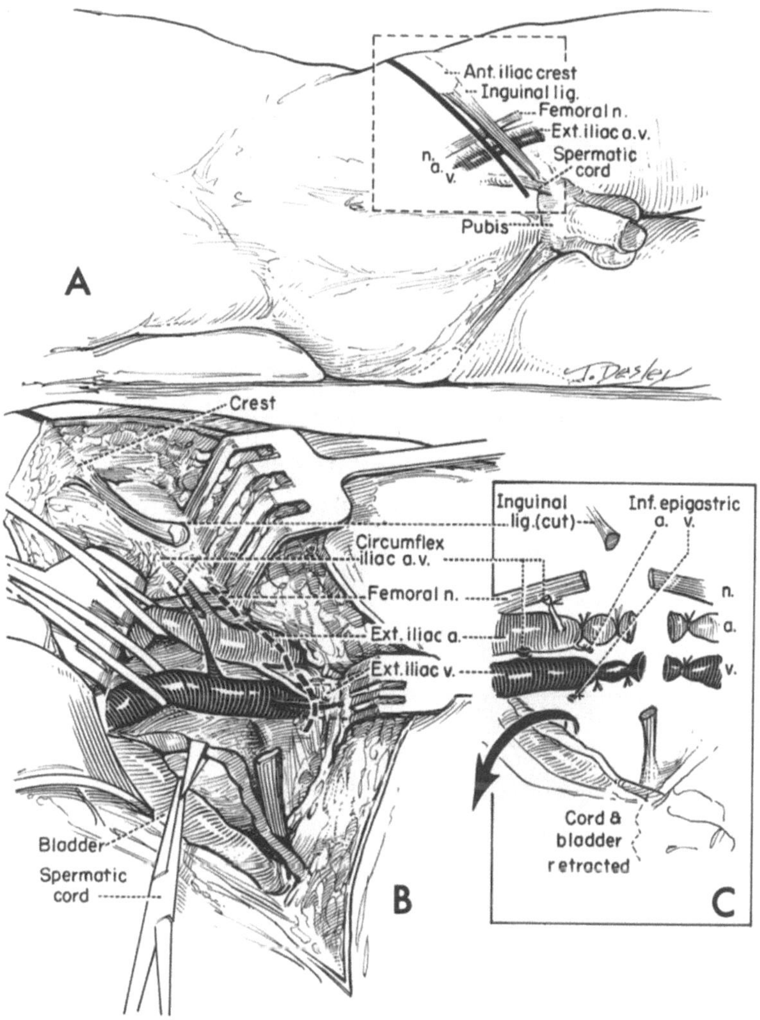

FIG. 2–15 Technique of hindquarter amputation. **A** Landmarks and superficial anatomy anteriorly. **B** Deep anatomy from the anterior approach. **C** Detail of ligation.

but also acts as a guide for the surgeon's finger when dissection is done in the perineum. In addition, a ureteral catheter on the side on which amputation is to be performed is helpful in allowing the ureter to be localized during the procedure; also, if the ureter is damaged during the procedure, it can be easily repaired over the catheter.

The patient is placed in a semisupine position at approximately a 45° angle with a sandbag under the shoulder; in this way, the patient can be rolled anteriorly or posteriorly to aid exposure. Gauze impregnated with petrolatum is inserted in the rectum, and both the anus and the navel are carefully draped from the operative field.

General Surgical Principles for Managing Tumors of the Upper End of the Femur

For most tumors of the hip, the patient is placed in the lateral position and a straight lateral incision is made. Even lesions of the region of the lesser trochanter can be approached through this lateral incision. However, for lesions involving the head of the femur, one might consider the use of an anterior curved incision such as a limited Smith-Peterson approach. It should be recognized, however, that if this approach is used for obtaining a biopsy specimen and if a subsequent resection

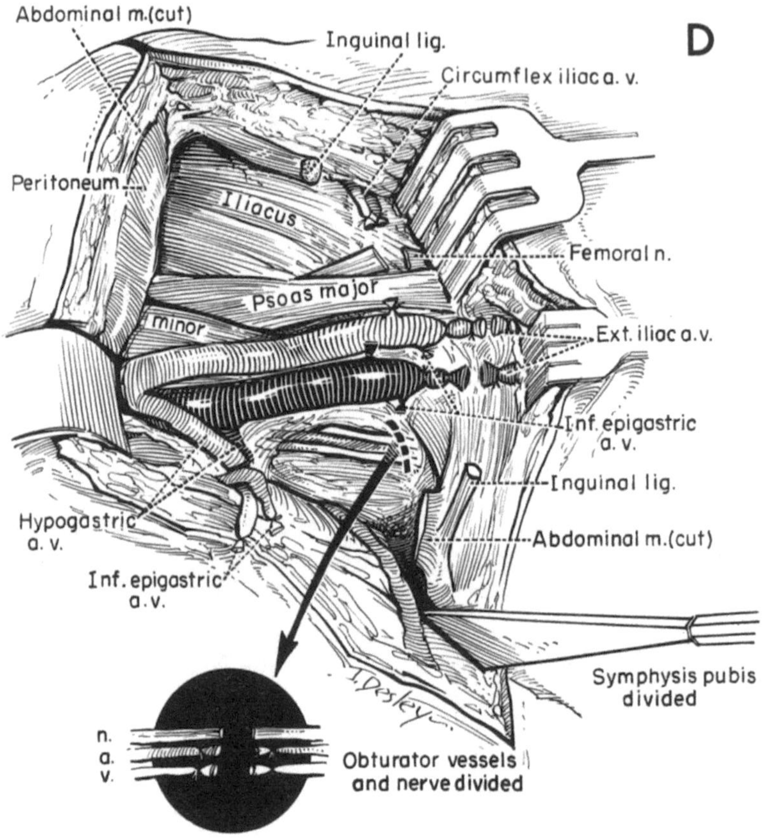

FIG. 2–15 *Continued* **D** Deep pelvic view of the sectioning of important structures.

of the upper end of the femur is indicated, placement of the biopsy incision may preclude a subsequent lateral approach. Therefore we seldom use this anterior incision when the roentgenographic appearance of the lesion is indicative of malignancy. Alternatively, the head of the femur may be biopsied through the lateral approach by taking a core of bone from the lateral aspect of the greater trochanter and extending the cut through the femoral neck to the head of the femur.

Some tumors in the proximal portion of the femur are amenable to resection and reconstruction using a custom-type total hip arthroplasty.[13] These tumors include low-grade malignant lesions such as chondrosarcoma, aggressive benign lesions such as giant cell tumors, and the occasional high-grade lesion that is small and entirely within the confines of the bone. In addition, metastatic lesions, particularly those with impending or established pathological fractures, are sometimes treated by this technique.

Obviously, the extent of the surgical resection depends on the exact location of the tumor and its extent and aggressiveness. The extent of the resection should be planned in advance of the surgical procedure. For high-grade tumors, generally, if the tumor is entered or even seen at the time of surgery, the procedure should be abandoned and hemipelvectomy considered. When a low-grade or indolent lesion is entered at surgery, the procedure might be continued with the realization that the lesion may recur locally.

The patient is positioned on the operating table in a straight lateral position, as for a routine total hip arthroplasty. A straight, lateral incision is utilized. Flaps are created anteriorly and posteriorly. The femoral vessels and femoral nerves are carefully retracted and protected. The gluteus minimus and gluteus medius muscles are divided proximal to their insertions on the greater trochanter. At this point, an intraoperative roentgenogram is obtained to define the level of intended division of

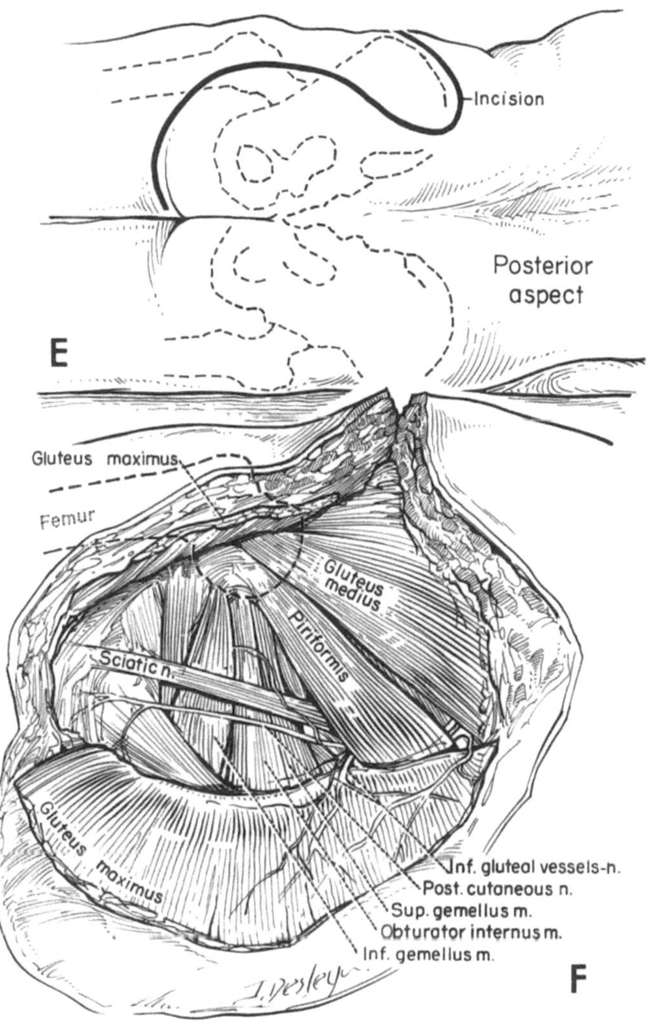

FIG. 2–15 *Continued* **E** Posterior incision. **F** The skin fascia and gluteus maximus are reflected from the buttock.

the femur distally. If the tumor is entirely within the confines of the bone, those muscles immediately overlying the bone on all aspects should be sacrificed. These muscles may be divided distally at the intended level of bone resection. A large bone-holding clamp may be placed over the end of the bone and the bone elevated. This maneuver greatly facilitates the subsequent dissection.

The vastus lateralis muscle is left attached to the bone; the anterior, medial, and posterior muscles are divided at the level of the hip joint. The hip joint capsule is then divided at the level of the acetabulum, and the entire specimen is delivered to the pathologist. The margins are immediately checked by frozen section study. The entire tumor specimen is divided longitudinally and then thoroughly inspected. If the margins are free of tumor on all aspects, the reconstruction can proceed. Reconstruction may be accomplished using a custom-type total hip prosthesis. If only a limited length of bone is sacrificed, a bipolar-type endoprosthesis may be utilized. For most situations, however, it is necessary to replace both the proximal femur and the acetabulum. The acetabulum is reamed in the usual manner to accept the acetabular component of a custom-type total hip arthroplasty. However, the acetabular component is positioned in a somewhat more horizontal position than is used for routine total hip arthroplasty. The component is placed in about 10° of anteversion.

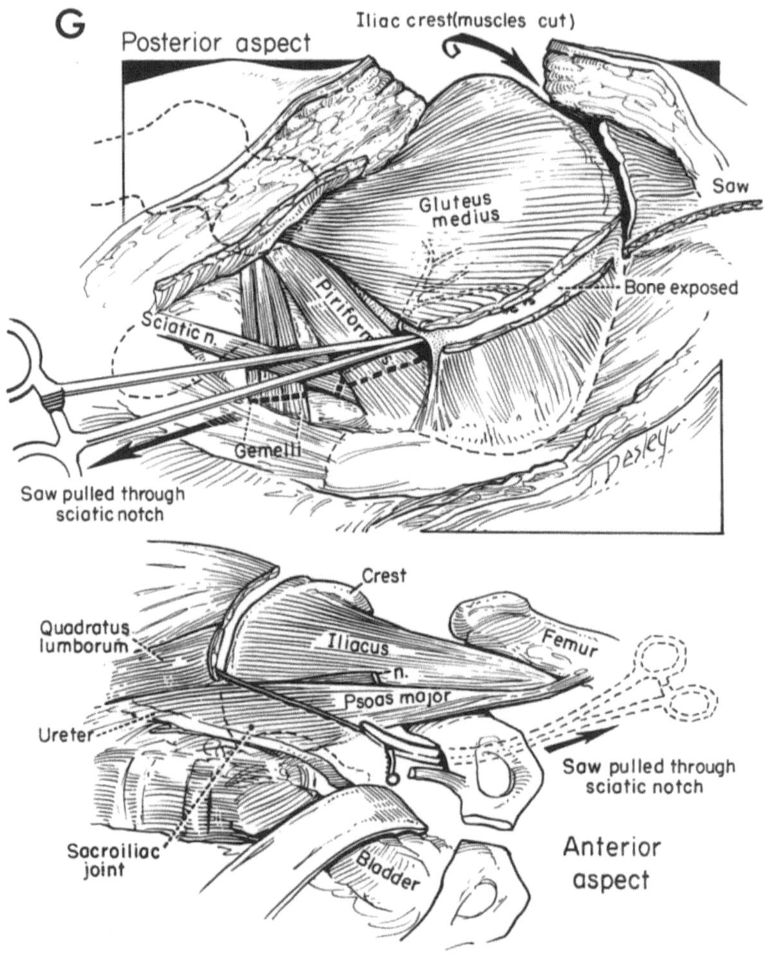

FIG. 2–15 *Continued* **G** Division of the posterior structures; one may use an osteotome or a power saw rather than a Gigli saw. *Top,* From the posterior aspect. *Bottom,* From the anterior aspect.

The medullary cavity of the remaining femoral shaft is then reamed to accept an appropriately sized custom-type femoral component. We use a femoral component with a stem that is approximately 15 cm long. If the stem is any longer than this, the curvature of the femur may cause problems when fitting the prosthesis. The femoral component is inserted in about 10° of anteversion; the hip may then be reduced and tested before the femoral component is cemented.

The appropriately sized prosthesis must be utilized in order to achieve adequate tension and minimize the possibility of subsequent dislocation. This requires that the femoral component be long enough so that the components can just barely be reduced. If there is any tendency for instability at this point, a longer femoral component is selected. Although it is desirable to have adequate tension, excessive lengthening may not be desirable and may in fact lead to a stretch palsy of the sciatic nerve.

In this regard, it is very helpful to have many different-sized components available at the time of surgery so that the appropriate length can be selected. It is not possible to make any modification at this point if one is relying on a single, custom-ordered prosthesis. The alternative is to mark the intended level of resection on a roentgenogram and send it to one of the many manufacturers that make such components and ask them to design and manufacture a prosthesis for the individual patient. This is a much less desirable approach, however, as one cannot always anticipate exactly where the resection will be; further-

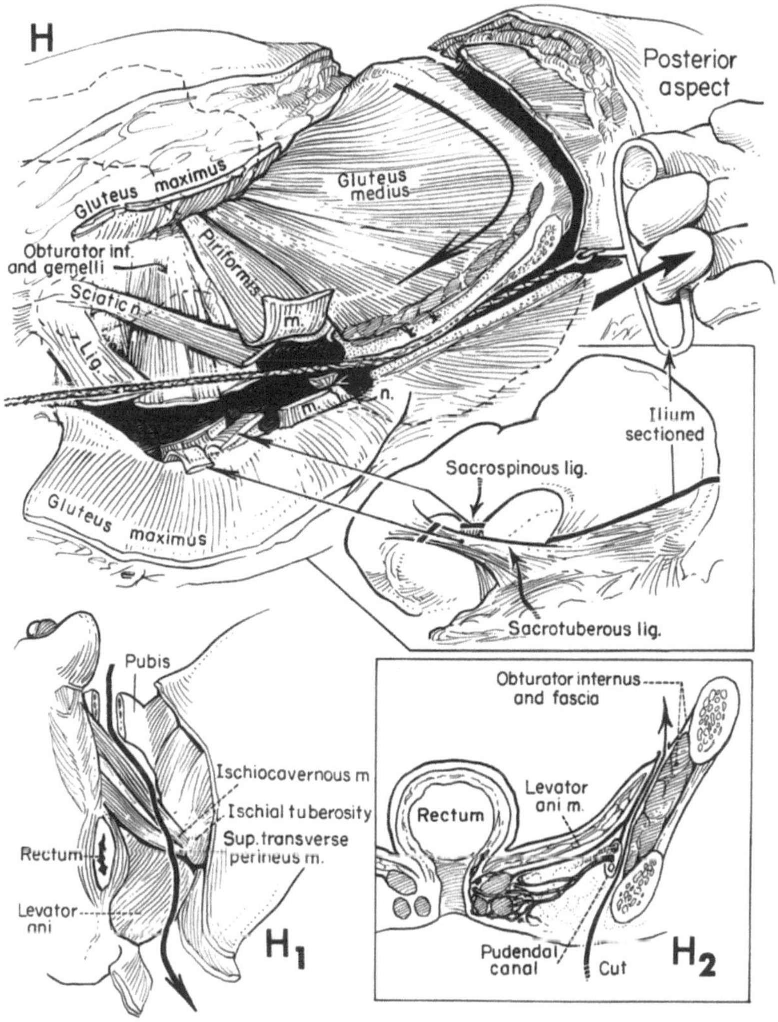

FIG. 2–15 *Continued* **H** Division of the ligaments in the peroneal portion, with details of the cleavage plane along the ischium.

more, the delay between the time of ordering the prosthesis and the time of delivery may cover several weeks. We have seen tumors that have grown considerably during a 2- to 3-week interval. Another choice is to perform the resection, measure the resected specimen, and order a prosthesis from this measurement. Neither of these choices is as satisfactory as having the components available at the time of the surgical procedure.

Once the femoral component is cemented in place and the hip is reduced, the muscle reconstruction obviously depends on the amount of muscle available. If possible, the abductor muscles are saved and are reattached to the tensor fascia lata. Results after this method of reconstruction seen to be much superior to those achieved by attempts at fastening the abductors to the metallic component itself. Although most patients treated in this manner have some abductor weakness, most can walk with surprisingly little difficulty by carrying a cane in the opposite hand. Most patients can ambulate with a minimally detectable limp.

Hemipelvectomy

Usually for hemipelvectomy an initial incision is made from the pubic tubercle to the anterosuperior iliac spine, parallel to the inguinal ligament (Fig. 2–15A). The incision is then extended laterally over the top of the iliac crest. The inguinal ligament is divided, and the abdominal muscles are detached and retracted medially. The spermatic

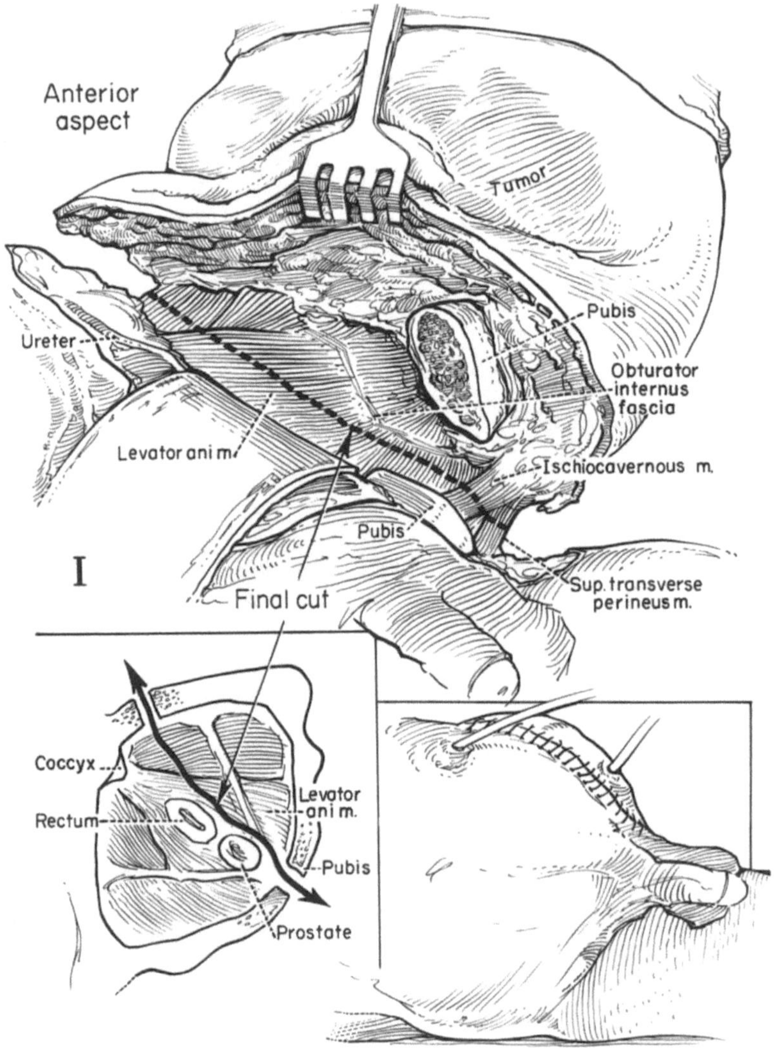

FIG. 2–15 *Continued* **I** Final severance of the limb. This may be done from anterior to posterior or from posterior to anterior. **Left inset** Cross section on the line of the cut. **Right inset** Closed incision with drains in place. (From Bickel, W. H., and Koch, M.: Amputations about the shoulder and about the hip. In *The Craft of Surgery,* 2nd ed., vol. 3. (Cooper, P., ed.) Boston, Little, Brown, 1971, pp. 1419–1438. By permission.)

cord is retracted medially (Figs. 2–15B and C). The iliac region is then explored, and any large palpable nodes are removed for immediate frozen section biopsy. The space of Retzius is then explored to determine if there is any tumor involvement. At this point, it usually can be decided if it is practical to continue with the procedure. If the situation is favorable, the iliac vessels are isolated. If the tumor is located so that the internal iliac vessels can be spared, the external iliac vessels are doubly ligated and their ends oversewn with 3-0 arterial silk (Fig. 2–15D). The rectus abdominis muscle is detached from the superior pubic ramus and symphysis. The soft tissues are dissected from all surfaces of the symphysis, a Gigli saw is passed under the symphysis, and the joint is divided. The abdominal contents can be retracted medially to expose the obturator nerve, artery, and vein, which are ligated and divided.

The hip is adducted and flexed, making the posterior portion of the buttock more prominent. The posterior flap is then created by extending the anterior incision over the iliac crest toward the midline and carrying the incision laterally and then distally to a point just beyond the greater trochanter (Figs. 2–15E and F). The incision then curves inferiorly around the gluteal fold and across the ischial tuberosity to join the previous incision anteriorly in the perineum. These incisions vary, depending on the location of the tumor. On occasion it is necessary to utilize an anterior thigh flap. In this situation the external iliac vessels are preserved and the femoral vessels ligated at the distal end of the anterior thigh flap.

When the standard approach is utilized, the gluteus maximus muscle is divided from its tendinous insertion to the femur and reflected with the skin flap to expose the posterior musculature. The

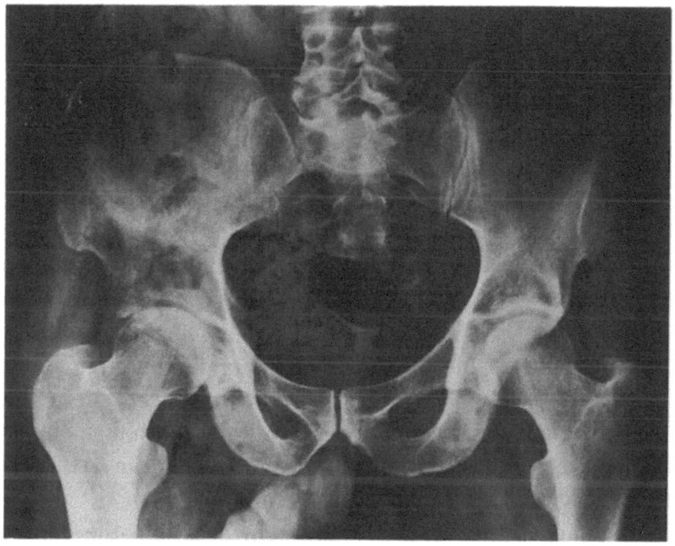

A

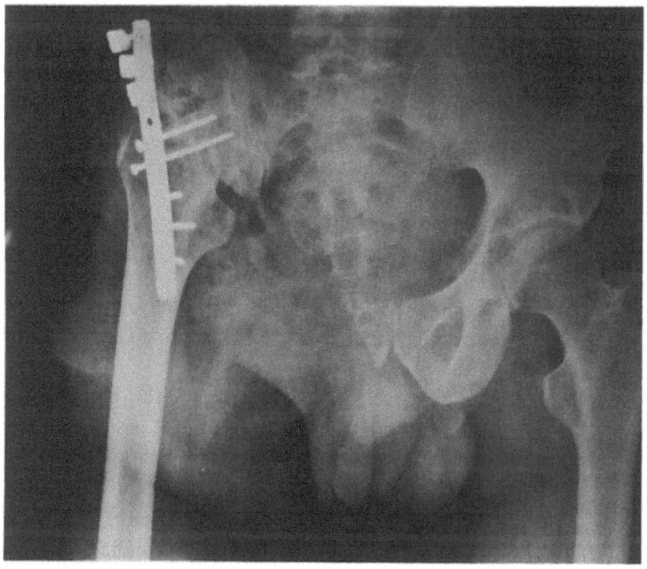

B

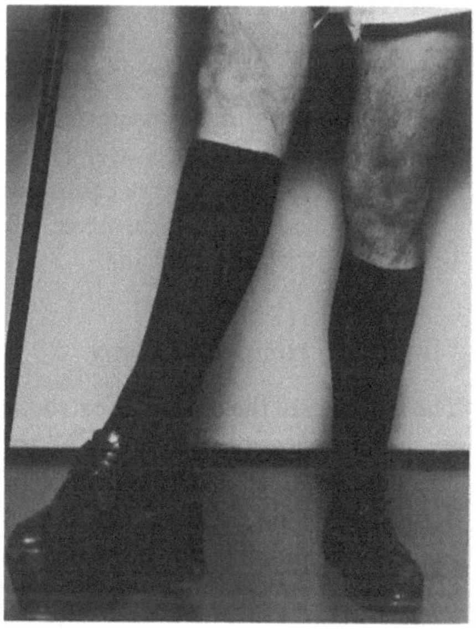

C

FIG. 2–16 **A** Grade 2 chondrosarcoma arising in the ilium adjacent to the superior aspect of the acetabulum. **B** Most of the right hemipelvis was resected along with the hip joint. The proximal femur was then arthrodesed to the remaining segment of the iliac bone. **C** The patient uses a lift on his shoe to compensate for leg-length inequality.

gluteus medius and gluteus minimus muscles, sciatic nerve, piriformis muscle, and other structures coming through the greater sciatic notch can be seen and, depending on the circumstances of the tumor, should be divided. The sciatic nerve is ligated with a heavy suture, as a vein is frequently found adjacent to the nerve. The nerve is pulled down as far as possible and cut with a sharp knife or razor blade. Depending on the level of the ilium to be divided, the soft tissues are then incised posteriorly and anteriorly along the line of intended transection (Fig. 2–15G). The vessels should be under good control before passing a Gigli saw through the sciatic notch. The bone can then be divided (Fig. 2–15H).

It may be necessary to disarticulate the sacroiliac joint of even to remove a portion of the sacrum. In this case the procedure must be modified. The femoral nerve and iliopsoas muscle are then divided in front of the sacroiliac joint. The sacrospinous and sacrotuberous ligaments and the piriformis muscle are then cut. At this point the entire hindquarter is loose except for a few muscle insertions or fibrous bands and the perineal muscles. The latter muscles are divided, and the ischiocavernous muscle is removed subperiosteally. Bleeding can be controlled by packing and suture ligation. The levator ani muscle is cut where it joins the fascia of the obturator internal muscle, and the hindquarter is lifted off. Careful hemostasis is then achieved, the flaps are fashioned, and the wound is closed in layers over Hemovac suction drains (Fig. 2–15I). A large compression dressing is then applied and held in place with a double-length 6-inch elastic bandage.

"Internal" Hemipelvectomy

The anatomy of the hip and the structures adjacent to the hip occasionally allow one to perform an adequate surgical procedure, resecting a portion of the pelvis or proximal portion of the femur (or both) without performing an actual hemipelvectomy. Such procedures are loosely referred to as "internal" hemipelvectomies. The surgical procedure needs to be tailored to the particular situation, and obviously no one technique is applicable in all situations. It is necessary to have a very thorough knowledge of the anatomy of this region as well as considerable surgical expertise and judgment to accomplish these procedures (Fig. 2–16).

No attempt is made here to describe each of the several types of procedure; rather, examples are cited. For a lesion of the ilium adjacent to the sacrum a fairly simple wedge excision may be done, with removal of as much ilium and sacrum as necessary to achieve a wide margin. The resulting defect can then be reconstructed by either bridging the gap with bone grafts or simply hinging the entire remaining hemipelvis at the sacroiliac joint and attempting to achieve an arthrodesis of the remaining ilium to the sacrum. For small lesions in the acetabulum with minimal soft-tissue extension, the entire acetabulum can be resected together with the entire hip joint, including the hip capsule, down to the intertrochanteric line. After such a resection, several reconstructive procedures have been utilized, including insertion of an entire hip allograft. However, the latter is still considered an experimental approach. It would probably be better to attempt an arthrodesis of the remaining proximal femur to the remaining pubis or to the ilium, depending on the amount of bone resected. Alternatively, the hip can simply be left flail; although the flail hip is probably less desirable than an arthrodesis, it is preferable to hemipelvectomy.

On occasion, the entire hemipelvis may need to be removed. In this situation, reconstruction necessitates either leaving the limb flail or attempting an arthrodesis to either the sacrum or the pubis. Again, these procedures are exceedingly difficult but may be gratifying if local control of the tumor can be achieved while preserving at least some of the function of the lower extremity.

References

1. Cadman, N. L., Soule, E. H., Kelly, P. J.: Synovial sarcoma: an analysis of 134 tumors. Cancer, 18:613, 1965.
2. Campanacci, M., Giunti, A., Olmi, R.: Giant-cell tumours of bone: a study of 209 cases with long-term follow-up in 130. Ital. J. Orthop. Traumatol., 1:249, 1975.
3. Dahlin, D. C.: *Bone Tumors: General Aspects and Data on 6,221 Cases,* 3rd ed. Springfield, Thomas, 1978, pp. 99–115.
4. Dahlin, D. C., Beabout, J. W.: Dedifferentiation of low-grade chondrosarcomas. Cancer, 28:461, 1971.
5. Dahlin, D. C., Coventry, M. B.: Osteogenic sarcoma: a study of six hundred cases. J. Bone Joint Surg., 49A:101, 1967.
6. Garrison, R. C., Unni, K. K., McLeod, R. A., et

al.: Chondrosarcoma arising in osteochondroma. Cancer, 49:1890, 1982.
7. Jaffe, H. L., Lichtenstein, L., Sutro, C. J.: Pigmented villonodular synovitis, bursitis and tenosynovitis: a discussion of the synovial and bursal equivalents of the tenosynovial lesion commonly denoted as xanthoma, xanthogranuloma, giant cell tumor or myeloplaxoma of the tendon sheath, with some consideration of this tendon sheath lesion itself. Arch. Pathol., 31:731, 1941.
8. Murphy, F. P., Dahlin, D. C., Sullivan, C. R.: Articular synovial chondromatosis. J. Bone Joint Surg., 44A:77, 1962.
9. Pritchard, D. J.: The surgical management of giant cell tumors of bone. Orthop. Surg. Weekly Update, 1:2, 1980.
10. Pritchard, D. J., Dahlin, D. C., Dauphine, R. T., et al.: Ewing's sarcoma: a clinicopathological and statistical analysis of patients surviving five years or longer. J. Bone Joint Surg., 57A:10, 1975.
11. Pritchard, D. J., Lunke, R. J., Taylor, W. F., et al.: Chondrosarcoma: a clinicopathologic and statistical analysis. Cancer, 45:149, 1980.
12. Reszel, P. A., Soule, E. H., Coventry, M. B.: Liposarcoma of the extremities and limb girdles: a study of two hundred twenty-two cases. J. Bone Joint Surg., 48A:229, 1966.
13. Sim, F. H., Chao, E. Y. S.: Hip salvage by proximal femoral replacement. J. Bone Joint Surg., 63A:1228, 1981.
14. Sim, F. H., Dahlin, D. C., Beabout, J. W.: Osteoidosteoma: diagnostic problems. J. Bone Joint Surg., 57A:154, 1975.
15. Strong, L. C., Herson, J., Osborne, B. M., et al.: Risk of radiation-related subsequent malignant tumors in survivors of Ewing's sarcoma. J. Natl. Cancer Inst., 62:1401, 1979.
16. Taylor, W. F., Ivins, J. C., Dahlin, D. C., et al.: Trends and variability in survival from osteosarcoma. Mayo Clin. Proc., 53:695, 1978.
17. Wright, P. H., Sim, F. H., Soule, E. H., et al.: Synovial sarcoma. J. Bone Joint Surg., 64A:112, 1982.

CHAPTER 3

Modified Hemipelvectomy Utilizing an Anteromedial Vascularized Myocutaneous Flap

JEFFREY J. ECKARDT

When the decision for hemipelvectomy has been made, careful attention must be paid to the condition of the soft tissue surrounding the hip, the buttocks, and the anterior thigh, as well as the vascularity to the area. The standard hemipelvectomy technique described by Banks and Coleman utilizes a large posterior flap which is brought anteromedially for closure. This vascularized myocutaneous flap consists primarily of the gluteus maximus and the skin and subcutaneous tissue that overlie the buttock and the proximal lateral portion of the thigh to just below the greater trochanter. It is vascularized by the superior and inferior gluteal arteries, which are the two distal branches of the posterior division of the internal iliac system. A variety of conditions may preexist which jeopardize the viability of this posterior flap, with wound dehiscence and skin necrosis having been reported to occur in 26 to 80% of hemipelvectomies done in this classic manner.

If the presence of tumor at the sciatic notch requires sacrifice of the superior and inferior gluteal vessels for oncological margins, or if they need to be sacrificed to maintain adequate hemostasis, the standard posterior flap may be substantially devascularized, jeopardizing primary wound healing. If a previous biopsy incision has been placed in the buttocks or over the greater trochanter, it must be assumed that these tissues are now contaminated with tumor and the biopsy tract must be surgically excised in continuity with the tumor as part of the operative procedure. This action may significantly decrease the tissue available for the posterior flap and compromise the closure. In certain instances, chronic infection of the proximal femur and pelvis may also be best managed with ablative amputation. The presence of a draining sinus in the buttock or over the greater trochanter may preclude the standard posterior flap incision which normally utilizes skin and subcutaneous tissue distal to the greater trochanter. Furthermore, decreased tissue viability as a result of previous extensive irradiation to the area of the buttocks and hip may prolong or jeopardize the healing process.

For the great majority of conditions which require hemipelvectomy, whether it be a tumor or an infectious process, the soft tissues over the anteromedial thigh are generally not involved. The presence of any of the above conditions which jeopardize the viability of the classic posterior myocutaneous flap would be an indication for utilizing an anteromedial flap based on the superficial femoral artery and vein. This vascularized myocutaneous flap may extend as far distal as the knee, and may include portions of the quadriceps and adductor musculature should oncological or infectious criteria permit their inclusion. This large vascularized myocutaneous flap can then be swung lateral and cephalad to cover large surgical defects which may extend well above the rim of the ilium.

Surgical Techniques

All patients undergoing hemipelvectomy must be adequately appraised of the indications as well as the magnitude of the surgery and the necessity for aggressive postoperative rehabilitation. Preoperative preparation includes a complete bowel preparation, vaginal preparation in women, and Foley catheterization. A ureteral stint on the involved side, especially if the patient has had previous radiation therapy or retroperitoneal surgery, has been found to be helpful in identifying the ureter. The entire extremity and flank should be included in the prepared area. The anus can be adequately excluded from the field by sterile draping if packed with a vaginal pack. Suturing the anus closed is not believed necessary. If there is an open, draining wound over the hip or buttock, it is first prepared, packed with surgical sponges soaked with Betadine, and covered with several layers of plastic drapes. This area is then included in the entire area that is prepared as the surgical field.

The skin incision for the standard anteromedial myocutaneous flap is depicted in Fig. 3–1. This incision can be easily modified depending on oncological requirements. In general, it starts in the area of the posterior iliac spine and extends up over the iliac crest to the anterior superior iliac spine. It is then directed distally to the knee and medially to the popliteal space. The femoral artery and vein may be isolated at the adductor hiatus and suture-ligated at this time. The posterior incision is then directed proximally, up the posterior aspect of the thigh, paralleling the buttock crease to meet the anterior incision at the posterior iliac spine.

The iliac vessels are exposed in a retroperitoneal manner (Fig. 3–2). The viscera are carefully retracted toward the midline, and attention is directed at identifying and protecting the ureter which may be more easily identified if a ureteral stint has been placed preoperatively. The internal iliac artery and vein are then identified and suture-ligated. The sartorius is transected proximally and allowed to be retracted with the anteromedial flap. The external iliac vessels are mobilized, and the profunda vessels may be tied at this time. If it has been determined preoperatively that a significant portion of the quadriceps and adductors may be retained with the flap, both the femoral nerve and profunda vessels may be retained. If they are to be excluded, the profunda vessels are suture-

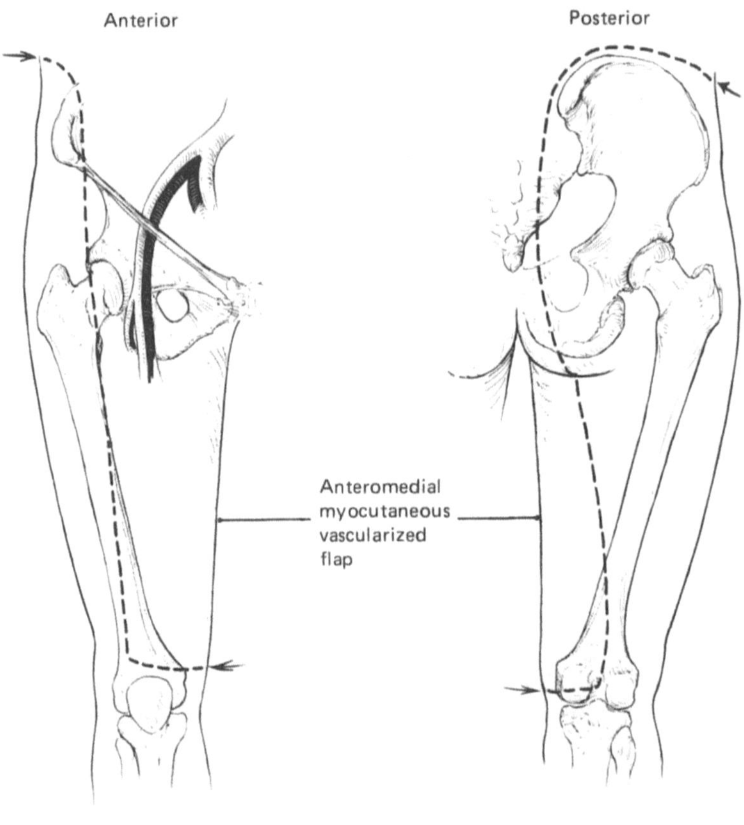

FIG. 3–1. Anteromedial myocutaneous vascularized flap skin incision. (Illustration by Gwynne Gloege, A.M.I.)

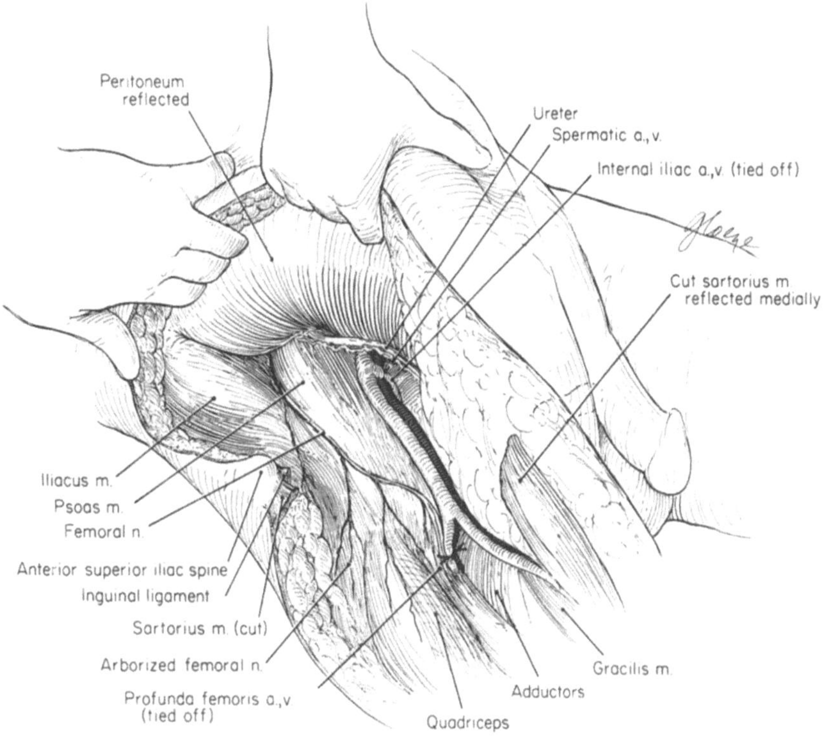

FIG. 3–2. Retroperitoneal dissection: ligation of the internal iliac and profunda vessels. (Illustration by Gwynne Gloege, A.M.I.)

ligated, and the femoral nerve is ligated prior to transection because it frequently carries a reasonably large vessel with it. The vascularized myocutaneous flap is further developed and taken distally to the knee.

Figure 3–3 depicts the vascularized anteromedial myocutaneous flap supplied by the superficial femoral artery and vein after the profunda vessels have been transected. Portions of the sartorius, gracilis, and adductors are retained with the flap. Placement of the pelvic osteotomies varies depending on the surgical indications for the hemipelvectomy. Anteriorly this may occur through the symphysis or the superior and inferior pubic ramus. If the osteotomy can be done through the superior and inferior pubic ramus, occasionally the obturator artery, vein, and nerve are retained with the flap. If the osteotomy is made at the symphysis, isolation of the obturator artery and adequate control of this vessel are important aspects of the procedure at this time.

Posteriorly the pelvis may be either disarticulated at the sacroiliac joint or osteotomies made through the ilium or sacrum. A Gigley saw is generally found to be most useful if the osteotomy is through the ilium and if the saw can be easily passed through the sciatic notch. Sacral osteotomies are more easily carried out with a combination of straight and curved osteotomes. The psoas muscle should be transected with a Bovie coagulation knife with careful attention to obtaining hemostasis from its retained proximal portion. The iliacus is retained with the hemipelvectomy specimen. The origin of the gluteal maximus is now incised with the coagulation knife, and the sacrotuberous and sacrospinous ligaments are identified and cut. The sciatic nerve requires ligation prior to transection in order to prevent excessive bleeding. The piriformis, levator ani, and coccygeal muscles are transected as the extremity is lifted away from the trunk.

Figure 3–4 depicts the surgical field following removal of the leg and hemipelvis. The osteotomy has been made at the symphysis pubis and the sacrum. The internal iliac vessels have been tied, as have the profunda vessels. The ureter has been protected. The psoas, gluteus maximus, and coccygeal muscles have been transected close to their origins. Portions of the adductors remain with the vascularized myocutaneous flap, which is now ready to be brought lateral and cephalad for closure (Fig. 3–5).

Prior to closure the wound is irrigated with copious amounts of irrigating fluid, and meticulous

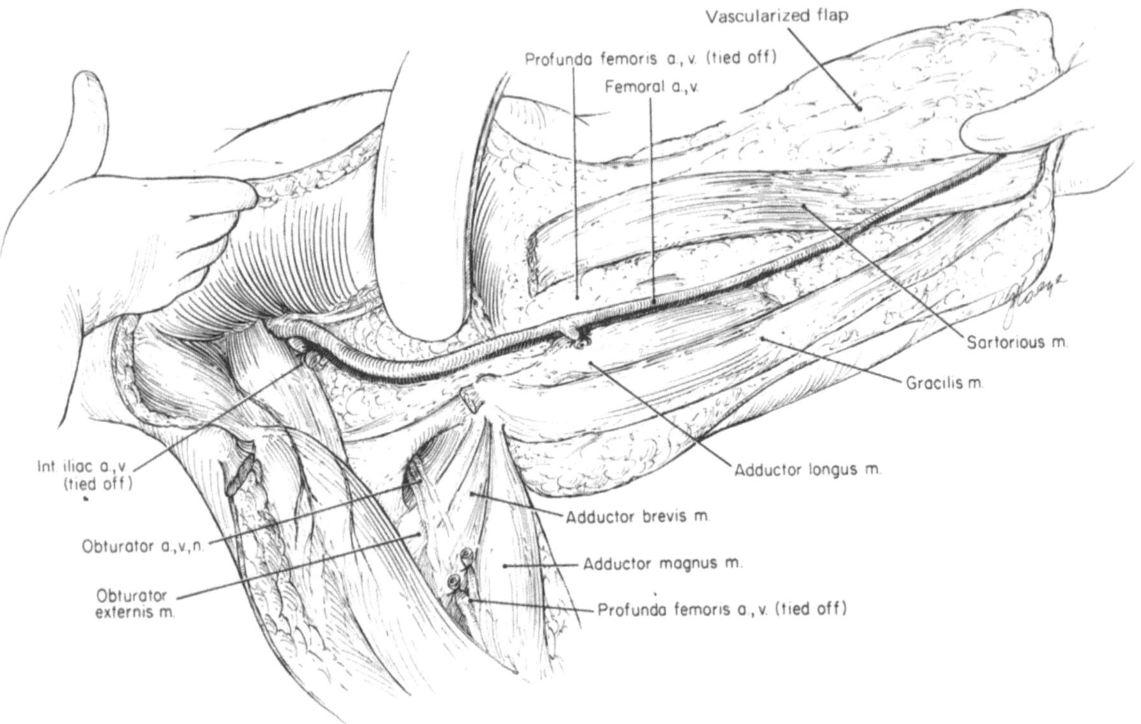

FIG. 3–3. Anteromedial flap development. The superficial femoral artery and vein have been transected at the level of the adductor hiatus, and the flap has been developed to the level of the knee. The internal iliac and profunda vessels have been tied off, and portions of the adductor musculature are retained with the vascularized flap. (Illustration by Gwynne Gloege, A.M.I.)

attention is paid to achieving hemostasis, particularly in the area of the hemorrhoidal and vesicular veins. The entire flap and vessels can now be rotated more than 90° without jeopardy. Two large drains are placed in the wound and are brought up through the abdominal musculature. The deep fascial tissues are approximated with heavy interrupted sutures, as are the subcutaneous tissues. Staples are routinely used for skin closure. The rectal pack is then removed, and the scrotum, which may have been sutured to the opposite thigh during preparation of the groin for surgery, is now released. A circumferential compressive dressing is applied. Postoperatively a nasogastric tube may be necessary if an ileus develops as a result of retraction on the peritoneal contents. A Foley catheter is generally required for several days, and the patient can be mobilized out of bed anywhere from the third to the fifth postoperative day. Perioperative antibiotics are routinely given for 48 to 72 hours. Circumferential Ace wrappings are helpful for abdominal support during the immediate postoperative period. Prior to discharge from the hospital the patient should be able to transfer and ambulate independently with a walker or crutches.

Illustrative Cases

A 67-year-old man had stage III chondrosarcoma arising in the left ilium (Figs. 3–6A to G). Figure 3–6A is an anteroposterior (AP) radiograph of the pelvis demonstrating the intrapelvic extension of the tumor which displaces the contrast-filled bladder to the opposite side. Figure 3–6B is a CT scan through the pelvis which reveals the large intra- and extrapelvic extension of the tumor with involvement at the sciatic notch. Figure 3–6C is a photograph of the pathological specimen illustrating intra- and extrapelvic extension of the tumor. Figure 3–6D is an intraoperative photograph similar to Fig. 3–3 just after development of the anteromedial vascularized flap, prior to resection of the hemipelvis and leg. Figure 3–6E is an intraoperative photograph of the flap having been

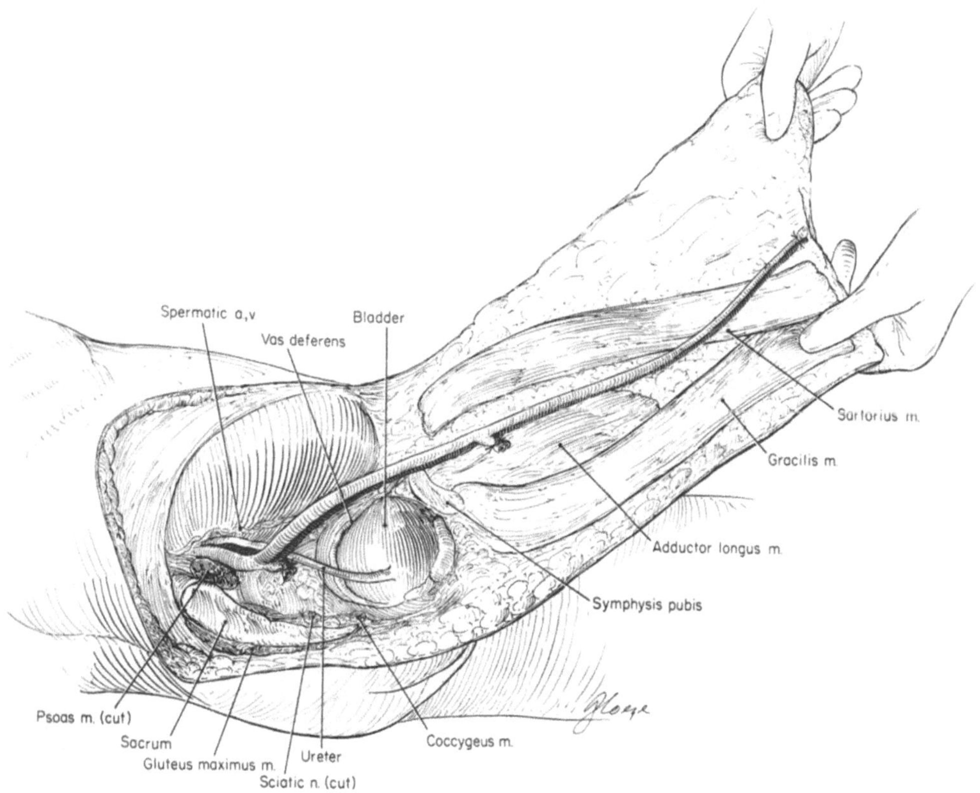

FIG. 3–4. Exposure following amputation of the hemipelvis with the vascularized flap ready for closure. The osteotomies have been through the symphysis pubis and the sacrum. The bladder and ureter have been protected. The psoas, gluteus maximus, and coccygeal muscles have been transected close to their origins. (Illustration by Gwynne Gloege, A.M.I.)

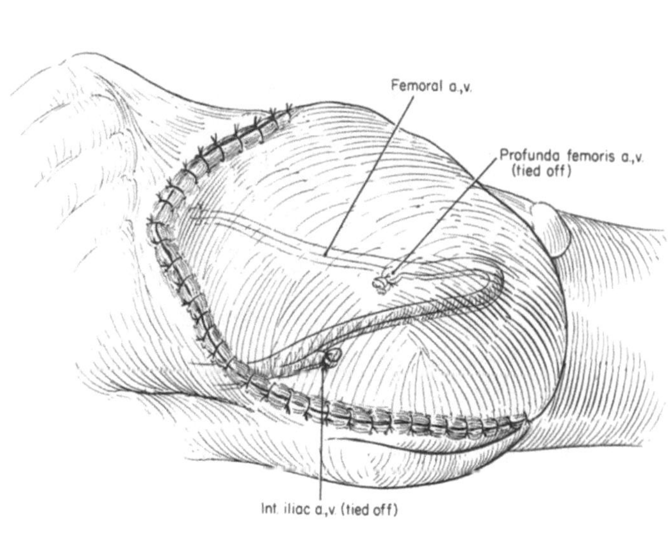

FIG. 3–5. Closure of the anteromedial vascularized flap, with the external iliac vessels rotated more than 90°. A pulse is palpable at the suture line. (Illustration by Gwynne Gloege, A.M.I.)

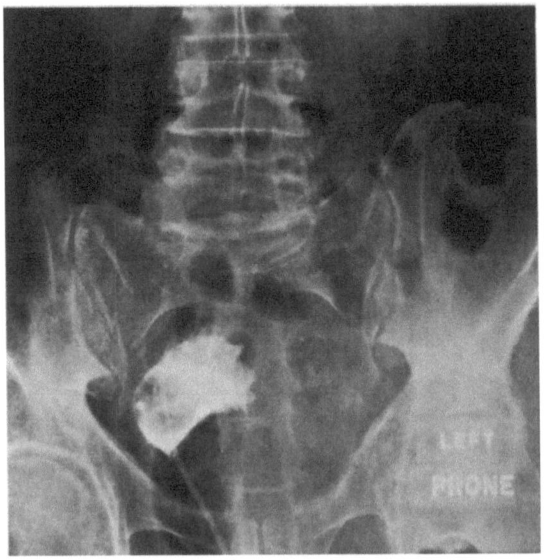

A

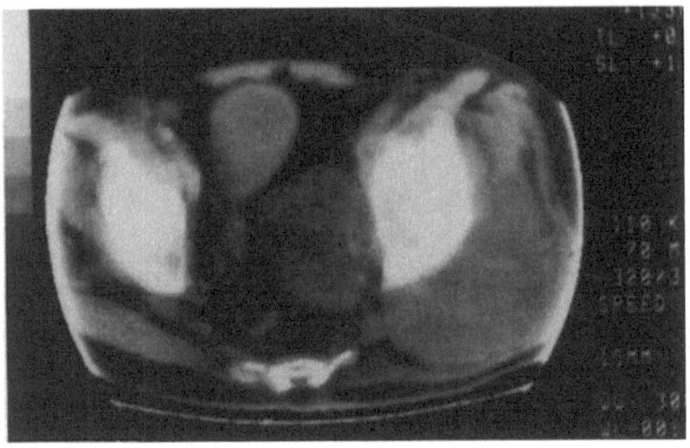

B

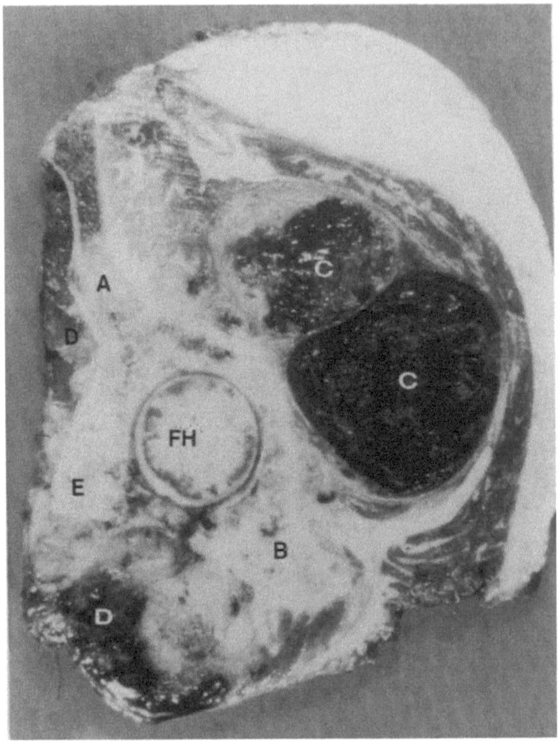

C

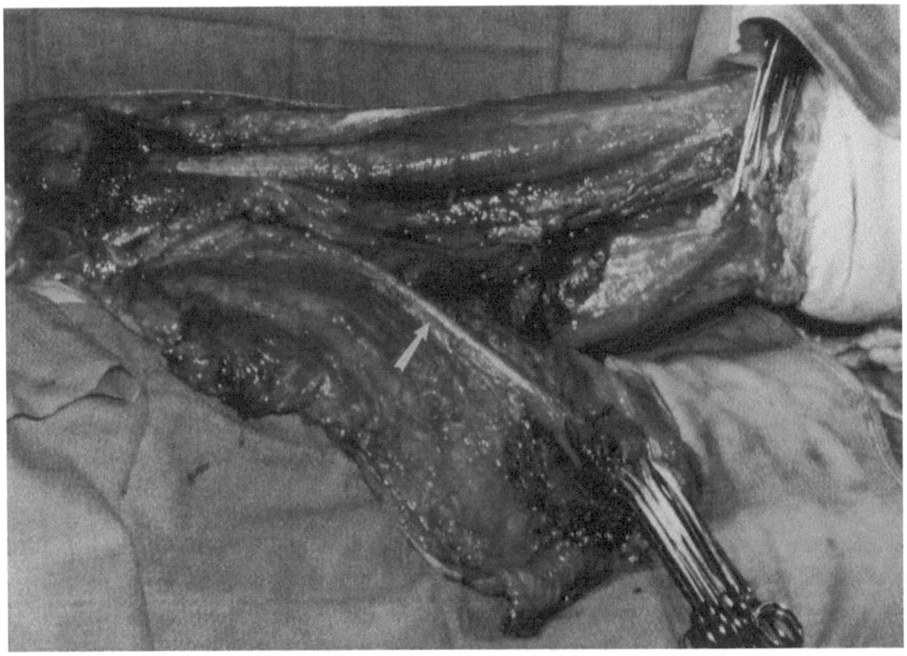

D

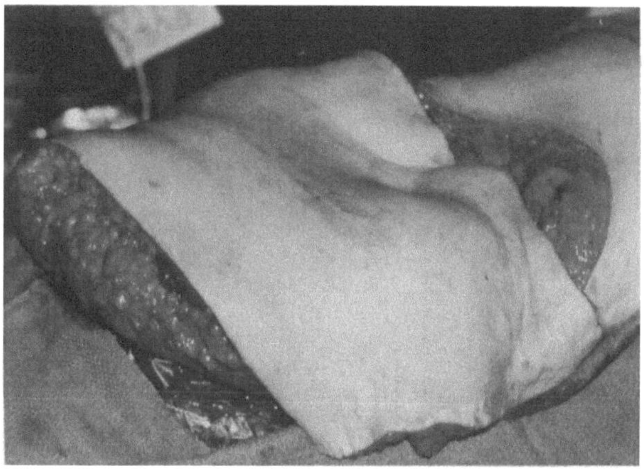

E

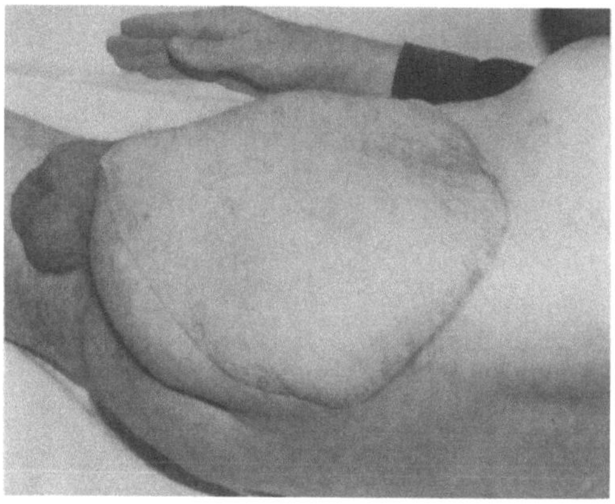

F

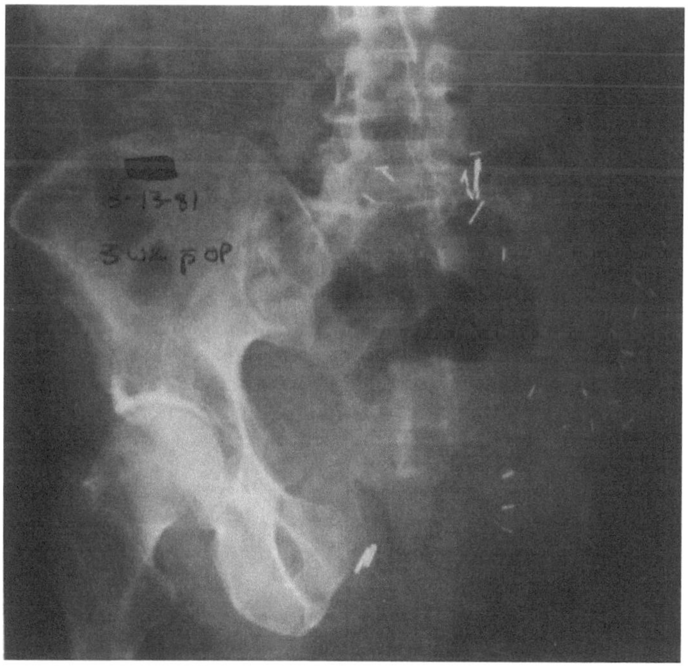

G

FIG. 3–6. **A** AP radiograph of a 67-year-old man with a large chondrosarcoma arising from the left ilium displacing the contrast-filled bladder to the opposite side. **B** CT scan through the pelvis revealing a large intra- and extrapelvic extension of the tumor with involvement at the sciatic notch. **C** Pathological specimen through the hip joint showing the intra- and extrapelvic extension of the chondrosarcoma. *FH*, femoral head; *A*, ilium; *B*, ischium; *C*, buttock, extrapelvic extension; *D*, intrapelvic extension; *E*, superior pubic ramus. **D** Intraoperative photograph (see Fig. 3–3) following development of the vascularized myocutaneous flap prior to resection of the hemipelvis and leg. The surgical clamps are on the superficial femoral artery and vein following transection at the adductor hiatus. *Arrow*, superficial femoral artery and vein. **E** Intraoperative photograph following flap rotation, prior to closure. **F** Clinical photograph 2 months after surgery revealing primary healing of the wound. **G** AP radiograph of the pelvis 3 weeks after surgery. The posterior osteotomy was through the sacrum and the anterior osteotomy through the symphysis pubis.

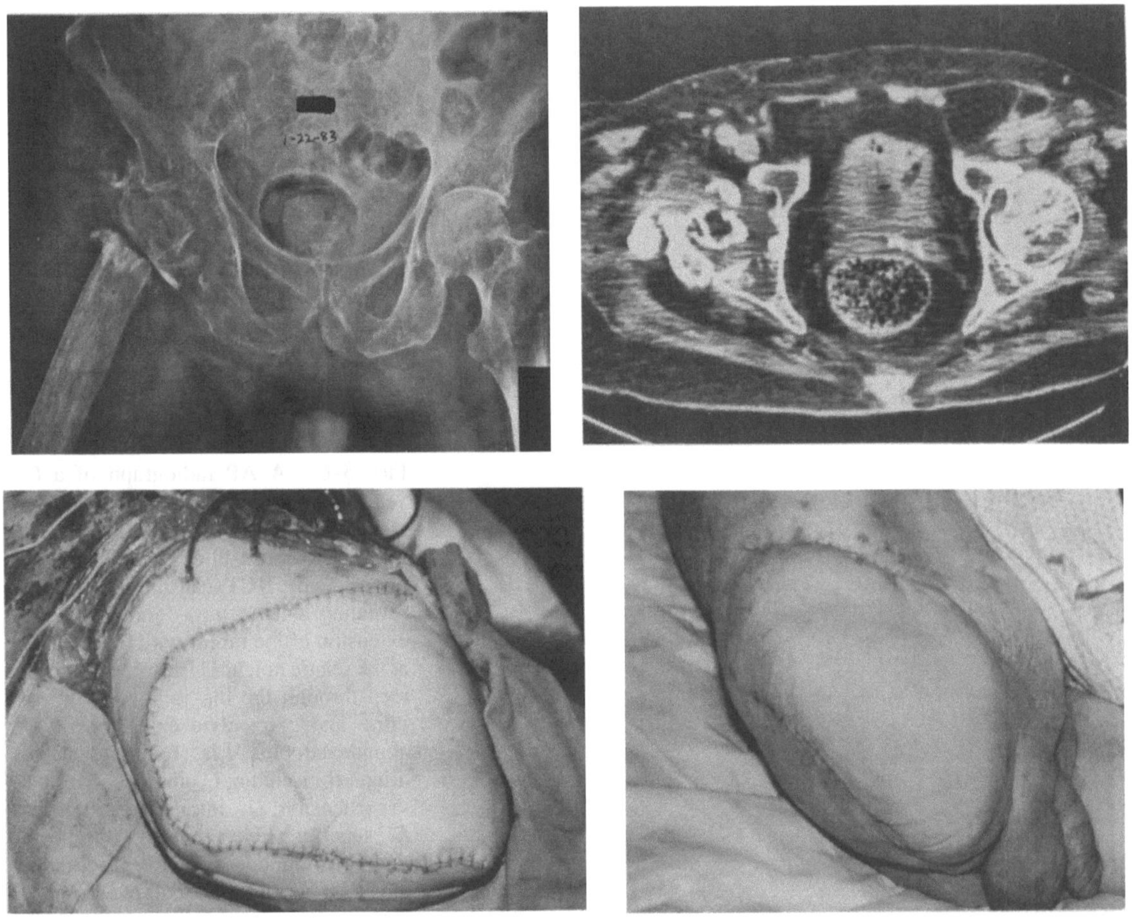

Fig. 3–7. **A** Radiograph of the pelvis of a 78-year-old man with acute and chronic *Pseudomonas* osteomyelitis involving the acetabulum and proximal femur. A significant portion of the proximal femur has been resorbed as a result of multiple débridement procedures, and the acetabular involvement by infection is suggested by the absence of the subchondral bone plate. **B** CT scan of the pelvis more clearly depicts destruction of the right acetabulum as a result of direct involvement of infection. **C** Intraoperative photograph immediately after closure (see Fig. 3–5). **D** This clinical photograph reveals primary wound healing at 6 weeks.

rotated and prior to closure. Figure 3–6F is a clinical photograph of the healed incision 2 months after surgery. A palpable pulse can be felt at the suture line. Figure 3–6G is the postoperative AP pelvic radiograph. The patient's rehabilitation was uneventful, though he succumbed to disseminated disease 17 months after surgery.

The second case is that of a 78-year-old man who developed *Pseudomonas* osteomyelitis of the right proximal femur and acetabulum following an open reduction and internal fixation of an intertrochanteric hip fracture. He presented 3 years from the time of his initial operation with a chronic draining sinus over the greater trochanteric area despite multiple hospitalizations for débridement and antibiotic treatment. His medical problems included chronic obstructive pulmonary disease, Felty's syndrome with a persistent leukopenia in the 1400/mm^3 range, obesity, and rheumatoid arthritis. His extremity was insensate, edematous, nonfunctional, and the hip was painful. The patient was bedridden because of the combination of the nonusable extremity and pain related to the open, draining sinus. Figure 3–7A is an AP pelvic radiograph revealing the extensive loss of the right femoral bone stock and acetabular sub-

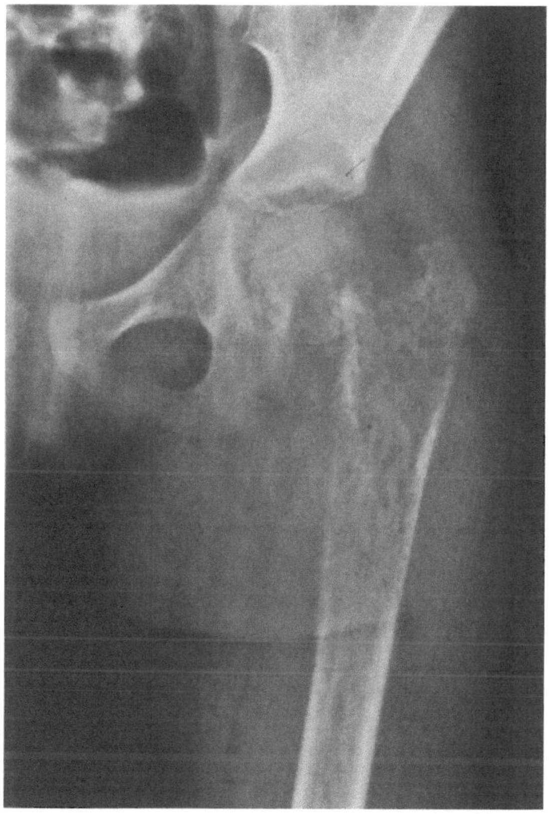

A

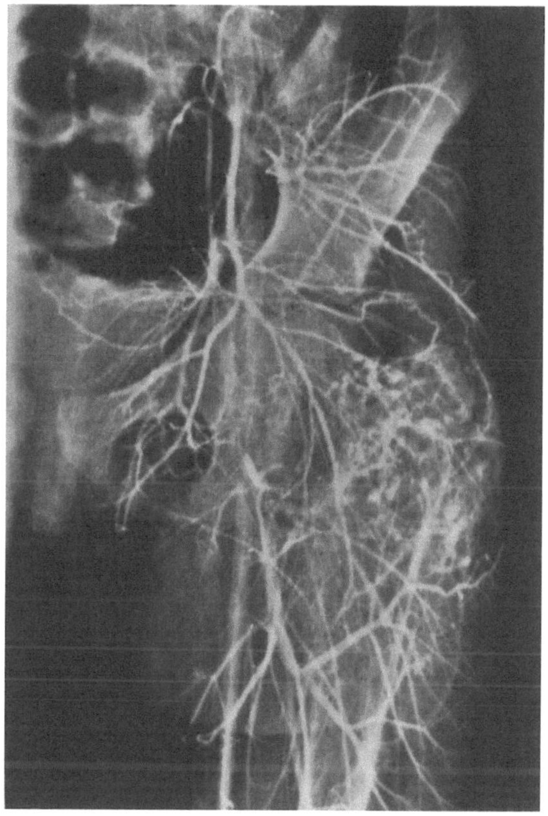

B

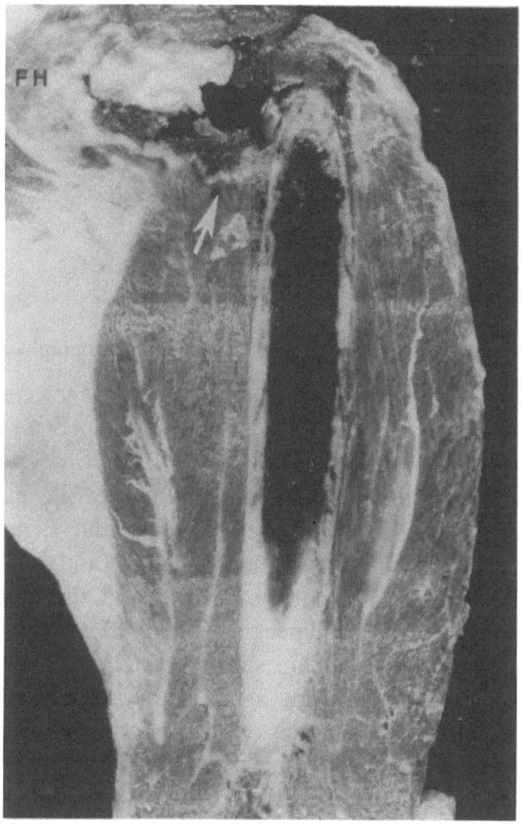

C

FIG. 3–8. **A** AP radiograph of the left hip with a telangiectatic osteosarcoma of the proximal femur. There is a pathological fracture of the femoral neck. **B** AP arteriogram reveals the tumor neovascularity. **C** This photograph of the pathological specimen demonstrates the extensive intramedullary extent of the telangiectatic osteosarcoma which is not fully appreciated on the plain radiographs. *FH,* femoral head; *arrow,* pathological fracture of the femoral neck.

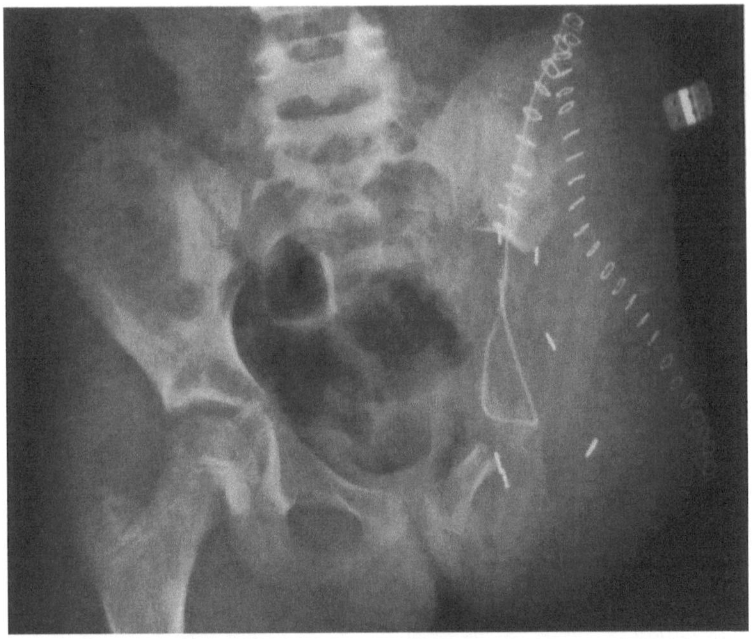

D

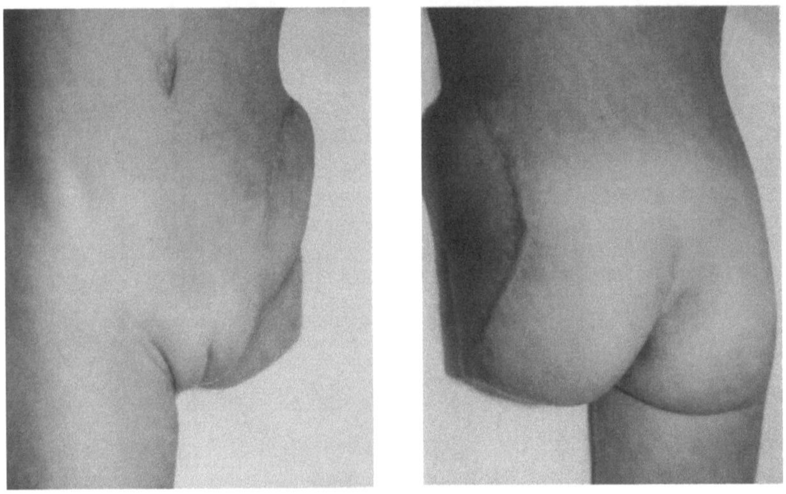

E F

FIG. 3-8 *Continued* **D** AP radiograph of the pelvis after hemipelvectomy. **E** and **F** Clinical photographs of the healed incision.

chondral bone plate. Figure 3-7B is a CT scan which more clearly reveals the acetabular involvement with chronic infection. Figure 3-7C is an intraoperative photograph following closure of the wound, and Fig. 3-7D shows the healed wound at 6 weeks. The patient was well 2 years from the time of his surgery.

The third case is that of a 6.5-year-old girl with a large telangiectatic osteosarcoma of the proximal femur complicated by a pathological fracture of the femoral neck. There was significant posterior extension of the tumor, and the biopsy site had been placed over the greater trochanter. Figure 3-8A is an AP radiograph of the left hip and proximal femur. A pathological fracture at this time involved the femoral neck. Figure 3-8B is an arteriogram of the left hip showing extensive tumor neovascularity. Figure 3-8C is the pathological specimen revealing the extensive intramedullary extent of the tumor which was not fully appreciated on the plain radiographs. Figure 3-8D is an AP radiograph of the pelvis following hemipelvectomy. Figures 3–8E and 3–8F are clinical photographs of the healed incision. Despite participation in postoperative polydrug chemotherapy, the patient succumbed to disseminated disease 13 months from the time of hemipelvectomy.

Comment

The modified hemipelvectomy utilizing a large anteromedial myocutaneous vascularized flap should be considered when large pelvic tumors, chronic draining sinuses, lateral or buttock biopsy incisions, or radiation fibrosis jeopardize the vascularity or viability of the posterior flap used in the classic hemipelvectomy described by Banks and Coleman. Because the size of the vascularized anteromedial myocutaneous flap is easily modified, the surgeon may resect tumors or lesions of the pelvis and proximal femur using good oncological principles without "skimping" on the margins because of soft tissue closure restraints.

Bibliography

1. Banks, S. W., Coleman, S.: Hemipelvectomy: surgical techniques. J. Bone and Joint Surg., 38A:1147, 1956.
2. Douglas, S., Jr., Razack, M., Holyoke, E. D.: Hemipelvectomy. Arch. Surg., 110:82, 1975.
3. Enneking, W. F.: *Musculoskeletal Surgery.* New York, Churchill Livingstone, 1983, pp. 515–518, 525–529.
4. Frey, C., Matthews, L. S., Benjamin, H., Fidler, W. J.: A new technique for hemipelvectomy. Surg. Gynecol. Obstet., 143:753, 1976.
5. Georgiade, N., Pickrell, K., Mequire, C.: Total thigh flaps for extensive decubitus ulcers. Plast. Reconstr. Surg., 17:220, 1956.
6. Gordon-Taylor, G., Wiles, P.: Interinnomino-abdominal (hind-quarter) amputation. Br. J. Surg., 22:671, 1935.
7. Higinbotham, N. L., Marcove, R. C., Casson, P.: Hemipelvectomy: a clinical study on 100 cases with 5-year follow-up on 60 patients. Surgery, 59:706, 1966.
8. Karakousis, C. P., Vezeridis, M. P.: Variance of hemipelvectomy. Am. J. Surg., 145(2):273, 1983.
9. Larson, D. L., Liang, M. D.: The quadriceps myocutaneous flap: a reliable, sensate flap for the hemipelvcctomy dcfect. Plast. Reconstr. Surg., 72(3):347, 1983.
10. Miller, T. R.: Hemipelvectomy in lower extremity tumors. Orthop. Clin. North Am., 8:903, 1977.
11. Mnaymneh, W., Temple, W.: Modified hemipelvectomy utilizing a long vascular myocutaneous thigh flap. J. Bone Joint Surg., 62A:1013, 1980.
12. Pack, G. T., Miller, T. F.: Exarticulation of the innominate bone and corresponding lower extremity (hemipelvectomy) for primary and metastatic cancer: a report of 101 cases with analysis of end results. J. Bone Joint Surg., 46A:91, 1964.
13. Pringle, J. H.: The interpelvic-abdominal amputation, with notes on two cases. Br. J. Surg., 4:283, 1916–17.
14. Sugarbaker, A. H., Chretien, E. A.: Hemipelvectomy for buttock tumors utilizing an anterior myocutaneous flap for quadriceps femoral muscle. Ann. Surg., 197(1):106, 1983.
15. Temple, W. J., Mnaymneh, W., Ketcham, A. S.: The total thigh and rectus abdominus myocutaneous flap for closure of extensive hemipelvectomy defects. Cancer, 50:2524, 1982.

CHAPTER 4

Septic Arthritis

MICHAEL N. JOLLEY, EDUARDO A. SALVATI,
AND PHILIP D. WILSON JR.

Infections of the hip can be categorized into three distinct forms depending on the patient's age: infantile, childhood, and adult forms.[58] The differences seen in each age group are due to anatomical variations in the vascular supply to the hip and to the differing suspectibility and immunological response to infection.[32]

Though the hip can be infected by contiguous spread of infection from adjacent sites or by direct inoculation (as during femoral venipuncture[32] or compound injuries), the most common mechanism is hematogenous spread.[5,7,12,20,69] In infants and children, because of their unique vascular anatomy, most infections of the hip begin as osteomyelitis in the proximal metaphyseal region of the femur, whereas in adults most infections begin with invasion of the synovium.[17,30,32,44,60] As the proximal metaphysis of the femur is for the most part an intracapsular structure, the metaphyseal osteomyelitis seen in infants and children soon spreads to the joint itself and becomes a suppurative arthritis.[17,18] Rarely, pyarthrosis of the hip results from a focus of infection on the acetabular side.[18]

Pyogenic arthritis of the hip is not equally distributed among all age groups, being most commonly seen in infants and young children.[12,17,18,60] Infection tends to strike rapidly growing bone and characteristically involves the metaphysis, whereas the synovium is a relatively more resistant structure.[60] For this reason and for others to be outlined, adults have relatively few primary infections of the hip.

Infants and Children

Etiological Considerations

In infants and children, the blood supply to the metaphysis is characterized by relatively sluggish flow near the epiphyseal plate, creating a favorable area for bacteria to lodge. The formation of a nidus of infection in this region is also favored by the fact that the afferent limb of the vascular loop lacks phagocytic lining cells, and the phagocytic cells in the efferent limb are functionally inactive.[60] As the loops do not anastomose, venous obstruction favors the spread of infection.[58,60]

In children, vessels do not penetrate the epiphysis from the metaphysis because the epiphyseal plate and bony epiphysis act as a vascular barrier. Only a limited number of intracapsular vessels supply the epiphysis at this stage, a developmental quirk fraught with hazards of ischemia.[43,57] This plate barrier begins to form at about 6 to 8 months of age and is usually established by about 18 months, the approximate age used to divide the infantile form of hip infection from the childhood form.[10,58] The adult form occurs after closure of the epiphysis.

In infants there is no barrier to transepiphyseal vessels. They penetrate almost to the surface of the epiphysis where they end in sinusoidal dilations.[10] These transepiphyseal vessels allow the passage of bacteria across the growth plate into the epiphysis and, because of their proximity to the articular surface, into the joint. This accounts for the early involvement of these structures in infections in infants, whereas in children[10,21] the isolation of the epiphysis affords it and the joint some degree of protection. Thus in an infant the infection usually enters the joint via the epiphysis, but in a child the joint is involved mainly through the metaphyseal cortical bone of the neck.[17,21,58]

Infants may also be more susceptible to infection owing to the transitory physiological hypofunction of their immune mechanisms.[32] The greater degree of damage seen in infants may be partially attributed to this decreased immune response that fails to check the spread of infection, once it is established.[32] The increased incidence of Gram-negative infections seen in infants may also be a result of this phenomenon.[49] However, it has been suggested that the problem may be a truly defective immune response rather than physiological hypofunction because some of these patients have a persistent degree of immunological deficiency as they age.[31,32]

In all age groups, once the infection is established, if left untreated it will lead to joint destruction. The pathophysiology of this destruction is not completely understood.[9,51] It was thought that cartilage destruction was due to proteolytic enzymes in pus, but now it appears that the cause is multifactorial, with mechanical and enzymatic components.[7,9,51]

With infection, the synovium becomes hyperemic, and its permeability increases. Fibrin enters the joint, causing clots that contribute to adhesions and pocketing of pus. Fibrin also adheres to cartilage, contributing to damage by impairing nutrient diffusion.[9] There is a decrease in the quantity and quality of hyaluronic acid production, with resulting loss of its lubricating effect, which increases the mechanical trauma to the joint.[7]

The cartilage is also subject to enzymatic breakdown. The matrix is attacked by several enzymes, including lysosomal enzymes from the leukocytes and synovium, and proteolytic enzymes produced by *Staphylococcus aureus.* Plasmin, a fibrinolytic enzyme derived from synovial cells and activated by kinases from *Staphylococcus* and *Streptococcus,* is also involved. With the matrix destroyed, the collagen fibrils that make up 90% of cartilage protein are subject to mechanical trauma in areas of direct cartilage-to-cartilage contact. The collagen is also attacked by collagenases derived from granulocytes or the synovium (*Clostridium* is the only bacterium with collagenase activity). The degradation of collagen may be the key step in this destructive process, and though bacteria initiate and act as a constant cause when present, the process can continue without them and occur even in sterile joints.[7,9,11,51]

Diagnosis

The clinical response to hip infection usually differs between infants and children. Infants may have minimal findings,[32,44] whereas children with infected hips classically are very ill, with systemic manifestations that may overshadow local signs. High fever, tachycardia, anorexia, and dehydration may be seen. Pain at rest, exacerbated by motion or weight-bearing and frequently referred to the knee, is common.[29,41] There can be extensive swelling of the thigh with obliteration of the inguinal crease, and often the affected limb is held in some flexion, abduction, and external rotation.[17,18] Soto-Hall et al. have shown that in this position the capsule has its greatest volume, and any change from this position increases the intracapsular pressure and therefore the hip pain.[56] The white blood cell count is usually elevated, with a large percentage of polymorphonucleocytes; the erythrocyte sedimentation rate (ESR) is increased; and there may be mild anemia.[17,18]

Early in the course of infection of the hip, x-ray films are of questionable value to the diagnosis, especially in children and adults.[35,63] Soft tissue changes, including a bulging capsule and the obturator sign, have been described as early signs of infection.[17,18,44] However, little value is placed on these soft-tissue changes by some,[3,32,35] as it has been shown that the so-called capsular swelling is a radiological artifact related to the position of the limb at the time the x-ray film is exposed.[3]

Destructive changes of bone are not usually seen before 10 days on x-ray films[53] because before a lytic process can be visualized 30 to 50% of the bone mineral must be removed. Likewise, new bone formation is not seen for approximately 10 days, as it takes that long for bone to mineralize enough to be seen on x-ray film.[10,12,60] Because of this lag effect, the amount of bone destruction seen on x-ray studies is considerably less than the actual amount of bone destruction present.[10]

Bone scans may be helpful in detecting infection before x-ray signs are apparent; however, scans are not specific for infection.[10,17,53,60] Gallium scans, indium-labeled polymorphonucleocyte scans, and three-phase scans appear to be the most sensitive and specific techniques in the diagnosis of bony infection.[22,33,37,46,61] A negative scan can be significant, as normal uptake is usually evidence against the presence of sepsis,[10] though early thrombosis of vessels in infection may temporarily cause a cold spot.[17]

The most important diagnostic test is aspiration of the joint. The fluid should be Gram-stained, cultured, and evaluated for cells, glucose, protein, and lactic acid.[48] Care must be taken when culturing the fluid.[26] Aerobic, anaerobic, fungal, and mycobacterial cultures should be prepared. They are plated and incubated as soon as possible and are maintained for up to 2 weeks in indicated situations in order to isolate the more fastidious organisms.[9,27,41] Because delay in diagnosis can have such untoward effects on the hip, it is recommended that if any suspicion of infection exists a hip aspiration be done.[17] Elevated lactic acid assays in synovial fluid are useful in the diagnosis of septic arthritis, and of particular diagnostic value in patients in whom antibiotic therapy was started before joint aspiration. Sequential measurements can be helpful in assessing the response of septic arthritis to treatment.[48] It has even been suggested that an exploratory arthrotomy, perhaps by arthroscopic means, may be warranted in uncertain cases.[44]

Even if the cultures and Gram stains of the aspirate are negative, it does not rule out completely septic arthritis.[1,11,12,40] Blood cultures improve the percentage of bacterial diagnosis by as much as 50 to 60%,[61] indicating the role that hematogenous spread plays in hip infections. Accordingly, patients should be evaluated for sources of infection elsewhere including ears, throat, skin, other joints, and, in infants, the umbilicus.[32] The highest yield of bacterial diagnosis in hip infections occurs when several sources including the hip, blood, and other foci are cultured.[12]

Bacteriology

Staphylococcus aureus is the most common bacterium isolated in infected hips in young people.[12,16,18,32,38,40,41,44,52,61] *Streptococcus*, other Gram-positive organisms, and Gram-negative microbes are also found but to a much lesser degree.[18,32,40,44,52] Nelson has pointed out in a study involving all joints that *S. aureus* is the main cause of septic arthritis in children over 2 years of age. *Hemophilus influenzae* is the most frequent pathogen in children from about 6 months to 2 years of age,[40] probably because the passive immunity against *H. influenzae* and other Gram-negative microbes acquired from the mother lasts about 2 to 3 months and then decreases, only to be restored to full levels by natural active immunization by 4 years of age.[10,62] *H. influenzae* tends to lodge primarily in the synovium, causing septic arthritis.[12,16] *H. influenzae* osteomyelitis is rare and seems to affect mostly the upper extremities.[12,40,52,60] Because most infections of the hip start as osteomyelitis in infants and young children, it is uncertain if *H. influenzae* is as important an etiological organism in infections of the hip as in other joints in the 6-month to 2-year-old age group. In an evaluation of several studies, it was not possible to determine if a significant percentage of hip infections in children age 6 months to 2 years were caused by *H. influenzae*.[16,18,21,35,40,44,62] However, in this age group the infection is less likely to be due to *Staphylococcus* than in older children.[16]

Treatment

Early treatment of infection of the hip is the key to a good result.[35,44,60] It can prevent damage to cartilage, prevent vascular problems, and eradicate osteomyelitis before large areas of necrosis are established and dissolution of the joint occurs. The usually recommended treatment for infection of the hip is surgical drainage in conjunction with bactericidal antibiotics, obtaining at least 1:8 peak bactericidal serum activity against the infecting organism.[16,17,30,32,44,52] With drainage and lavage, the joint is cleared of destructive enzymes, fibrin clots, cellular debris, and bacteria. Antibiotic effectiveness is enhanced by surgical decompression. Purulent exudates retard bacterial growth and dormant bacteria are able to survive locally in the presence of otherwise bactericidal levels of antibiotics.[9,11]

Antibiotics should *not* be given before a diagnosis is made and cultures obtained. Antibiotics can alter the clinical picture, causing a delay in diagnosis and adequate treatment.[63] The likelihood of identifying the offending organism is decreased, especially from blood cultures.[35] As many as half of the cultures can be negative,[18] though one report indicated that the likelihood of identifying the organism from the joint did not appear to be decreased.[35]

Once cultures have been obtained from the hip, blood, and other appropriate sources, the antibiotic treatment should be started empirically based on the Gram stain if possible, or the statistically most likely offending organism.[17,18,41] Usually a penicillinase-resistant penicillin (or a cephalosporin) should be started. If Gram-negative organisms are suspected, an aminoglycoside antibiotic can be added. In children 6 months to 2 years of age, where the organism may be *H. influenzae,* ampicillin may be indicated. Once definitive culture and sensitivity results are available, the antibiotic regimen can be modified accordingly.[17,41]

Antibiotics should be administered for 4 weeks or longer if there is evidence of bone infection.[5,17,32,44,52,60,64] If a shorter course is given, many infections recur, especially if *Staphylococcus aureus* or Gram-negative organisms are the cause.[12,21,47] The antibiotics may be given parenterally only[12] or parenterally followed by an oral course.[17,52,64] Once a definitive course of antibiotics has been given, discontinuation is guided by the general assessment of the patient's clinical and laboratory findings.[37] The while blood cell count should be normal and the ESR normal or decreasing. A persistently elevated ESR is a sign of continued infection.[1,5,28,41] The patient should be afebrile and the wound healed without drainage, swelling, erythema, or tenderness.

In theory, if infection of the hip is diagnosed before any significant inflammation, necrosis, suppuration, or increased intracapsular pressure occurs, antibiotics alone may be sufficient treatment.[16] However, rarely does such a situation present itself, and the uncertainty involved in choosing such treatment and the potentially disastrous consequences of an inadequately treated pyogenic arthritis of the hip mitigates against such a course.

Although repeated aspiration of the hip has been described,[13,19,35] it is not recommended as a method of treatment either. The hip is relatively inaccessible, so repeated successful aspirations can be difficult and painful. Aspiration is also unable to adequately evacuate and decompress the hip, nor is it able to break up loculations, remove fibrin clots, or débride the joint successfully.[7,9,17,44] More severe sequelae also occur with higher frequency in patients treated with aspiration.[21,29,63]

Surgical drainage of the infected hip is an integral part of treatment. If metaphyseal osteomyelitis is diagnosed early, before spreading from the bone into the joint, extracapsular bone decompression by the lateral approach is recommended.[17] Should the joint itself be involved, an anterior, medial, or posterior approach can be used. If the posterior approach is chosen, care must be taken to open the capsule near the acetabular labrum in a "T" fashion and incise along the middle of the neck. Avoid incising laterally (to protect the medial circumflex artery), superiorly, or inferiorly as the retinacular vessels can be injured.[17] Closure can be done without drains after partially excising the capsule[32,44] or with closed suction irrigation for 2 to 3 days. Both methods have their proponents and appear to heal with equally good results.[18,35]

Postoperatively the hip is splinted in slight abduction, flexion, and neutral or slight external rotation until the soft-tissue healing is complete. Traction, perhaps followed by a spica cast, is recommended for a few weeks.[17,32,35,44] The traction and immobilization help stabilize the hip, contain the femoral head, and reduce the deformity.[32] Advocates of traction believe that, in addition, it reduces the joint pressure and allows early motion to help cartilage lubrication and recovery.[17]

Sequela

Of all the joints affected by pyogenic arthritis, the hip has the highest incidence of unsatisfactory results.[16] Delay in diagnosis and treatment is one of the major contributors to poor results.[16,17,32,35,44] Other factors that can adversely affect the outcome include the presence of osteomyelitis in the femoral head and neck,[17,35] *Staphylococcus* infection,[35] inadequate treatment,[35] and a younger age.[17] However, if a rapid diagnosis is made and early treatment instituted, the outcome in young children is just as good as in older groups, thereby eliminating age as an adverse factor.[21,35]

Complications can be disastrous in a child with an infected hip. There can be complete or partial destruction of the femoral head and/or epiphyseal plate leading to varying growth disturbances and deformities of the hip and involved limb.[10,17] The hip can dislocate, become stiff and painful, and ankylose,[16] resulting in chronic osteomyelitis with persistent drainage. All sequelae are not immediately obvious. Children thought to be normal after apparently successful treatment and discharge from the hospital have returned with residual joint damage.[21] It is important therefore to thoroughly and adequately treat these children and follow them until skeletal maturity.

Avascular necrosis of the capital femoral epiphysis is one of the complications seen after hip infections (Fig. 4–1). Though vascular insult can occur at any age, it is most prevalent in the child from about 2 to 10 years of age because of the tenuous blood supply at that stage of development.[57]

The blood supply to the femoral head can be interrupted either intra- or extracapsularly at the level of the trochanter. Kemp and Lloyd-Roberts believed that the most common site of onset of infection in the hip is in the trochanteric area.[30,32] The branches of the circumflex vessels form a circle around the distal attachment of the hip capsule that lies near the trochanter. They can be compromised by compression or thrombosis secondary to the sepsis. A sterile intracapsular effusion often accompanies the osteomyelitis but, if not treated quickly, becomes a pyarthrosis as the infection spreads into the joint. The increased intracapsular pressure from the effusion or pus can occlude and thrombose the retinacular vessels.[17,18,30] Furthermore, if the joint should dislocate as a result of excess pressure, there can be further vascular embarrasment due to stretching, compression, or kinking of the vessels.[17,59] The blood supply to the hip can also be interrupted iatrogenically during surgical decompression of the hip. As stated previously, care must be taken to avoid surgical injury to the intracapsular posterosuperior and posteroinferior retinacular vessels as well as the medial circumflex artery.

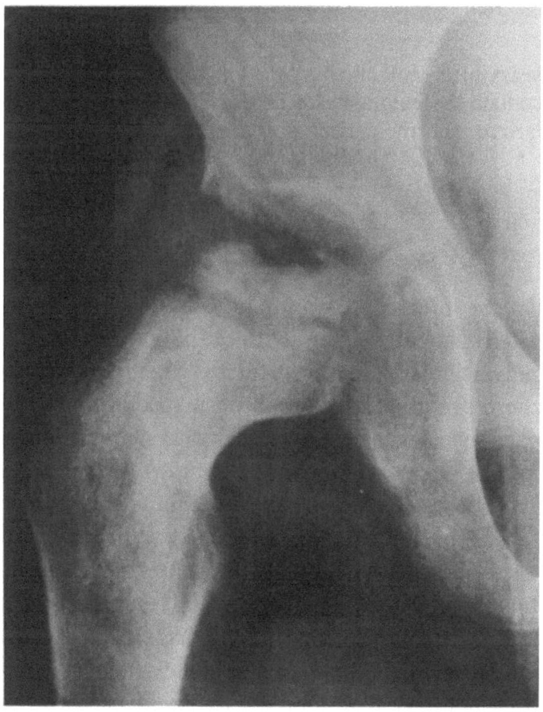

FIG. 4–1 Right hip of a 5-year-old boy 1 year after an infection. The hip had dislocated and was treated with incision, drainage, antibiotics, traction, and then spica casting. Note the irregularity and increased density of the femoral head with bony destruction and erosion of the acetabulum as well.

In children, the x-ray signs of avascular necrosis are usually not seen for 6 to 8 weeks, but the diagnosis can be suspected clinically by the continuing irritability of the hip.[32] The ischemia produces an x-ray picture very like that of Legg-Perthes' disease (during the early part of this century it was thought that Legg-Perthes' disease was infectious in origin).[30] There can be segmental or total head involvement. If the ischemia is segmental, the subsequent course of healing and ensuing deformity resembles that of Legg-Perthes' disease.[30,32] However, if the ischemia is total, the situation is not analogous to Legg-Perthes' disease with whole head involvement because decreased range of motion with partial ankylosis and deformity is often seen.[32]

The recommended treatment for avascular necrosis secondary to hip infection is maintaining mobility and containment of the head as in Legg-Perthes' disease[18,32] (Figs. 4–2A and B). A corrective osteotomy may be indicated to obtain coverage,[32] at the intertrochanteric or iliac level. Morrey et al. described two children with painful avascular necrosis who obtained relief of pain after subtrochanteric osteotomies but lost considerable motion of the hip.[35]

Lloyd-Roberts has grouped the avascular necrosis seen in the infected hip into aseptic and septic forms.[32] The septic form results from direct attack of the head by infection and can generally be seen on x-ray studies within 2 to 3 weeks of onset. It results in much worse damage to the epiphysis with sequestration, ankylosis, or severe deformity and usually has a poor result.[30,32]

Another complication of vascular etiology seen after hip infection in infants and children is coxa magna. However, rather than being secondary to ischemia, it has been postulated to be due to in-

A 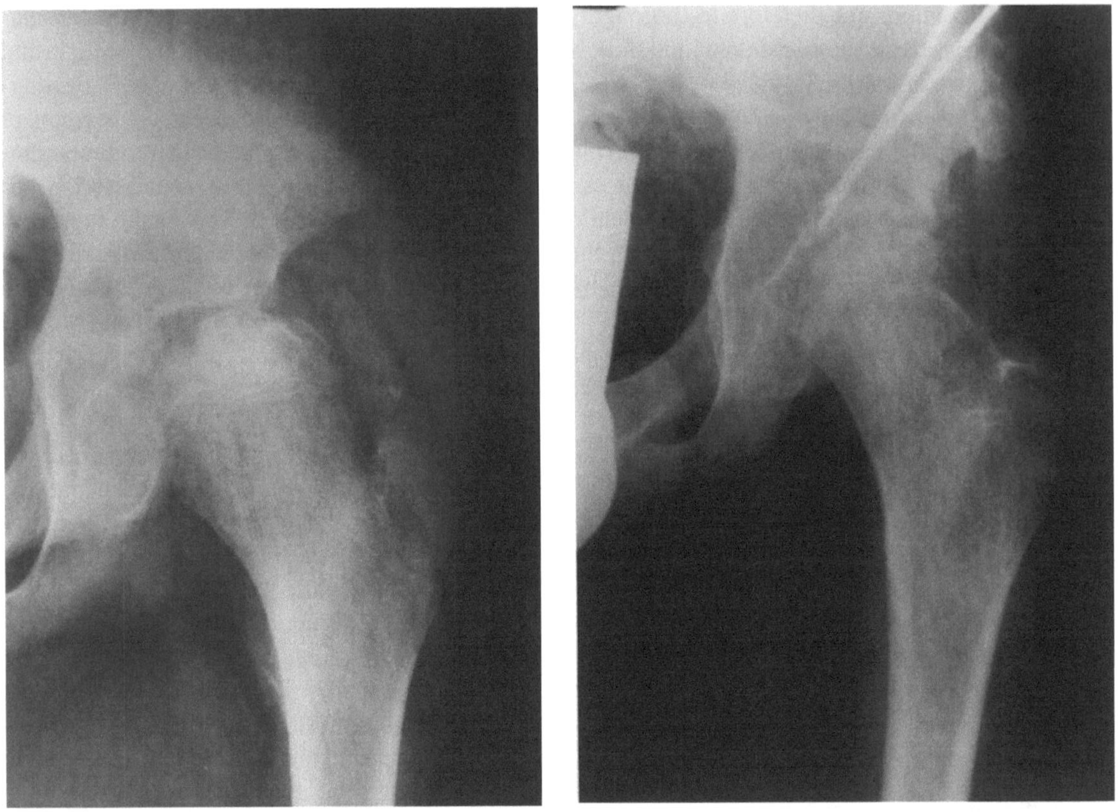 B

FIG. 4–2 **A** Left hip of a 10-year-old boy 14 months after septic arthritis. Note the loss of joint space and subluxation. The sclerotic, deformed capital femoral epiphysis is consistent with avascular necrosis. **B** Four years after innominate osteotomy performed to help contain the femoral head. The femoral head has revascularized, and the patient is asymptomatic.

creased blood flow. The infectious process causes an increase in vascularity and blood flow to the area with consequent stimulation of growth to the femoral head.[30,35,58]

Adults

Infections of the hip in adults are most commonly seen after surgical procedures to the hip. They present a severe problem, especially following prosthetic arthroplasty. In contrast, primary hip joint infections are relatively rare in adults, and in several studies of bacterial arthritides the hip was not the most commonly affected joint.[1,5,26,34] Twenty cases were seen over a 10-year period at Robert Jones and Agnes Hunt Orthopaedic Hospitals in Great Britain,[5] and 26 cases in 20 years at the Mayo Clinic.[28]

The infected virgin hip is seen in elderly debilitated patients, often with a high incidence of polyarticular involvement.[28,29,41,65] Frequently there are associated predisposing conditions that can be categorized as local or systemic factors.

The local factors include prior joint disease such as osteoarthritis[1] or avascular necrosis.[19] A hip aspiration or injection can directly inoculate bacteria into the joint. Injected steroids may inhibit local defense mechanisms.[7] Trauma may produce a hemarthrosis that predisposes to sepsis. However, at least in hemophiliacs, hemarthrosis does not appear to increase the incidence of pyarthrosis.[5,20]

The systemic factors associated with bacterial arthritis are often debilitating to the patient and increase their susceptibility to infection. They include chronic illnesses such as diabetes, alcoholism, nephrotic syndrome, cirrhosis, cancer, certain gastrointestinal diseases, ochronosis, rheumatoid arthritis, and other collagen diseases.[1,26,34] Patients with rheumatoid arthritis may be more susceptible owing to hypocomplementemia,[26,27] and patients with cancer and gastrointestinal disorders have a generalized lowering of their immune defense mechanisms.[27] Other associated factors include a focus of infection elsewhere[5,34], steroid, radiation, and cytotoxic therapy[26,68], recent surgery[68]; and heroin addiction.[34] Patients with advanced neurological diseases can be particularly susceptible to hip joint infections from decubitus ulcers.[14]

Pathogenesis

Most cases of septic arthritis of the hip in adults are hematogenous in origin, with the organisms often spreading from a focus of infection elsewhere and lodging initially in the synovium.[1,26,28,46] The synovium appears to be an ideal tissue for infection to localize for the following reasons: (1) the endothelium of synovial blood vessels is phagocytic; (2) the vessels in the synovium are uniquely permeable to circulating microorganisms, especially when the joint is abnormal to begin with[1]; (3) diffusion into the joint occurs readily as the vessels are very close to the joint space; (4) bacteria gain access to synovial fluid more easily than to spinal fluid, aqueous humor, or urine.[0]

The hip's venous system drains into Batson's veins around the bladder, prostate, uterus, and rectum. Retrograde flow occurs with increased intraabdominal pressure, such as coughing and straining.[5] This retrograde flow can be responsible for hip joint infections in the presence of bacteremia as a result of intraabdominal or pelvic trauma or surgery, especially involving genitourinary or pelvic instrumentation.[42,55]

The arterial supply to the hip sends ramifications through the capsule and synovium as well as into the bone via the nutrient vessels. In adults the metaphyseal and epiphyseal vessels have anastomosed. As a result, bacteria entering via the nutrient arteries can lodge very close to the articular cartilage and easily spread infection into the joint.[58] However, hematogenous osteomyelitis in this area in an adult is rare, except in addicts,[41,58,60] unlike in children where the metaphysis has enhanced susceptibility for infection owing to its unique circulation.[26,58,60]

Microorganisms can also gain access to the hip by direct spread from infections at other sites.[8] Intraabdominal and retroperitoneal abscesses can spread to the hip along the iliopsoas muscle. The thinnest portion of the hip capsule is where the iliopsoas crosses the hip, between the iliofemoral and iliopubic ligaments.[55] At this site, occasionally, there is a communication between the intraarticular space and the iliopsoas bursa. Direct inoculation of bacteria into the hip during diagnostic or therapeutic procedures is another method of entry. Penetrating wounds, if not treated initially with antibiotics, surgical irrigation, and débridement, can lead to pyarthrosis.[45,69]

Diagnosis

Because hip infections in adults are infrequent, they are often missed and the diagnosis is made late.[5,29] The patient's symptoms may be attributed to some preexisting condition such as rheumatoid arthritis or osteoarthritis, and the delay in diagnosis adversely affects the outcome.[28,29] It is imperative, therefore, that a careful examination be done and a high index of suspicion be maintained.

The work-up of adult hip infections as well as the clinical and radiological findings are essentially the same as those discussed previously for children, with some exceptions. Though systemic signs of sepsis including chills, fever, tachycardia, and malaise may be present, the course, especially in elderly debilitated patients (like infants), can be more insidious with a relatively low-grade systemic and local response.[1,5,55] External signs of inflammation are rare in adults.[49] The peripheral white blood cell count may or may not be elevated, though there is usually an increase in polymorphonuclear cells. Bacteremia with positive blood cultures may be seen in acutely ill patients and often portends a poor prognosis.[29]

As indicated in the previous section, x-ray films are not very useful in the early diagnosis of acutely infected hips. They are often normal or not specific for the first week or two, though occasionally loss of cartilage space may be seen before the end of a week.[1,5] In general, the classic x-ray signs of infected joints, including narrowing of the joint space, subchondral erosion, resorption, and osteoporosis, appear after a few weeks, and destructive changes of the femoral head and acetabulum are seen in the late stages of the disease.[5,28,67] Occasionally, gas is seen in the unviolated joint as a result of glucose metabolism by either *Escherichia coli* or *Clostridium welchii.*[2,34]

Bacteriology

The most commonly cultured organism in adult hip infections is *Staphylococcus aureus*, appearing in 40 to 75% of infections.[1,5,7,26–28,47] Other less commonly seen Gram-positive organisms include *Streptococcus*, anaerobic *Streptococcus*, and *Pneumococcus*.[5,6] The incidence of gonococcal Gram-negative infections is rising.[26,27,34,41] *E. coli* accounts for about one-third of Gram-negative infections, and those patients with Gram-negative pyarthrosis tend to have the worst results.[26,34]

There are many reports in the literature of infected adult hips secondary to uncommon organisms such as *Serratia*,[68] *Pseudomonas*,[28] *Proteus*,[28] *Hemophilus influenzae*,[47] *Bacterium alkaligenes*,[5] *Clostridium welchi*,[2,5] diphtheroids,[5] and *Salmonella*.[26]

These rare infections usually occur in hosts who are debilitated from diseases such as diabetes, carcinoma, or alcoholism or in those whose immune response has been blunted by steroids or immunosuppressive therapy. They are also seen in patients who are on antibiotics. In these cases, the new pathogens usually are resistant to the antibiotic. However, the increased incidence of infection caused by Gram-negative bacteria and organisms of low pathogenicity may also be due in part to better collection and culturing techniques.[41]

Treatment

Infection of the hip was once a disastrous occurrence, with severe disability and even death a common sequelae. With the advent of antibiotics, the possibility of not only curing the infection but maintaining motion and function was realized. The keys to successful results are the rapid diagnosis and early, adequate treatment of the pyarthrosis.

In the acute situation, open surgical drainage and lavage in conjunction with appropriate parenteral bactericidal antibiotics is advised.[5,11,26,28] Most antimicrobial agents easily diffuse into infected joint spaces and bone. Bactericidal levels in synovial fluid have a linear relation to bactericidal serum activity. In synovial fluid, antibiotic levels are substantially higher in infected joints than in noninfected joints. Bone levels of most antibiotics approximate 10 to 30% of serum levels, readily traversing capillary membranes. Repeated aspiration is not recommended as a method of treatment for reasons outlined previously.

The hip can be drained via most standard approaches, though the posterior approach offers the possibility of dependent drainage. Based on the extent of the infection and destruction found at surgery, several alternatives to closure are possible. These include incomplete closure of the capsule and overlying muscle and skin, leaving the capsule open or marsupializing it, with or without drains, or packing the wound open. Closed-suction irrigation appears to offer a better alternative to leaving the joint open, especially in the acute situation. It helps decompress and clear the joint, dilutes and flushes away bacteria and necrotic debris, and at least in children improves the results of treatment.[11] It is not without problems, however, including leakage, blockage, difficulty regulating flow, and absorption of the irrigating fluid. The possibility of retrograde contamination and secondary infection exists, as does the possibility of interference with cartilage nutrition in extended use, so most authors recommend limiting its use to 2 to 3 days.[17,26,27,41,45] One study has shown that suction irrigation does not perfuse the whole joint, and these authors recommended distention by periodic clamping and release of the outflow tube.[24]

The instillation of antibiotics into the joint, whether by intraarticular injection or suction irrigation, has been debated in the past, though most authorities believe that it is not indicated now.[9,26,52] It has been shown in many studies that the synovium, especially when inflamed, is highly permeable to virtually all antibiotics in adequate serum concentrations, negating the need for direct instillation.[9,27,39,50] It has also been shown that antibiotics are irritating to the joint when injected directly intraarticularly, and they have been implicated in postinfectious synovitis.[1] However, this synovitis, which occurs after the infection has been controlled and the synovial fluid is once again sterile, may be more directly the result of the infection itself.[51] Parenteral antibiotics should be used for at least 4 weeks if the infection involves soft tissues and 6 weeks or longer if it involves bone, especially in rheumatoid and debilitated patients, to prevent recurrence.[47]

In those cases where joint destruction has occurred and the infection has penetrated the bone because of either late diagnosis or failure of previous therapy, most authors recommend extensive débridement, including excision of necrotic, devitalized, and granulation tissue and removal of

A
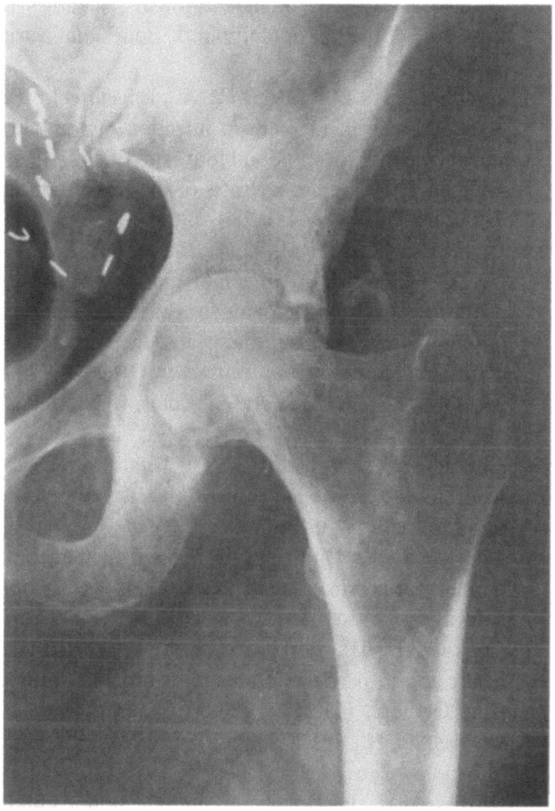

B
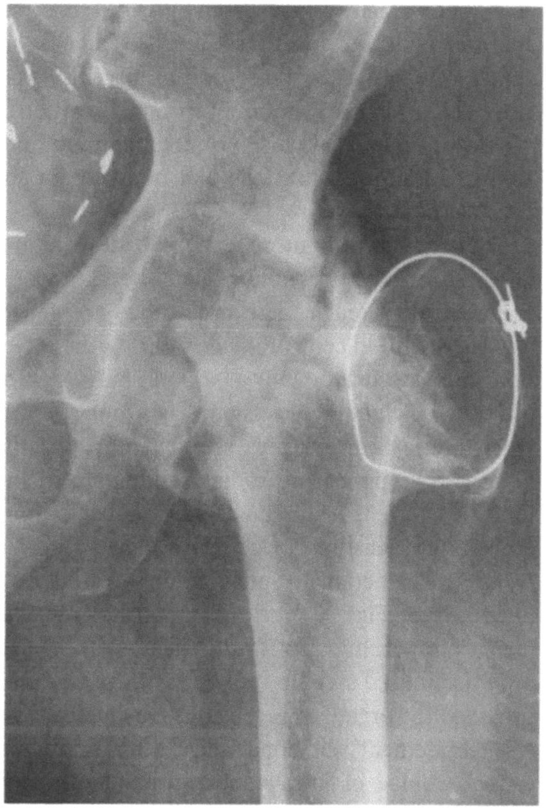

C
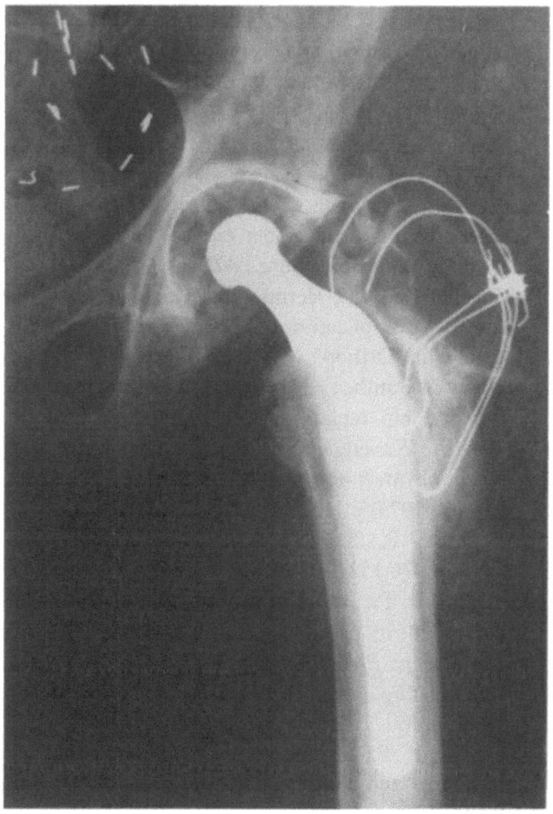

FIG. 4–3 **A** Left hip of a 58-year-old woman with lymphoma who developed *Salmonella* pyarthrosis after treatment with chemotherapy. **B** The hip was resected, and **C** 10 months later the patient had a total hip replacement. At the time, all cultures were negative. The result has been successful.

all foreign bodies. If enough bone stock is left, the procedure is followed by immobilization either in traction or in a spica cast, with the hope that the joint will ankylose. Best results occur in patients who go on to bony or fibrous ankylosis, provided it is in a good functional position.[28] However, bony ankylosis is not common, and those with hip mobility could also have pain and be severely disabled.[5,28,54]

In patients with more extensive destruction, Girdlestone-type resection has been recommended.[26,54] Though these procedures are generally successful in controlling and curing the infection, they are functionally disabling. Salvage procedures including excision arthroplasty or trochanteric arthroplasties are generally unsatisfactory. The patient often has residual pain, the limb is shortened and unstable, requiring some ambulatory assistive device.[28,67]

For the functionally unacceptable results outlined above (Figs. 4–3A to C), total hip replacement is now being offered to patients with healed hip infections. Total hip replacement can be done, provided the organism is sensitive, adequate surgical débridement was done, and after a minimum 6-week course of intravenous antibiotic therapy produced at least 1:8 peak bactericidal serum levels. The results in most cases are encouraging; however, recurrence of infection is seen in some cases, especially those done in hips with a history of certain infections (*Pseudomonas, Streptococcus* group D, *Proteus,* and *Escherichia coli*)[4] or infections due to resistant microbes. Currently, extensive clinical and basic research is being conducted to establish the proper pre- and postoperative evaluation and treatment, the proper timing of surgery, and the role of antibiotic-impregnated acrylic cement to better define the indications and improve the results of total hip replacement in the treatment of infected hips.[4,6,15,23,25,26,36,41,49,66,67,5a]

Acknowledgment

The authors wish to thank Nan Weinerman for technical assistance in the preparation of this chapter.

References

1. Argen, R. J., Wilson, C. H., Wood, P.: Suppurative arthritis. Arch. Intern. Med., 117:661, 1966.
2. Bliznak, J., Ramsey, J.: Emphysematous septic arthritis due to Escherichia coli. J. Bone Joint Surg., 58A:138, 1976.
3. Brown, I.: A study of the "capsular" shadows in disorders of the hip in children. J. Bone Joint Surg. 57B:175, 1975.
4. Buchholz, H. W., Elson, R. A., Engelbrecht E., et al.: Management of deep infection of total hip replacement. J. Bone Joint Surg., 63B:342, 1981.
5. Bulmer, J. H.: Septic arthritis of the hip in adults. J. Bone Joint Surg., 48B:289, 1966.

5a. Callaghan, J. J., Salvati, E. A., Brause, B. D., Rimnac, C. M., Wright, T.: Reimplantation for salvage of the infected hip: Rationale for the use of gentamicin-impregnated cement and beads. In: *The Hip Society, Proceedings of the Thirteenth Open Scientific Meeting of The Hip Society.* St. Louis, C. V. Mosby, 1985, p. 65.

6. Cherney, D. L., Amstutz, H. C.: Total hip replacement in the previously septic hip. J. Bone Joint Surg., 65A:1256, 1983.
7. Clawson, D. K., Dunn, W. A.: Management of common bacterial infections of bones and joints. J. Bone Joint Surg., 49A:164, 1967.
8. Cooke, C.P., III, Levinsohn, E. M., Baker, B. E.: Septic hip in pelvic fractures with urologic injury. Clin. Orthop., 147:253, 1980.
9. Curtiss, P. H., Jr.: The pathophysiology of joint infections. Clin. Orthop., 96:129, 1973.
10. Curtiss, P. H., Jr.: Bone and joint infection in childhood. Instr. Course Lect., 26:14, 1977.
11. Dale, D., Akeson, W., Amiel, D., et al: Lavage of septic joints in rabbits: effects of chondrolysis. J. Bone Joint Surg., 58A:393, 1976.
12. Dich, V. Q., Nelson, J. D., Haltalin, K. C.: Osteomyelitis in infants and children. Am. J. Dis. Child., 129:1273, 1975.
13. Eyre-Brook, A. L.: Septic arthritis of the hip and osteomyelitis of the upper end of the femur in infants. J. Bone Joint Surg., 42B:11, 1960.
14. Freehafer, A. A., Herndon, C. H.: Infection of the hip as a complication of advanced neurologic disease. Clin. Orthop., 64A:135, 1969.
15. Fremont-Smith, P.: Antibiotic management of septic total hip replacement: a therapetuic trial. In: *The Hip Society, Proceedings of the Second Open Scientific Meeting of The Hip Society.* St. Louis, Mosby, 1974, p. 301.
16. Gillespie, R.: Septic arthritis of childhood. Clin. Orthop., 96:152, 1973.
17. Griffin, P. P.: Acute septic arthritis of the hip in childhood: its pathogenesis and treatment. In: *The Hip Society, Proceedings of the Seventh Open Scientific Meeting of The Hip Society.* St. Louis, Mosby, 1979, p. 89.
18. Griffin, P. P., Green, W. T.: Hip joint infections in infants and children. Orthop. Clin. North Am., 9:123, 1978.
19. Habermann, E. T., Friedenthal, R. B.: Septic arthri-

tis associated with avascular necrosis of the femoral head. Clin. Orthop., 134:325, 1978.
20. Houghton, G. R.: Septic arthritis of the hip in a hemophiliac. Clin. Orthop., 129:223, 1977.
21. Howard, J. B., Highgenboten, C. L., Nelson, J. D.: Residual effects of septic arthritis in infancy and childhood. JAMA, 236:932, 1976.
22. Howie, D. W., Savage, J. P., Wilson, T. G., Paterson, D.: The technetium phosphate bone scan in the diagnosis of osteomyelitis in childhood. J. Bone Joint Surg., 65A:431, 1983.
23. Hughes, P. W., Salvati, E. A., Wilson, P. D., et al: Treatment of subacute sepsis of the hip by antibiotics and joint replacement: criteria for diagnosis with evaluation of twenty-six cases. Clin. Orthop., 141:143, 1979.
24. Jackson, R. W., Parsons, C. J.: Distension-irrigation treatment of major joint sepsis. Clin. Orthop., 96:160, 1973.
25. Jupiter, J. B., Karchmer, A. W., Lowell, J. D., Harris, W. H.: Total hip arthroplasty in the treatment of adult hips with current or quiescent sepsis. J. Bone Joint Surg., 63A:194, 1981.
26. Kelly, P. J.: Bacterial arthritis in the adult. Orthop. Clin. North Am., 6:973, 1975.
27. Kelly, P. J.: Infections of bones and joints in adult patients. Instru. Course Lect., 26:3, 1977.
28. Kelly, P. J., Martin, W. J., Coventry, M. B.: Bacterial arthritis of the hip in the adult. J. Bone Joint Surg., 47A:1005, 1965.
29. Kelly, P. J., Martin, W. J., Coventry, M. B.: Bacterial (suppurative) arthritis in the adult. J. Bone Joint Surg., 52A:1595, 1970.
30. Kemp, M. B. S., Lloyd-Roberts, G. C.: Avascular necrosis of the capital epiphysis following osteomyelitis of the proximal femoral metaphysis. J. Bone Joint Surg., 56B:688, 1974.
31. Kuo, K. N., Lloyd-Roberts, G. C., Orme, I. M., et al: Immunodeficiency and infantile bone and joint infection. Arch. Dis. Child., 50:51, 1975.
32. Lloyd-Roberts, G. C.: Pyogenic arthritis of the hip. In: *Hip Disorders in Children.* Butterworths, 1978. p. 91–118.
33. Maurer, A. H., Chen, D. C. P., Camargo, E. E., et al: Utility of three-phase skeletal scintigraphy in suspected osteomyelitis: concise communication. J. Nucl. Med., 22:941, 1981.
34. Meredith, H. C., Rittenberg, G. M.: Pneumoarthropathy: an unusual radiographic sign of gram negative septic arthritis. Radiology, 129:642, 1978.
35. Morrey, B. F., Bianco, A. J., Rhodes, H. K.: Suppurative arthritis of the hip in children. J. Bone Joint Surg., 58A:388, 1976.
36. Muller, M. E.: Preservation of septic total hip replacement versus Girdlestone operation. In: *The Hip Society, Proceedings of the Second Open Scientific Meeting of the Hip Society.* St. Louis, Mosby, 1974, p. 308.
37. Nade, S.: Acute haematogenous osteomyelitis in infancy and childhood. J. Bone Joint Surg., 65B:109, 1983.
38. Nade, S.: Acute septic arthritis in infancy and childhood. J. Bone Joint Surg., 65B:234, 1983.
39. Nelson, J. D.: Antibiotic concentrations in septic joint effusions. N. Engl. J. Med., 284:349, 1971.
40. Nelson, J. D.: The bacterial etiology and antibiotic management of septic arthritis in infants and children. Pediatrics, 50:437, 1972.
41. Nelson, J. P.: Musculoskeletal infection. Surg. Clin. North Am., 60:213, 1980.
42. Nicholson, J. T., Sherk, H. H., Christides, S., et al: Hip sepsis complicating pelvic fractures and urologic trauma. Clin. Orthop., 76:21, 1971.
43. Ogden, J. A.: Changing patterns of proximal femoral vascularity. J. Bone Joint Surg., 56A:941, 1974.
44. Patterson, D. C.: Acute suppurative arthritis in infancy and childhood. J. Bone Joint Surg., 52B:474, 1970.
45. Patzakis, M. J., Dorr, L. D., Ivler, D., et al: The early management of open joint injuries. J. Bone Joint Surg., 57A:1065, 1975.
46. Propst-Proctor, S. L., Dillingham, M. F., McDougall, I. R., Goodwin, D.: The white blood cell scan in orthopaedics. Clin. Orthop., 168:157, 1982.
47. Raff, M. J., Dannaher, C. L.: Hemophilus influenzae septic arthritis in adults. J. Bone Joint Surg., 56A:408, 1974.
48. Riordan, T., Doyle, D., Tabaqchali, S.: Synovial fluid lactic acid measurement in the diagnosis and management of septic arthritis. J. Clin. Pathol., 35:390, 1982.
49. Salvati, E. A., Chekofsky, K. M., Brause, B. D., Wilson, P. D., Jr.: Reimplantation in infection. Clin. Orthop., 170:62, 1982.
50. Schurman, D. J., Hirschman, P. H., Nagel, D. A.: Antibiotic penetration of synovial fluid in infected and normal knee joints. Clin. Orthop., 136:304, 1978.
51. Schurman, D. J., Mirra, J., Ding, A., et al: Experimental E. coli arthritis in the rabbit. J. Rheumatol., 4:118, 1977.
52. Scoles, P. V., Aronoff, S. C.: Antimicrobial therapy of childhood skeletal infections. J. Bone Joint Surg., 66A:1487, 1984.
53. Scoles, P. V., Hilty, M. D., Sfakianakis, G. M.: Bone scan patterns in acute osteomyelitis. Clin. Orthop., 153:210, 1980.
54. Slowick, F. A.: Purulent infections of the hip joint: an analysis of sixty cases. N. Engl. J. Med., 212:672, 1935.
55. Smith, W. S., Ward, R. M.: Septic arthritis of the hip complicating perforation of abdominal organs. JAMA, 195:170, 1966.
56. Soto-Hall, R., Johnson, L. H., Johnson, R. A.: Variations in the intra-articular pressure of the hip joint

in injury and disease. J. Bone Joint Surg., 46A:509, 1964.
57. Trueta, J.: The normal vascular anatomy of the human femoral head during growth. J. Bone Joint Surg., 39B:358, 1957.
58. Trueta, J.: The three types of acute hematogenous osteomyelitis. J. Bone Joint Surg., 41B:671, 1959.
59. Wainwright, D.: Some problems in the treatment of disorders of the hip joint in various age groups. Proc. R. Soc. Med., 52:864, 1959.
60. Waldvogel, F. A., Medoff, G., Swartz, M. N.: Osteomyelitis: a review of clinical features, therapeutic considerations and unusual aspects. N. Engl. J. Med., 282:198, 1970.
61. Waldvogel, F. A., Vasey, M.: Osteomyelitis: the past decade. N. Engl. J. Med., 303:360, 1980.
62. Wall, J. J., Hund, D. D.: Acute hematogenous pyarthrosis caused by Hemophilus influenzae. J. Bone Joint Surg., 50A:1657, 1968.
63. Watkins, M. B., Samilson, R. L., Winters, D. M.: Acute suppurative arthritis. J. Bone Joint Surg., 38A:1313, 1956.
64. Wilkowske, C. J., Hermans, P. E.: Actions and uses of antimicrobial agents in the treatment of musculoskeletal infections. Orthop. Clin. North Am., 6:1129, 1975.
65. Willkens, R. F., Healey, L. A., Decker, J. L.: Acute infectious arthritis in the aged and chronically ill. Arch. Intern. Med., 106:104, 1960.
66. Wilson, P. D., Jr.: Total hip replacement in management of the infected hip. In: *The Hip Society, Proceedings of the Second Open Scientific Meeting of The Hip Society.* St. Louis, Mosby, 1974, p. 313.
67. Wilson, P. D., Jr., Aglietti, P., Salvati, E. A.: Subacute sepsis of the hip treated by antibiotics and cemented prosthesis. J. Bone Joint Surg., 56A:879, 1974.
68. Yosowitz, G. M.: Serratia arthritis of the hip. Clin. Orthop., 85:122, 1972.
69. Zamani, M. H., Brooker, A. F.: Osteomyelitis and septic arthritis in the adult hip. Orthop. Rev., 7:71, 1978.

CHAPTER 5

Fractures and Fracture Dislocations

DANA C. MEARS AND HARRY E. RUBASH

Since Callisen first described a central acetabular fracture in 1788,[9] the optimal form of management has remained controversial. Admittedly, there is a consensus that a minimally displaced acetabular fracture without dislocation of the femoral head has an excellent prognosis when it is managed nonoperatively by bed rest or by a short period of traction followed by a variable period of a partial weight-bearing gait.[2,26] To attain reproducibly good results in the management of most intraarticular fractures it is generally agreed that perfect restoration of the alignment of the articular surfaces is highly desirable if not essential. Although this principle is rigorously accepted for most intraarticular fractures, it has remained controversial in the case of the displaced acetabular fracture. At first glance this exception is nonsensical. A review of the proponents of the nonoperative and the operative schools, however, provides an explanation for this controversy.

Conservative Treatment

It is solely of historical interest that some workers[21] espoused hip spica cast immobilization for variable periods of several weeks as a suitable form of management.[18] Without the provision for an accurate reduction of a displaced acetabular fracture or of early posttraumatic restoration of joint mobility, cast immobilization is recognized as a wholly unsuitable technique. Cutaneous or skeletal traction[20,28] remains widely employed to the present time.[2,17,26] Multiple traction pins can be inserted into the greater trochanter and the distal femur or the proximal tibia. In this way, the principal vector of the distraction can be directed to correct proximal and medial displacement of the femoral head and acetabulum, respectively. Early active motion exercises of the hip joint can be undertaken and continued for the variable period of distraction, frequently 9 to 12 weeks. Many authors suggested that under the influence of skeletal traction applied to the femur, and of the presumably intact capsule of the hip joint, the acetabular fragments are realigned reproducibly in an anatomical configuration. This concept of "ligamentotaxis," as defined by Vidal, may apply to minimally displaced and minimally comminuted fractures. For the more comminuted and displaced acetabular insults, skeletal traction permits moderately anatomical realignment of the femoral head. A critical assessment of follow-up radiographs indicates that the acetabular fragments tend to unite in their malaligned configuration with the formation of a fibrous or fibrocartilaginous lining. Subsequently, when full weight-bearing ultimately is restored, this pseudoarticular surface generally undergoes rapid deterioration.

Some authors have acknowledged that, whereas significant displacement of the superior or weight-bearing portion of the acetabulum fails to respond satisfactorily to skeletal traction, comparable displacement of the residual portions of the acetabulum is favorably influenced by this technique. Although successful results following skeletal traction applied to uncomminuted fractures of the medial wall with modest displacement have been documented, more recent reports have indicated a substantial incidence of failure with late traumatic arthritis.[19,21]

Two other patterns of acetabular fracture were

widely recognized for their failure to respond to nonoperative management. In the presence of loose osteochondral fragments interposed between the traumatized acetabulum and femoral head, rapid onset and progression of traumatic arthritis can be anticipated. Also, in the presence of a displaced acetabular fracture with a concomitant displaced pelvic ring fracture, nonunion and/or malunion of both the acetabular and pelvic ring disruptions is likely to follow.

Surgical Treatment

In 1912 Vaughn[28] provided the first American report of a central acetabular fracture managed by open reduction. In 1943 Levine[12] heralded the use of internal fixation for the treatment of a central acetabular fracture. In 1948 Armstrong[1] suggested that certain markedly displaced and comminuted central acetabular fractures possessed such a high rate of anticipated failure after resort to the available methods of treatment that primary arthrodesis was advised. In 1954 Westerborn[29] documented equally disappointing results following the use of conservative therapy and therefore recommended a primary cup arthroplasty for the reconstruction of a central acetabular fracture/dislocation.

During the ensuing years several authors such as Pennal reported the use of open reduction and internal fixation. Levine,[12] Urist,[27] Elliott,[4] and Judet et al.[7] recorded the use of various modes of fixation including screws, plates, and Hage's pins. Although isolated cases of successful surgical intervention were reported, there was a general dissatisfaction with operative management. As LeTournel acknowledged in 1950, given the available radiological views of the pelvis, surgeons could not identify the disrupted segment of the acetabulum. On more than one occasion, distinguished hip surgeons undertook a posterior surgical approach to the acetabulum and failed to observe any evidence of traumatic disruption. To their chagrin, a second anterior surgical exposure was necessary. Even when the fracture was visualized, with the then-available techniques of reduction and stabilization failure to achieve and maintain a satisfactory congruent reduction was exceedingly common.

This environment provided the stimulus to initiate basic studies on acetabular disruption. Okelberry[16] and Knight and Smith[8] described the mechanisms of acetabular disruption and provided a practical classification of central acetabular fractures. These workers studied anteroposterior radiographs of acetabular fractures and attempted to correlate specific fracture lines with the radiological findings. Meanwhile, Judet et al.[7] initiated their pioneering studies on the pelvis. For his dissertation, LeTournel applied lead wires to a cadaveric pelvis and undertook various radiological views. For the first time most of the specific anatomical features of the pelvis were documented. Two novel oblique radiological views were developed.

With this knowledge, the French School was able to identify the anatomical origin of displaced fracture fragments. Next they studied various surgical approaches to the disrupted acetabulum. With a posterior and/or anterior exposure they were able to visualize and reduce virtually all fracture patterns. They devised special bone-holding forceps and curved bone plates that greatly facilitated the immobilization. As a culmination of their extraordinarily productive research on the acetabulum by 1964, Judet et al.[7] recommended an open reduction and internal fixation for all displaced acetabular disruptions. In 1981 these authors reported 568 cases of acetabular fractures that were managed by an open reduction. In their follow-up of 2 to 21 years 74% of the cases showed very good results with a normal hip, 6% of the results were good, and 5% were fair. In this series a perfect initial postoperative radiographic reduction was consistent with an 85% very good result and a 7.6% good clinical result.[11] Thus late follow-up of acetabular disruptions treated by an open reduction and internal fixation supported the contention that a satisfactory outcome can be anticipated if the initial fracture reduction is perfect. The converse, however, is also true. If the initial postoperative reduction is imperfect, symptomatic traumatic arthritis can be anticipated.

During the past decade Pennal and Massiah,[20] Tile,[24] and other workers confirmed certain of the observations documented by Judet and coworkers.[7] They acknowledged that a successful open reduction and stabilization of a displaced acetabular fracture generally culminated in a very good late result. Many of these workers were troubled by the complexities of the exposure, reduction, and stabilization of the various comminuted acetabular fractures, or even of the transverse fracture patterns. These surgeons cautiously recommended an open reduction for a limited variety of simple acetabular fractures. For the more complex variants with the anticipated technical complexities, they recommended consideration for skeletal traction.

By 1980 in the United States there was a dilemma for the rational management of a displaced acetabular fracture. Nonoperative methods were advised for minimally displaced fractures or for complex comminuted and displaced injuries. Operative treatment was advised only for relatively simple but displaced fractures which failed to undergo an adequate reduction under the influence of skeletal traction. The crux of the optional form of management rested on a preoperative assessment of the technical feasibility of a surgical procedure. Several surgeons studied simpler methods to expose, reduce, and stabilize these complex acetabular reductions. Ruedi (personal communication, 1981), LeTournel,[10] Senegas and Yates,[23] and Mears and Rubash[15] devised simplified extensile surgical exposures.

Superior reduction forceps and the availability of more malleable plates further simplified the surgical procedure. On this basis, Mears and Rubash[15] reaffirmed the observation of Judet et al. that operative methods were preferred treatment for virtually all displaced acetabular fractures. In the following sections the surgical anatomy of the pelvis, the principles of the surgical approach, open reduction, and internal fixation are discussed.

Surgical Anatomy

Surgical treatment of an acetabular fracture requires not only knowledge of the anatomy of the relevant fracture pattern but also consideration of the osseous supports that buttress the acetabulum and which provide the sites for anchorage of the internal fixation devices.

An inspection of the lateral aspect of the innominate bone reveals two columns of bone (Fig. 5–1). The strong posterior, or ilioischial, column extends from the central portion of the obturator foramen through the middle of the acetabulum. It then courses posteriorly to the greater sciatic notch and inferiorly to the ischial tuberosity. Its thick surfaces are easily recognized as sites for solid anchorage of internal fixation. It is triangular in its overall configuration and possesses internal, lateral, and posterior surfaces. The internal surface

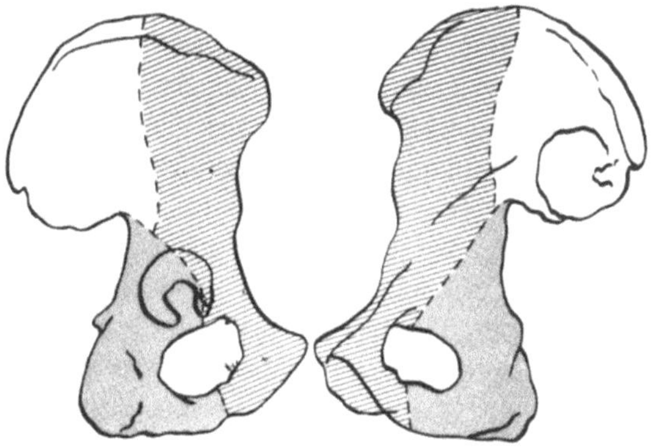

FIG. 5–1 Outer and inner views of the innominate bone show the iliac wing (*white*), anterior column (*lined*), and posterior column (*shaded*).

comprises a quadrilateral area on the inner aspect of the body of the ischium.

The anterior, or iliopubic, column extends from a confluent point on the obturator foramen. From the acetabulum it courses inferiorly to the anteroinferior iliac spine and anteriorly to the pubic symphysis. The anterior column possesses iliac and acetabular portions and the superior pubic ramus. A so-called dome region receives contributions from the anterior and posterior columns and constitutes the crucial superior weight-bearing portion of the acetabulum. Comminution, and especially residual displacement of the dome fragment, is of great prognostic importance. The remainder of the lateral ilium comprises the superior aspect of the sciatic notch and the posterior aspect of the iliac wing. Numerous acetabular fractures propagate into the lateral ilium. In such cases an open reduction and internal fixation of the ilium are required during surgical reconstruction of the acetabulum itself. The sacroiliac joint is located medial to the posterolateral portion of the ilium. *Many complex acetabular fractures are complicated by an ipsilateral sacroiliac disruption which requires surgical stabilization as part of the acetabular reconstruction.*

The contour and structure of the innominate bone is related to the forces which are transferred from the lower end of the vertebral column and relayed to the femur. Three trabecular systems identified as sacral-acetabular, sacral-pubic, and sacroischial subsections are related to the anterior and posterior columns, the lateral ilium, and the sacroiliac joint. The apex of the bony trabeculae forms a thickened area directly inferior to the sacroiliac joint, which protects it from fracture when the acetabulum is traumatically disrupted. Several studies[6] have examined the intimate local variations in the mechanical properties of the acetabulum and adjacent pelvis by the application of finite element analysis. From such data computerized models of the hip joint have been prepared which predict the physiological transmission of weight-bearing forces through the pelvis.

In addition to its relation to the acetabulum and hip joint, the pelvic ring provides protection for certain intraabdominal viscera and the adjacent neurovascular structures including the external and internal iliac, pudendal, obturator, and gluteal arteries. In the area of the iliac fossa approximately 1 cm anterior to the articular surface of the sacroiliac joint and 1 cm above the iliopectineal line a principal nutrient artery to the ilium enters the bone. Numerous other branches from the external iliac and obturator arteries form a highly vascular network which supplies the ilium. In the middle of the gluteal area of the iliac wing, a large nutrient artery enters the mid-section of the lateral ilium directly superior to the acetabulum. Despite the presence of this extensive anastomotic blood supply to the pelvis and acetabulum, excessive stripping of the soft tissues from the fracture can lead to avascular necrosis with a considerable predilection for nonunion, malunion, and osseous infection.

Mechanisms of Acetabular Fractures

From an examination of pedestrians struck by cars or victims of motor vehicular accidents, the principal mechanisms of acetabular injuries have been determined.[9] Most fractures of the acetabulum are provoked by forces applied to (1) the greater trochanter along the axis of the femoral neck; (2) the front of the flexed knee along the axis of the femoral shaft; (3) the plantar surface of the foot of a seated individual in whom the ipsilateral hip and knee are extended; or rarely (4) the posterolateral aspect of the lumbosacral regions. A few attempts to recreate acetabular fractures experimentally in fresh cadaveric specimens have been complicated by the need to provide the influence of postural muscular forces, intraabdominal pressure, and the physiological intraosseous hydrostatic pressure demonstrable in living bone. The studies are rendered still more difficult by the need to recreate the vector and the velocity of the provocative force and to determine the fracture pattern, the degree of comminution, and the propensity for remote disruption of the pelvic ring.

Displacement of the crucial dome, or weight-bearing portion of the acetabulum, has been generally acknowledged as a particularly sinister injury with a propensity for severe traumatic arthritis unless an anatomical reduction is achieved. The more recent observations by Judet and LeTournel have confirmed a poor prognosis when residual acetabular displacement was left uncorrected. These workers observed that acetabular malalignment secondary to a "step-off" of greater than 1 to 2 mm, a loss of sphericity, and segmental impaction in any portion of the acetabular bone contribute heavily to late traumatic arthritis.[11]

Another controversy focused on the degree of acetabular congruity that would be achieved by the use of skeletal traction applied along the axis of the principal displacement in an attempt to achieve an accurate closed reduction. Most workers agree that many simple displaced fractures are satisfactorily realigned by the application of such a closed reduction with the use of skeletal traction. Previously, a closed reduction was believed to facilitate an accurate reduction of more complex comminuted and displaced injuries. More recent observations, however, have generally refuted this hypothesis. With the degree of capsular disruption that has been documented for a typical comminuted fracture, it appears that skeletal traction provides a reduction of the femoral head but not of the comminuted acetabular fragments. Many of the comminuted fragments, especially in the dome region, undergo marked rotational displacement which is amenable only to surgical correction.

A third controversy has focused on the incidence of avascular necrosis of the femoral head or chondrolysis of the femoral head following an acetabular fracture managed by closed or open methods. Some previous workers suggested that the provocative force had a considerable likelihood to initiate such late complications. From the more recent observations by LeTournel[10] and Rubash and Mears[22] it appears that avascular necrosis of the femoral head and chondrolysis of the hip joint secondary to an acetabular fracture are extremely uncommon complications. Admittedly, if the capsular blood supply to the femoral head is completely disrupted at the time of an open reduction or if there is a concomitant femoral neck fracture, avascular necrosis may be anticipated. The most common cause of chondrolysis following an acetabular fracture is when an open reduction is accompanied by a screw which violates the articular surfaces of the hip joint.

Radiological Assessment of the Acetabulum

With the complex three-dimensional anatomical configuration of the innominate bone, accurate radiological interpretation of an acetabular fracture necessitates the application of a series of special radiological views and, supplementary computed tomography (CT). An accurate three-dimensional image of the fracture pattern is perceived by scrutiny of these various views and delineation of the fracture lines on a life-size pelvic model. This detailed assessment provides crucial information concerning the configuration of the fracture, the integrity of the acetabular dome and the quadrilateral surface, the degree of displacement, and the presence of loose interarticular osteochondral fragments. The CT scan also permits detection of an ipsilateral or contralateral fracture of the pelvic ring, especially an unstable disruption of the sacrum which is not readily identified by scrutiny of conventional radiographic views.

The development of computed body tomography has led to revolutionary changes in the evaluation of complex bony architecture, especially with MPR (multiplane reconstruction). With this system, images can be visualized in planes other than the single scan plane. It possesses all of the benefits of transaxial CT imaging and it provides additional information that is especially helpful for the characterization of various complex fracture patterns.

More recently, by the use of special discs and software, shading algorithms have been prepared which provide an accurate 3-D view of a pelvic or acetabular fracture. The method is particularly helpful for documentation of rotational displacement. Recent reviews by Mears and Rubash[22] describe this technique and its application to the pelvis and acetabulum. Currently, 3-D CT is the optimal method for preoperative assessment as well as postoperative review of open reduction. The scatter artifact allied with the presence of metal implants is relatively modest. The method, along with magnetic resonance imagery (MRI) permits the definition of soft tissues. The latter method is of limited value to study bone.

Five radiological views are needed to adequately assess an acetabular disruption: a standard anteroposterior view of the whole pelvis, the 45° inlet and the tangential outlet projections of the pelvic ring, and two oblique pelvic views taken at 45° to the coronal plane (Fig. 5–2). The anteroposterior radiograph of the acetabulum reveals six fundamental radiological landmarks, which are seen in Fig. 5–2A. These are the borders of the anterior and posterior walls of the acetabulum, the teardrop, the roof, the ilioischial and iliopectineal lines, and the pelvic inlet (i.e., the brim of the true pelvis). The pelvic inlet view demonstrates posterior migration of a hemipelvis accompanying a sacroiliac disruption and central migration of an acetabular fracture (Fig. 5–2B). The pelvic outlet view provides a detailed assessment of the obturator ring (Fig. 5–2C). The obturator oblique view shows the pelvic brim (anterior column), the posterior border of the acetabular articular surface, the obturator foramen, and the iliac wing, which is seen in section. In addition, the junction of the anterior and posterior columns, which defines the roof or the dome of the acetabulum, is visible (Fig. 5–2D). The iliac oblique radiograph reveals the posterior border of the iliac bone, the posterior column, the anterior border of the acetabulum, and an outline of the iliac wing (Fig. 5–2E). Even when applied to the acutely injured patient, computed tomography has become an invaluable tool to facilitate a three-dimensional appraisal of the disrupted pelvis and acetabulum. Five coronal sections of the pelvis are studied (Fig. 5–3). The most superior section demonstrates the sacroiliac joints and the iliac wings. A scan taken approximately 4 cm inferior to the first one reveals the ilium at the level of the anteroinferior iliac spine and the diamond-shaped bony masses formed by the junction of the anterior and posterior columns which support the crucial acetabular roof. The tip of the coccyx is evident in this view. A scan taken approximately 1 cm further inferior to the previous one which approximates the level of the sacroiliac notch demonstrates the circular cross-section of

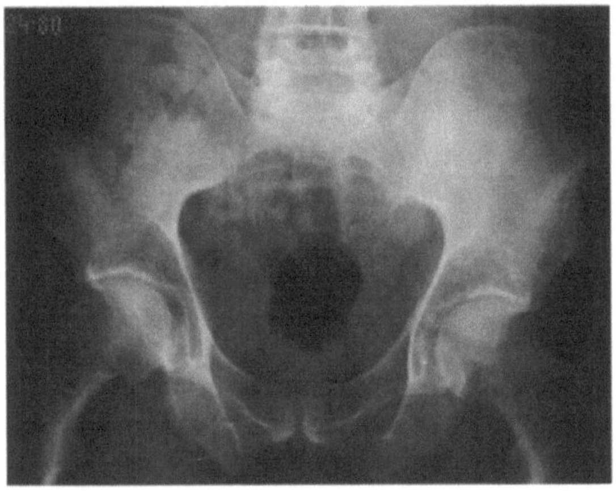
A

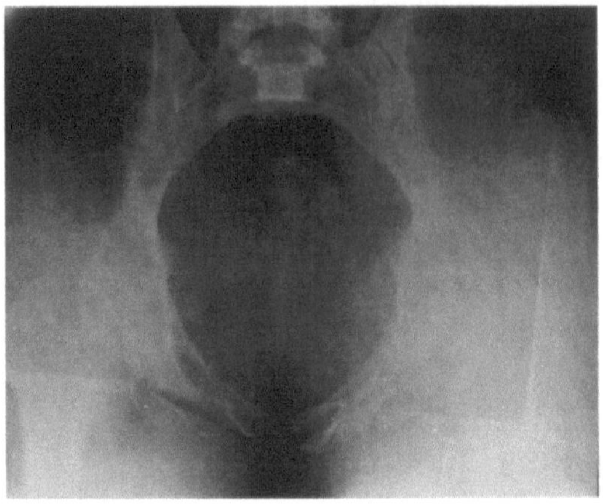
B

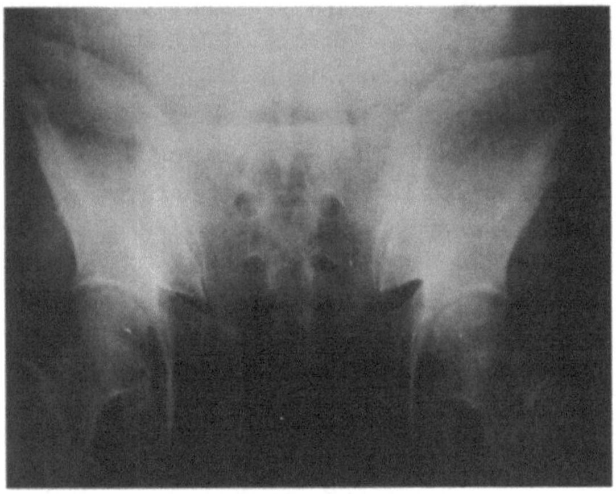
C

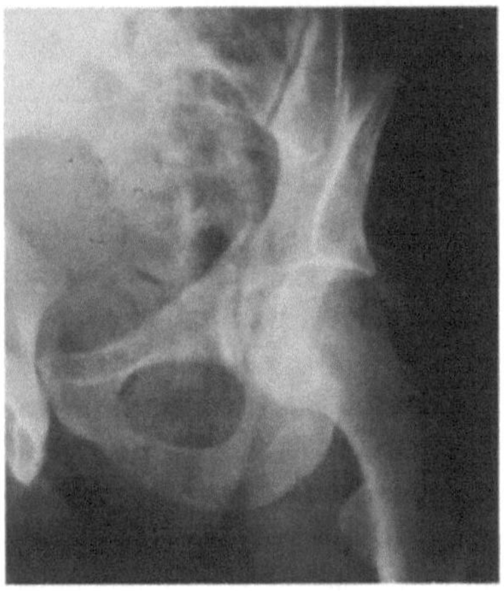
D

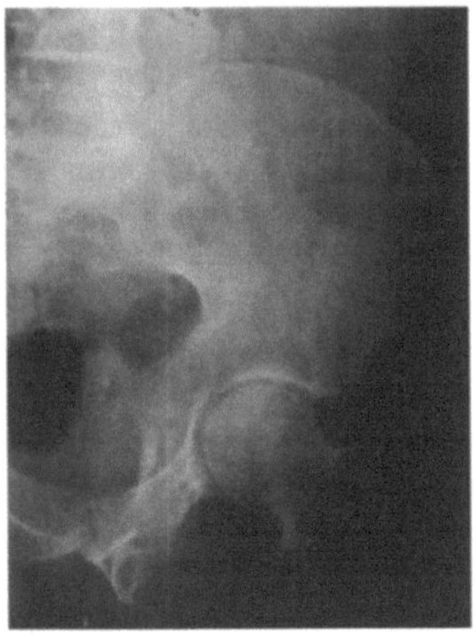
E

FIG. 5–2 Five radiographic views of the pelvis. **A** Anteroposterior view. **B** Pelvic inlet view. **C** Pelvic outlet view. **D** Obturator oblique view. **E** Iliac oblique view.

the acetabular dome region. A scan taken 1.5 cm more caudal to the last transects the mid-acetabular region to reveal the triangular cross-sections of the anterior and posterior columns and the femoral head with its central depression at the level of the ligamentum teres. The most inferior section reveals the inferior pubic ramus and the ischial tuberosity as well as the femur at the level of the greater trochanter. Further elaboration of the radiological views and the CT scans is provided under the classification of specific acetabular fracture patterns.

Previously a variety of classification schemes were devised in an attempt to provide accurate prognostication referable to the type of fracture, the degree of damage of the weight-bearing surface, the amount of displacement, and the presence of complicating factors such as a concomitant pelvic ring disruption. Although such classification schemes, including those by Cauchoix and Truchet,[3] Pennal et al.,[19] and Tile,[24] may have facilitated prognostication following the application of skeletal traction, they were not sufficiently detailed to permit a detailed scrutiny of the injury to define the optimal surgical approach and the site(s) for application of internal fixation. About 20 years ago LeTournel initiated a radiological and anatomical study of the pelvis in which lead strips were applied to a disarticulated pelvic model. Multiple radiological views were prepared and studied. Specific regions of the pelvis were identified and correlated with fracture lines that appeared in a wide variety of acetabular and pelvic ring disruptions. Anatomical preparations were then undertaken by LeTournel to elucidate the optimal surgical exposures for the foremost fracture patterns.

From this classic investigation a classification system of acetabular fractures was developed which segregates the disruptions according to the anatomical site(s) of involvement. This system, currently employed by the authors, provides a rational basis for planning the surgical exposure, the technique of reduction and fixation, and, not least, the degree of difficulty which can be anticipated at the time of surgery.

Judet and co-workers[7] recognize five simple patterns of acetabular disruption: fractures of the posterior wall or "lip"; fractures of the posterior column; fractures of the anterior wall; fractures of the anterior column; and transverse fractures. These authors also identified several complex acetabular disruptions, including at least two of the elementary forms. Examples include a fracture of the posterior column and posterior wall, a transverse and posterior column fracture, a fracture of the anterior column or anterior wall associated with a hemitransverse posterior fracture, a both-column fracture, a T-shaped fracture, and an associated acetabular and pelvic ring fracture. An example of the last group would be an acetabular fracture accompanied by a sacroiliac disruption and a diastasis of the symphysis pubis. The dome portion of the acetabulum is recognized as a principal superior, weight-bearing area. In the several fracture patterns where the dome region is violated, the roof may constitute an anterior or posterior column fragment or a separate piece. In any event, the preoperative planning necessitates adequate exposure of the dome to permit accurate reduction and stabilization.

Simple Fracture Patterns

Posterior Wall Fracture

A posterior wall fracture (Fig. 5–4) creates a "lip" fragment which arises from the posterior articular surface, often as part of a posterior dislocation of the hip joint. Fractures of the posterior wall constitute approximately 30% of all acetabular fractures. The major weight-bearing portion of the posterior column is undisturbed. Usually the displaced wall fragment remains vascularized by its residual attachment to the capsule of the hip joint. The stability of such a hip joint is related to the size of the wall fragment(s) and to its site of origin as a posterior fragment, a posterosuperior fragment, or a posteroinferior fragment. The presence of the posterosuperior fragment is indicative of the least stable hip and the posteroinferior fragment of the most stable hip. In the typical fracture pattern on the anteroposterior radiograph, the femoral head is dislocated posteriorly and a displaced wall fragment is displaced cephalad of it. All of the other acetabular landmarks are intact. The obturator oblique view provides the optimal estimate of the size of the displaced wall fragment and the position of the femoral head. The iliac oblique view confirms the integrity of the posterior border of the innominate bone, the anterior border of the acetabulum, and the iliac wing.

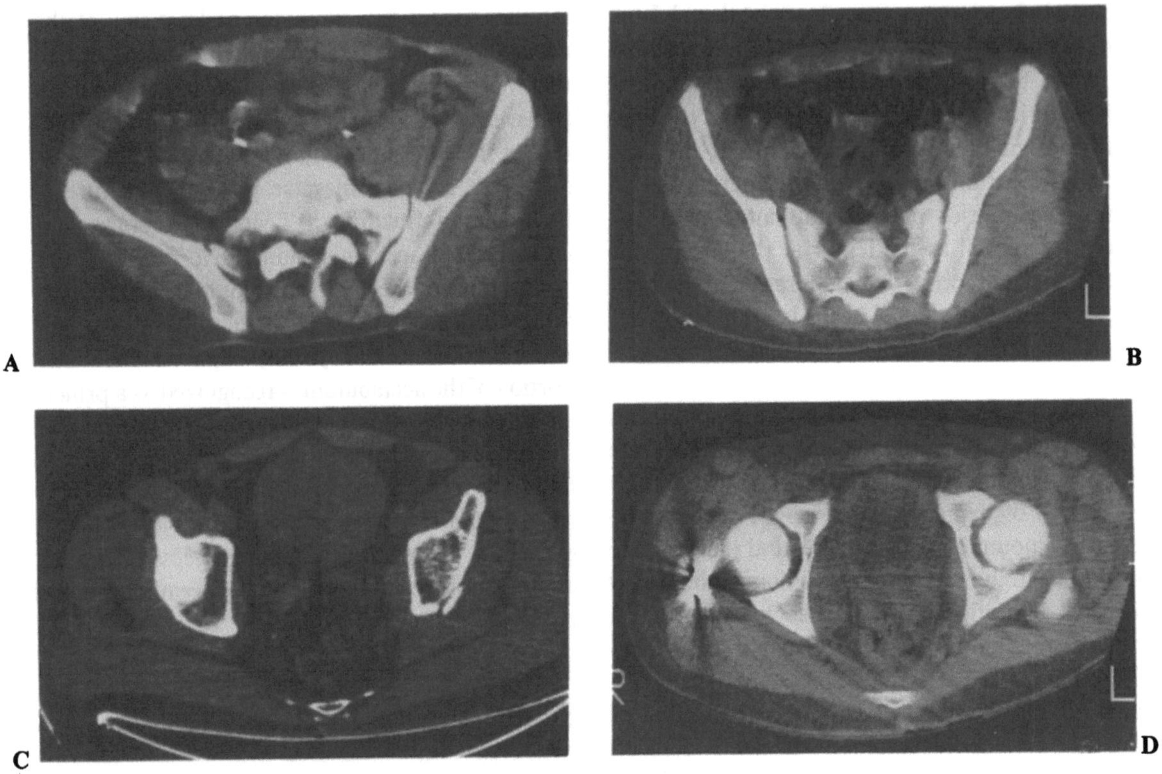

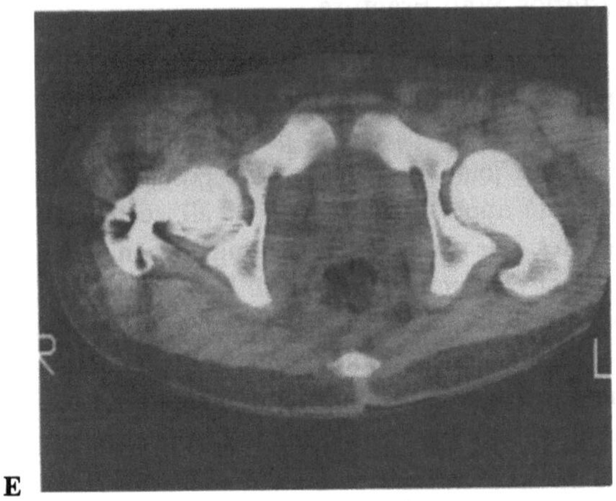

FIG. 5–3 Computed tomography provides five coronal sections of the pelvis and acetabulum. **A** Iliac wings and sacroiliac joints. **B** Sacroiliac joints and sacrum. **C** Acetabular roof or dome. **D** Medial acetabular wall and hip joint. **E** Rami and symphysis.

Posterior Column Fracture

Posterior column fractures (Fig. 5–5) constitute approximately 5% of all acetabular fractures. Most fractures of the posterior column are simple disruptions in which the entire posterior column migrates inward and posteriorly and the adjacent thickened portion of the acetabular roof remains intact. Usually the femoral head follows and remains congruent with the posterior column fragment so that all or almost all of the posterior capsule remains intact. Radiologically, in the anteroposterior view the femoral head is displaced inward and encroaches on the outline of the pelvic inlet. The ilioischial line is superimposed on the displaced fracture fragment. The acetabulum and the teardrop maintain their normal positions. The obturator oblique view confirms the integrity of

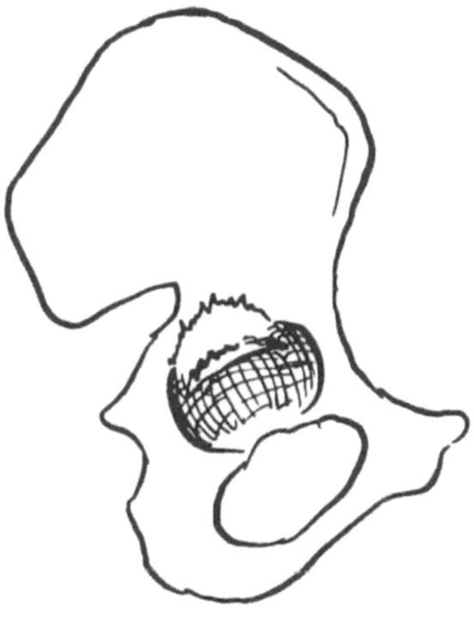

FIG. 5–4 Posterior wall fracture with a lip fragment.

the iliopectineal line (innominate line and the anterior column). The iliac oblique view confirms the preservation of the column and the acetabular roof.

Anterior Wall Fracture

Fractures of the anterior wall (Fig. 5–6) constitute approximately 2% of all acetabular fractures. This injury, first defined by LeTournel in 1968, is analogous to a posterior wall fracture. An anterior wall fracture results in displacement of a portion of the anterior articular surface along with a large part of the middle third of the anterior column (i.e., a portion of the iliopectineal line). In the anteroposterior radiographic view, the medial displacement of an isolated segment of the iliopectineal line along with the anteriorly dislocated femoral head is evident. Usually the teardrop is displaced medially and maintains its normal relation with the displaced anterior column segment. The unbroken ilioischial line and the preservation of the posterior border of the acetabulum confirm the integrity of the posterior column. The crucial obturator oblique view clearly reveals the displaced anterior wall fragment. The iliac oblique view confirms the integrity of the posterior border of the posterior column.

Anterior Column Fracture

An uncommon acetabular injury, the anterior column fracture (Fig. 5–7) has a fracture line which extends from the iliopubic ramus inferiorly to any cephalad point as far posterior as the mid-portion of the iliac crest. Frequently the femoral head is dislocated anteriorly to approximate the position of the displaced anterior column fragment. The most significant radiological feature shared with an anterior wall fracture is the integrity of the posterior column documented in the anteroposterior and iliac oblique views. The obturator oblique view confirms the displacement of the anterior column and the disruption of the iliopectineal line. An anterior column fracture is characterized by

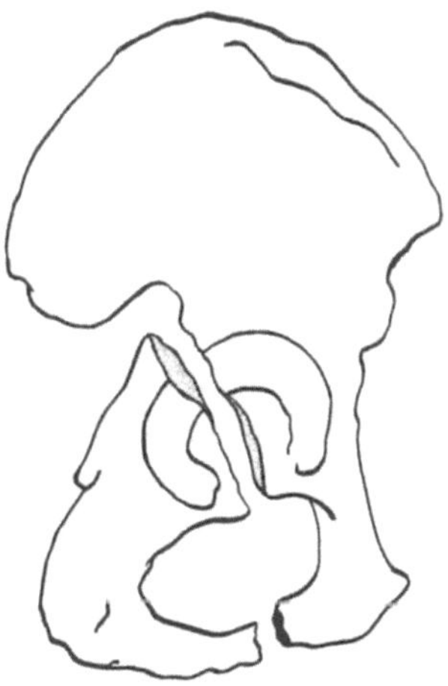

FIG. 5–5 Posterior column fracture.

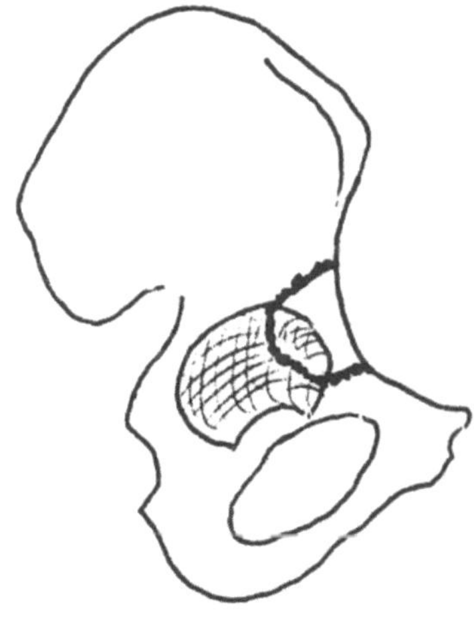

FIG. 5–6 Anterior wall fracture.

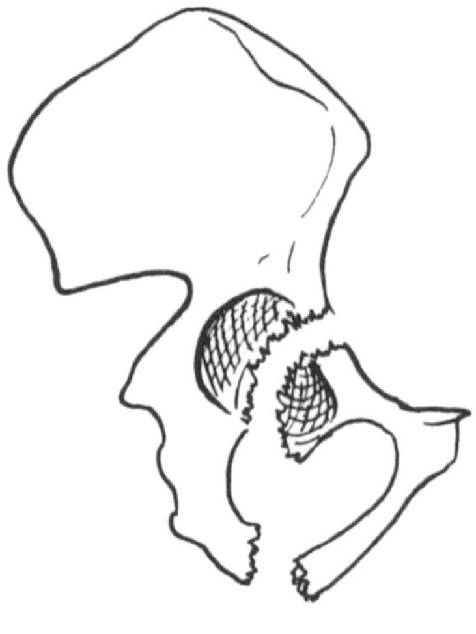

FIG. 5–7 Anterior column fracture.

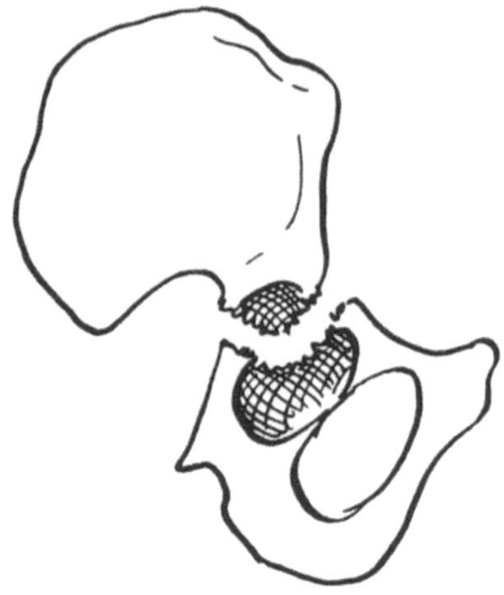

FIG. 5–8 Transverse fracture.

the site in the superior portion of the ilium where the fracture exits from the bone. In the extreme case, the fracture line extends superiorly to the mid-portion of the iliac crest.

Transverse Fracture

Transverse fractures (Fig. 5–8) represent approximately 9% of all acetabular disruptions. They divide the innominate bone into superior and inferior segments consisting of the ilium and the ischium and pubis, respectively. The upper and lower segments of the divided columns remain intact with respect to one another. The acetabulum can be disrupted at all levels including the junction of the roof and the cotyloid fossa, juxtatectal portion of the roof, transtectal portion of the roof, and rarely through the cotyloid fossa violating the horns of the infratectal portion of the acetabulum. The fracture line progresses in one plane, although the obliquity of that plane is highly variable. Frequently central displacement of the femoral head is documented along with medial displacement of the ischiopubic acetabular fragment. An anteroposterior radiographic view confirms most of the salient features of the injury. The fracture line disrupts all of the vertically oriented pelvic structures (e.g., the innominate and ilioischial lines, the anterior and posterior columns, and the borders of the acetabulum). In all of the transverse fracture patterns an undamaged segment of the acetabular roof remains intact with the iliac wing fragment. The obturator oblique view clearly shows the orientation of the fracture line and the integrity of the obturator foramen. The iliac oblique view shows the posterior portion of the fracture line including the site where it exits from the acetabulum.

Complex Fracture Patterns

Each of the complex fracture patterns identified in the classification scheme represents a combination of at least two of the elementary forms previously described.

Posterior Column and Posterior Wall Fracture

The combination of a posterior column and posterior wall fracture (Fig. 5–9) occurs in 3% of acetabular fractures and must be differentiated from the pure posterior column fracture. When the posterior column and posterior wall lesions are associated, usually the posterior wall fragment is large and possesses an extensive articular cartilaginous surface which requires accurate reduction and rigorous stabilization to restore adequate stability and a congruent acetabular surface. Whereas the posterior column fracture usually shows minor

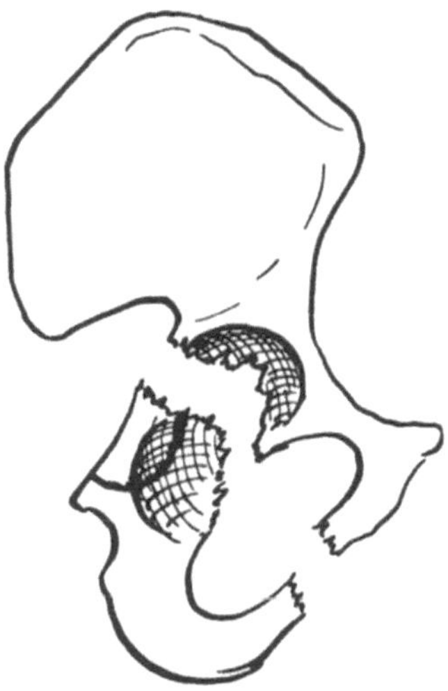

FIG. 5–9 Posterior wall with a posterior column fracture.

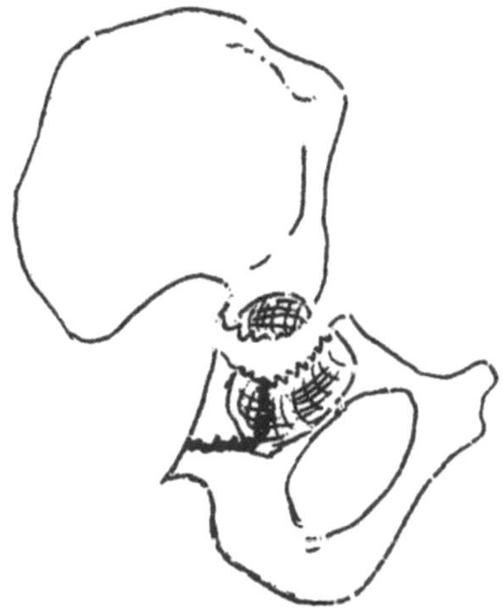

FIG. 5–10 Transverse fracture with a posterior wall fracture.

rotational displacement, the crucial posterior wall fragment generally is completely displaced and markedly rotated, often by 180°. The injury represents one pattern of a posterior fracture dislocation of the hip. The posterior wall fracture is visible on the anteroposterior and especially the iliac oblique views. The landmarks of the anterior column are intact on the obturator oblique view.

Transverse and Posterior Wall Fracture

The association of a transverse fracture with a fracture of the posterior wall (Fig. 5–10) occurs frequently, in approximately 20% of acetabular fractures. Here the combination of a transverse and a posterior wall fracture can be produced by either central dislocation or posterior dislocation of the femoral head. When a posterior dislocation occurs, the transverse fracture represents a propagation of the posterior wall disruption. In this instance the crucial posterior wall fracture dictates the instability of the femoral head. In the presence of a central dislocation the displaced transverse fracture component provides the principal source of instability of the femoral head, and the posterior wall fracture is an accessory lesion. With the posterior type of fracture dislocation, in the anteroposterior radiographic view the femoral head projects behind the roof of the acetabulum. One or more posterior wall fragments may be evident. The iliac oblique and anteroposterior views show disruption of the vertical landmarks of the acetabulum consistent with a transverse fracture. In the obturator view, however, the obturator ring is intact. In the presence of a central fracture/dislocation in the anteroposterior radiographic view, the medial displacement of the femoral head and its loss of congruity with the residual portion of the acetabular roof is evident. The more subtle posterior wall fracture is best seen in the iliac oblique view.

Associated Anterior and Posterior Hemitransverse Fracture

The association of an anterior and a posterior hemitransverse fracture (Fig. 5–11) comprises an anterior wall or column fracture together with a posterior column fracture. This injury constitutes about 5% of all acetabular fractures. The posterior column fracture is comparable to the posterior half of a transverse fracture. Usually relatively minor posterior displacement is seen. The name hemitransverse is derived from the presence of one-half of a transverse fracture component. The anterior displacement of the femoral head which accompanies this fracture pattern is similar to that documented in the pure anterior wall or column

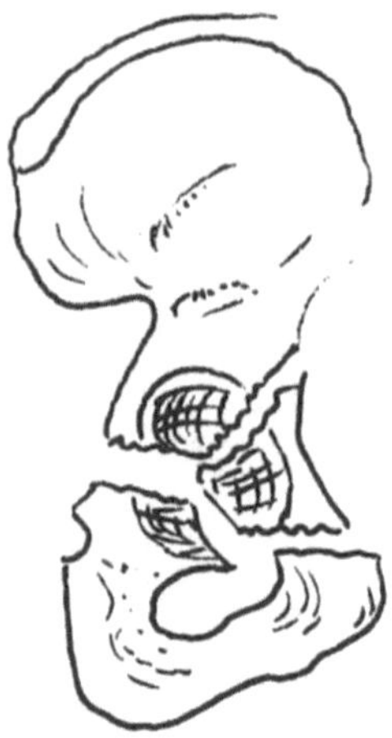

FIG. 5–11 Associated anterior wall and posterior hemitransverse fracture.

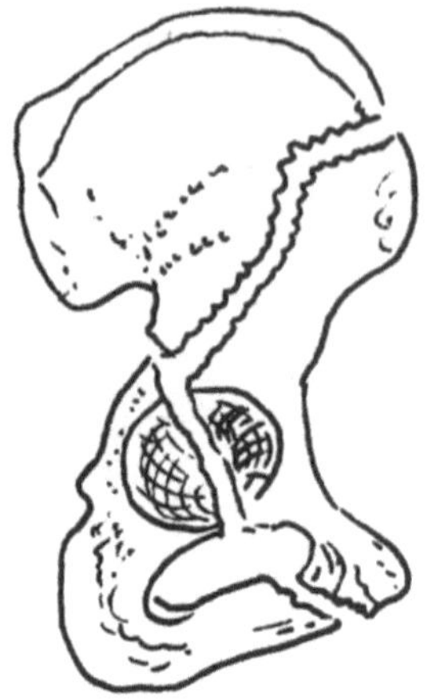

FIG. 5–12 Both-column fracture.

fracture. The anterior wall and column fractures along with the typical anteriorly displaced femoral head are most easily recognized by scrutiny of the anteroposterior and obturator oblique views. Subtle radiographic features differentiate this injury from a T-type fracture or a both-column fracture. In a T-type fracture the anterior column is displaced at a variable level but the plane of the upper fracture is identical to that of the pure transverse fracture. In the both-column fracture no sector of the acetabular roof remains in place.

Both-Column Fracture

An associated both-column fracture (Fig. 5–12) refers to an acetabular disruption in which the anterior and posterior columns sustain discrete injuries. Historically, the term "central acetabular fracture" was employed to characterize this fracture. More recently this term has been loosely applied to any pattern of acetabular disruption in which the femoral head is centrally displaced. These comminuted fractures comprise the most complex acetabular injuries and account for about 20% of the acetabular disruptions. The anterior and posterior columns, along with their respective adjacent segments of articular surface, are separated from one another. Only a small piece of the iliac wing remains attached to the sacrum at the ipsilateral sacroiliac joint. These fragments are often highly comminuted; the presence of numerous osseous fragments which do not possess any articular surface is a characteristic of this injury.

The posterior part of the fracture complex including its displacement is similar to a simple posterior column fracture. The principal posterior column fragment is detached superiorly by a fracture which begins at a variable level on the posterior border on the pelvic bone in the area of the greater sciatic notch and extends inferiorly. Occasionally, secondary fracture lines in the posterior column are seen. The anterior column is often separated by a fracture which begins confluent with the fracture of the posterior column and extends across the iliac wing to the iliac crest or the anterior border of the iliac bone. Anterior comminution of these fractures can be anticipated. The articular surface is disrupted into several large, irregular osteochondral fragments. Central dislocation of the femoral head is a constant feature. Unlike a T-type fracture, no iliac portion of the acetabular roof remains undisplaced. The discrete iliac fracture fragment often rotates markedly and may be displaced secondarily at the sacroiliac or at an adjacent fracture of the posterior ilium or the sacrum. In the crucial systematic review of the pelvic radiographs, the central displacement of the femoral head often with an accompanying portion of the acetabular roof is evident in the anteroposterior view. A large medially displaced ilioischial fragment and an iliac fracture line which violates the iliac wing to reach the anterior margin or the iliac crest are identified. In the obturator oblique view the separate anterior column is clearly seen, as is secondary comminution and an anterior wall fracture. Superior to the centrally displaced acetabular roof a characteristic spur of bone indicative of both a column fracture and the pattern of the iliac disruption can be seen. The iliac oblique view demonstrates a fracture of the posterior column as well as the iliac fracture line. The anterior iliac fracture fragment with a portion of the articular roof is tilted so that it remains congruent with the femoral head. The presence of the central dislocation of the femoral head, the iliac wing fracture, and the spur sign permit radiological distinction of a both column fracture from a T-type fracture, an anterior column and posterior hemitransverse fracture, and an associated transverse fracture with comminution of the iliac wing. Unlike a both-column fracture in all of these latter examples, an articular segment of acetabulum remains attached to the iliac wing.

T-Shaped Fracture

The T-shaped fracture (Fig. 5–13) is documented in approximately 6% of acetabular fractures and often presents a radiographic problem in diagnosis. The fracture has a transverse component with a vertical component combined with displacement of the femoral head. The transverse component may occur at the various levels previously described for a simple transverse fracture. The vertical component may exit anteriorly, directly inferiorly, or posteriorly depending on the vector of the provocative force.

The radiologic characterization of this injury is comparable to the recognition of a transverse fracture. In the anteroposterior and the obturator and iliac oblique views, all of the vertically aligned landmarks are violated by the displaced transverse limb of the fracture. Although difficult to recognize, the vertical limb of the T-type fracture is best seen on the obturator oblique view, although it may be evident in the AP view. The iliac oblique view clearly shows the posterior part of the transverse fracture limb. Usually the iliac wing is uninvolved, although a stable disruption of the ipsilateral sacroiliac joint is not uncommon.

Complex Pelvic Injury

Acetabular and Pelvic Ring Fracture

A separate category is an acetabular fracture complicated by other disruptions of the pelvic ring which the authors identify as a complex pelvic injury (Fig. 5–14). The concomitant fractures in the pelvic ring can occur on either side of the ring and at one or several sites including the contralateral acetabulum. Other authors[25] have classified pelvic ring fractures according to the direction of the provocative force, the degree of posterior pelvic instability, and the sites of disruption. The direction of the provocative force may be anteroposterior, lateral, or vertical. Virtually all of the acetabular fractures with supplementary pelvic

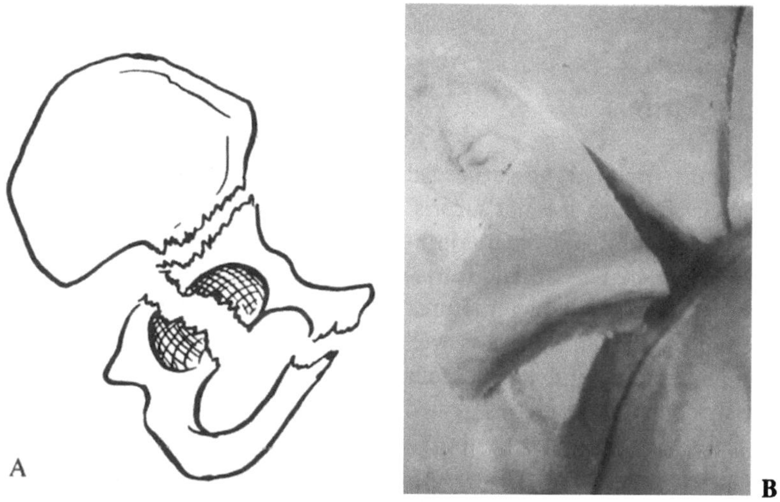

FIG. 5–13 **A** T-shaped fracture. **B** Intraoperative close-up photograph reveals a displaced dome fragment complicating a T-fracture. The femoral head is in the lower right corner.

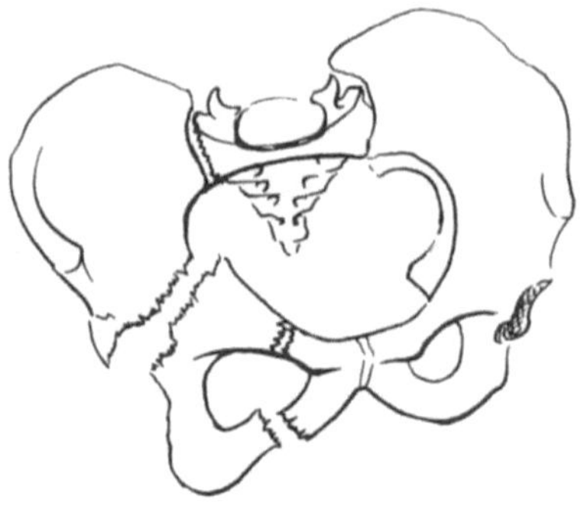

FIG. 5–14 Complex pelvic injury with a transverse acetabular fracture, ipsilateral rami fractures, and sacroiliac disruptions.

disruption are variants of lateral compression injuries. Previously, about 10% of all acetabular fractures were characterized as a complex disruption. With the more recent availability of routine computed tomography, probably a more accurate figure is 20 to 25%. The larger incidence is related to stable and minimally displaced ipsilateral or contralateral sacroiliac disruptions and sacral fractures difficult to recognize in conventional radiographs but readily distinguishable on a CT scan. In addition to the conventional radiographic studies for recognition of the acetabular fracture, the inlet and outlet views are crucial for discerning posterior or superior displacement of the pelvic ring disruption. *Routine computed tomography of the pelvic ring is strongly recommended to characterize posterior pelvic ring violations as to their site(s) and degree of instability.*

Systemic Manifestations

With the violence of the traumatic force needed to provoke an acetabular fracture, it is not surprising that accompanying fractures and visceral injuries are frequently encountered. Associated injuries to the ipsilateral extremity, including fracture/dislocations of the foot, ankle, and knee, as well as tibial and femoral fractures and ligamentous injuries to the knee are common. In a series treated at Presbyterian University Hospital, approximately 40% of the patients presented with associated skeletal injuries to the ipsilateral extremity and 50% presented with some associated skeletal injury to the face, extremities, chest, or spinal column.

Associated visceral injuries occurred in approximately 10% of patients. Examples of these included cerebral concussion and contussion, hemopneumothorax, and rupture of an abdominal viscus or the urinary bladder. Vascular injuries occurred in 1% of the patients. This included one patient with a laceration of the superior gluteal vessel which was entrapped in the upper part of the posterior column fracture. In a second patient with an associated pelvic ring fracture there was a rupture of the internal iliac artery at the site of takeoff of the obturator artery. In general, vigorous preoperative resuscitation has not been necessary with the isolated acetabular fractures. Patients have been treated by a standard multiple trauma protocol which is provided elsewhere.[14]

Although an acetabular fracture is generally accompanied by an intraperitoneal hematoma of variable size, surgical exploration of the abdomen to evacuate the hematoma is rarely necessary. The newest 3-D modelling techniques will become a great advancement in detecting hematomas, their location and their size. Approximately 10% of the patients with acetabular fractures have demonstrated physical findings consistent with a *sciatic nerve injury.* Many of the sciatic palsies are relatively minor and are recognized only by a careful initial clinical examination. Whereas the severity of the sciatic damage is highly variable, the highest incidence and greatest severity of nerve palsies is documented in patients who present with posterior wall and column fractures provoked by a posterior dislocation of the femoral head. In contrast, medial displacement of the femoral head that accompanies a transverse, or T-type, fracture is unlikely to be associated with a sciatic nerve palsy. Accompanying lacerations and complete transection of the sciatic nerve appear to be remarkably uncommon. During several operative interventions we have observed displacement of the sciatic nerve into the fracture line of the posterior column without any apparent nerve damage. Impalement by osseous fragments or hemorrhage of the nerve appear to be the principal sources of neurological injury. In the series of patients reported by LeTournel,[11] approximately 75% of the patients who underwent early posttraumatic exploration of the sciatic nerve for a palsy recovered near-normal or normal nerve function.

Management of the Patient

Because a high percentage of the patients who present with fractures of the acetabulum are multiple trauma victims, it should be self-evident that a rigorous diagnostic protocol and the immediate availability of resuscitative measures are essential. The principal features of the initial resuscitation are outlined in Fig. 5–15. At the site of the accident, restoration of a suitable airway and administration of intravenous fluids are undertaken. Severe hypovolemia is optimally managed by the application of a MAST suit (military antishock trousers) which requires careful deflation in the emergency room or operating room; otherwise precipitous return of hypotension may ensue upon removal of the pneumatic garment. In the emergency room arrangements are made for appropriate blood replacement, and the diagnostic protocol is initiated. Space precludes a full discussion of the protocol, so only the salient features are reviewed here.

After control of the airway and of bleeding is achieved, a systematic approach to the central nervous system, digestive tract, and excretory system function is undertaken. Once the patient has been stabilized other skeletal injuries are evaluated. Concomitant limb injuries as well as injuires to the sciatic nerve are relatively common and influence the timing and extent of the initial intervention. Thus a complete physical examination with attention to skeletal injuries and neurological and vascular competency of the extremities is of great importance. After the physical examination and stabilization of the patient, appropriate radiographs are obtained including an anteroposterior pelvic view, 45° pelvic inlet and outlet views, and

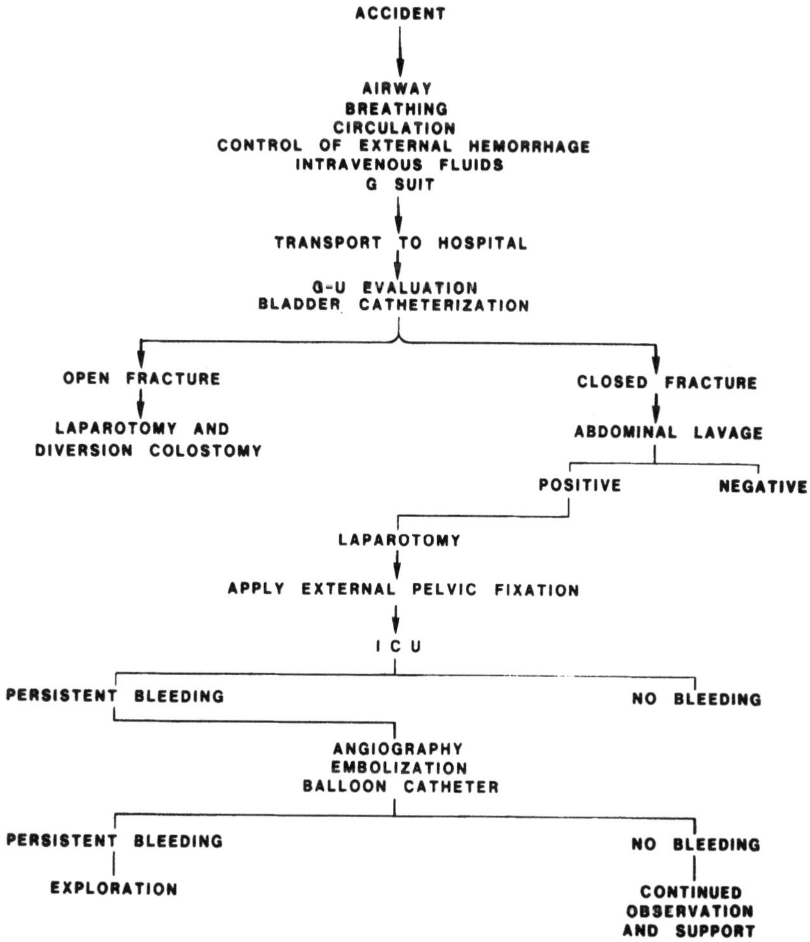

FIG. 5–15 Control of hemorrhage in a patient with a pelvic fracture. The principal features of initial resuscitation are illustrated.

45° obturator oblique and iliac oblique views of both hips. Computed tomography of the pelvis follows frequently as an extension of a scan necessitated by the presence of a closed head injury or of intra-abdominal trauma. Once a multiple trauma victim requires a scan of one organ, little supplementary time is expended by an ancillary examination of the pelvis. Serial cuts are taken through the sacroiliac joints, sacrum, acetabular roof, hip joints, and rami. Once the complete radiographic protocol is completed, careful scrutiny of the entire sequence is undertaken so that the plan for management of the acetabular fracture can be prepared.

In the presence of a dislocated femoral head, apart from a central fracture dislocation, immediate reduction of the femoral head using a closed or open method is crucial so that the risk of avascular necrosis of the femoral head is minimized. The relative merits of closed versus open reduction remain somewhat controversial and are reviewed shortly. When skeletal traction is employed during the early therapeutic period, a traction pin is inserted into the distal femur or proximal tibia. The optimal timing for an open reduction, however, remains a controversial issue. An initial period of skeletal traction lasting 24 to 48 hours provides an opportunity to ensure the hemodynamic and respiratory stability of the patient and to carefully plan the operative approach. In certain instances skeletal traction provides a satisfactory reduction so that an open reduction is unnecessary. After 48 hours of skeletal traction has been employed, a more prolonged period of traction is unlikely to lead to further improvement in the reduction unless the vector of the traction is altered. After 24 hours of longitudinal traction, in the presence of persistent medial displacement of the femoral head, a supplementary greater trochanteric traction pin can be applied in an attempt to correct this deformity. In our experience this supplementary measure affords a poor likelihood of an adequate reduction. If the greater trochanteric pin is used for more than a few days, a high risk for a pin track infection arises, which might compromise the possibility of undertaking an open reduction.

For the past 4 years, in the presence of a displaced acetabular fracture we have attempted to undertake early operative intervention, generally on the day of presentation of the patient. Early surgical intervention has the advantage of simplified exposure of the fracture fragments. The hematoma is readily removed to expose clean fracture surfaces. Granulation tissue which rapidly invades the pelvic hematoma obliterates the fracture surfaces and enhances the difficulties associated with anatomical reduction. With the improvements in reduction techniques, the previous advantages of preoperative skeletal traction are minimized. With the improvements in surgical exposure of the pelvis and acetabulum, the previous risks of excessive blood loss in the trauma victim have been greatly lessened. The average duration of the surgical procedure has been substantially shortened.

When surgery is deferred more than a day after the accident, the patient with an acetabular fracture and especially the multitrauma victim has a considerable chance of developing a pulmonary or urinary tract infection, thromboembolic problems, decubiti, or other complications of enforced recumbency. These complications greatly enhance the mortality and morbidity of the initial traumatic insult. Once a complication has occurred, reconstructive surgical procedures may have to be deferred for a week or more, by which time acetabular reconstruction becomes much more difficult. With such a delay in surgery the anticipated incidence of postoperative ectopic bone formation greatly increases. Provided that appropriate resources for acetabular reconstruction are available, early surgical intervention therefore appears to be the optimal goal. When the femoral head is dislocated in an anterior, posterior, or superior direction, emergency reduction of the femoral head is indicated, preferably with primary repair of the acetabulum.

Indications for Surgical Intervention

Whatever the indication for an open reduction of an acetabular fracture, the essential goals of surgical management are accurate restoration of the articular surface combined with solid fixation so that the benefits of early postoperative mobilization can be realized. Until recently, with the limitations of available operative approaches, techniques of reduction, and internal fixation of acetabular disruptions, widespread resort to surgical methods could not be recommended. With the striking improvements that have been documented in both the diagnostic and therapeutic aspects of operative management, a major change in the role of surgery has occurred. Admittedly, some experience with the improvements is required before routinely successful results can be anticipated. Nevertheless, with the available surgical armamentarium and the potential for referral of acetabular fracture victims to appropriate surgical centers by rapid air transportation, most patients who present with an acetabular disruption should have access to the optimal type of therapeutic protocol for virtually any type of fracture.

The specific indications for surgical intervention of an acetabular fracture remain controversial. Nevertheless, the authors recommend the following considerations.

1. Where there is evidence of a loose interposed osteochondral fragment on the conventional radiographs or the CT scans, arthrotomy with removal of the loose fragments is necessary. In most instances, simultaneously, an open reduction and internal fixation are undertaken.

2. When the acetabular fracture is accompanied by an anterior, posterior, or superior dislocation of the femoral head, an accurate closed or, if necessary, open reduction of the femoral head is indicated. It would be best if both the reduction of the femoral head and reconstruction of the acetabular fractures were done at the same time. Careful planning is very important to accomplish such a demanding task.

3. When a simple displaced acetabular fracture is not accurately reduced after 24 to 48 hours of skeletal traction, operative intervention is indicated. A more prolonged period of traction is unlikely to provide further improvement in the reduction. Both longitudinal traction with a distal femoral or proximal tibia skeletal pin and lateral traction with a supplementary greater trochanteric pin are applicable. The greater trochanteric pin should not be employed for more than a few days. With the inevitable marked osteoporosis of the cancellous intertrochanteric region, a more prolonged period of use favors loosening of the pin and a possible pin track infection.

The precise amount of displacement that is deemed unacceptable remains unclear. The amount depends on its location within the acetabulum and the degree of acetabular incongruity with respect to the femoral head. A step-off in the crucial weight-bearing acetabular roof has the poorest prognosis, whereas a comparable magnitude of displacement through the inferior aspect of the medial wall is less likely to culminate in symptomatic traumatic arthritis. Substantial loss of acetabular congruity and malrotation of a large dome fragment is associated with a poor prognosis.

4. Most displaced comminuted acetabular fractures such as an anterior and posterior column injury or a T-fracture merit early consideration for open reduction and internal fixation. When skeletal traction is applied to such an injury for definitive management, accurate restoration of the acetabular anatomy is rarely achieved. Skeletal traction employs "ligamentotaxis" whereby the force of distraction is transmitted from the femoral head via an adequately intact capsule to the displaced acetabular fragments. In the presence of free displaced acetabular fragments or marked comminution or extensive capsular disruption, skeletal traction is unlikely to be effective.

5. Certain patients with multiple traumatic insults merit an open reduction and internal fixation of their acetabular disruption. In the presence of an unstable pelvic ring fracture, operative stabilization of both the acetabulum and the pelvic ring is essential to avoid problems of malunion or nonunion which are almost inevitable. In the presence of a displaced acetabular fracture and a displaced ipsilateral sacroiliac disruption or iliac fracture, skeletal traction is compromised by the absence of a stable base for the acetabulum. Because the force of distraction tends to further displace the pelvic ring disruption, operative intervention is indicated. In the presence of multiple appendicular fractures as well as an acetabular fracture, generally an open reduction and internal fixation of all the osseous insults is needed to avoid the complications of prolonged recumbancy which are very likely to ensue.

6. A relative indication for an open reduction and internal fixation is a displaced acetabular fracture where skeletal traction provides an accurate closed reduction. With operative immobilization, early discharge from the hospital with a touch-down gait becomes possible. The role of surgery in this situation depends on the skill of the surgical team and the statistical likelihood for the stabilization of the accurate open reduction with stable internal fixation.

Contraindications to Operative Intervention

Certain absolute or relative contraindications to open acetabular reduction and stabilization do exist.

1. Marked senile or other pathological origin of osteoporosis is the foremost contraindication.

When severe, osteoporosis precludes effective fixation of the bone. In sedentary individuals over age 50, careful radiographic scrutiny for evidence of osteoporosis is strongly recommended prior to operative intervention.

2. The presence of open and contaminated wounds adjacent to the hip contraindicates acetabular reconstruction, at least until the wound has been adequately débrided and the cutaneous envelope has been restored.

3. Marked comminution of displaced acetabular fragments is a relative contraindication. Prior to the onset of surgery, the surgical team must evaluate whether they possess the experience and resources to realistically achieve an accurate open reduction and stable fixation. If such a goal is clearly unrealistic, consideration for referral to a suitable trauma center or a closed method of treatment is preferred. Perhaps 50% of displaced acetabular fractures are comminuted so that the results of closed methods predictably are disappointing. The realistic hope for a good result of treatment is if the patient undergoes an open reduction and internal fixation by an experienced surgical team.

4. When the patient's general condition is unstable hemodynamically or from other points of view, acetabular reconstruction is at least temporarily contraindicated.

Surgical Approach

Once an acetabular fracture has been rigorously characterized as to the region and extent of the acetabular disruption, adequate visualization of the fracture zone is carefully planned. The fracture lines are drawn on a pelvic model to fully clarify the optimal surgical exposure. Previously an uncomminuted fracture involving a discrete posterior or anterior portion of the acetabulum was adequately visualized by resort to the then available incisions. Inadequate visualization, however, was a frequent and formidable problem when a fracture violated anterior and posterior portions of the acetabulum or other adjacent areas of the hemipelvis. In such instances the use of an anterior and a posterior incision was employed, although the technical difficulties were nearly unsurmountable. Once the anterior portion of a fracture had been exposed, reduced, and stabilized, manipulation and fixation of the posterior portion through the second incision was immeasurably complicated by the first stage of the operation. Attempts were made to devise truly extensile exposures that would permit adequate visualization of even the most complex acetabular fractures. During the past decade several incisions have been developed which largely solve the previous problems. One example is the long lateral longitudinal transtrochanteric approach which permits satisfactory visualization of a transverse acetabular disruption. This approach does not permit reconstruction of the anterior column including the superior ramus or the medial wall of the acetabulum. Another example, the Senegas,[23] or modified Ollier, approach has similar assets and comparable liabilities. LeTournel[10] designed an iliofemoral approach which provides excellent exposure of the lateral ilium, acetabulum, and anterior and posterior columns. With its surgical division of the origins and insertions of the gluteus medius and gluteus minimus along the iliac crest and the greater trochanter, respectively, it limits the blood supply of these vital hip abductors to the superior gluteal vessels. Those vessels are sometimes damaged as part of the initial traumatic insult or at the time of surgery; in such a case, unless a satisfactory microvascular reanastomosis is achieved the hip abductors undergo catastrophic ischemic necrosis.

A triradiate incision with osteotomy of the greater trochanter has been developed which permits a relatively rapid and safe extensile exposure of the lateral ilium and acetabulum and the anterior column but with a diminished risk of devascularization of the principal hip abductors. The greater trochanter can be reattached with lag screws to permit early functional restoration of abductor function.

Examples of suitable exposures for virtually all types of acetabular fractures are presented in the following sections.

Anterior Approach

The fractures suitable for an isolated anterior exposure include anterior wall fractures and anterior column fractures. The ilioinguinal approach (Fig. 5–16) described bv LeTournel and Judet[11] offers extensive access to the internal portion of the iliac bone, the anterior rami and symphysis, and the pelvic cavity. The patient is placed in a supine position with the ipsilateral extremity draped

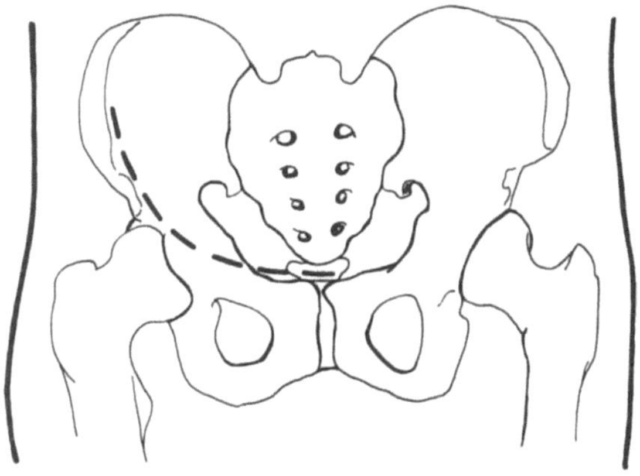

FIG. 5–16 Cutaneous incision for the ilioinguinal approach.

freely. A fracture table can be utilized, although it is unnecessary. The cutaneous curvilinear incision is made along the anterior two-thirds of the iliac crest, which extends across the anterosuperior iliac spine to the midline approximately two fingerbreadths above the public symphysis. The muscles of the abdomen are sharply incised from the iliac crest and are elevated along with the iliacus muscle from the inner aspect of the ilium. The aponeurosis of the external oblique is incised from the anterosuperior iliac spine to the midline, passing 2 cm above the superficial ring of the inguinal canal. The lateral cutaneous nerve of the thigh is identified medial to the anterosuperior spine and carefully protected. The inferior portion of the aponeurosis of the external oblique is elevated and retracted inferiorly to expose the conjoint tendon and the origin of the internal oblique and transversus abdominus muscles. The conjoint tendon is separated from the inguinal ligament at its tendinous zone of origin, which facilitates the repair of the inguinal canal. In the presence of bilateral ramus fractures or bilateral anterior column fractures, the incision is extended as a bilateral ilioinguinal approach to permit visualization of the entire disrupted segment. At this level the adjacent psoas muscle sheath is closely adherent to the inguinal ligament.

To gain access to the extraperitoneal space, the iliopsoas muscle is mobilized through a transverse incision in the iliopsoas sheath. By finger dissection the medial surface of the psoas fascia is separated from the adjacent femoral sheath. The fascia is divided down to the iliopectineal eminence and progressively along the brim of the pelvis. The iliopsoas muscle, the femoral nerve, and the lateral cutaneous nerve of the thigh are isolated in a broad sling or a Penrose drain. A vascular tape is placed around the spermatic cord in a male patient or the corresponding round ligament in a female patient. When necessary the symphysis pubis is visualized by incising the rectus abdominis musculature from its insertion on the pubis.

Finally, the external iliac vessels are isolated with blunt finger dissection. The vessels and their accompanying deep lymphatics are encircled by a third sling or a Penrose drain. An anatomically aberrant retropubic anastomosis between the external vessels and the obturator artery is carefully identified and ligated. In this way the structures passing under the inguinal ligament are isolated so that they can be mobilized transversely to provide access to the entire segment of underlying pelvic bone.

One or two Steinmann pins are driven into the posterior pelvis in the area of the posterior ilium adjacent to the sacroiliac joint and serve as abdominal retractors. Medial retraction of the iliopsoas provides access to the entire internal aspect of the ilium from the sacroiliac joint to the iliopectineal eminence. Outward retraction of the iliopsoas and inward retraction of the external iliac vessels provides access from the iliopectineal eminence to the mid-portion of the superior pubic ramus including the entire quadrilateral surface. Lateral retraction of the external iliac vessels accompanied by medial retraction of the spermatic cord provides visualization of the whole superior pubic ramus. Lateral retraction of the spermatic cord provides visualization of the symphysis. Although a limited portion of the posterior column can be visualized through the greater sciatic notch, an adequate open reduction of a low posterior column or a wall fracture is not possible by resorting to this exposure.

Following this approach a meticulous soft tissue repair is essential. After the insertion of a suction drain into the iliac fossa, the abdominal musculature is reconstructed to the level of the gluteal fascia using sturdy interrupted sutures. For repair of the inguinal canal the posteror wall is reconstituted by reattaching the internal oblique and transversalis fascia to their detached distal portions. Upon repair of the rectus abdominis and conjoint tendon, the transversalis fascia is sutured as far laterally as possible. The spermatic cord or round ligament is placed into the reconstituted canal, and the aponeurosis of the external oblique is resutured. A suction drain is placed into the retropubic space before its closure.

Another suitable exposure for an anterior column fracture is a modified Smith-Petersen approach in which the muscles on the inner wall of the ilium are elevated. LeTournel has further improved this approach and renamed it the iliofemoral approach (Fig. 5–17). Here the inferior extent of the incision from the level of the anterosuperior iliac spine follows the sartorius along its medial border, and the musculature on the external face of the iliac wing is preserved. The anterior abdominal musculature is incised from the iliac crest, and the iliac fossa is exposed by elevating the iliacus muscle. The cutaneous, or external, branch of the lateral femoral cutaneous nerve of the thigh is divided. To provide greater access to the anterior column the iliopsoas tendon can be incised. In this way the iliofemoral approach provides visualization of the iliac crest, the superior portion of the anterior column, and the superior pubic ramus but not the symphysis. Posteriorly, exposure of the ilium to the sacroiliac joint is possible including a limited access to the inner wall of the true pelvis and the quadrilateral surface. During this exposure, the femoral nerve and vessels as well as the preserved branches of the lateral cutaneous nerve of the thigh are carefully protected. Subsequently, a routine anatomical closure is undertaken including, when necessary, a repair of the psoas musculature.

Finally, a similar exposure to the anterior column as in the iliofemoral approach can be obtained using the anterior limb of the Y, or triradiate, approach, which is discussed under Extensile Acetabular Approaches, below. In this Y exposure, however, the lateral femoral cutaneous nerve of the thigh can be retracted. A curvilinear incision is made from the greater trochanter across the anterosuperior spine. The muscular attachments on the anterior iliac crest including the origin of sartorius are incised. The myofascia of the tensor fascia is incised along the line of the cutaneous incision. The anterior border of the tensor fascia lata is incised from the adjacent fascia and reflected posteriorly with the abductors after the trochanter is osteotomized. The direct head and, if necessary, the indirect head of the rectus femoris are incised from the anteroinferior spine, and the adjacent lateral ilium and the muscles are reflected in an anterior direction. The musculature on the inner aspect of the ilium is elevated. When necessary, the interval on the medial aspect of the iliopsoas can be developed to expose the superior pubic ramus. This extension of the incision is undertaken similar to that done during a comparable development of the iliofemoral approach. Likewise the incision does not permit visualization of the symphysis. For the closure, the rectus femoris and sartorius are reattached to the pelvis using large sutures inserted into 2-mm drill holes in the bone. The fascia tensor fascia is carefully repaired.

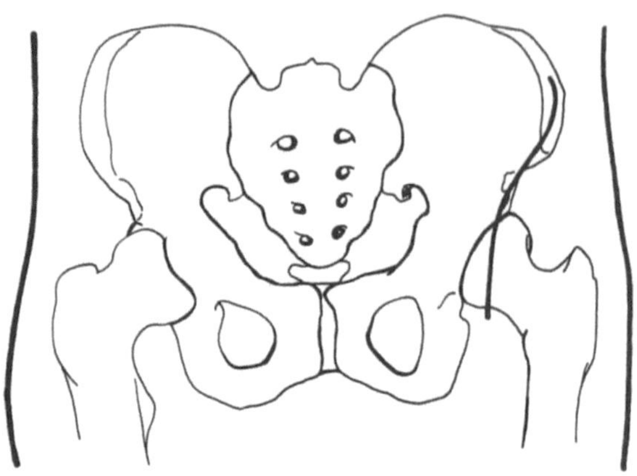

FIG. 5–17 Cutaneous incision for the iliofemoral approach (i.e., modified Smith-Petersen approach).

Posterior Approach

Of the numerous posterior approaches previously utilized to expose fractures of the acetabulum, the combination of a Langenbeck approach and a Kocher approach, described as the Kocher–Langenbeck approach, provides adequate access for a wide variety of fractures of the posterior wall and posterior column (Fig. 5–18). (See Acton, R. K.: Surgical approaches to the hip, in *Surgery of the Hip Joint,* Vol. I, R. G. Touzo (ed.). Philadelphia, Lea & Febinger, 1973, p. 109, Figure 4–29, for a comprehensive review of these exposures and for his extensile lateral approach; page 102, Figures 4.21–4.26.) The operation is performed with the patient lying prone or, preferably, in a posterolateral position. If a fracture table is used in combination with a supracondylar traction pin, the knee is maintained in at least 45° of flexion to avoid excessive distraction on the sciatic nerve. The incision extends from the superior border of the greater trochanter toward the posterosuperior iliac spine. Although it usually terminates within 6 to 8 cm of the posterosuperior spine, it can be ex-

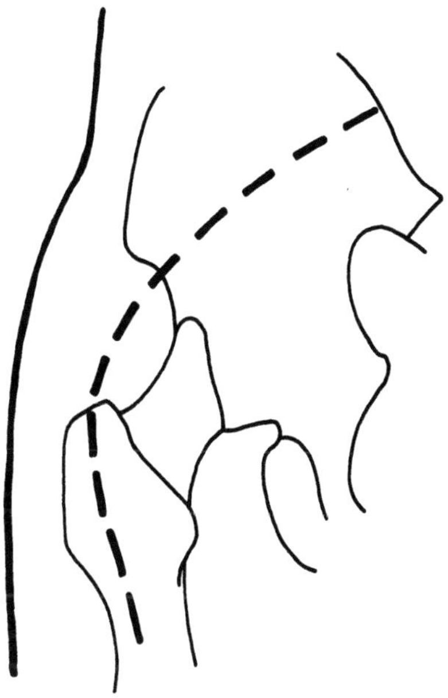

FIG. 5–18 Cutaneous incision for the Kocher–Langenbeck approach.

tended directly to the spine. The incision can be extended distally along the outer surface of the thigh for approximately 6 to 10 cm.

The superficial fascia is divided in line with the cutaneous incision for the entire length of the incision. The gluteus maximus is bluntly split in line with its fibers. The branch of the inferior gluteal nerve to the upper part of the gluteus maximus is carefully protected to avoid paralysis of the corresponding part of the muscle. This hazard increases with more superior and medial extension of the dissection. The sciatic nerve is identified by following the inferior border of the quadratus femoris muscle in a medial direction. When necessary, removal of impaling bone fragments or neurolysis of the sciatic nerve is performed. Occasionally the tendinous insertion of the gluteus maximus on the femur is incised to facilitate exposure of the inferior pubic ramus distal to the ischial tuberosity. The piriformis, obturator internus, and gemellae are incised from the greater trochanter and retracted medially, where they provide protection for the sciatic nerve. The posterior column is visualized to the ischial tuberosity where the origin of the semimembranosus is sharply elevated. Subperiosteal elevation of the gluteus minimus and gluteus medius is undertaken on the posterior and lateral ilium. The muscles can be retracted by insertion of smooth Steinmann pins in the ilium 2.5 and 5.0 cm, respectively, above the roof of the greater sciatic notch. At the level of the greater sciatic notch, the superior gluteal nerve and gluteal vessels are identified and carefully protected.

The exposure provides access to the entire posterior column medial to the greater and lesser sciatic notches, the ischial spine, and, by finger dissection, the inner wall of the pelvis. Incision of the sacrospinous ligament or osteotomy of its adjacent osseous insertion on the ischial spine augments exposure of the inner wall of the pelvis, although it compromises a substantial pelvic ligamentous support. By inferior dissection the ischiopubic ramus can be followed for at least 5 cm beyond the ischial tuberosity. Further lateral extension of the incision can be achieved by osteotomy and elevation of the greater trochanter.

Prior to closure of the incision a drain is inserted into the posterior wound adjacent to the bone. The short external rotators are reattached to their fibrous remnants on the posterior trochanteric crest. Finally, the myofascia and subcutaneous tissues are closed. If the greater trochanter is osteotomized, it is reattached with two 6.5 mm long threaded cancellous lag screws anchored in the calcar femoralis.

Extensile Acetabular Approaches

If there is involvement of both the anterior and posterior columns, a transverse acetabular fracture, or a T-shaped fracture, more extensive visualization of the lateral ilium, rami, and acetabulum generally is required. Previously, various authors have employed separate anterior and posterior approaches to permit complete visualization of the fracture. An example is the use of a Kocher–Langenbeck posterior approach with an iliofemoral or ilioinguinal anterior approach. Whether the two approaches were performed at one operation or sequentially with a few intervening days, this method possesses considerable shortcomings. Frequently the reduction and fixation of one portion of the fracture greatly complicates the later attempt to reduce and stabilize the other part of the fracture. Subsequently, several workers[5,24] (T. Ruedi, personal communication, 1981) developed truly extensile approaches to the acetabulum, most of which are transtrochanteric routes.

Senegas popularized a modified Ollier approach.[23] See *Surgery of the Hip Joint,* Volume I, Chapter 4, page 99, Figures 4–18 and 19. The surgical incision extends from the posterosuperior iliac spine to the mid-portion of the greater trochanter anteriorly around the anterior and medial aspect of the thigh and inferior to the middle of the superior pubic ramus (Fig. 5–19). The posterior incision splits the gluteus maximus muscle, osteotomizes the greater trochanter, and proceeds anteriorly to transect the tensor fascia lata to the level of the femoral sheath. The superior portion of this flap is extended to expose the superior aspect of the acetabulum. Next, the short external rotators are detached from their insertions on the greater trochanter. Sufficient exposure of the posterior column is undertaken to provide complete visualization of the fracture. In addition, detachment of the rectus femoris from the anteroinferior iliac spine and the superior acetabulum is undertaken to expose the origin of the superior ramus. This exposure is hampered by its limited access to the anterior column, which impedes attempts to reduce and stabilize those fractures which violate this region.

A second transtrochanteric lateral approach employs a straight lateral longitudinal incision extending distally from the superior iliac crest across the mid-point of the greater trochanter to a variable level on the lateral aspect of the femur (Fig. 5–20). The tensor fascia and the myofascia of the gluteus maximus are split in line with the incision. The greater trochanter is osteotomized for proximal reflection of the gluteus minimus and gluteus medius. To augment anterior visualization the tensor fascia lata and gluteus minimus are sharply incised from their origins on the iliac crest in line with the incision. Although this extension inevitably violates the nerve supply to the tensor fascia lata, it provides exposure of a fracture of the anterior iliac crest. Posterior exposure is enhanced by splitting the gluteus maximus muscle in line with its fibers and sharply reflecting the short external rotators from the proximal femur. The supplementary posterior exposure is comparable to that described for the Kocher–Langenbeck approach. This exposure also provides inadequate visualization of a complex acetabular fracture that violates both posterior and anterior columns.

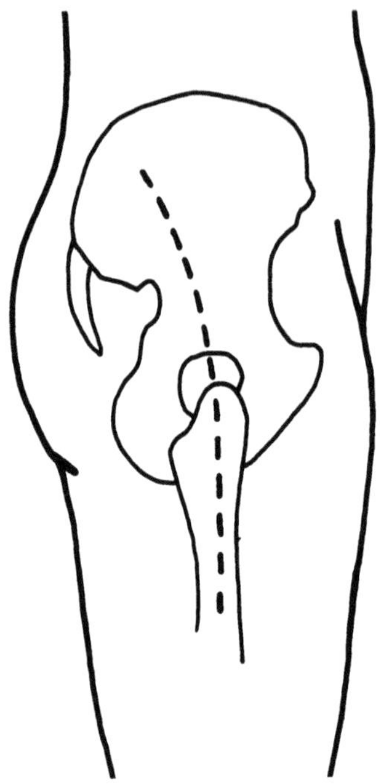

FIG. 5–20 Lateral cutaneous incision for the lateral transtrochanteric approach.

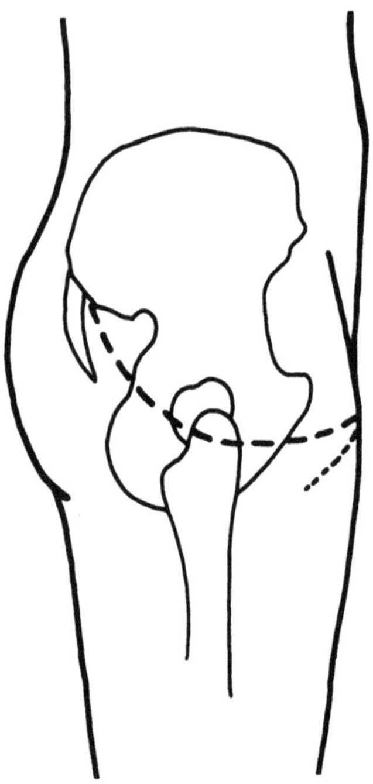

FIG. 5–19 Cutaneous incision for the Senegas (modified Ollier) approach.

LeTournel and Judet[11] devised a so-called extended iliofemoral approach as a posterior enlargement of the previously described iliofemoral procedure (Fig. 5–21). The patient is placed in a lateral position, preferably on a fracture table although a standard operating table can be used. If a supracondylar traction pin is employed for longitudinal

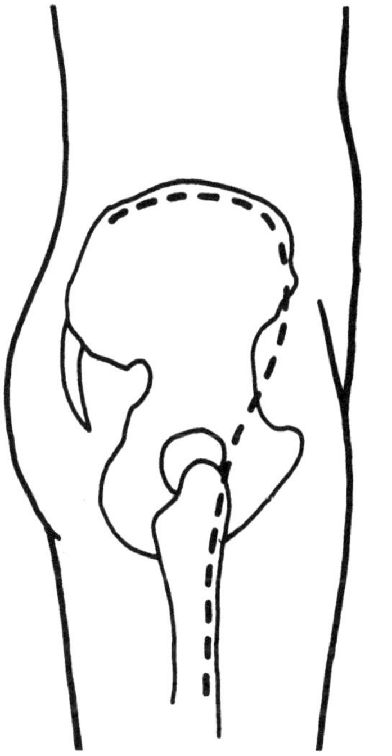

FIG. 5–21 Cutaneous incision for the extended iliofemoral approach.

traction, the knee is flexed at 45° to protect the sciatic nerve. The incision, in the form of an inverted J, starts at the posterosuperior iliac spine and follows the iliac crest to the anterior iliac spine. Then it continues distally halfway down the anterior thigh toward the outer border of the patella. The gluteal fascia is incised and the musculature progressively detached from the iliac wing. The dissection continues anteriorly to the tensor fascia lata. The branches of the lateral cutaneous nerve of the thigh are rigorously protected at a level superior to the greater trochanter, and the fascia lata is split.

Continuing posteriorly, the tendons of the gluteus minimus and gluteus medius are incised near their insertions on the greater trochanter to permit subsequent repairs of the tendons. A massive flap of tissue which includes the tensor fascia lata, gluteus medius, and gluteus minimus together with their neurovascular bundles is elevated from the outer aspect of the ilium and retracted posteriorly.

To visualize the posterior surface of the hip, the insertions of the short external rotators are incised and the muscles are reflected posteriorly for protection of the sciatic nerve. Access to the inner aspect of the pelvis is achieved through the lesser sciatic notch by incising the bursa under the obturator internus. The entire posterior column distal to the ischial tuberosity is exposed by sharp dissection. When necessary, circumferential capsulotomy around the rim of the acetabulum is performed to inspect the hip joint. The exposure visualizes the external aspect of the ilium and the entire posterior column. By reflecting the origins of the sartorius and rectus femoris and elevating the iliacus, the anterior column can be visualized to the iliopectineal eminence. Further anterior extension is hampered by the iliopsoas musculature, although visual or tactile access to the superior pubic ramus is possible to within 5 cm of the midline. The simple anatomical closure starts with reattachment of the short external rotators to the greater trochanter. When necessary, suction drains are inserted anteriorly and posteriorly. Next the gluteus medius and gluteus minimus along with tensor fascia lata are repaired near the greater trochanter and reattached to the iliac crest and the adjacent abdominal musculature. When utilizing this approach the structures at particular risk include the lateral cutaneous nerve of the thigh, the sciatic nerve, and especially the superior gluteal neurovascular bundle. If the last structures are compromised, the massive abductor flap is devitalized to create a formidable complication.

The triradiate incision is a modification of a surgical approach which Charnley initially employed for total hip joint replacement. Currently the authors use the triradiate approach to provide extensile exposure of the acetabulum, anterior and posterior columns, lateral ilium, and pelvic brim (Fig. 5–22). In certain instances, initially the anterolateral limb or the posterolateral is employed. If supplementary exposure is needed, the additional limb of the incision is made to provide an extensile exposure.

Under general anesthesia, the patient is placed in a full lateral position on a conventional operating table. Routine preparation and draping are undertaken from the anterior to the posterior midlines, including the ipsilateral extremity. The extremity is fully exposed to permit intraoperative manipulation. The superficial landmarks for the incision are the anterosuperior iliac spine, posterosuperior iliac spine, and greater trochanter. The longitudinal limb of the triradiate incision extends distally from the greater trochanter for a distance of about 6 to 8 cm. The proximal extensions of the incision course in the anterosuperior and pos-

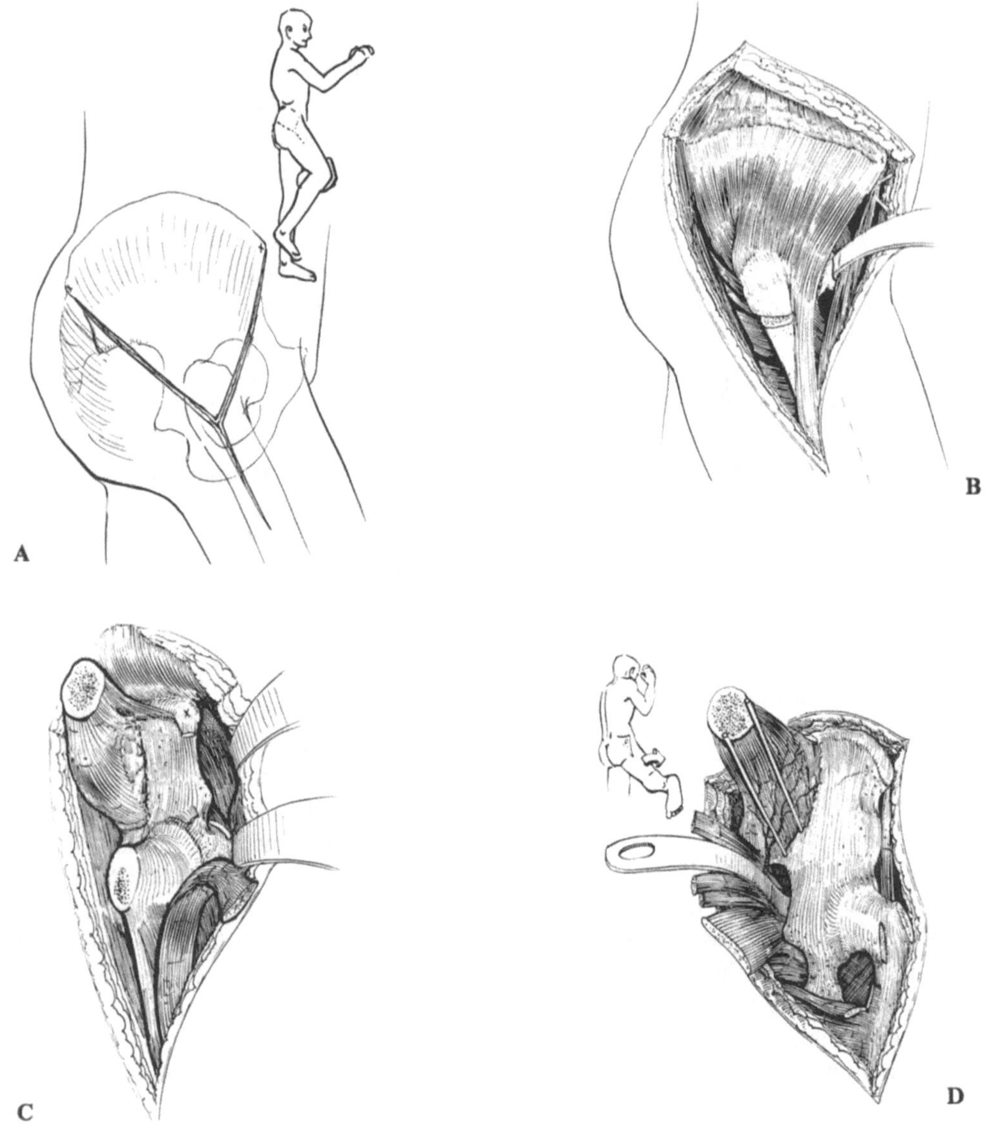

A B C D

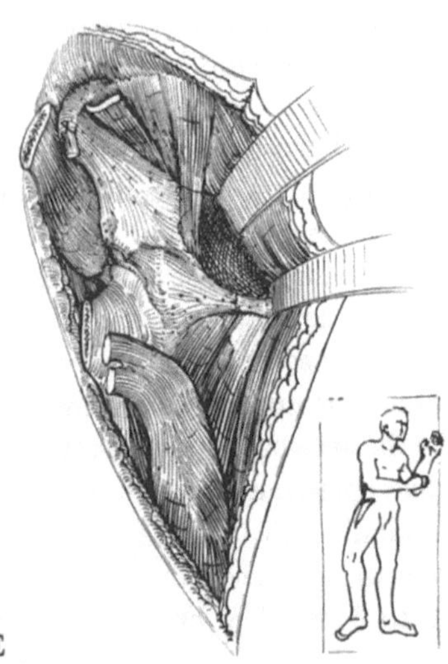

E

FIG. 5–22 Cutaneous incision and exposures of the acetabulum using the triradiate incision. **A** Cutaneous incision. **B** Trochanteric osteotomy. **C** Elevation of the tensor fascia lata, gluteus minimus, and gluteus medius musculature from the lateral ilium, as well as flexion of the reflected head of the rectus and sartorius. **D** Retraction of the tensor and glutei with Steinmann pins and exposure of the posterior column from the greater sciatic notch to the ischial tuberosity. **E** Elevation of the iliacus musculature reveals the intrapelvic portion of the ilium and anterior column.

terosuperior directions, respectively. The angle formed by the superior limbs is about 120°. The anterosuperior limb continues across the anterosuperior iliac spine, and the posterosuperior limb projects toward the posterosuperior iliac spine. The distal longitudinal limb of the incision is extended down to the fascia lata, which is divided longitudinally. This fascial incision continues parallel to the anterior and posterior cutaneous incisions.

For exposure of the anterior column the fascia lata and myofascia of tensor fascia lata are incised from the anterosuperior spine to the greater trochanter. The anterior border of the tensor fascia lata muscle is sharply incised from its fascia so that the entire muscle can be retracted superiorly and posteriorly along with the cutaneous flap. The origins of the tensor fascia lata and the gluteus minimus are incised from the iliac crest. Subperiosteal elevation of the gluteus medius and gluteus minimus is undertaken from anterior to posterior and distally to the capsule of the hip joint.

Through the posterior limb of the incision proximal to the greater trochanter, following the incision of the myofascia of the gluteus maximus, the muscle is bluntly split in line with its fibers. On the lateral aspect of the proximal femur the interval between the gluteus medius and the vastus lateralis is identified, and a transverse incision is made in the periosteum. Using an oscillating saw or osteotome, the greater trochanter with the attached gluteus medius and gluteus minimus is osteotomized and reflected craniad. With curved heavy scissors, working from proximal to distal and anterior to posterior, the gluteus medius and gluteus minimus are sharply elevated from the capsule of the hip joint. The capsule is carefully preserved. The dissection continues to the greater sciatic notch where the superior gluteal vessels are identified. Next the short external rotators of the hip are incised from their insertions to the proximal femur, distal to the mid-portion of the quadratus femoris. They are reflected in a posterior direction to visualize the underlying posterior column and the adjacent capsule of the hip joint. With the gluteus medius and gluteus minimus reflected superiorly, the lateral pelvis and roof of the acetabulum are approached by elevating the periosteum. Using sharp and blunt dissection the posterior column is exposed, starting at the greater sciatic notch. Blunt Hohmann-type retractors are carefully inserted into the greater sciatic notch to maintain the exposure of the posterior column. The abductor muscle mass is anchored superiorly and posteriorly using two Steinmann pins inserted into the ilium 2.5 and 5.0 cm, respectively, above the roof of the greater sciatic notch. The distal portion of the posterior column is observed to the level of the ischial tuberosity by sharp incision of the origin of the hamstring muscles. The ridge on the ischial tuberosity may be trimmed with a rongeur to facilitate the application of a plate along the posterior column. The sacrospinous ligament can be incised to facilitate palpation of the inner wall of the ilium. This maneuver is discouraged as it compromises one of the few stabilizing elements that is preserved in many acetabular fractures.

Exposure of the Sacroiliac Joint

As part of the exposure of the anterior column, often it is necessary to extend the dissection medially to the iliopectineal eminence and posteriorly to the sacroiliac joint (Fig. 5–22C). The anterior limb of the cutaneous incision is continued 6 to 8 cm medial to the anterosuperior iliac crest. A plane is developed between the abdominal musculature and the flexors of the hip to expose the inner table of the ilium. The iliacus muscle is elevated from the inner table of the ilium and retracted medially. The exposure continues posteriorly to expose the sacroiliac joint. A curet is employed to remove callus or loose fracture fragments from the sacroiliac joint. By manipulating the ilium, an accurate reduction of the sacroiliac joint is achieved. Stabilization of the joint is undertaken by inserting two 6.5-mm cancellous lag screws with washers through the superficial surface of the ilium 2.5 and 5.0 cm, respectively, above the roof of the greater sciatic notch into the ala of the sacrum. When an ipsilateral sacroiliac dislocation complicates an acetabular fracture, the reduction of the former is the foundation for rebuilding the latter. Unless the ilium is anatomically realigned, accurate reduction of the acetabular fracture becomes excessively difficult or, more often, impossible. In addition to exposure of the sacroiliac joint, the inner wall of the ilium and the quadrilateral surface of the acetabulum can be approached to expose medially displaced acetabular fragments. In addition, a plate can be applied along the iliopectineal line for stabilization of a fracture of the anterior column and the superior pubic ramus (Fig. 5–23).

When the capsule is intact it is incised sharply from its origin around the acetabular rim to permit access to the hip joint. In the presence of a posterior wall fracture, the osteochondral fragment with its adjacent capsule is reflected to expose the hip joint. If necessary, the adjacent intact capsule is incised from its origin until sufficient exposure of the hip joint is achieved. Following the exposure of the adjacent parts of the pelvis, visualization of the hip joint is necessary in order to identify and remove loose interposed osteochondral fragments, to verify the presence of an anatomical reduction, and to observe and remove misdirected screws which violate the joint.

For closure of the triradiate incision, a suction drain is inserted and the lower extremity is positioned on a stand with about 30° of abduction of the hip joint. The two Steinmann pins are removed from the ilium to permit reattachment of the origins of the gluteus muscles and the tensor fascia lata to the iliac crest. The capsule of the hip joint is reattached to the origin of the indirect head of the rectus femoris and to the ilium. Both of the previous repairs may be facilitated by the use of sutures inserted through 2-mm drill holes in the ilium. The greater trochanter is accurately reduced and temporarily immobilized with a tenaculum forceps. Two 6.5 mm long threaded cancellous screws with washers are used to secure the greater trochanter. To resist cut-out, the screws are secured to the cortical bone of the medial wall of the femur in the calcar femoralis, adjacent to the lesser trochanter. In the presence of mildly osteoporotic bone a supplementary figure-of-eight 18-gauge tension band wire is employed (see Volume I, Chapter 4, page 97, Figure 4–16F). If the bone is moderately osteoporotic, a "hook" plate [Synthes Ltd. (U.S.A.), Wayne, PA] is used to reattach the greater trochanter. An apical stitch is used to reconstruct the three fascial edges superficial to the greater trochanter. Then the three fascial limbs of the incision are repaired followed by closure of the subcutaneous and cutaneous layers.

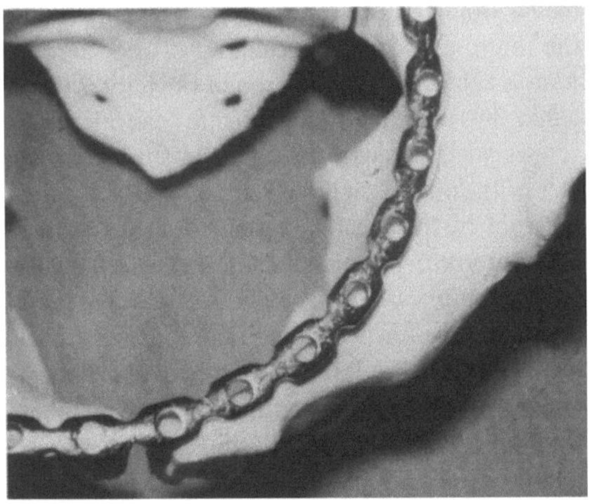

FIG. 5–23 Curved LeTournel plate applied along the iliopectineal line and across the symphysis of a model pelvis.

Management of Specific Acetabular Fracture Patterns

Minimally Displaced Fracture

After adequate radiological confirmation including computed tomography, a minimally displaced fracture is managed by the application of skeletal traction to the ipsilateral extremity. Usually the patient is comfortable within a period of 1 to 3 days when physical therapy with active and passive assisted motion exercises of the hip and progressive resistance exercises of the limbs are initiated.

Generally, 6 weeks after injury, bed-to-chair transfers and a touchdown gait are encouraged. following a radiographic assessment to document satisfactory and unchanged alignment. Twelve weeks after injury sufficient radiographic evidence of fracture repair is anticipated so that progression to a full weight-bearing gait and unlimited activities can be encouraged.

Fracture Dislocation of the Hip Joint

A traumatic posterior or anterior dislocation of the hip joint necessitates a reduction of the femoral head as an emergency procedure. If the capsule of the joint remains taut around the dislocated femoral head for more than a few hours, the blood supply of the femoral head is jeopardized and avascular necrosis is likely to ensue. Previously the relative merits of closed versus open reduction of the hip joint have been controversial. Admittedly, in the absence of any associated fracture a closed reduction is a satisfactory method of treatment. In many instances acetabular rim or femoral head fragments or avulsion fractures from either end of the ligamentum teres are interposed between the acetabulum and the reduced femoral head. Rapid and severe destruction of the hip joint is provoked by such abrasive wear. Some workers[5] have recommended an open reduction of all traumatic dislocations of the hip joint to prevent this disastrous and avoidable complication. The open reduction is accompanied by a thorough inspection and irrigation of the joint to remove all debris. With the widespread availability of computed tomography[13] the detection of intraarticular osteochondral fragments after a closed reduction will help the decision making process of future care. In the presence of a displaced acetabular fracture, radiologically demonstrable interposed osteochondral fragments, or a failed closed reduction, an open reduction is necessary.

Displaced Acetabular Fractures

The indications for an open reduction were outlined in a previous section. Preoperative longitudinal skeletal traction applied for 24 to 48 hours may provide a partial reduction to lessen the amount of correction that is needed at the time of surgery. The partial closed reduction achieved by skeletal traction used to be an important ancillary measure; however, with the improvements in techniques of open reduction it no longer appears to be a major factor.

Similarly, to facilitate the open reduction, especially when an ilioinguinal or iliofemoral approach is employed, LeTournel and Judet[11] advocated the use of intraoperative skeletal traction. Longitudinal skeletal traction is applied through a distal femoral traction pin to a special orthopedic table. The knee is rigorously maintained in a flexed position to minimize the likelihood of a postoperative sciatic nerve palsy. A large pad positioned in the groin pushing toward the affected side may be used to apply a lateral force on the proximal femur for the correction of central migration. Whereas such external aids facilitate gross realignment of the hip joint, they may hamper the final stages of the open acetabular reduction. They necessitate special expensive apparatus, and unless used carefully they may be associated with a greater incidence of sciatic nerve palsy.

Another innovation has been the development of superior methods of intraoperative reduction. Following an appropriate extensile exposure for complete visualization of the fracture, special bone-holding forceps are applied to the principal bone fragments. A unicortical 3.2-mm drill is made in the fragments for the application of large tenaculum bone-holding forceps [Synthes Ltd. (U.S.A.), Wayne, PA] (Fig. 5–24). Alternatively, 4.5-mm cortical screws, or in softer or more osteoporotic bone long, threaded 6.5-mm cancellous

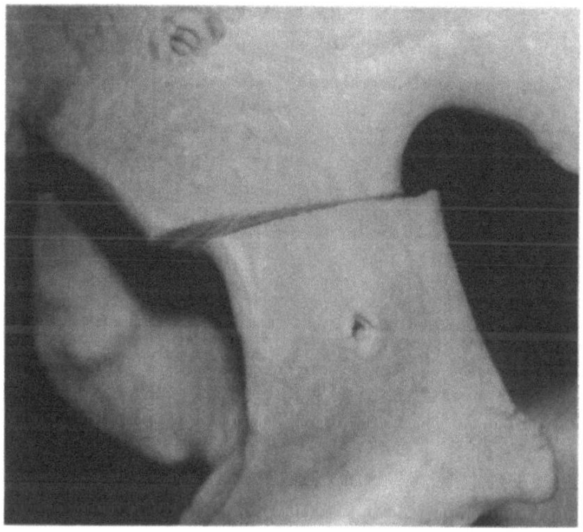

A

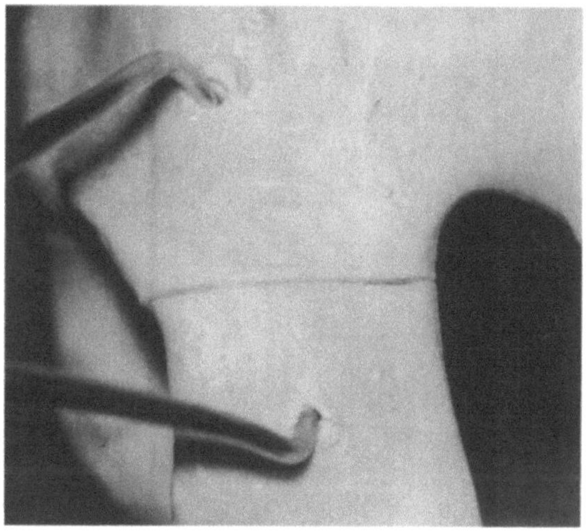

B

FIG. 5–24 Application of tenaculum bone-holding forceps to reduce a displaced posterior column fracture in a pelvic model. **A** Prior to reduction 3.2 mm unicortical drill holes are made in the bone fragments. **B** The pointed ends of the forceps are inserted into the drill holes to manipulate and immobilize the osseous fragments.

screws, are inserted into the principal bone fragments. The screw heads protrude 5 to 10 mm above the surface of the bone (Fig. 5–25). Farabeuf–Lambotte forceps are applied to a pair of screws. Generally at least two pairs of forceps of either type are required. When the broad interdigitating fracture surfaces are interlocked in a maldisplaced position, a small osteotome is carefully positioned in the fracture line and manipulated to separate the fragments. The bone-holding forceps are then used to realign and approximate the fracture fragments. Another helpful ancillary technique is the use of a 3.5-mm reconstruction plate as an aid to reduction. For example, for a posterior column fracture, a plate of appropriate length, usually six to nine holes, is selected (Fig. 5–26). Using a plate simulator and contouring device, the plate is contoured as accurately as possible even though the fracture remains malaligned. The plate is anchored to the ischial tuberosity and the adjacent portion of the posterior column inferior to the fracture using 3.5-mm cortical screws. A tenaculum forceps is applied to the terminal hole in the most superior portion of the plate. The other pointed end of the forceps is placed around the exposed iliac crest or into a unicortical 3.2-mm drill hole in the lateral ilium. Separate tenaculum forceps can be used to correct overriding with posterior and medial displacement of the inferior fracture fragment. The second forceps is positioned with one pointed end in the greater or lesser sciatic notch and the other on the superficial surface of the anterolateral ilium. Medial or posteromedial displacement of the posterior column also can be corrected by inserting a bone hook into the greater sciatic notch to apply a lateral or anterolateral corrective force to the displaced osseous fragment. After the fracture is realigned the first forceps applied to the reconstruction plate is used to compress the fracture. The remainder of the 3.5-mm cortical screws are inserted into the posterior column plate.

When the femoral head is lodged firmly in a medially displaced position, a femoral distractor [Synthes Ltd. (U.S.A.), Wayne, PA] is used to disengage it. The two 4.5-mm stabilizing pins are inserted into the lateral ilium and the osteotomized surface of the greater trochanter, respectively. Pelvic reduction forceps are available which provide considerable mechanical advantage. The device is applied to a pair of cancellous screws which are first inserted with a transverse alignment with respect to the fracture (Fig. 5–27). Obliquely aligned screws do not permit application of the forceps to the screw heads. As it is currently designed, the pelvic reduction forceps is difficult to satisfactorily apply and is the least valuable method of those previously described.

Judicious application of a bone hook is helpful

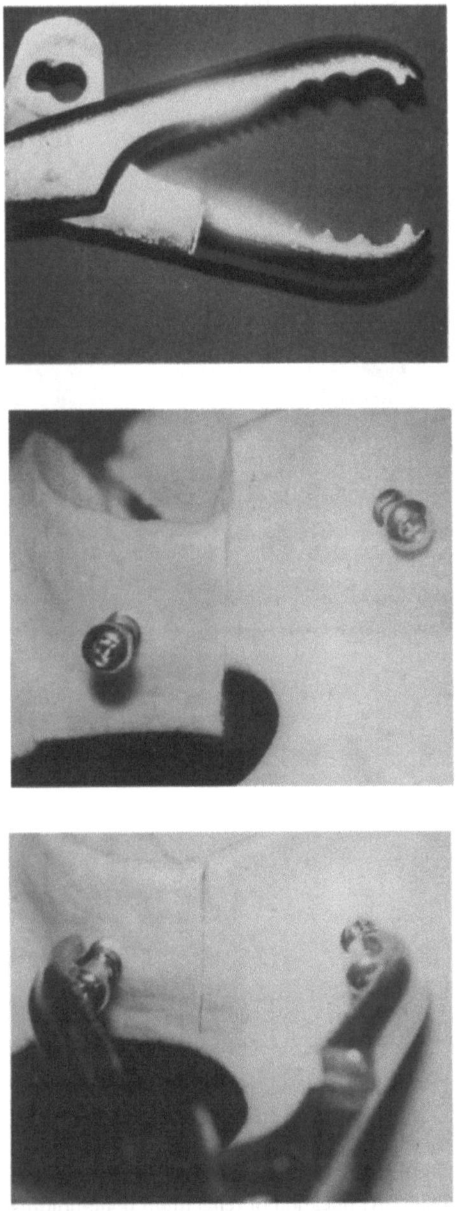

A

B

C

FIG. 5–25 Use of Farabeuf–Lambotte forceps to reduce an acetabular fracture. **A** Farabeuf–Lambotte forceps. **B** Insertion of 4.5-mm cortical screws into the osseous fragments. **C** Application of the forceps to reduce and immobilize the fracture.

FIG. 5–26 Application of a 3.5-mm reconstruction plate to the posterior column. **A** The optimal contour of the plate to fit the bone. **B** Use of the special plate-contouring device.

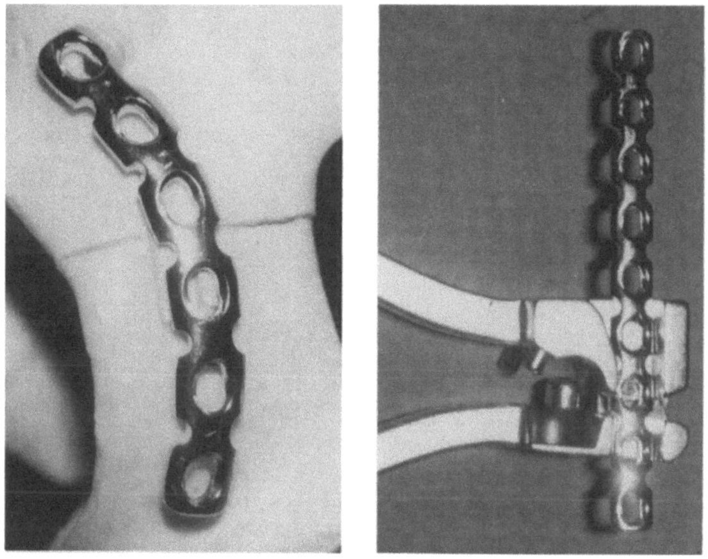

A B

to achieve an accurate reduction of several fracture patterns. With a posterior column or transverse fracture, the bone hook can be placed around the posterior column into the sciatic notch. It permits lateral and anterior manipulation of the posterior column. It may facilitate realignment of the anterior column by insertion into the obturator foramen. It may be applied to the inner wall of the acetabulum to correct medial displacement. Whenever the bone hook is applied to the pelvis, great care is needed to avoid the obvious risk of neurovascular injury.

With any of the bone-holding forceps applied to an acetabular fracture, the site for application of the device requires careful selection. Once the forceps are applied in a particular orientation, compression should provide accurate realignment of the fracture. Also, the site of attachment of the forceps or femoral distractor cannot interfere with the optimal site for application of lag screws or a fixation plate. With the limited bone stock available, a comprehensive plan is essential. Nevertheless, with this armamentarium virtually all patterns of acute acetabular fractures can be accurately reduced.

When the principal acetabular fragments are displaced in three planes, an anatomical reduction is notoriously difficult to achieve. A technique of staged approximation of the fracture fragments has been particularly helpful for us. Rather than a single manipulation to correct the several deformities in different orientations, a series of maneuvers is performed, each of which is designed to correct the malalignment in one particular plane. For example, a typical transverse acetabular fracture shows medial and posterior displacement of the inferior fragment and a supplementary rotational malalignment.

To achieve the reduction, first, by use of the tenaculum forceps or the Farabeuf–Lambotte forceps, applied to a pair of screws secured in the principal osseous fragments, the rotational error is readily corrected. Next the same bone-holding forceps are manipulated to correct the posterior displacement of the inferior fragment. Usually these two steps are most readily accomplished by application of the forceps across the anterior column disruption. A second forceps may be applied to the posterior column disruption. To correct the residual medial displacement, a bone hook is inserted into the greater sciatic notch so that its pointed end engages the medial wall of the inferior fragment. At this stage, before any attempt to rigorously approximate the fracture fragments and thereby obliterate the fracture gap, a Kirschner wire is inserted transversely across the anterior half of the fracture (Fig. 5–28). A suitable 3.5-mm reconstruction plate of six to eight holes, depending on the site where the fracture violates the posterior column, is selected. The plate is contoured using a plate simulator and a bending tool, and is anchored to the ischial tuberosity with two 3.5-mm cortical screws. A tenaculum bone-holding forceps is applied to the proximal end of the plate

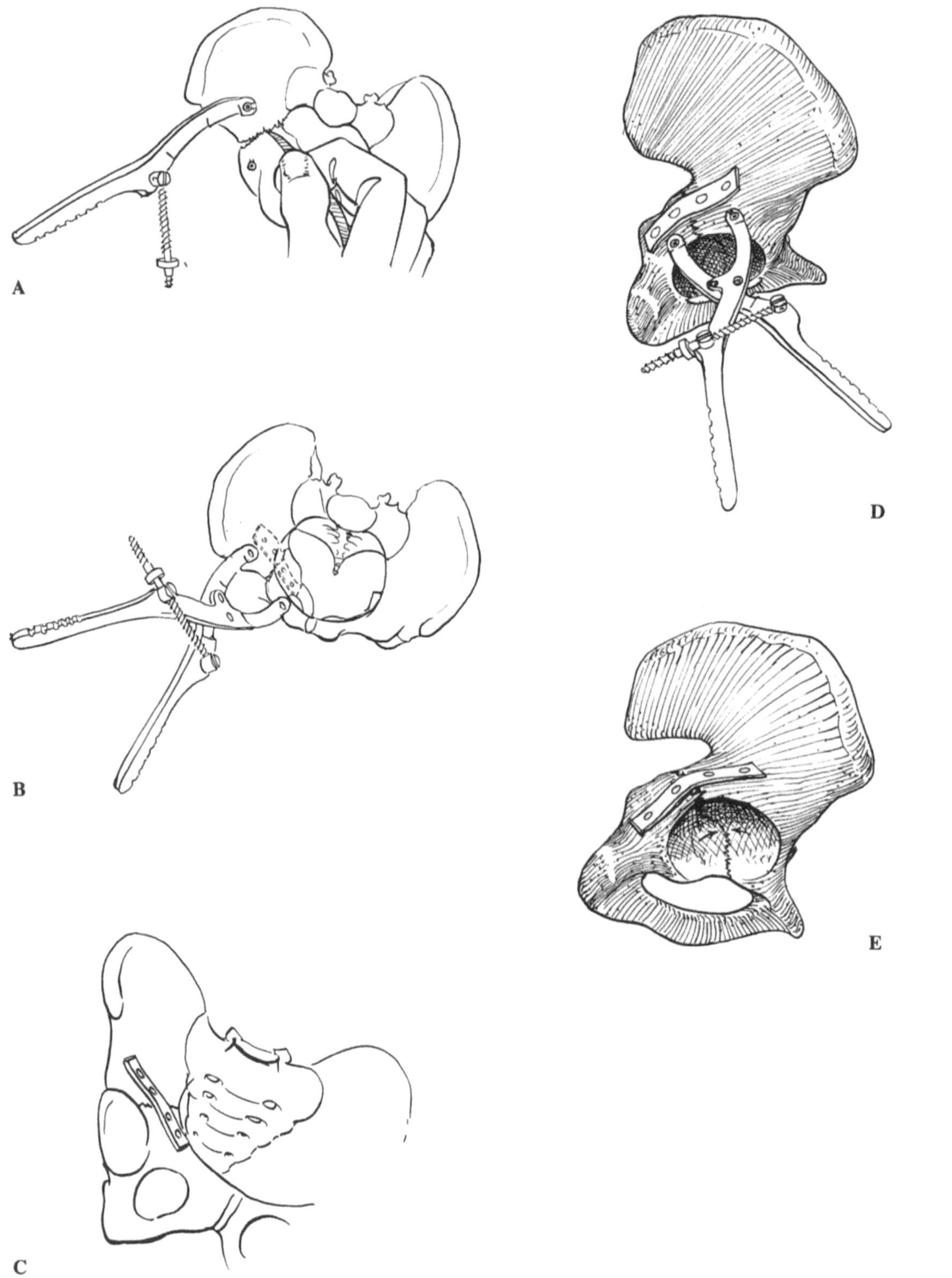

FIG. 5–27 Use of the pelvic reduction forceps to reduce anterior and posterior columns, respectively. **A** Application of the separate jaws of the forceps to two cortical or 6.5-mm cancellous screws inserted on either side of the anterior column disruption. **B** Manipulation of the fracture fragments. The device is carefully applied so that the optimal site for application of the anterior column plate is not obscured. **C** The plate is applied to the fracture, and the forceps with the two screws is removed. **D** and **E** Application of the pelvic forceps to a posterior column fracture for reduction and plate fixation.

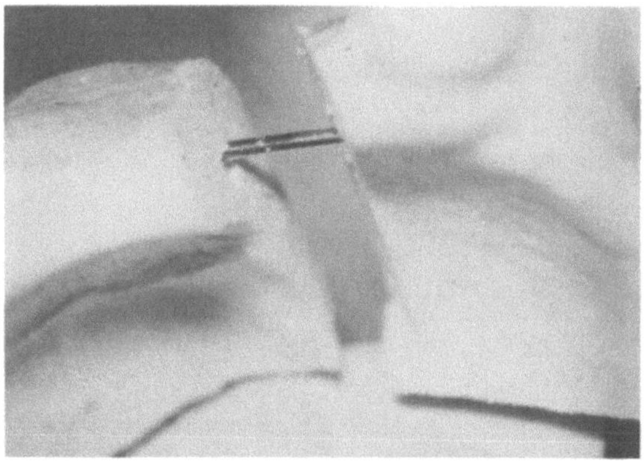
A

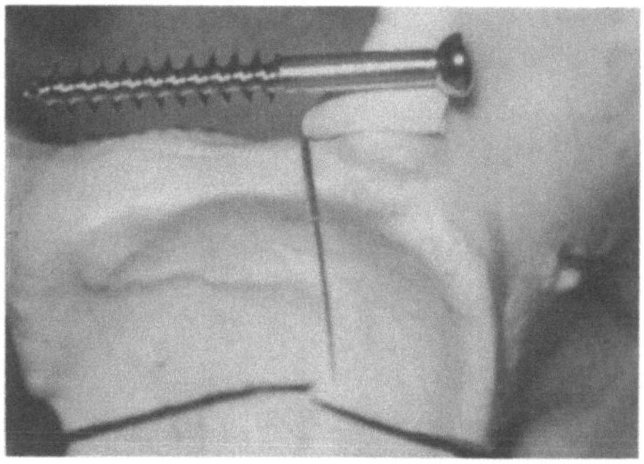
B

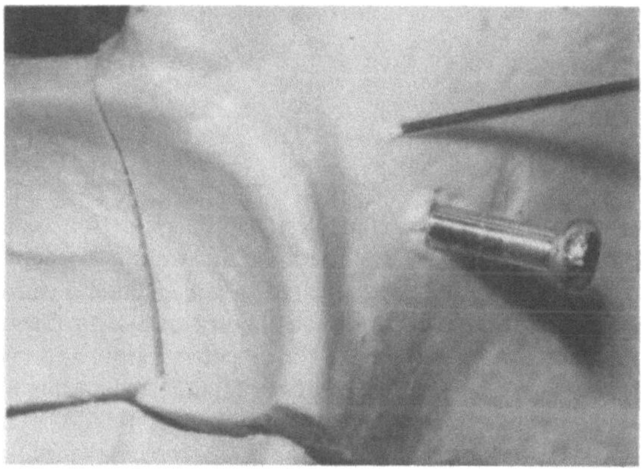
C

FIG. 5–28 Application of the staged reduction technique for a simulated anterior column disruption in a transverse, or T, fracture is shown. **A** After provisional realignment of the anterior column, a Kirschner wire is inserted across the disruption, and a tenaculum forceps is applied to the bone fragments. While a power tool is used to rotate the "K" wire, the tenaculum forceps is tightened so that the osseous fragments are approximated. **B** A lengthy 6.5 mm long threaded cancellous screw is used to secure the anterior column. **C** The screw is introduced along the lateral iliac ridge about 3.0 cm superior to the acetabular rim.

and around the iliac crest. After it has been tightened, a power tool is reapplied to the Kirschner wire. When the power is applied to rotate the Kirschner wire, the bone-holding forceps is tightened to rigorously approximate the fracture. The femoral head is inserted into the acetabulum, and the area is carefully scrutinized to confirm the presence of a congruent acetabular reduction. Then the residual screws are applied to the plate on the posterior column and a 6.5 mm long thread cancellous lag screw with a washer is introduced across the anterior column. A trial range of motion of the hip is performed. Finally, the Kirschner wire and the bone-holding forceps are removed.

Sequential Reduction of the Fracture

In the presence of a comminuted acetabular fracture complicated by an ipsilateral sacroiliac fracture/dislocation and iliac comminution, the proper sequence in the reduction technique is crucial to permit accurate realignment of the articular surface itself (Fig. 5–29). With the patient positioned in a lateral position, usually widening of a displaced ipsilateral sacroiliac joint corrects itself spontaneously. Residual rotational displacement of the sacroiliac joint is reduced primarily so that the principal or posterior portion of the ilium is anatomically realigned. When a Kocher–Langenbeck, triradiate, or extended iliofemoral incision is used, the sacroiliac joint can be palpated through the greater sciatic notch. With the latter two incisions, even when malalignment has been present for a few weeks, anterior exposure of the sacroiliac joint provides the opportunity to débride and accurately realign the joint. The joint is immobilized by the insertion of two or three 6.5-mm cancellous lag screws applied 3 and 6 cm, respectively, above the roof of the greater sciatic notch. The second stage in the sequence of reduction is a displaced iliac fracture. A tenaculum or Farabeuf–Lambotte forceps is employed for the iliac reduction. The optimal stabilization is achieved using one 3.5-mm reconstruction plate along the iliac crest and one

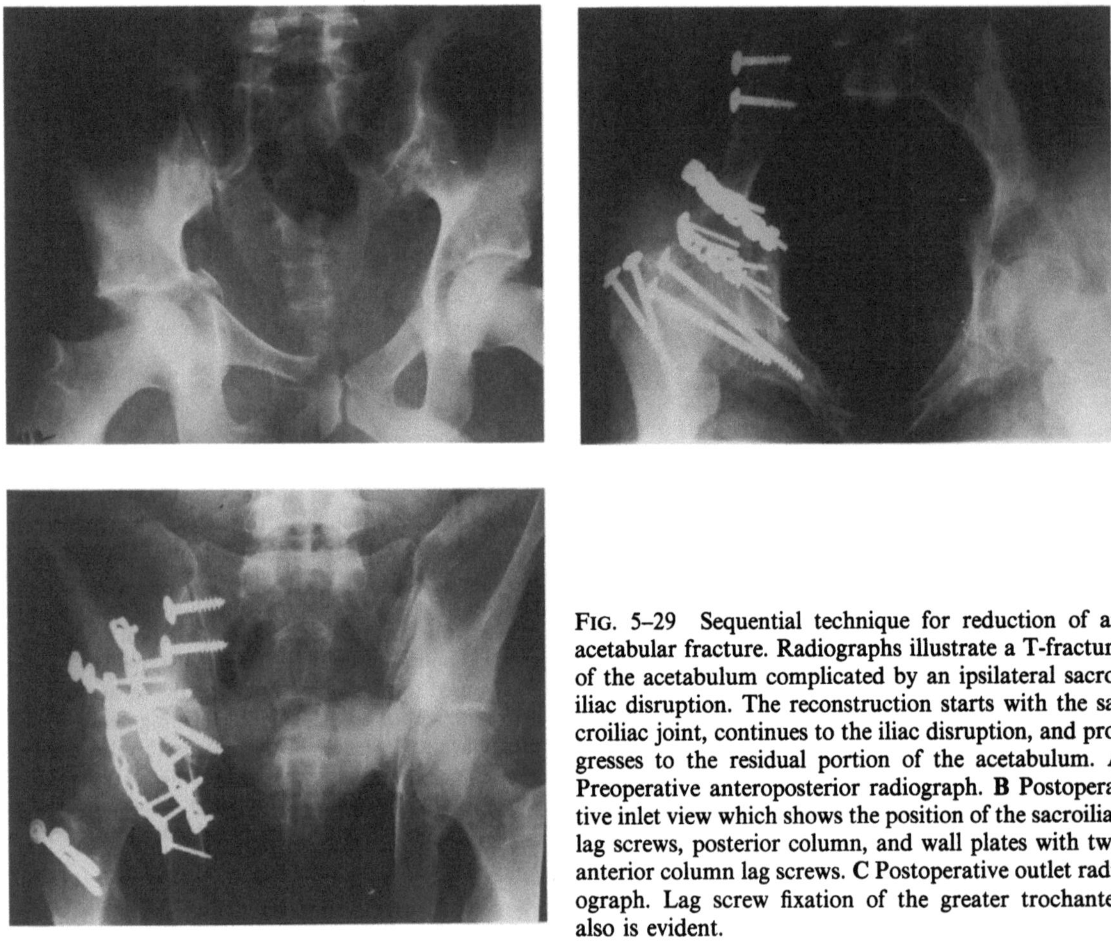

A B C

FIG. 5–29 Sequential technique for reduction of an acetabular fracture. Radiographs illustrate a T-fracture of the acetabulum complicated by an ipsilateral sacroiliac disruption. The reconstruction starts with the sacroiliac joint, continues to the iliac disruption, and progresses to the residual portion of the acetabulum. **A** Preoperative anteroposterior radiograph. **B** Postoperative inlet view which shows the position of the sacroiliac lag screws, posterior column, and wall plates with two anterior column lag screws. **C** Postoperative outlet radiograph. Lag screw fixation of the greater trochanter also is evident.

or two four- or five-hole supplementary plates on the lateral iliac surface. In the presence of marked iliac comminution, which is commonly encountered, multiple short plates may be necessary to adequately stabilize the bone. Once the ilium is reduced, at least one portion of the acetabular roof of highly variable size is anatomically situated. Clearly, in the presence of an acetabular fracture uncomplicated by an ipsilateral sacroiliac dislocation or an iliac fracture, the initial stage of the open reduction starts from this point.

A posterior wall fracture accompanying a posterior dislocation of the hip joint is reduced by the use of tenaculum forceps. It can be provisionally stabilized with Kirschner wires. In the presence of dense bone and a fragment which extends toward the greater sciatic notch, immobilization with two 4.0-mm cancellous lag screws is possible (Fig. 5–30). When the fragment is osteoporotic or large or when it is primarily an articular fragment, a superior method of stabilization is the use of a second 3.5-mm reconstruction plate. The plate buttresses the fragment so that the principal screw fixation is achieved in the ischial tuberosity and the lateral ilium, superior to the acetabulum. In this way the likelihood for inadvertent insertion of a screw into the hip joint is minimized. Short unicortical screws are inserted through the plate to immobilize the wall fragment itself. When a posterior column fracture is complicated by a posterior wall fragment (Fig. 5–31), initially the wall fragment is displaced to permit visualization of the hip joint and accurate reduction of the posterior column. After internal fixation of the posterior column with a reconstruction plate, the wall fragment is reduced, provisionally stabilized with Kirschner wires, and firmly buttressed with a second reconstruction plate.

FIG. 5–30 Open reduction internal fixation of a posterior wall fracture. **A** and **B** Sites for introduction of screws. **C** Preoperative anteroposterior radiograph of a typical case. **D** Postoperative obturator oblique radiograph.

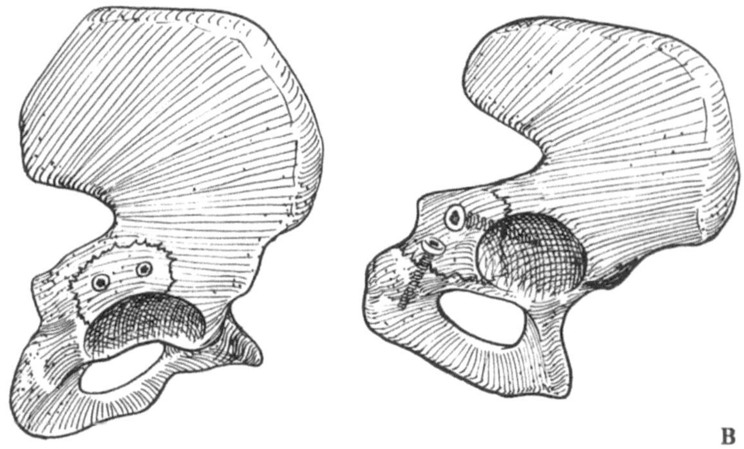

A B

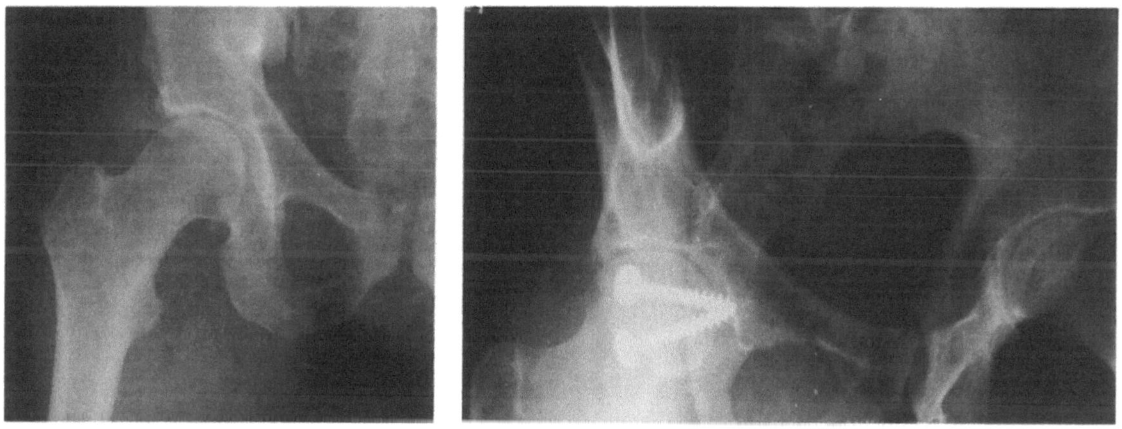

C D

The same general principles are followed for the relatively uncommon isolated anterior column and wall fractures (Fig. 5–32). For an isolated anterior or posterior column fracture, a supplementary lag screw greatly augments the effectiveness of the fixation. For a transverse fracture, the preferred method of fixation is a long anterior column 6.5-mm cancellous lag screw accompanied by a posterior column reconstruction plate (Fig. 5–33).

For the reduction of a T-fracture or other comparable associated comminuted variants, the anterior column is first reduced with respect to the residual acetabular "roof" portion of the ilium. Elimination of any visible "step-off" at the fracture site is essential. A more subtle aspect of the reduction is restoration of the congruity of this portion of the acetabulum with respect to the radius of curvature of the femoral head. Usually the anterior column shows medial displacement of its inferior portion so that the radius of the curvature of the acetabulum is greater than that of the femoral head. An accurate restoration of the acetabular surface is achieved by a multistaged procedure (Fig. 5–29). First, using tenaculum-type bone-holding forceps, the iliac and pubic fragments are aligned so that there is no step-off between them. A small Kirschner wire is inserted across the fragments. A bone hook is applied around the inferior aspect of the anterior column to correct any residual medial displacement. Then a tenaculum bone-holding forceps is applied across the anterior column fracture to irradicate any residual fracture gap. At this stage the femoral head provides the template to judge the accuracy of this phase of the reduction. Next, a 6.5-mm cancellous screw 80 to 90 mm in length is inserted into the lateral ilium about 3 cm superior to the acetabulum in the lateral ridge of bone. Using a similar technique, the posterior column or ischial fragment is then reduced with respect to the iliac and pubic fragments. Afterward, comminuted fragments, especially those around the rim of the acetabulum,

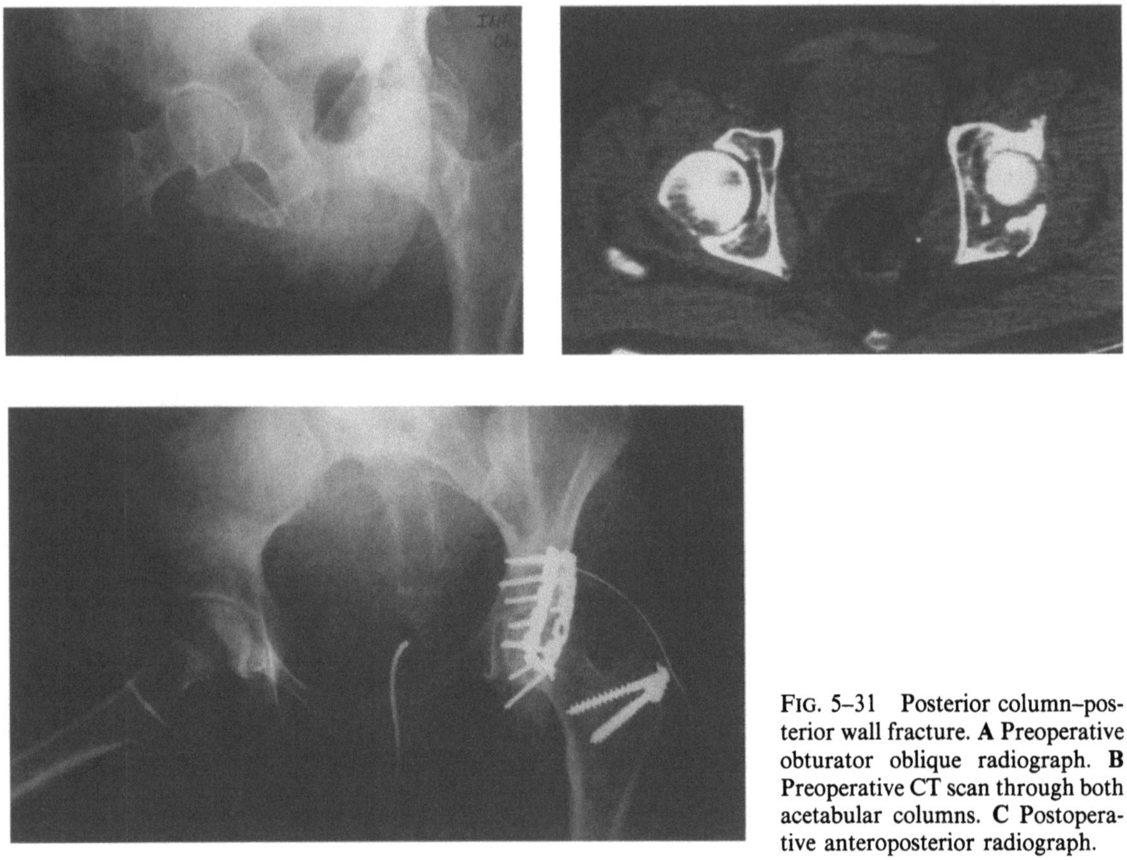

FIG. 5–31 Posterior column–posterior wall fracture. **A** Preoperative obturator oblique radiograph. **B** Preoperative CT scan through both acetabular columns. **C** Postoperative anteroposterior radiograph.

are reduced and temporarily maintained using small Kirschner wires. The posterior column fracture and, when present, rim fragments are stabilized by the application of appropriately contoured 3.5-mm reconstruction plates. When the posterior or anterior columns are comminuted, the use of the 4.5-mm reconstruction plate or the LeTournel plate (Howmedica, Inc., Rutherford, NJ) with 4.5-mm cortical screws is preferred. Application of the 4.5-mm plate is facilitated by use of the AO flexible drilling tapping and screwing apparatus, which enables the surgeon to utilize obscure plate holes for the insertion of screws into the plate which otherwise could not be inserted unless a more extensile exposure was used. Bending the plates is complicated by the three-dimensional contours of the posterior and anterior columns. The 3.5-mm reconstruction plate is readily contoured when the associated contouring press is employed (Fig. 5–26). After the pelvic fracture has been reduced and stabilized by internal fixation, intraoperative radiography or image intensification is used to confirm the adequacy of the reduction, the absence of screws in the hip joint, and a suitable location of an anterior column lag screw.

Preferred Sites for Acetabular Fixation

With the complex multiple contours, variable structure, and thickness of the innominate bone, careful pre- and intraoperative scrutiny of a simulated pelvic model is needed to identify the optimal sites available for the application of plates and screws. Grossly, the innominate bone has inner and outer cortical walls separated by a layer of cancellous bone. From the level of the dome of the acetabulum to the most posterior portion of bone, the cortical and cancellous layers show progressive thickening. From the level of the anterosuperior iliac spine posterior to the level of the sacroiliac joint, the iliac crest provides dense, thick bone highly suitable for the application of plates

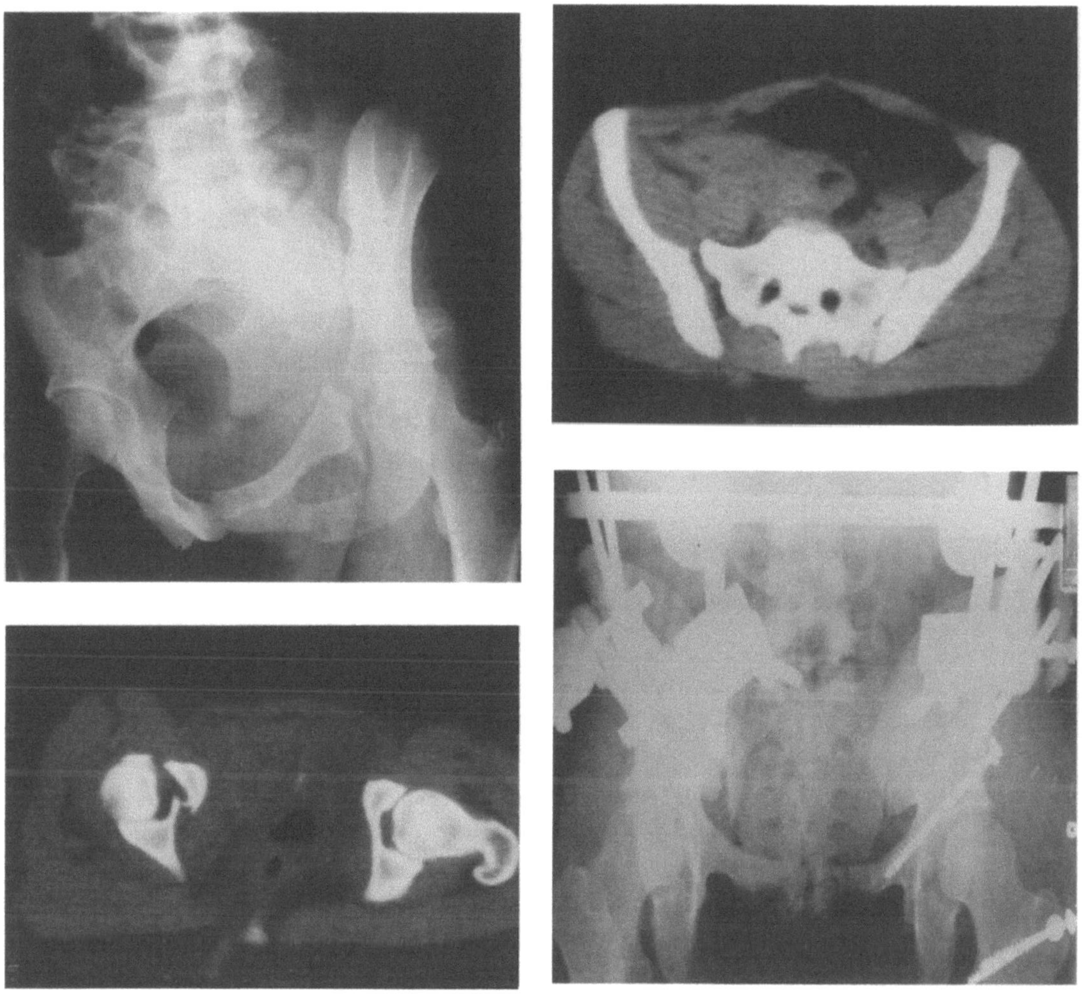

FIG. 5–32 Anterior column fracture complicated by an unstable ipsilateral sacroiliac dislocation. **A** Obturator oblique radiograph of anterior column disruption. **B** CT scan through the sacroiliac joint. **C** CT scan through the anterior column disruption. **D** Postoperative anteroposterior radiograph with lag screw fixation of the anterior column and Pittsburgh triangular frame to stabilize the pelvic ring.

and screws to both the inner and the outer walls. Transversely across the ilium from the roof of the greater sciatic notch to the dome of the acetabulum and extending 1 cm superior to this line is a region of thick cortical bone. Fracture lines infrequently violate this tough zone of bone. On the medial surface of the iliac bone at the level of the iliopectineal line and extending anteriorly along the true pelvic inlet, thick cortical bone suitable for plate and screw fixation is encountered. A final area of dense cortical bone extends from the level of the anterosuperior iliac spine inferiorly to the level of the pubic tubercle. The superior surface of the superior ramus and the anterior surface of the anterior column are appropriate for the application of plates and screws. The remaining areas of the ilium provide thin cortical bone and thickened areas of cancellous bone. Although cancellous screws can be used in these areas, they require careful orientation so that the greatest surface area of bone is available for anchorage. One broad horizontally oriented strip of cancellous bone extends from the level of the anteroinferior iliac spine to the level

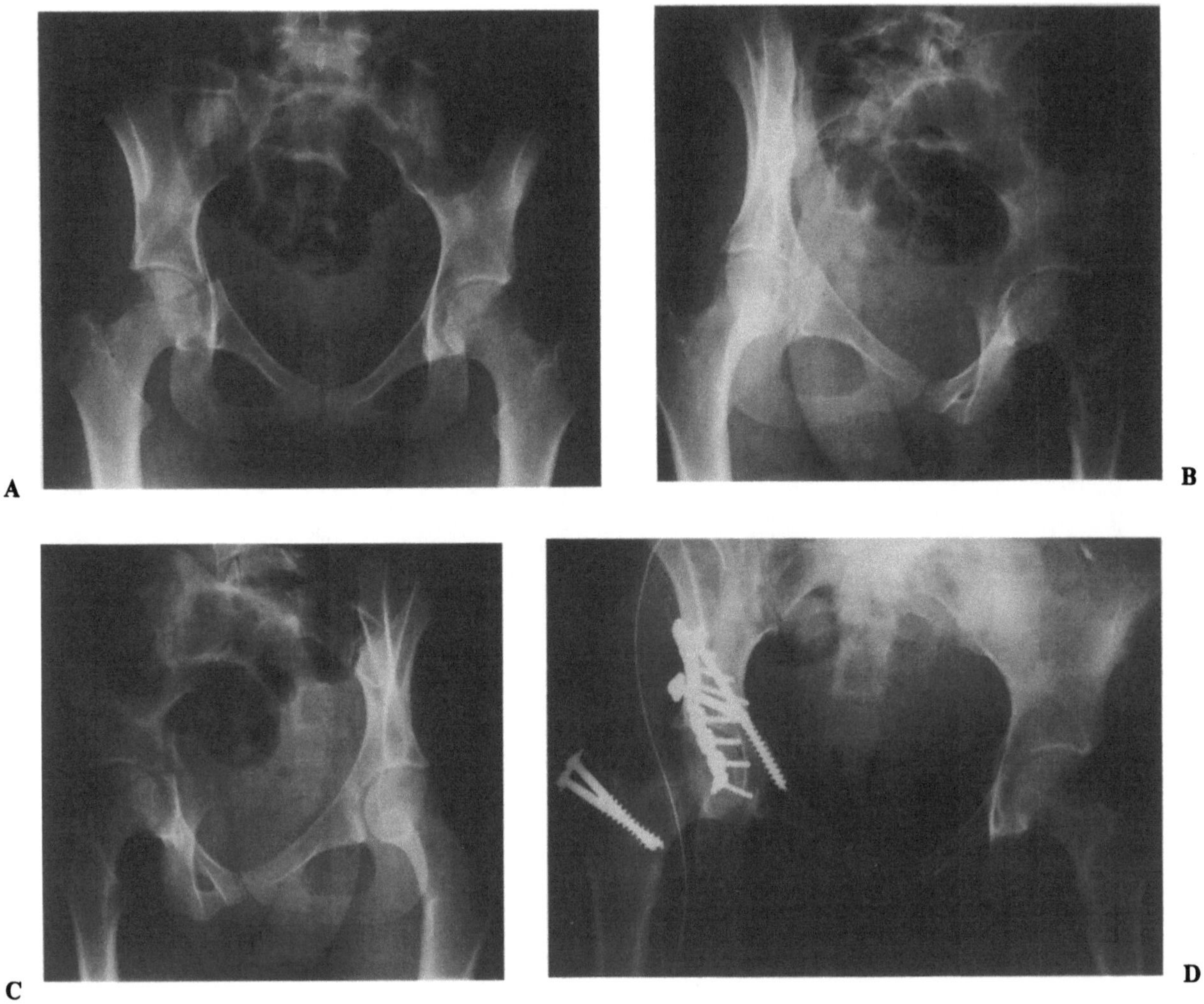

FIG. 5–33 Radiographs present a simple transverse fracture. **A** Anteroposterior view. **B** Obturator oblique view. **C** Iliac oblique view. **D** Postoperative anteroposterior view.

of the sciatic notch. This area traverses the ilium immediately superior to the dome of the acetabulum. A second area courses from the level of the inferior-most aspect of the posterior wall and extends distally along the posterior column to the level of the ischial tuberosity. This is the site for the application of a plate to the posterior column.

Fixation of the anterior column is often accomplished by inserting a long 6.5-mm cancellous screw from the level of the superior acetabulum through the inferior aspect of the inferior iliac spine into the cancellous bone of the superior pubic ramus. The screw is introduced about 3 to 4 cm above the acetabulum on the posterior aspect of the superior gluteal ridge, which corresponds to the sites of origin of the tensor fascia lata and of the gluteus medius and gluteus minimus.

The newly available canulated screws are preferred for this application. After an accurate open reduction has been achieved under image intensification, an appropriate guide pin is inserted along the axis of the superior pubic vamus. A cancellous screw typically of 90 to 100 mm in length is threaded over the guide pin. The thread length of the screw should be at least 32 mm. Alternately a lengthy 4.5 mm cortical screw can be employed. Prior to the reduction of the fracture, a 4.5 mm gliding hole is prepared by entry into the superior gluteal ridge. The appropriate exit site for the hole is confirmed on the fracture surface. Then the fracture is reduced and provisionally stabilized with bone forceps. A 3.2 mm drill sleeve is inserted into the gliding hole. The thread hole is prepared with a 3.2 mm drill bit. After the use of a depth gauge, the top screw is inserted. This method also provides an accurate direction for the screw.

Special Problems Encountered in Acetabular Reconstruction

With the enormous variability of acetabular fracture patterns that have been documented, inevitably peculiar technical problems arise during the surgical reconstructive procedures. A few of the more frequently encountered problems deserve special consideration.

Comminution

When a complete radiographic series and CT scans of many acetabular fractures are reviewed in view of the high-energy dissipation of the time of injury, it is surprising how few of the disruptions show a significant degree of comminution. Most of the fracture patterns consist of two or three large osseous fragments. Admittedly, one or two small, free osteochondral remnants may be interposed between the femoral head and acetabulum and represent a potentially catastrophic source of abrasive wear. Although these free fragments require removal, generally they do not pose a problem in acetabular reduction and fixation. When a part of the acetabulum or the adjacent pelvis is highly comminuted, the degree of technical difficulty encountered during the acetabular reconstruction increases rapidly. In rare instances generalized comminution of virtually the entire acetabulum may preclude any realistic hope for effective surgical reconstruction. In these unusual cases, skeletal traction accompanied by early mobilization of the hip in traction remains the optimal therapeutic option. The various patterns of regional comminution are now considered.

Comminution of the posterior wall is the most commonly encountered problem. This crucial portion of the acetabulum requires rigorous buttressing to prevent a late loss of reduction. In most cases a posterior column or a transverse fracture is accompanied by comminution of the posterior wall (Fig. 5–34 and 5–35). In these instances the posterior column is reduced and stabilized by a 3.5-mm reconstruction plate. The wall fragments are reduced and provisionally stabilized by Kirschner wires. Then a second 3.5-mm reconstruction plate is applied around the acetabular rim to buttress the posterior wall. Both plates are secured distally to the ischial tuberosity and proximally to the ilium. If the entire width of the posterior column is comminuted, the medial and principal weight-bearing portion is stabilized with a more rigid 4.5-mm LeTournel plate. Prior to its application this plate requires accurate contouring so that it matches the contour of the anatomically reduced posterior column. Otherwise, at the time of application of the plate an accurate reduction is lost as the bone fragments subside to approximate the faulty contour of the plate. Depending on the degree of comminution of the posterior wall, a second LeTournel plate is applied to more comminuted fractures or a 3.5-mm reconstruction plate is applied to a less comminuted one. Unless the reduced fragments are inherently stable under the impetus of compression afforded by the relatively flexible reconstruction plate, the use of the more rigid LeTournel plate is indicated.

Anterior comminution usually provides a less demanding technical problem than a comparable magnitude of posterior comminution. In most instances the anterior comminution involves the adjacent nonarticular portion of the superior pubic ramus. With the modest weight-bearing support provided by this structure, provided that stable reconstruction of the remainder of the acetabulum is achieved, the superior pubic ramus can be ignored or stabilized by lag screws introduced through the lateral ilium (Fig. 5–36). If the comminution propagates from the superior pubic ramus to the adjacent anterior articular surface, anterior fixation is required. The long anterior column lag screw cannot be employed in these instances, so an anterior column buttress plate is needed. A surgical exposure of the anterior column and the iliopectineal line is undertaken. With the lesser mechanical demands, generally a 3.5-mm reconstruction plate applied to the anterior column suffices. If the acetabular fracture is complicated by multiple sites of pelvic ring disruption, stabilization of the anterior column with a 4.5-mm LeTournel plate is preferred (Fig. 5–37). Exposure of the

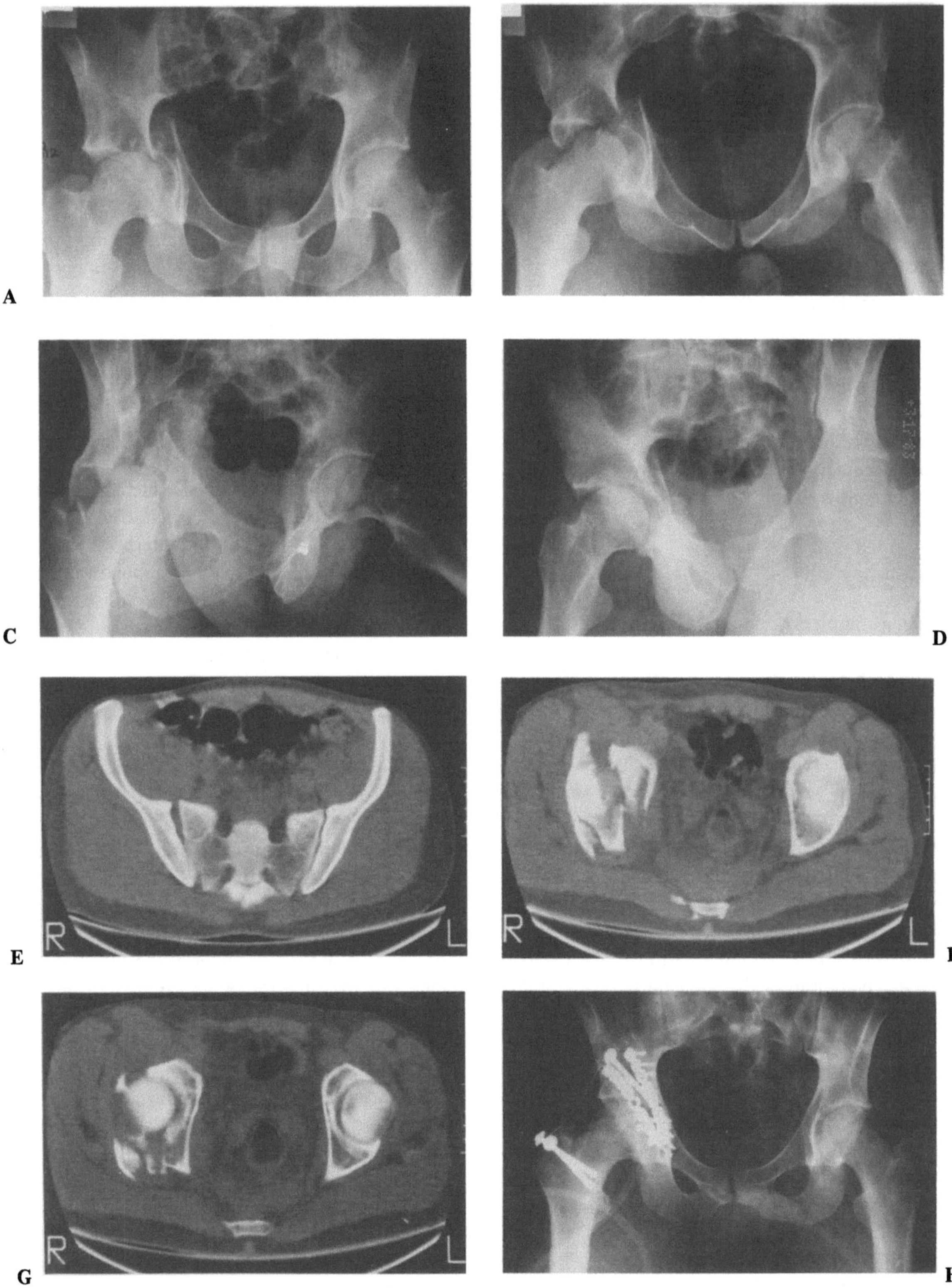

FIG. 5–34 Transverse fracture complicated by a dome fragment. **A** Anteroposterior radiograph. **B** Inlet view. **C** Obturator oblique view. **D** Iliac oblique view. **E** CT scan shows the ipsilateral stable sacroiliac disruption. **F** CT scan shows the dome fragment and posterior wall fragment. **G** CT scan shows comminution of the posterior wall. **H** Postoperative anteroposterior radiograph with an anterior column lag screw and the posterior column with posterior wall plates. Lag screw fixation of the greater trochanter is evident.

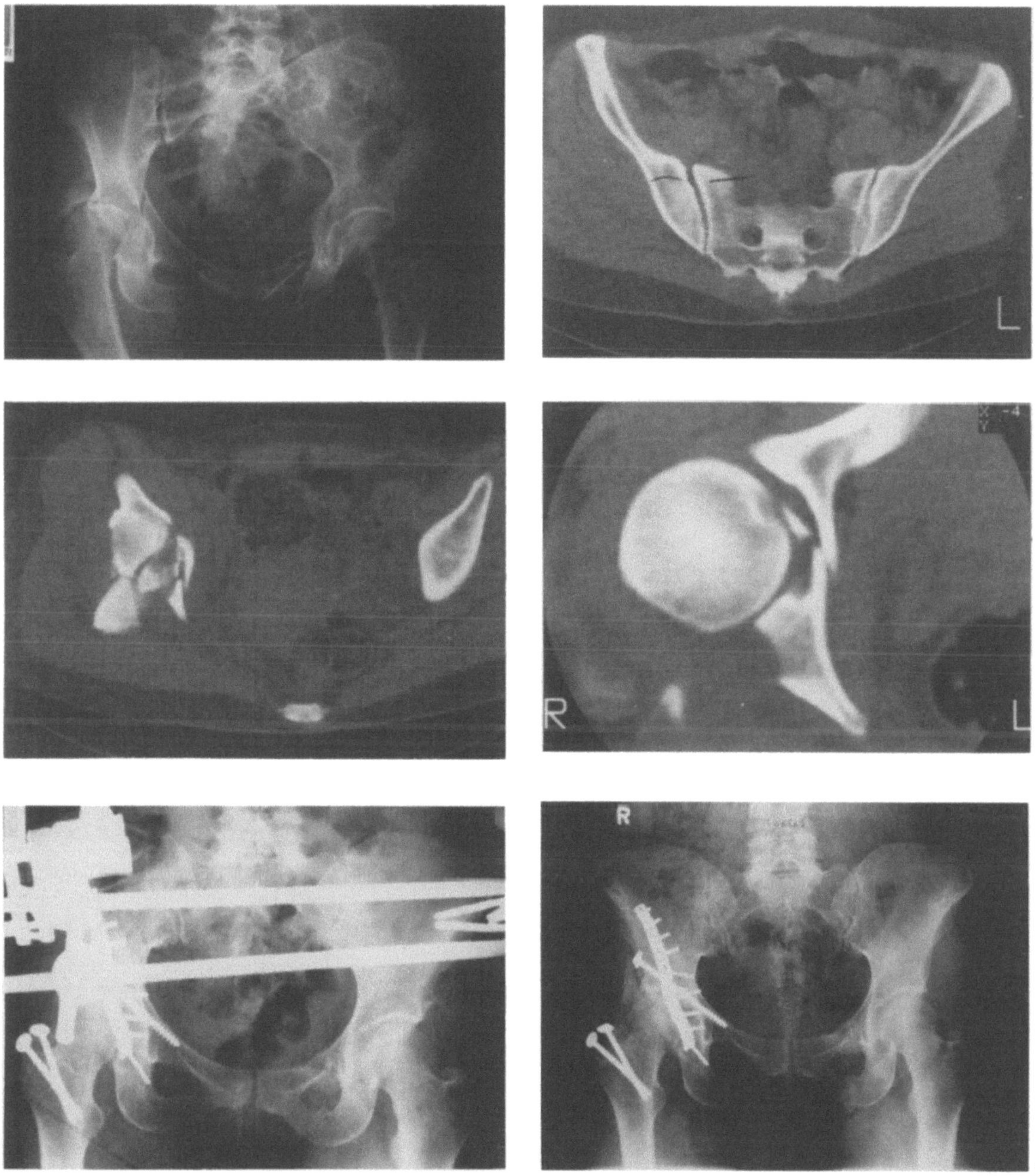

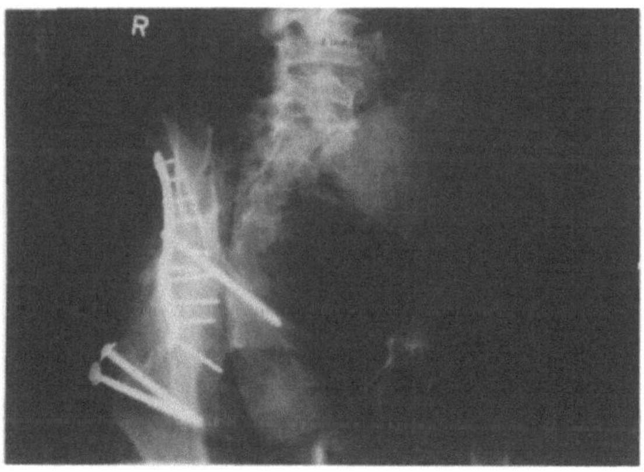

FIG. 5–35 T-fracture complicated by pelvic ring disruption. **A** Obturator oblique radiograph showing ipsilateral sacroiliac disruption, the transverse portion of the T-fracture with a posterior wall fragment, and contralateral rami disruptions. **B** CT scan with an ipsilateral stable sacroiliac disruption. **C** CT scan with comminution of the dome region. **D** CT scan of the central acetabulum reveals the T disruption. **E** Anteroposterior postoperative radiograph with a triangular frame for stabilization of the pelvic ring and internal fixation of the acetabulum. **F** Anteroposterior radiograph taken 3 months later when the external frame has been removed. **G** Obturator oblique postoperative radiograph shows the position of the anterior column lag screw.

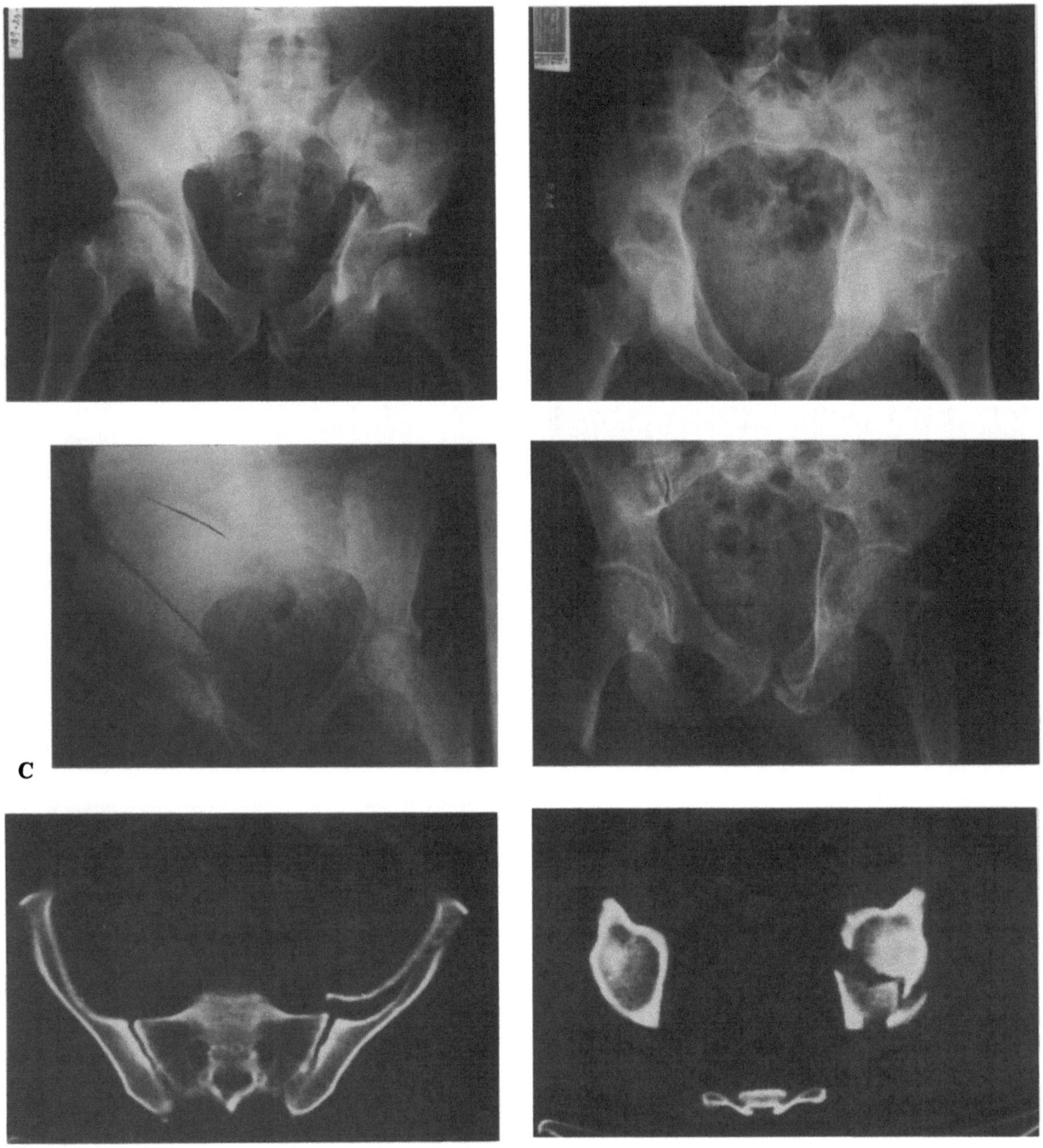

A B C D E F

Fig. 5–36 T-fracture with associated iliac and anterior wall comminution. **A** Anteroposterior radiograph. **B** Inlet view. **C** Obturator oblique view. **D** Iliac oblique view. **E** CT scan shows a section through the superior iliac wing. **F** CT section through the dome region shows the T-fracture with a posterior wall fragment. **G** CT section through the central acetabular region shows the anterior column and wall fragments.

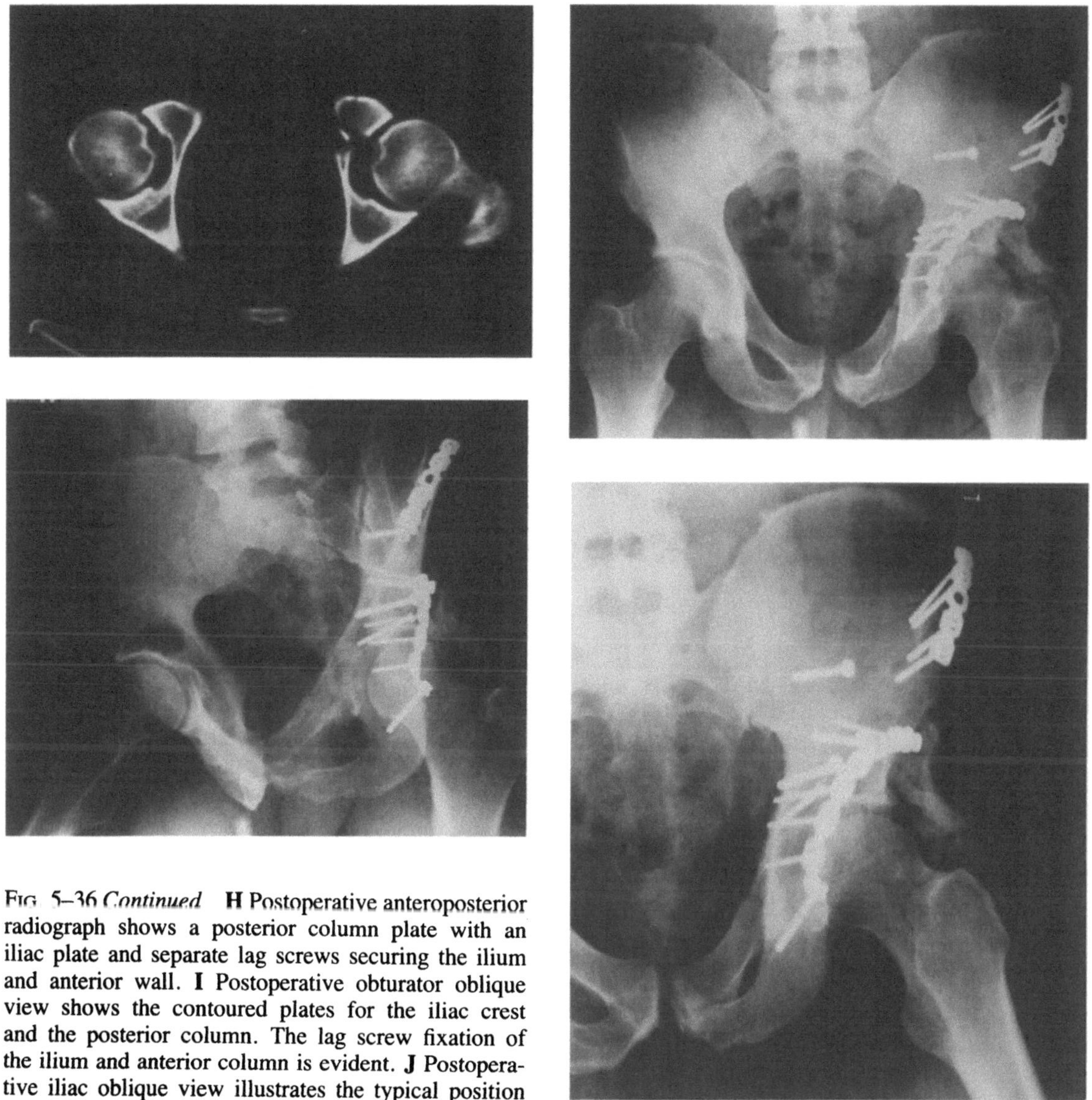

G H I J

FIG. 5–36 *Continued.* **H** Postoperative anteroposterior radiograph shows a posterior column plate with an iliac plate and separate lag screws securing the ilium and anterior wall. **I** Postoperative obturator oblique view shows the contoured plates for the iliac crest and the posterior column. The lag screw fixation of the ilium and anterior column is evident. **J** Postoperative iliac oblique view illustrates the typical position for ectopic bone formation superior to the lateral ilium.

anterior column medial to the symphysis pubis may be required so that the involved hemipelvis is adequately stabilized.

Central comminution poses a potential problem for restoration of effective mechanical support for the femoral head and as a source of recurrent free osteochondral fragments. If the central comminution pertains primarily to the inner pelvic table, stabilization is the principal concern, whereas comminution of the articular surface of the acetabulum inevitably provides a source of loose intraarticular fragments. To buttress the medial wall of the acetabulum a 3.5-mm reconstruction plate can be applied from the posterior column across the medial wall to the anterior column. The technique is undertaken by resort to a triradiate incision with extensive visualization of the medial wall. The plate requires extensive contouring so that it spans the fracture zone. The fixation screws can be anchored solely in the anterior and posterior columns.

At the time of subluxation or dislocation of the femoral head to inspect the zone of central comminution, loose osteochondral fragments are removed and carefully preserved. The principal structural sites of the fracture are reduced and

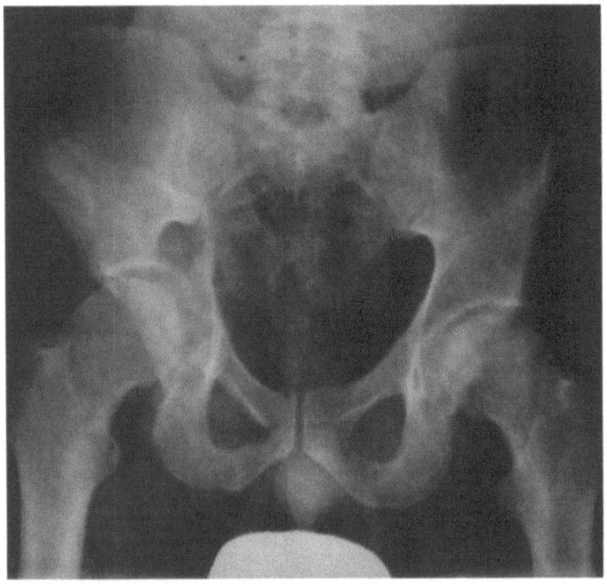
A

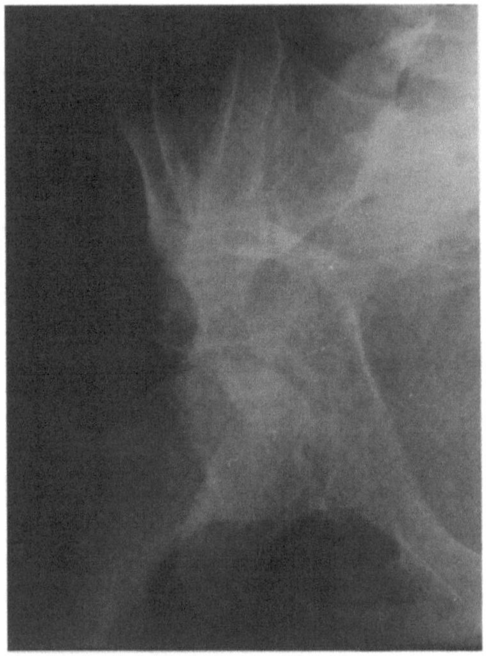
B

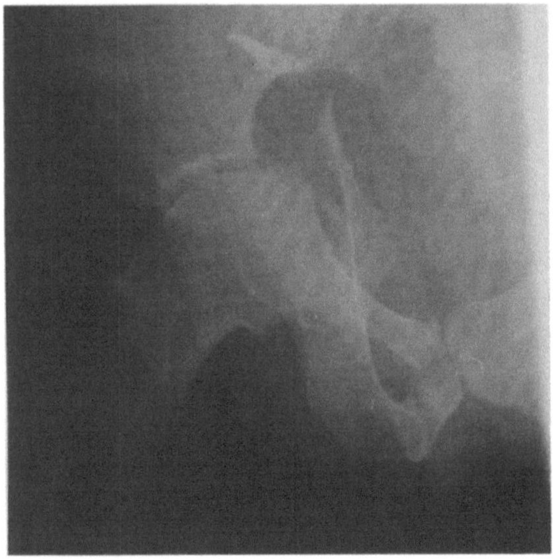
C

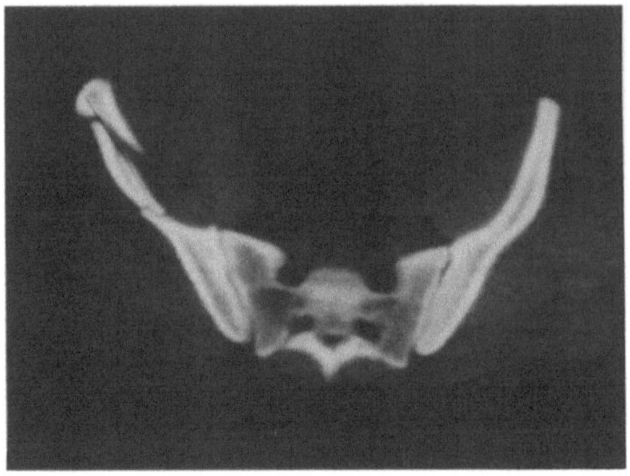
D

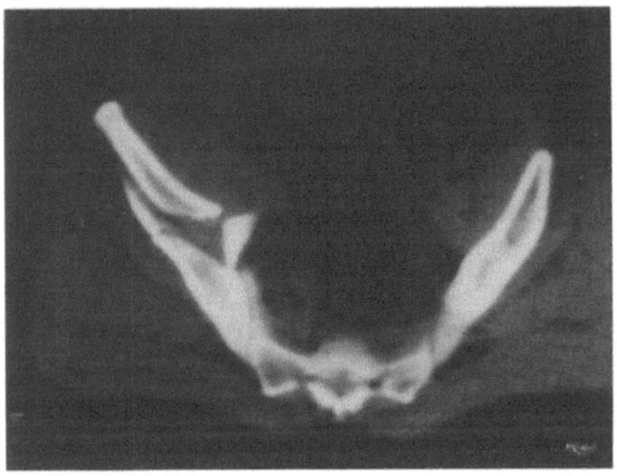
E

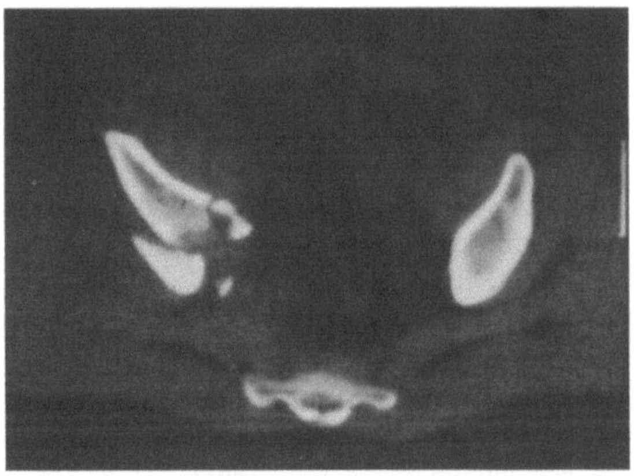
F

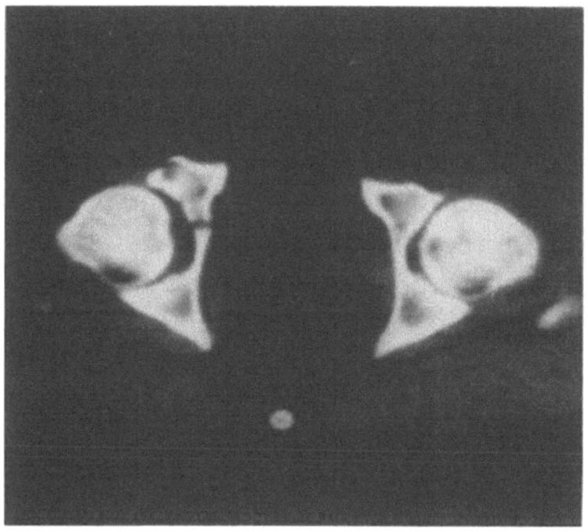

G

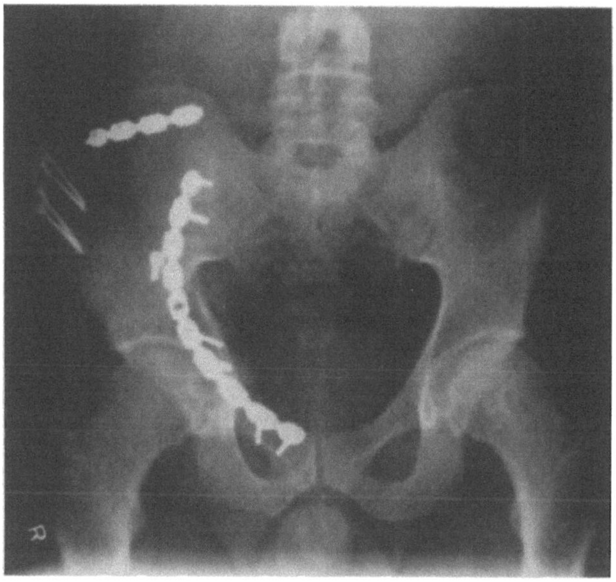

H

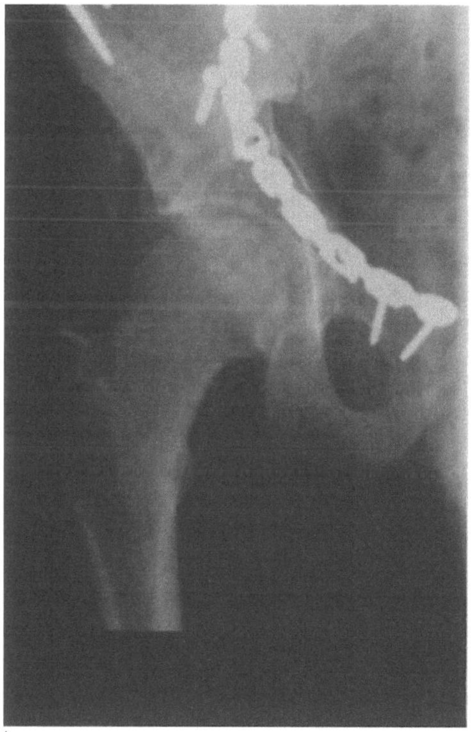

I

Fig. 5–37 Both-column fracture with two anterior column fracture lines. **A** Anteroposterior x ray. **B** Obturator oblique view. **C** Iliac oblique view. **D** CT scan shows exit of fracture through the iliac crest. **E** CT scan shows mid-iliac comminution. **F** CT scans through the superior dome regions show the both-column disruptions. **G** CT scan through the mid-acetabular region shows the T-component of the fracture. **H** Postoperative anteroposterior radiograph shows the anterior column plate and iliac plate with an iliac lag screw. **I** Close-up postoperative anteroposterior radiograph highlights the anterior column plate.

stabilized. The central acetabular region is then reinspected. Small voids (1 to 2 mm) along the fracture line are packed with autologous cancellous bone graft. The graft is impacted so that the material is unlikely to migrate into the joint space. The exposed surface of the graft is prepared so that it is about 0.5 mm below the articular surface. Larger voids can be obliterated in the same way. Great care is taken to impact the graft material. When large, free osteochondral fragments (greater than 1 cm per edge) are encountered, an attempt is made to restore the fragment anatomically. In most cases, at the time of reduction of the rest of the acetabulum, the free fragment can be accurately reduced so that it does not require supplementary fixation. Still larger central fragments are optimally secured using 4.0-mm cancellous lag screws. One or two screws are inserted through the appropriate portion of the pelvis into the fragment. The tip of the screw is buried in the fragment at least 3 mm away from the articular surface.

Extensively comminuted fractures may present with separation of the inner wall from the outer wall of the pelvis. Accurate reduction of the articular surface is essential. With marked comminution of the inner pelvic wall, the use of a buttress plate fixation is needed. Part of the inner wall is not accessible for plate fixation. Large amounts of cancellous bone graft are applied to these regions. Early postoperative active and passive motion exercises are encouraged, but in these instances a significant degree of weight-bearing is deferred for 12 weeks, until the comminuted zone has consolidated.

Impaction of the Articular Surface

At the time of injury part of the articular surface which bears the brunt of the injury may be impacted toward the inner wall of the pelvis. Generally the cancellous bone interposed between the inner and outer wall is compressed, without distortion of the adjacent cortical surfaces. As Judet and LeTournel first described, by using a narrow curved osteotome applied to the interposed and compressed cancellous layer, the inner osteochondral surface can be carefully elevated to restore congruency between the femoral head and the acetabulum. Finally, morsalized cancellous bone graft is applied to the cancellous bone to restore its volume to anatomical proportions. This technique is readily applied to a small, peripheral part of the acetabulum, although it becomes much more difficult to undertake for large, centrally depressed zones.

Osteoporosis

Ultimately severe generalized osteoporosis wholly precludes effective internal fixation. Preoperative radiographic scrutiny is crucial to determine the degree of osteoporosis, especially in elderly patients. In sedentary individuals more than 70 years of age, particular concern about osteoporosis is needed. If markedly osteopenic bone is evident, generally skeletal traction is the preferred method of treatment. In less severe cases, alteration of the fixation technique may be helpful. The use of larger screws greatly augments the stability achieved in osteoporotic bone. By replacing the 3.5-mm reconstruction plate with a LeTournel plate, 4.5-mm cortical screws can be used. Rarely, a 4.5-mm Dynamic Compression (DC) Plate is needed so that 6.5-mm cancellous screws can be employed. The larger screws provide a much greater risk for a screw to inadvertently enter the hip joint. Another supplementary measure is the use of methyl methacrylate cement to augment the osteoporotic bone. Dowels of cement can be inserted at appropriate sites in the pelvis so that the screw holes are prepared in the cement. Special care is needed so that free molten cement is not extruded into the hip joint. In the osteoporotic cases, reattachment of the greater trochanter is undertaken using a hook plate or a tension band wiring.

Postoperative Care: General Principles

When the acetabular reconstruction reveals the presence of extensive contusion of muscle or when considerable intraoperative bleeding is documented, bilateral split Russell's traction is employed for 48 hours after surgery. Otherwise, a passive motion machine is applied to the patient's bed in the operating room for the immediate initiation of gentle continuous passive motion exercises to the hip. Initially a 60° arc of hip flexion—of 20° to 80°—is undertaken. Subsequently the arc is increased by about 20° per day. On the first or second day after surgery the patient is encouraged to undertake bed-to-chair transfers. The patient undergoes physical therapy with active motion exercises of the hip and progressive resistance exercises of the lower extremity. Quadriceps and hip abductor strengthening exercises are particularly important. Within 4 days after surgery gait training as touchdown with the use of crutches is begun. Generally the patient is discharged within 1 week after surgery.

Serial radiographs are obtained 1, 6, and 12 weeks after surgery. Usually at the 6-week postoperative visit a 50% weight-bearing gait is initiated. Full weight-bearing is deferred for 10 to 12 weeks after surgery and depends on the degree of acetabular comminution and osteoporosis as well as the technique of surgical stabilization. Progressive resistance exercises are strongly encouraged for at least 1 year after surgery. Generally, when an extensile surgical exposure has been employed, a gluteus medius lurch is evident for 4 to 6 months after surgery. Supplementary exercise programs are helpful to overcome the muscle weakness. Whenever possible, swimming is initiated 2 to 3 weeks after surgery.

Clinical Results

A review of 97 patients with 100 fractures of the acetabulum managed by open reduction and internal fixation was undertaken. All of these patients were involved in high-velocity injuries resulting from vehicular accidents to pedestrians or passengers, motorcycle accidents, industrial accidents, sporting injuries, or falls from great heights. The average age of this population was 38 years with a 2:1 ratio of male to female patients. The age distribution shows a peak incidence between the ages of 20 and 40 years. Eight other patients presented with minimally displaced unilateral acetabular fractures and were treated nonoperatively with traction and early range-of-motion exercises. The latter group is not included in the subsequent discussion.

The distribution of acetabular injuries according to the classification system of Judet and LeTournel is presented in Table 5–1. In this series, 45 patients sustained other musculoskeletal injuries including fractures of the upper and lower extremities and spinal injuries. One patient presented with a concomitant femoral neck fracture which was treated with open reduction and internal fixation at the time of the acetabular reconstruction. Ten patients sustained a traumatically induced sciatic nerve injury. Eight of the patients presented with foot drop, and two of the patients had supplementary weakness of the gastrocnemius and soleus muscles. One patient presented with extensive macroscopic injury to the femoral head. Forty-five of the patients sustained a pelvic ring disruption which complicated their acetabular fracture.

TABLE 5–1 Classification of Acetabular Fractures Managed by Surgical Reconstruction

Fracture	%
Simple fractures	
Posterior wall	2
Posterior column	6
Anterior wall	1
Anterior column	1
Transverse	36
Associated fractures	
T-shaped	28
Posterior column + posterior wall	3
Transverse + posterior	3
T-shaped + posterior	2
Anterior column + posterior hemitransverse	3
Both-column	15

The pelvic ring disruptions included sacroiliac dislocations, sacral fractures, and various anterior pelvic ring injuries. Four patients had bilateral displaced acetabular fractures. Urological injuries were documented in 16 patients with 9 ruptures of the bladder and 7 urethral injuries. A vascular injury to a major branch of the internal iliac artery was documented by arteriography in one patient with bilateral acetabular fractures, an open diastasis of the symphysis, and bilateral sacroiliac dislocations.

At present, the average follow-up in this series is 5 years with a range of 4.5 to 8.5 years. The triradiate incision was used in all but eight of the operative cases. In the other eight cases, one anterior column fracture and one anterior wall and anterior column fracture were exposed using an ilioinguinal approach. Two posterior wall and four posterior column fractures were exposed using a Kocher–Langenbeck posterior incision. For stabilization of the fractures, reconstruction, LeTournel, and DC plates were employed with supplementary lag screws. The overall clinical results were assessed using the Harris hip scale system, which includes an evaluation of pain, function, range of motion, and deformity. The results were graded as follows: poor, less than 70 points; fair, 70 to 80 points; good, 80 to 90 points; excellent, 90 to 100 points. At the time of this review the overall average Harris hip rating for the entire series was 81 points. When examining this series with respect to the first 50 fractures versus the second 50 fractures, 65% of the first 50 patients had a rating of more than 75 points whereas 75% of the second 50 patients possessed a rating of more than 90 points. In an assessment of the simple fractures, 80% of the patients had a Harris hip scale rating of more than 80 points. Among patients who sustained a complex fracture, only 60% had a rating of more than 80 points.

The accuracy of the surgical reduction was assessed in a study of postoperative radiographs. In the first 50 cases that were managed, 40% of the fractures were considered to be absolutely anatomical reductions. In the second group 90% were considered to be anatomical reductions with less than 1 mm of displacement. Generally a poor clinical result followed an imperfect reduction. In addition, less satisfactory reductions were noted in the more complex fracture patterns.

There were no deaths during the pre- or postoperative period in this series. There were four postoperative superficial wound infections of the hip joint which resolved uneventfully. One deep wound infection was managed by serial débridement and intravenous antibiotics. Ultimately a hip fusion was successfully performed, and the drainage ceased.

No patients developed iatrogenically induced sciatic nerve palsies. Of the 10 patients who sustained a sciatic nerve palsy of traumatic origin, eight achieved a full spontaneous recovery.

One patient underwent a late loss of reduction probably related to an extremely comminuted fracture and osteoporotic bone. Subsequently, this patient was lost to follow-up and was considered to have a poor result. There were no nonunions and no cases of implant failure. In five cases screws partly disengaged spontaneously, although this was solely a radiographic finding without clinical significance. There was one case of avascular necrosis of the femoral head. This patient sustained a concomitant fracture of the ipsilateral femoral neck and was treated with open reduction internal fixation of both the femoral neck and the acetabulum. At the time of surgery extensive disruption of the capsule of the hip joint was noted. Following severe painful collapse of the femoral head, a total hip replacement was undertaken uneventfully. Approximately 8 months after surgery one patient developed early traumatic arthritis with marked limitation of motion and hip pain. His acetabular radiographs revealed residual displacement of the fracture fragments of more than 2 mm and marked loss of the joint space. Subsequently a hip fusion was performed without difficulty.

Ectopic bone formation in the periarticular area occurred in 60% of the patients. The predilection for ectopic bone formation appeared to be related to deferral of the surgery for 1 to 3 weeks after the time of the injury and to extensive pelvic comminution. Three of the patients had exuberant ectopic bone formation in the capsular and hip abductor mechanism which was associated with hip pain and substantial limitation in the range of hip motion. All of the patients underwent acetabular reconstruction about 3 weeks after their injuries by resort to an extensile exposure. About 1 year later one of the patients underwent removal of the ectopic bone followed by a course of disodium edriodronate. After surgery the hip rating of the patient improved by 10 points. In most cases in which postoperative radiographs showed evidence of limited deposits of ectopic bone, no clinical symptoms or signs have been documented to implicate undesirable side effects.

At present, 60% of the patients have been able to return to their original occupation. This group includes heavy laborers, carpenters, and patients who spend a majority of their time on their feet such as physicians and a pharmacist. The average time off from the initial accident to the return of gainful employment has been 8 to 12 months.

Discussion

A discussion of acetabular fractures would not be complete unless a comparison between the results of open and closed treatments is addressed. From previous reports in the orthopedic literature, the results following the use of traction employed to manage a simple acetabular fracture are moderately good. In such simple fractures where capsular attachments are spared, traction may permit acceptable realignment of the articular surface and a satisfactory outcome. Probably the best examples include a mildly displaced uncomminuted transverse acetabular fracture and some simple disruptions of the posterior or anterior column. In the presence of marked comminution of the central or dome region of the acetabulum, especially when there is extensive capsular disruption, the application of skeletal traction is unlikely to provide an anatomical reduction. A great likelihood for an unsuccessful outcome of treatment is thereby created. More recently, from the clinical reports of LeTournel and Judet[11] and Mears and Rubash,[22] by resorting to improved surgical exposures, reduction techniques, and fixation methods a variety of comminuted acetabular fractures can be effectively managed by operative techniques, thereby providing a 90% likelihood of a good or excellent result. From the series of nearly 700 cases undertaken by the former authors, it appears that patients who rapidly achieve a painless mobile hip following acetabular reconstruction tend to maintain the good result for many years.

Undoubtedly there is a "learning curve" for this type of surgery. The progressive improvement documented in the quality of the results attained by Mears and Rubash[22] in part confirms this impression. Provided truly anatomical reduction is achieved, even in the presence of comminution the results appear to be remarkably good.

The irony is the particular need and indication for surgery in the more comminuted and displaced fractures where the technical difficulties are more demanding than in the simpler fractures but where the results of nonoperative treatment are poor. If the acetabular fracture is accompanied by an unstable pelvic ring disruption, the results anticipated from skeletal traction are abysmal, so that open reduction and internal fixation of the acetabulum with internal or external fixation of the pelvic ring is indicated.

Following the use of an extensile approach to the acetabulum the most frequently encountered complication is radiographic evidence of ectopic bone formation (e.g., 60% of cases), although only 10% of these patients complained of pain or stiffness which could be related to the presence of the heterotopic mineralization. Avascular necrosis of the femoral head was documented solely in one case where a concomitant ipsilateral femoral neck fracture was present. A deep wound infection complicated one case (1%) and culminated in a hip fusion.

The acetabular reconstruction is most easily performed within a few days after the injury and before granulation tissue invades the fracture site. Previous workers recommended a 24-hour period of preoperative skeletal traction to provide a partial reduction and thereby simplification of the open reduction. In our experience, with the availability of more extensive surgical exposures and especially of improved methods of open reduction, preoperative or intraoperative skeletal traction is rarely of any significant benefit as a method to simplify the open reduction. Intraoperative skeletal traction provides a small (6%) but increased risk of iatrogenically induced sciatic nerve palsy. When reconstructive surgery is deferred for 3 weeks after injury, the technical difficulties encountered in an attempted anatomical open reduction are greatly increased. This surgical impediment is associated with poorer anticipated clinical results, generally less accurate reductions, and increased susceptibility to extensive symptomatic ectopic bone formation. The principal contraindications to an open reduction are osteoporosis and generalized comminution to a degree which precludes a reasonable likelihood of achieving stable fixation. In the presence of moderately severe osteoporosis and/or comminution, some modification of the surgical technique such as the use of larger buttress plates and screws is recommended.

With the innovations in acetabular reconstruction and the corresponding improvements documented in postoperative results, it seems that the present indications for surgery compare favorably with the generally accepted indications for surgery on other displaced appendicular intraarticular fractures.

References

1. Armstrong J. R.: Traumatic dislocations of the hip joint: review of one hundred and one dislocations. J Bone Joint Surg., 30B:430, 1948.
2. Carnesale, P. G., Stewart, M. J., Barnes, S. N.: Acetabular disruptions and central fracture-dislocations of the hip. J. Bone Joint Surg., 57A:1054, 1975.
3. Cauchoix, J., Truchet, P.: Les fractures articulaire de la hanche (col excepté). Rev. Chir. Orthop., 37:266, 1951.
4. Elliot, R. B.: Central fractures of the acetabulum. Clin. Orthop., 7:189, 1956.
5. Epstein, H. C.: Posterior fracture-dislocations of the hip. J. Bone Joint Surg., 56A: 1103, 1974.
6. Jacob, H. A., Nugger, A. H., Dretschi, C.: Mechanical function of subchondral bone as experimentally determined on the acetabulum of the human pelvis. Biomechanics, 9:625, 1976.
7. Judet, R., Judet, J., LeTournel, E.: Fractures of the acetabulum: classification and surgical approaches for open reduction, J. Bone Joint Surg., 46A:1615, 1964.
8. Knight, R. A., Smith, H.: Central fractures of the acetabulum. J. Bone Joint Surg., 40A:1, 1958.
9. Lansinger, O.: Fractures of the acetabulum: a clinical, radiological and experimental study. Acta Orthop. Scand. [Suppl.], 165, 1977.
10. LeTournel, E.: Acetabular fractures: classification and management. Clin. Orthop., 151:81, 1980.
11. LeTournel, E., Judet, R.: *Fractures of the acetabulum.* New York, Springer-Verlag, 1981, pp. 327–335.
12. Levine, M. A.: A treatment of central fractures of the acetabulum. J. Bone Joint Surg., 25:902, 1943.
13. Mack, L. A., Harley, J. D., Winquist, R. A.: CT of acetabular fractures: analysis of fracture patterns. Am. J. Radiol., 138:407, 1982.
14. McMurtry, R., Walton, D., Dichensen, D., et al: Pelvis disruption in the polytraumatized patient: a management protocol. Clin. Orthop., 151:23, 1980.
15. Mears, D. C., Rubash, H. E.: Extensile exposure of the pelvis. Contemp Orthop., 6:21, 1983.
16. Okelberry, A. M.: Fractures of the floor of the acetabulum. J. Bone Joint Surg., 38A:441, 1956.

17. Pearson, J. R., Hargodon, E. J.: Fractures of the pelvis involving the floor of the acetabulum. J. Bone Joint Surg., 44B:550, 1962.

18. Peet, M. M.: Fractures of the acetabulum with intrapelvic displacement of the femoral head. Ann. Surg., 70:296, 1919.

19. Pennal, G. F., Davidson, J., Garside, H., Plewes, J.: Results of treatment of acetabular fractures. Clin. Orthop., 151:115, 1980.

20. Pennal G. F., Massiah, K. A.: Nonunion and delayed union of fractures of the pelvis. Clin. Orthop., 151:124, 1980.

21. Rowe, C. R., Lowell, J. D.: Prognosis of fractures of the acetabulum. J. Bone Joint Surg., 43A:30, 1961.

22. Mears, D. C., Rubash, H. E.: *Pelvic and acetabular fractures*. Thorofare, N.J., Slack Inc., 1986, pp. 429–486.

23. Senegas, J., Yates, M.: Complex acetabular fractures: a transtrochanteric lateral approach. Clin. Orthop., 151:107, 1980.

24. Tile, M.: Fractures of the acetabulum. Orthop. Clin. North Am., 11:481, 1980.

25. Tile, M.: Pelvic fractures: operative versus nonoperative treatment. Orthop. Clin. North Am., 11:423, 1980.

26. Tipton, W. W., D'Ambrosia, R. D., Garrett, R. P.: Nonoperative management of central fracture-dislocations of the hip. J. Bone Joint Surg., 57A:888, 1975.

27. Urist, M. R.: Fractures of the acetabulum. Ann. Surg., 127:1150, 1948.

28. Vaughn, G. T.: Central dislocations of the femur. Surg. Gynecol. Obstet., 15:249, 1912.

29. Westerborn, A.: Central dislocations of the femoral head treated with mold arthroplasty. J. Bone Joint Surg., 36A:307, 1954.

CHAPTER 6

Management of Wounds of the Hip Joint

JOSEPH H. MOLL

Anatomically, the hip joint is deeply seated and well protected by the heavy musculature of the thigh and buttock; therefore wounds of this joint are relatively infrequent.

Less than 5% of all joint wounds involve the hip.[13,19] The relative infrequency of such injuries and the unfamiliarity with the devastating sequence of events subsequent to hip joint wounding all too often lead to inadequate initial evaluation and treatment. Results have been poor and the evolution of effective treatment slow[2,6,19,21] (Table 6–1). Exclusive of the events of armed conflict, wounds of the hip joint are infrequently encountered in civilian gunshot injuries and occasionally are associated with crushing or penetrating injuries in industrial and vehicular accidents. Despite their low overall incidence, they are very important injuries.

Ballistic Considerations

Missiles inflict damage to tissues by piercing, lacerating, and contusing the penetrated tissue medium. A traveling projectile develops varying magnitudes of kinetic energy owing to the velocity of the mass of the missile. The kinetic energy imparted to tissue upon impact is related to the square of the velocity of the missile. In high-velocity missile wounding, exceeding 2000 feet per second (FPS, Table 6–2), the magnitude of kinetic energy transfer to tissue is tremendous, and a peculiar sequence

TABLE 6–1 Missile Wounds of the Hip Joint: Evolution of the Results of Treatment

Time Period	Investigators	No. of Cases	Morbidity (%) Sepsis	Morbidity (%) Ankylosis	Mortality (%)
American Civil War (1861–65)	Otis & Huntington	386	—	—	85
Franco-Prussian War (1870–71)	Von Lagenbeck	132	—	—	77
World War I (1916)	British official medical history	—	—	—	60
World War II (1940–45)	Ellis	44	38.6	29.5	—
World War II (1946)	Carney, Fitts Kirby (China, Burma, India theatre)	11	100	45	18
World War II (1947)	Urist	29	33	75 (>25% hip disability)	—
Korean War (1953)	Thompson & Omer	24	68	54	—
Vietnam War—Brooke General Hospital (1965–70)	Moll	29	38	34	—

TABLE 6–2 Ballistics of Common Cartridges

Caliber	Bullet Weight (grains)	Velocity Muzzle	FPS 100 Yards	Energy Muzzle	Ft-Lb 100 Yards
Civilian rifles					
.22 (short, high velocity)	29	1125	920	81	54
.22 (long rifle)	40	1145	975	116	84
.220 Swift	48	4410	3490	1800	1300
.22 Hornet	45	2690	2030	740	410
.243 Winchester	100	3070	2790	2090	1730
.30 M1 Carbine	110	1980	1540	960	580
.30–30	170	2200	1890	1860	1350
.375 H & H	300	2550	2280	4330	3460
Military rifles					
M-16 .223 (5.56 mm)	55	3250	2869	1289	1004
M-14 .308	110	3340	2810	2730	1930
7.62 mm (AK-47)	122	2350	2047	1496	1134
Pistols (hand guns)					
32 Colt New Police	100	680	635	100	80
357 Magnum	158	1550	1380	845	665
38 Special	158	1090	1030	415	370
45 Automatic	230	850	810	370	335

Sources: National Rifleman, March 1968; *Shooter's Bible of Handguns;* and *Aberdeen R & D.*

of events creates extensive tissue damage.[5] A temporary pulsatile cavity many times exceeds the size of the missile tract, creating varying degrees of tissue injury and necrosis at some distance to the missile tract (Fig. 6–1). The secondary missile effect of bone fragments may penetrate vital structures, including joints. The temporary pulsatile cavity at subatmospheric pressure for exceedingly brief periods of time sucks in contaminants and foreign material from the exterior of the wounded extremity.[10] Missiles are also prone to follow erratic pathways after penetrating the body surface (Fig. 6–2). Wounds above the level of the knee and wounds of the lower abdomen and pelvis not uncommonly involve injury to the hip joint either by secondary missile effect of bone spicules or by fragmentation of the missile upon striking bony surfaces. A suspicion of hip joint violation must be entertained when missile wounds are apparent in these areas.[12]

In vehicular or industrial accidents where crushing or penetrating injuries of the pelvis are incurred, involvement of the hip joint may occur from displaced and penetrating bone fragments, particularly from the inner surface of the acetabulum. They are often associated with contamination from lower-bowel injury.

Evaluation and Initial Management of Wounds of the Hip

Clinically, a high index of suspicion of hip joint injury is indicated in penetrating missile injuries involving the thighs, buttocks, and lower abdomen. Clinical findings of interpelvic or intraabdominal injury may shroud the typical clinical findings of injury to the hip joint (Fig. 6–3). In injuries to the thigh and buttock, pain, tenderness, bleeding, and edema at the wound site are self-evident. Initial evaluation shortly after wounding may show little evidence of intraarticular involvement when one considers the classic findings of loss of hip motion, pain in the region of the hip joint, or referred pain to the knee. These findings are overshadowed by findings incident to the wound site itself. Seldom is good range of passive or active motion of the hip obtainable in the face of such injuries. Gentle attempts at hip rotation by the examiner may reveal signs of hip pain and confirm suspicions of intraarticular injury in the lesser-injured, alert, cooperative patient.

Systematic evaluation and treatment of the patient with a wound of the hip joint generally fall into three parameters: general, regional, and local.

General Involvement

Missile wounds of the hip joint are associated with massive degrees of soft-tissue and bone involvement. Extensive hemorrhages and embolic phenomena are not uncommon. The pulmonary effects of nonthoracic trauma are clinically manifested in a patient with a high-velocity injury to the hip or buttock who is restless or slightly obtunded. Low arterial blood oxygen tensions on blood gas analyses confirm the perfusion deficit.[15] It may take hours or days before confirmatory radiographic pulmonary opacification becomes evident. Treatment must be initiated promptly for adequate tissue perfusion and oxygenation. Adequate transfusion to restore blood volume is mandatory. Arterial blood oxygenation through adequate pulmonary oxygenation (whether it be by nasal catheter or pressurized through an endotracheal or tracheostomy tube) must be instituted promptly and continued until arterial blood gases reflect normal oxygen tensions in room air. Tetanus immunization must be undertaken in the combat patient, and toxoid boosters are routinely given. For civilian injuries, passive immunization and the initiation of active immunization should be instituted.

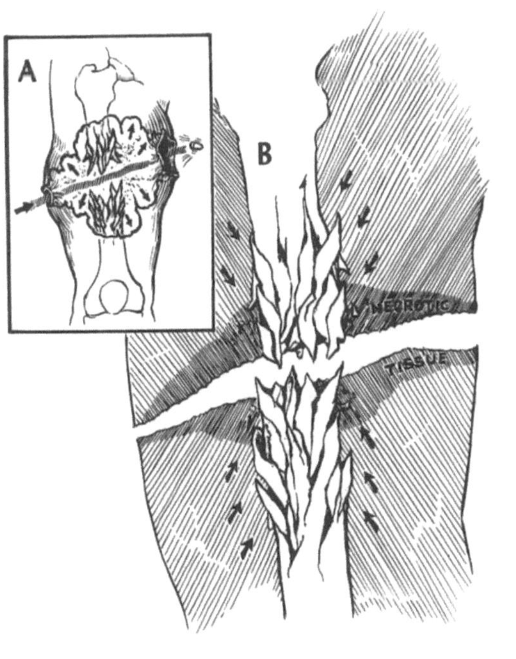

FIG. 6–1 A Cavitational effect of high-velocity missile wounding. Instantaneous centripedal dispersion of energy, missile fragments, and secondary missiles of bony tissue many times exceeds the magnitude of the wound tract. B Found at débridement.

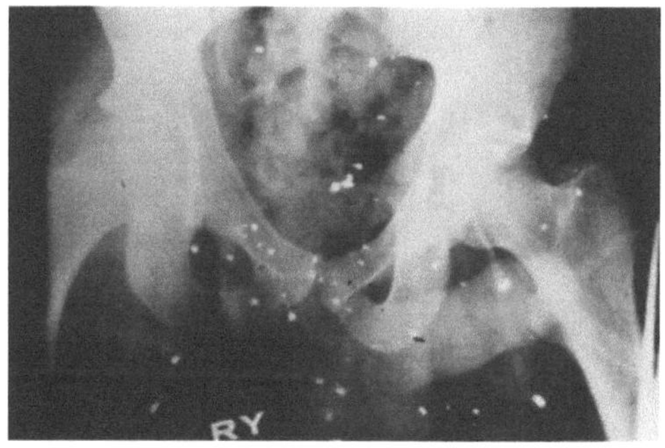

FIG. 6–2 Widespread dispersion of missile fragments violates the hip joint after initial penetration.

Regional Involvement

Injury to the pelvic viscera with penetrating injuries of the hip joint are frequent[19] (Fig. 6–4). Bladder catheterization and rectal digital and proctoscopic examination are indicated for evidence of urethral, bladder, or bowel involvement. X-ray examinations by contrast studies, cystourethrograms, and intravenous pyelograms are indicated and should be done at the time of initial biplane x-ray examination for evaluation of the osseous damage and spread of fragments. Diverting colostomy is essential for lower-bowel injuries with associated injuries to the pelvis or hip joint. Computed tomography (CT) scanning, when available, of the pelvis is an invaluable aid in determining the presence and location of intraarticular osseous or metallic fragments. Sciatic nerve injury occurs in approximately one-third of the cases of missile injury[2,21] and a brief but thorough neurological examination must be performed. Most important is concise and accurate documentation of the level of injury and the nerve involved. Failure to document initial neurological findings adequately often confuses subsequent serial testing when attempting to decide whether the lesion at time of injury was complete or incomplete.

Local Involvement

Local evaluation consists in thorough evaluation of the wound site and the hip joint. It is integral with the surgical treatment of the wound. The evaluation and treatment of an injury to the hip joint embody the principles of débridement and arthrotomy.[8,11,20] Adequate incision to expose normal tissue about the wound tract is mandatory.

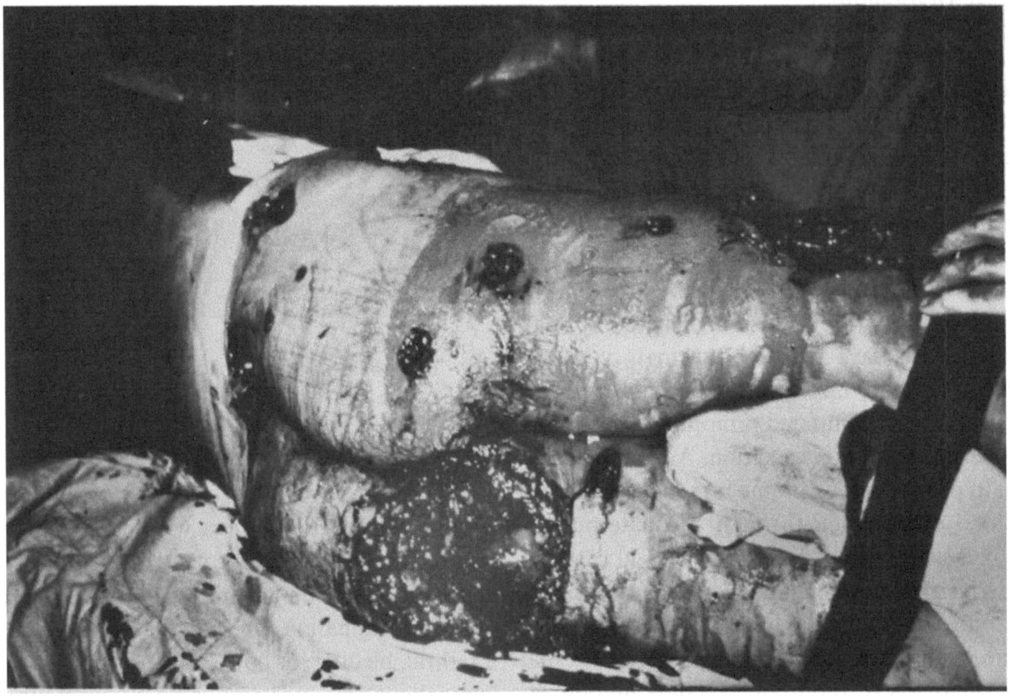

Fig. 6–3. Extensive multiple wounds from a mine explosion, violating both hip joints and causing rectal and bladder injury. Only systematic general, regional, and local evaluation can diagnose hip joint involvement with this type of wounding.

When investigating the depths of the wound through an adequate incision, direct involvement of the hip joint may be encountered (Figs. 6–5 to 6–8). An arthrotomy (including liberal capsular incision, thorough exploration of the joint to remove all particulate matter, and thorough lavage of the hip joint) is a necessary and direct method of evaluating the presence and extent of injury to the joint. If after thorough débridement of the missile tract hip joint involvement is not encountered but is still suspected because of the clinical findings or spread of missile or bone fragments seen on x-ray films, a formal hip arthrotomy through an electively placed posterior incision is indicated and should not be delayed to "see how the hip does." Only in this manner can the question of hip joint involvement be answered. The overlooked hip wound is the common denominator of sepsis, ankylosis, and permanent loss of hip function.

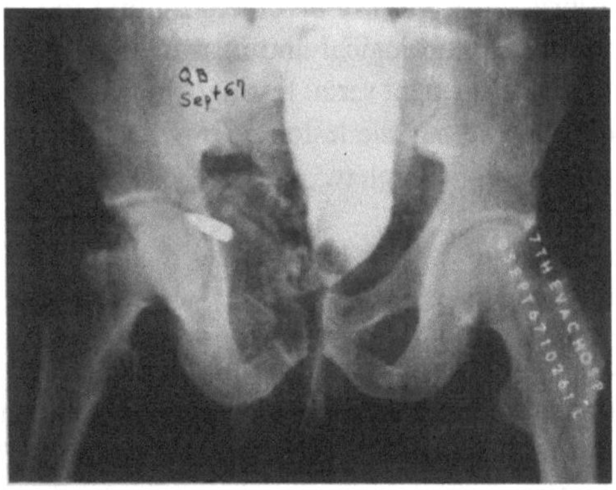

Fig. 6–4 Gunshot wound which entered through the lower right buttock and penetrated the pelvis, injuring the bladder and violating the right hip joint through to the acetabulum.

After initial débridement and arthrotomy, the wound should never be closed. Should the wound be extensive or posteriorly or perineally located, colostomy is performed immediately following débridement (Fig. 6–9). Rigid polyethylene catheter drains to the joint capsule provide better insurance against sealing off of wounds by the heavy musculature of the thigh and buttock than do soft Penrose drains. The wounds are dressed with gauze and fluffs, and the extremity is stabilized by skeletal traction. These wounds should be routinely reinspected no longer than 4 days after initial

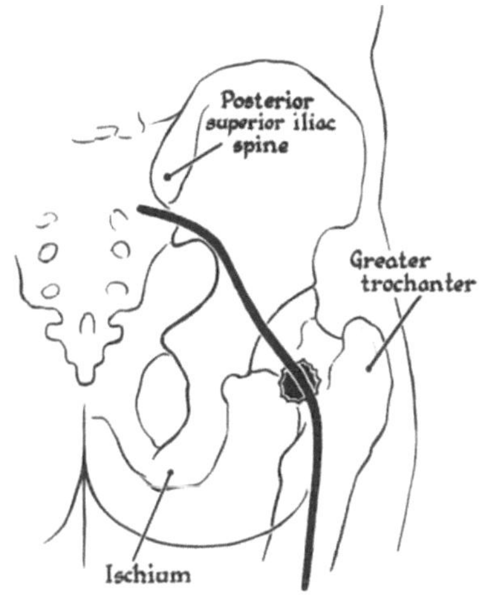

FIG. 6–5 Posterior gluteus-splitting (or, for wide exposure, gluteus medially reflecting) incision is utilized for elective arthrotomy or, with buttock wound débridement, for visualizing the hip joint.

wound surgery and at any time that bleeding, inordinate wound pain, fever, odor, or drainage develops. Surgical reexamination of the débrided wound is its entirety to ensure adequacy of débridement, lavage, and drainage is all-important to initial uncomplicated wound healing. Redébridement and dressing change are performed if indicated by the presence of residual tags of necrotic tissue within the wound.

Judicious delayed wound closure is performed only when the wound appears beefy red and healthy. The object of wound surgery is to obtain uncomplicated healing, and no physiological basis mandates wound closure 4 days after wounding. The wound is reexamined surgically as frequently as necessary and closed only when the wound bed appears healthy. Delayed closure over suction

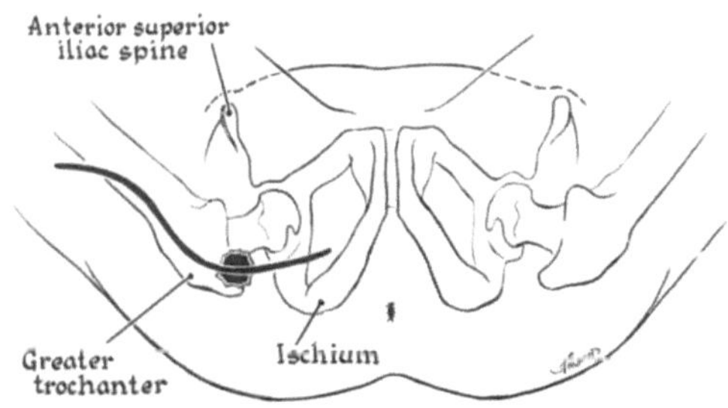

FIG. 6–6 Medial (Ludloff) approach to the hip joint utilized to débride lower quadrant buttock or medial thigh wounds and to obtain adequate hip joint exposure.

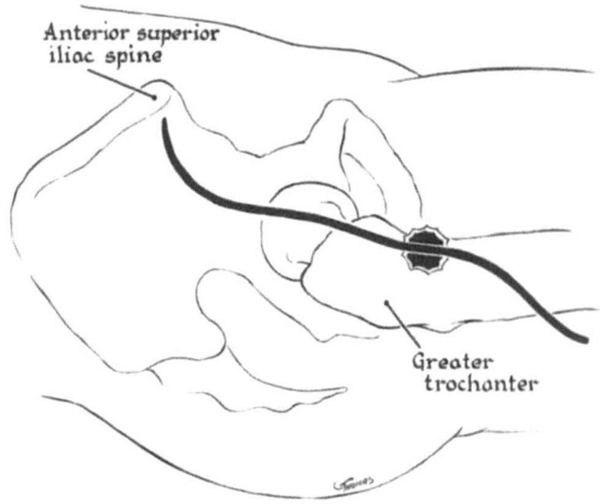

FIG. 6–7 Hip joint arthrotomy incision developed in débriding lateral wounds in the region of the trochanter. Approach developed in the interval between the tensor fascia femoris and the gluteus medius.

drainage has proved useful in reducing the formation of hematomas, but injudicious premature suture closure over suction drainage or suction irrigation has led to skin closure and healing over smoldering deep sepsis, resulting in joint destruction and chronic osteomyelitis, which greatly jeopardize later reconstructive surgery.[4]

Classification of Joint Injuries

A meaningful classification of joint injuries should contain both therapeutic and prognostic considerations. The primary therapeutic considerations are: When is a joint injured? What surgical ap-

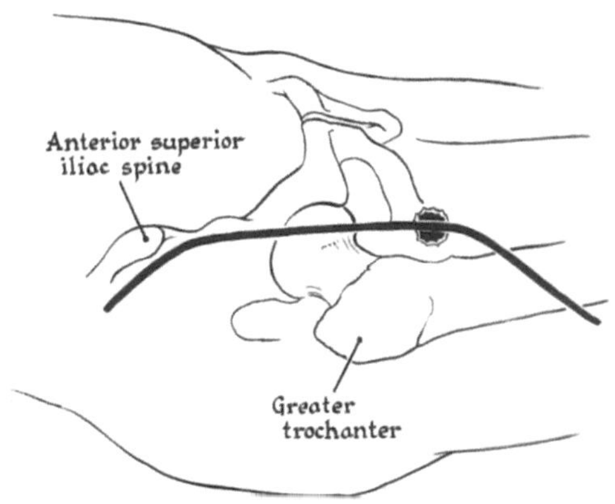

FIG. 6–8 Anterior iliofemoral approach used in débriding anterior upper thigh or groin wounds. Also useful in arthrotomy for anterior pelvic wounds involving the hip joint from the inner pelvic wall.

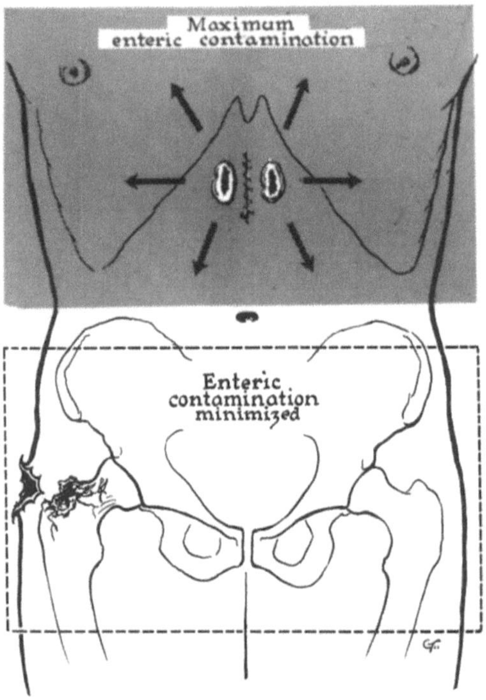

FIG. 6–9 Diverting colostomy placed as high as possible in the upper abdominal quadrants effectively diminishes enteric contamination of the perineum and buttocks and precludes fecal fistula development in continuity with the bony pelvis and hip joint.

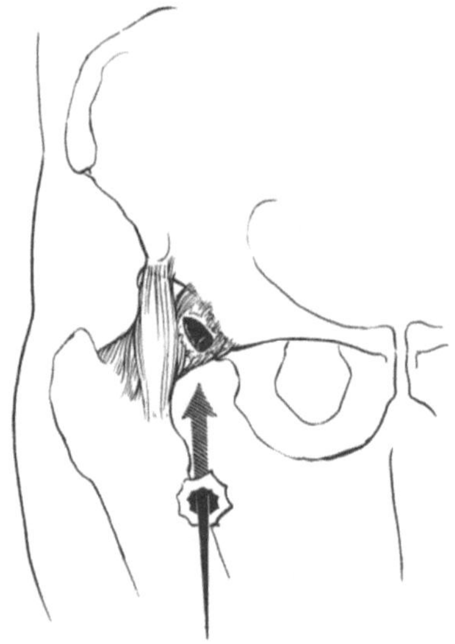

FIG. 6–10 No or minimal singular articular surface injury.

proach for arthrotomy is indicated? The prognostic implications should lead one to consider the techniques of initial treatment which best provide a basis for uncomplicated wound healing and which permit further reconstructive surgery. The following classification, based on that of Thompson and Omer, elucidates these factors[19] (Figs. 6–10 to 6–14).

Penetrating or Perforating Wounds with No or Minimal Singular Articular Injury

Penetrating or perforating wounds of the hip joint with no or minimal singular articular injury offer the best prognosis for functional recovery (Figs. 6–15 and 6–16). A wound situated in the anatomical region of the joint or x-ray discovery of foreign bodies in the region of the joint mandates wound débridement and arthrotomy. However, this type of joint violation may occur from a wound at a distance (thigh, buttock, or abdomen); and even though the display of metallic fragments or bone spicules on x-ray films invades the region of the joint, an optimistic wait-and-see attitude is all too often adopted. Deffer and Sellman have noted that during the Vietnam conflict, in a series of 85 joint wounds, only 10% of the hip joint wounds were treated by initial arthrotomy.[4] Vigorous and appropriate treatment of only the accompanying wound, including antibiotic therapy, masks joint sepsis until hip motion is lost and joint destruction is apparent on x-ray films. The slightest suspicion

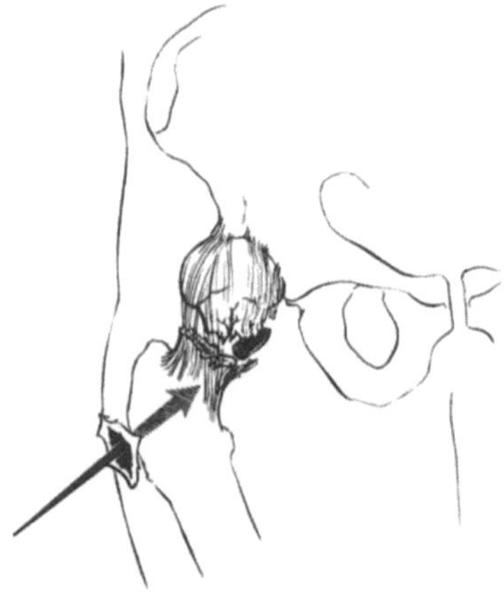

FIG. 6–11 Injury to the femoral head or neck.

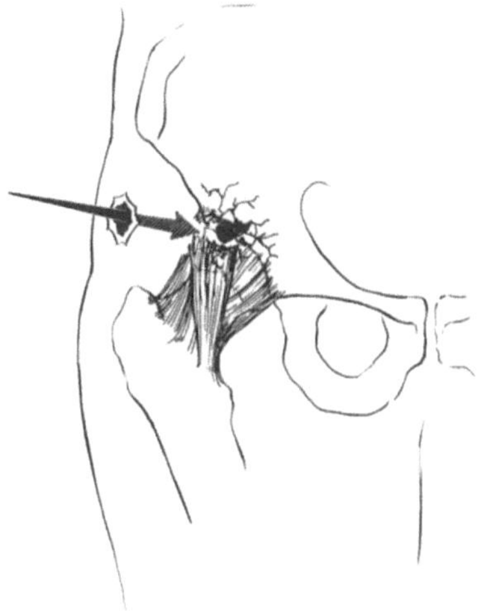

FIG. 6–12 Biarticular injury to the superior femoral head and acetabular surface.

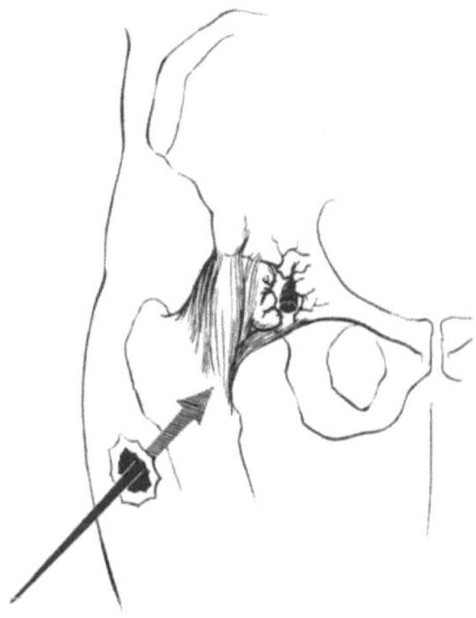

FIG. 6–13 Biarticular injury to the inferior medial femoral head and acetabulum.

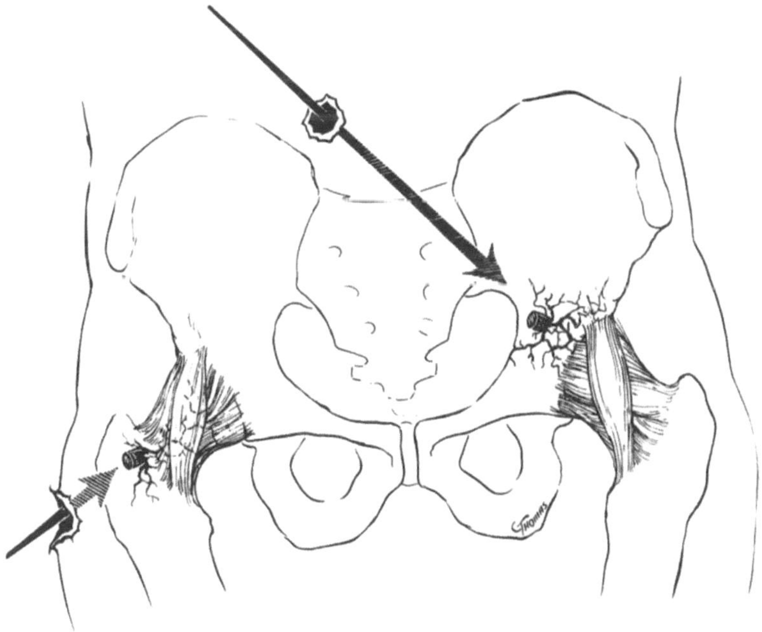

FIG. 6–14 Involvement of the hip joint from extraarticular missile fractures with extension into the joint.

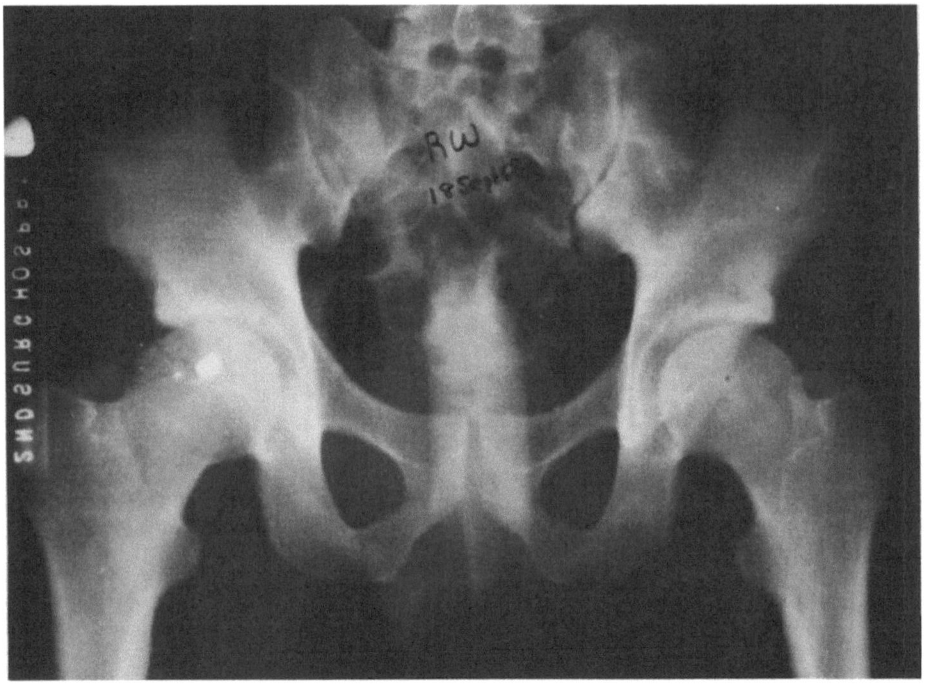

FIG. 6–15 Gunshot wound of the joint with a low-velocity missile round embedded in the superior femoral head.

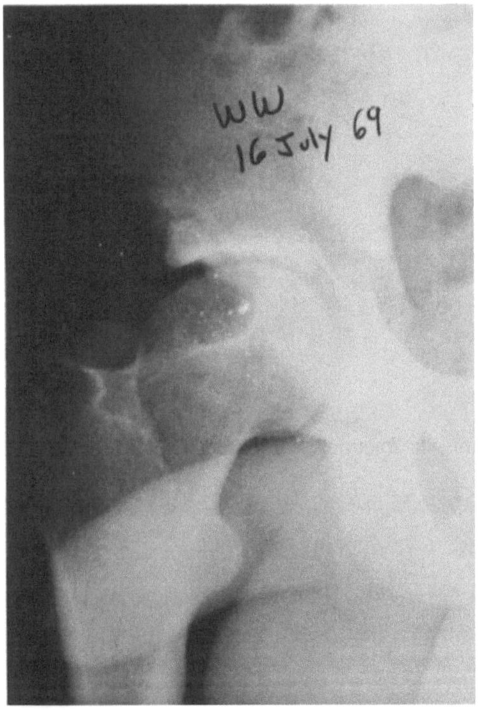

FIG. 6–16 Same patient as in Fig. 6–15. Normal hip function following arthrotomy.

of joint involvement by (1) localization of the wound on the thighs, buttocks, or lower abdomen, (2) the deduced pathway of the fragments based on the patient's position at the time of injury or the location of the entrance and exit wounds, or (3) even the suggestion of hip involvement by missile or bone fragment spread is an indication for a thorough formal arthrotomy.

Penetrating or Perforating Wounds with Singular Articular Surface Injury

Hip joint wounds with penetrating or perforating wounds with a singular articular surface injury are less common than biarticular injuries. They have a favorable prognosis for return of function, depending on the location and magnitude of the joint surface injury. As with all joint wounds, the optimum return of function is dependent on the avoidance of sepsis.

Isolated Femoral Head or Neck Injury Injury to the nonweight-bearing surface of the femoral head is compatible with satisfactory function (Figs. 6–17 and 6–18). Defects which compromise as

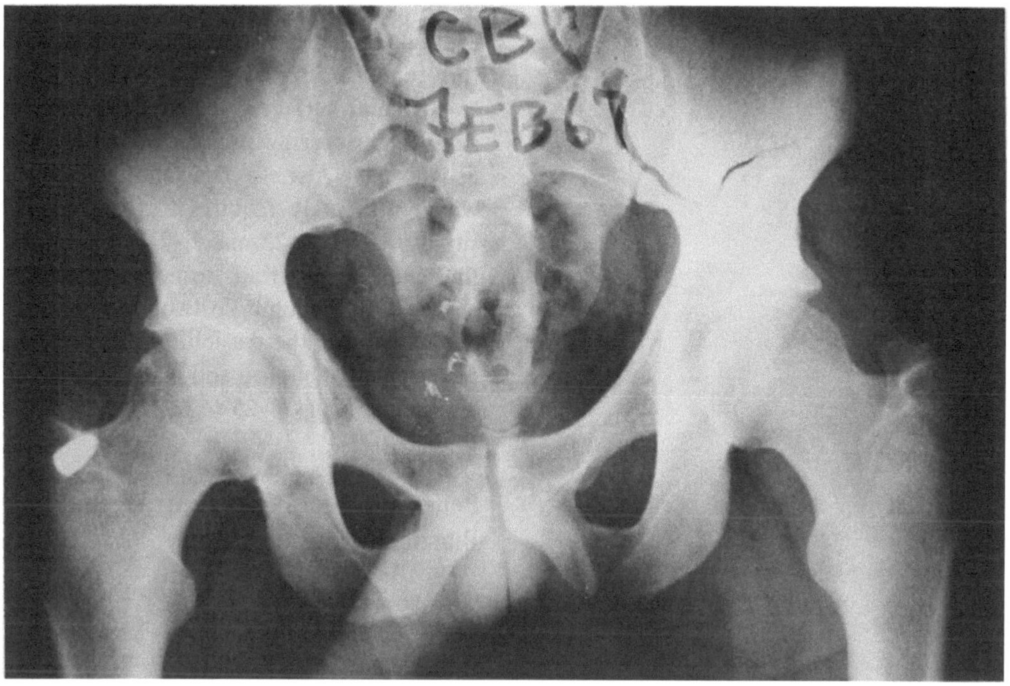

FIG. 6–17 Minimal articular and femoral head damage from a fragment wound. Cystic defect is filled with a corticocancellous tibial graft.

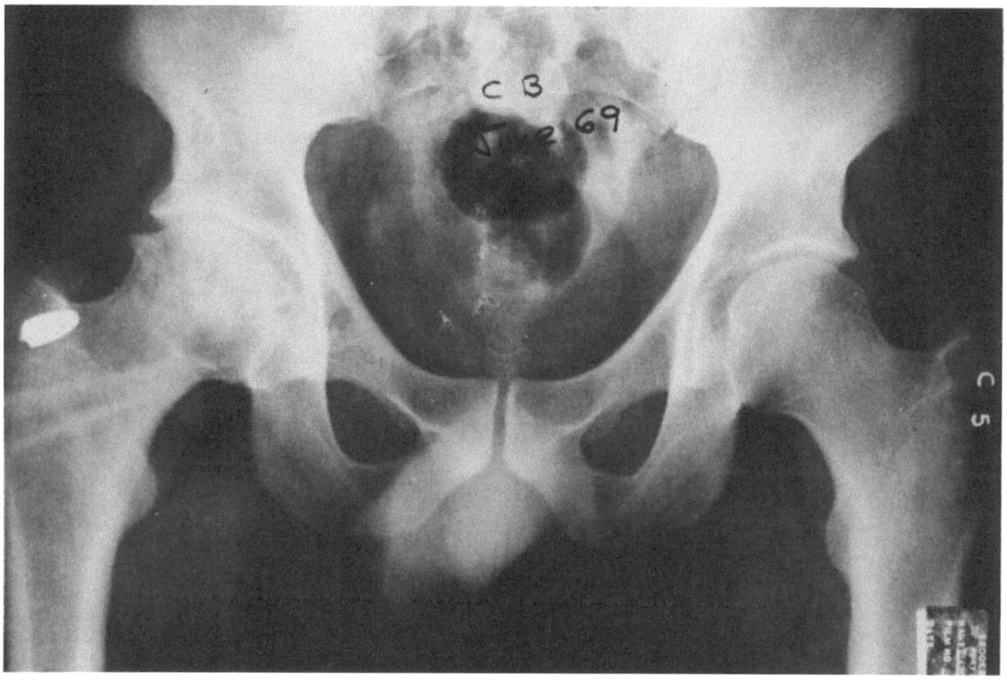

FIG. 6–18 Same patient as in Fig. 11–17. Full recovery of function.

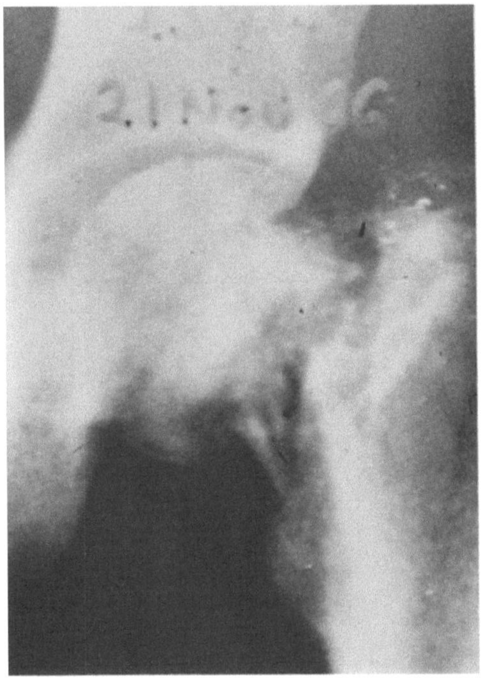

FIG. 6–19 Gunshot wound of the upper thigh with comminuted fracture of the femoral neck.

much as 40% of the femoral head on its inferior medial aspect are compatible with good hip function. Comminuted fractures of the femoral neck, sparing the articular surfaces, usually result in ischemia to the femoral head, but if sepsis is averted reconstructive surgery can restore satisfactory function (Figs. 6–19 to 6–22).

Articular surface defects on the anterior superior weight-bearing portion of the femoral head usually give rise to degenerative joint disease which ultimately requires further reconstructive surgery (Figs. 6–23 and 6–24). Comminution of the femoral head leads to necrosis, collapse, and ankylosis of the joint. Postwound sepsis, of course, severely limits the feasibility and success of any reconstructive efforts, and arthrodesis is the only alternative (Figs. 6–25 to 6–27).

Penetrating or Perforating Wounds with Biarticular Surface Injury

Approximately 50% of hip joint wounds produce damage to both sides of the joint surface. Prognosis depends on the location of the articular injury and the magnitude of the injury. Only relatively minor biarticular injuries are compatible with a return of satisfactory hip function.

Superior Femoral Head and Acetabular Surface Injuries This pattern of joint injury (Figs. 6–28 to 6–30) is associated with a poor prognosis even in the absence of postwound sepsis. The injured

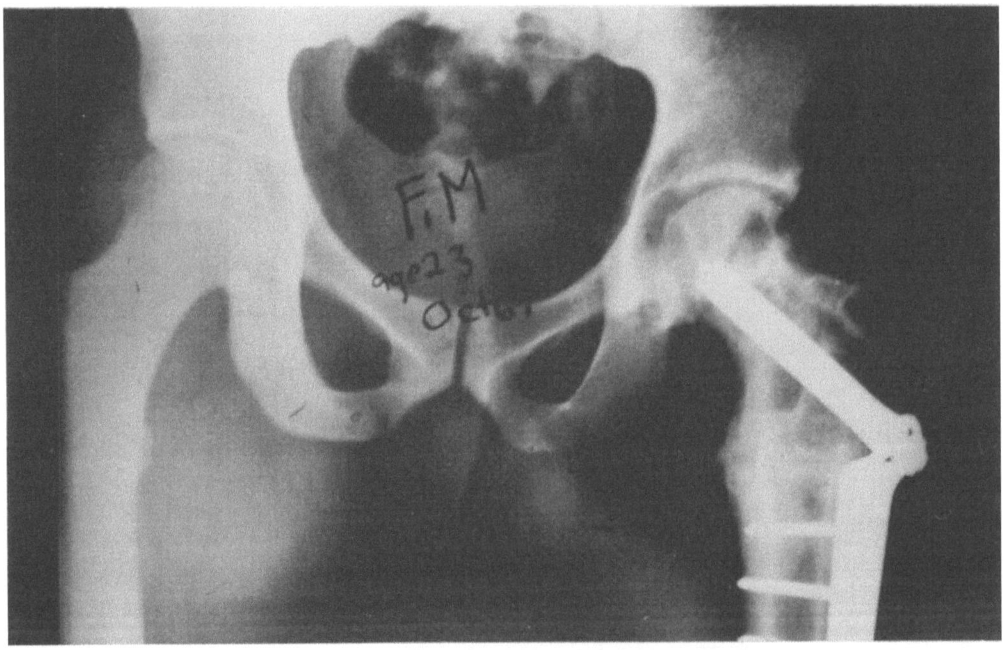

FIG. 6–20 Same patient as in Fig. 6–19. Uneventful wound healing following arthrotomy and débridement; valgus osteotomy and bone grafting followed wound maturation.

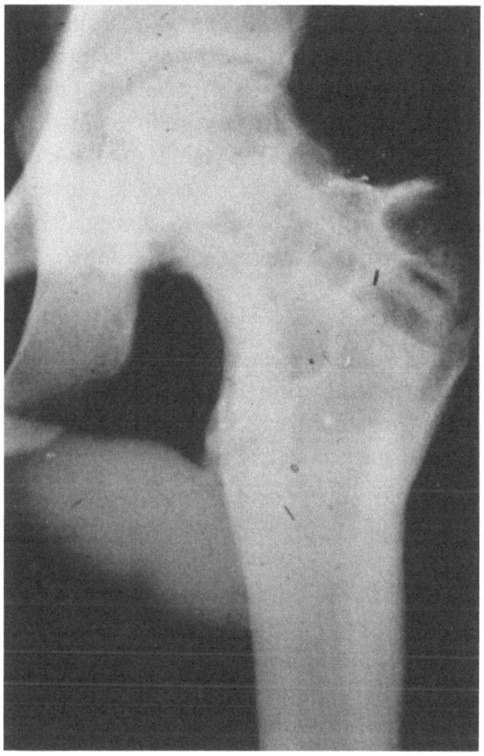

FIG. 6–21 Same patient as in preceding figures. Biopsy evidence of aseptic necrosis of the femoral head at the time of internal fixation removal, treated after tibial grafting.

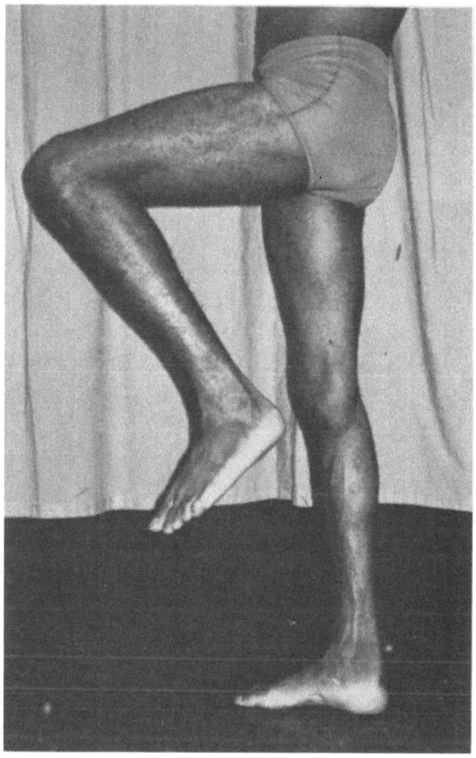

FIG. 6–22 Same patient as in preceding figures. Eventual full range of motion and good hip function.

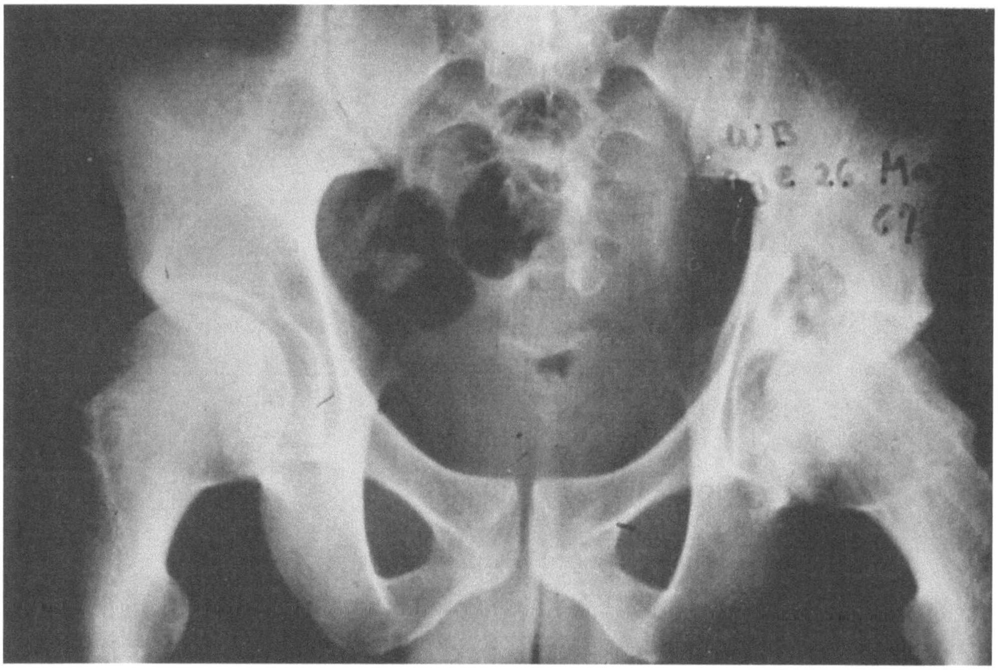

FIG. 6–23 Gunshot wound of the hip with uneventful healing following débridement and arthrotomy. Cystic defects in the femoral head are treated by tibial graft.

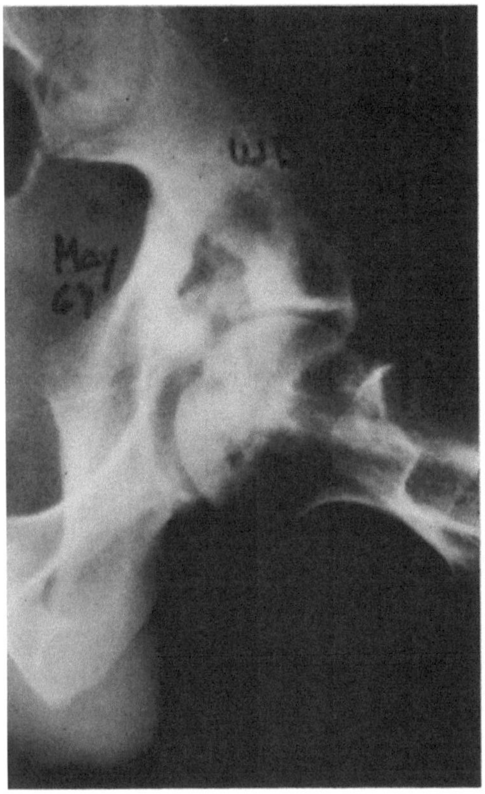

FIG. 6–24 Same patient as in Fig. 6–23. An acetabular cyst developed which will require further reconstructive surgery.

femoral head migrates superiorly and laterally in the acetabular defect. The joint is unstable and painful when weight-bearing is attempted. The hip abductor musculature or its nerve supply also incurs considerable injury, which further compounds the insult to hip stability. Abductor injury often precludes the prospect of hip arthroplasty, and such injuries have been managed by rather early arthrodesis after wound healing and maturation.

Inferior Medial Femoral Head and Acetabular Injuries Intact hip joints with this pattern of injury are much less common than those with superior joint injury. Patients incurring direct injury to the inferior and medial aspect of the hip joint in most instances also incur injuries of the femoral artery, femoral nerve, and/or sciatic nerve. Although vascular repair is often successful,[16] this pattern of injury has been noted in hip disarticulation amputees and occasionally in those with above-knee amputations resulting from unsuccessful artery repair (Figs. 6–31 to 6–33). Seven of the nine patients seen with hip joint and sciatic nerve injury at Brooke General Hospital from 1965 to 1970 had this type of joint injury, and one patient had femoral nerve injury. The prognosis for recovery of hip function is poor

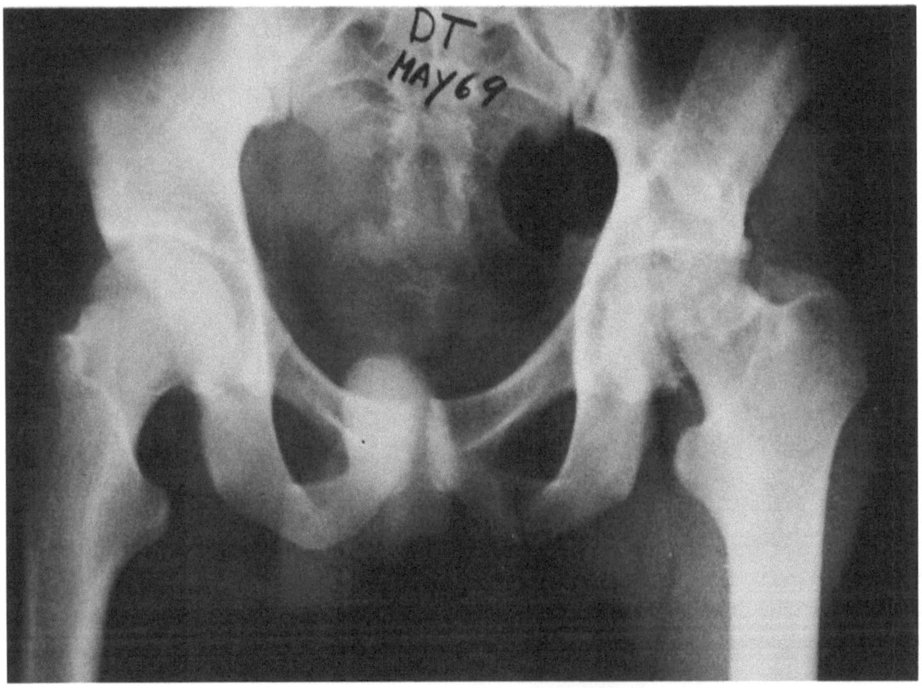

FIG. 6–25 Gunshot wound of the hip with superior femoral neck and head damage.

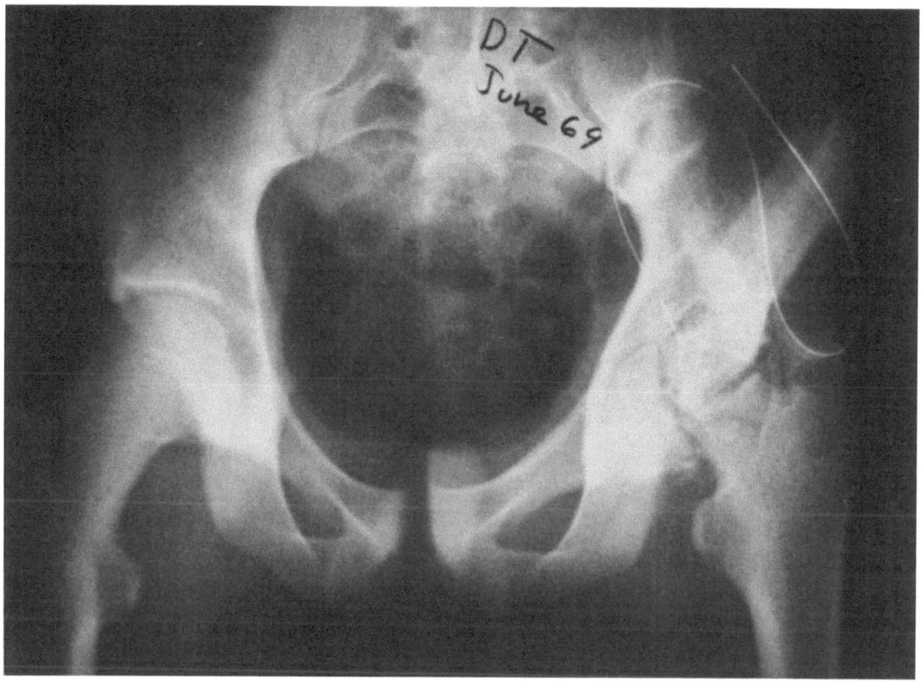

FIG. 6–26 Same patient as in Fig. 6–25, one month later.

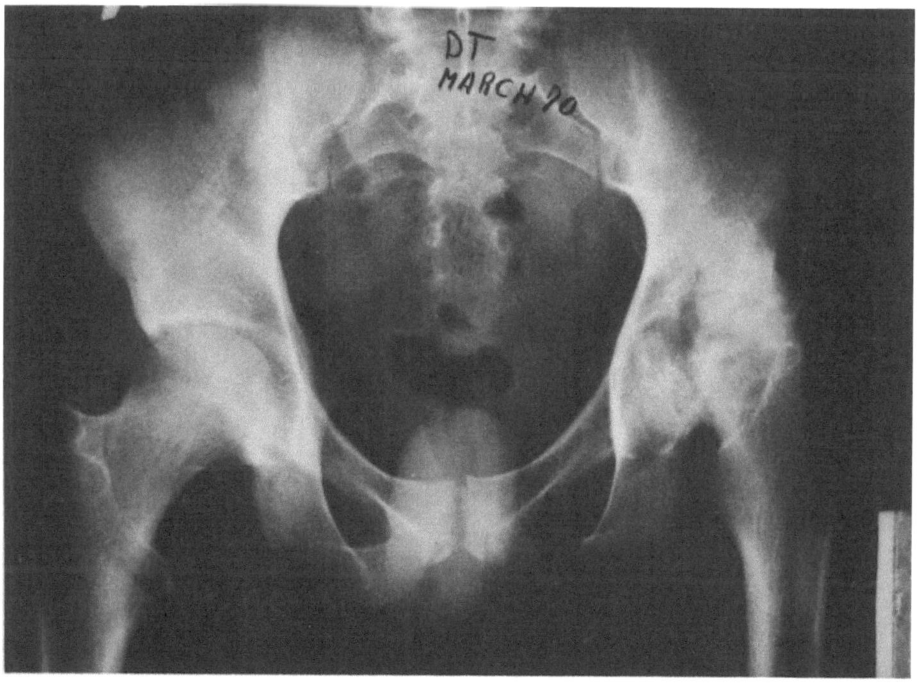

FIG. 6–27 Same patient as in preceding two figures. No formal arthrotomy, sepsis, and spontaneous ankylosis obtained in a weight-bearing spica cast.

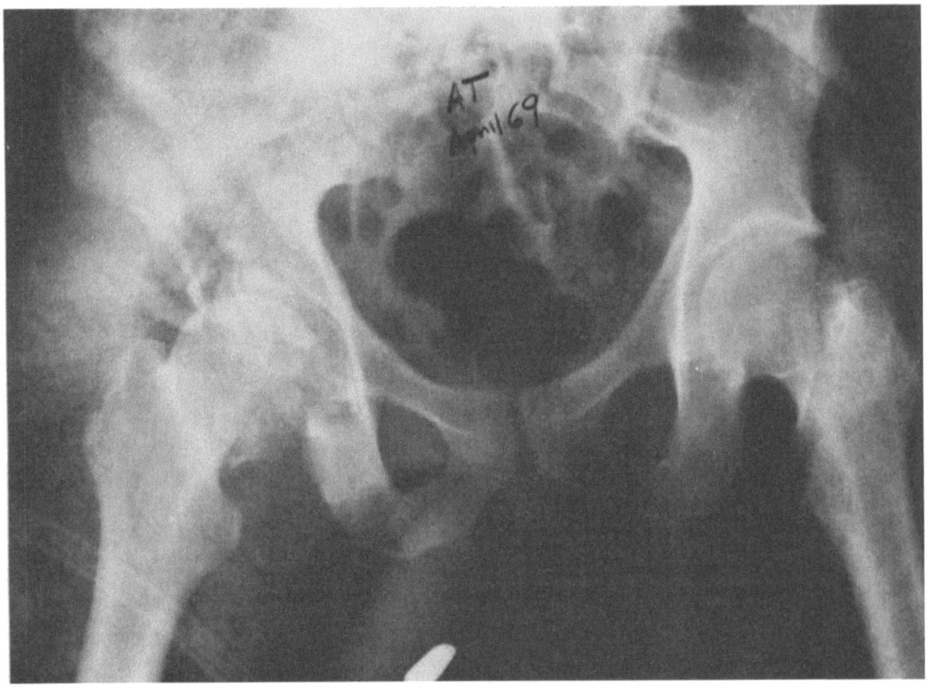

FIG. 6–28 Gunshot wound of the hip with extensive superior biarticular injury.

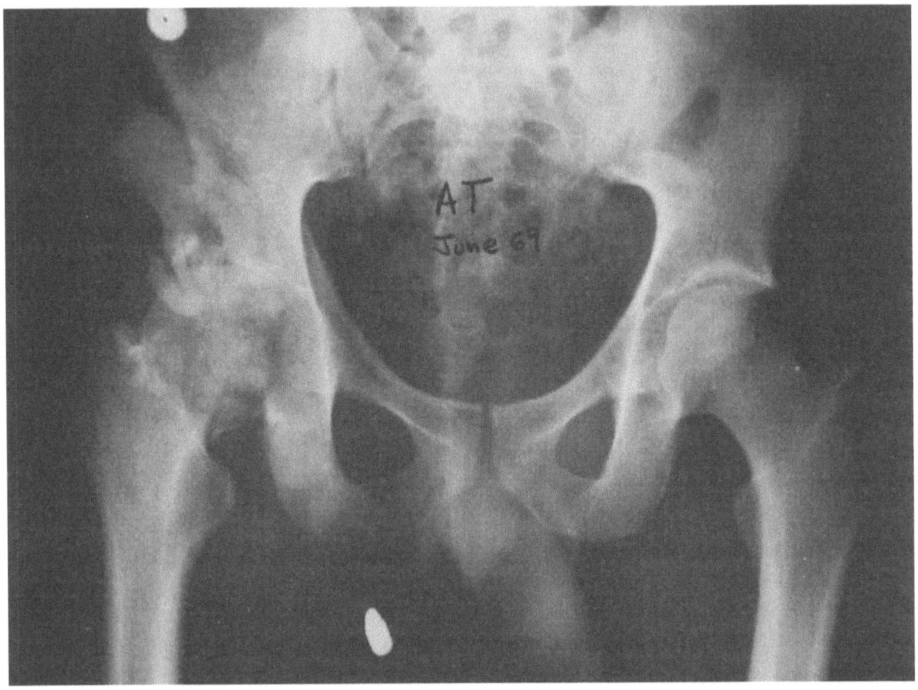

FIG. 6–29 Same patient as in Fig. 6–28. Uneventful wound healing.

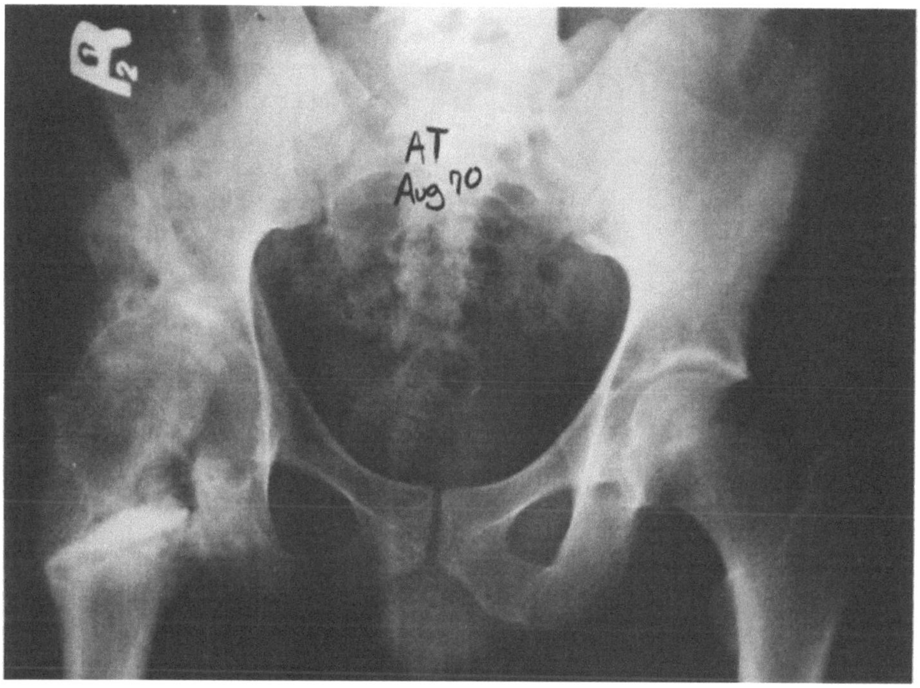

FIG. 6–30 Same patient as in preceding two figures. Superior migration of the femoral head with painful ankylosis treated by ischial-femoral arthrodesis.

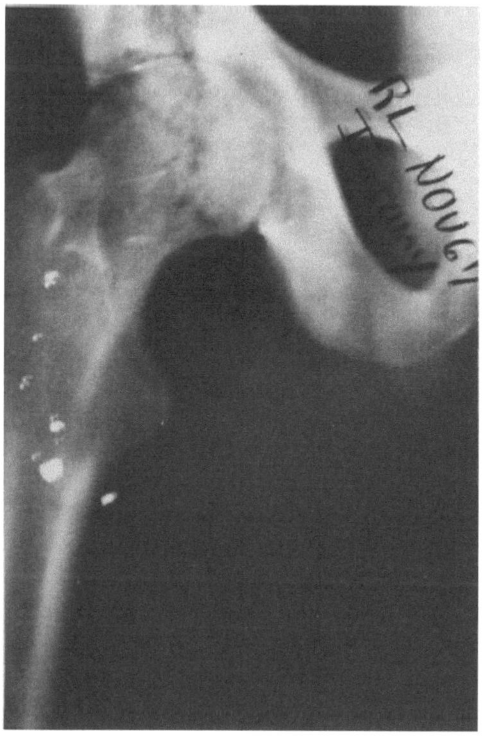

FIG. 6–31 Anteromedial high-velocity gunshot wound of the hip with femoral artery disruption and biarticular inferior medial joint injury.

except in the unusual minor joint wound which involves neither artery or nerve. Ankylosis or surgical arthrodesis has resulted in profound impairment of extremity function with sciatic nerve injury but in lesser impairment of function with femoral nerve injury.

Indirect Involvement of the Hip Joint from Adjacent Extracapsular Pelvic or Proximal Femoral Fractures

The prognosis for hip joint function with indirect hip involvement from adjacent extracapsular pelvic or proximal femoral fractures is generally good, provided the initial treatment is based on the recognition of joint violation (Figs. 6–34 to 6–36). Articular surface damage is often minimal, and the only appreciable threat to future hip joint function is postwound sepsis.

Adequate wound débridement, hip arthrotomy, diverting colostomy, and judicious delayed wound closure are the keys to success. All patients who developed joint sepsis and ensuing ankylosis in this group did so because these basic principles were not followed.

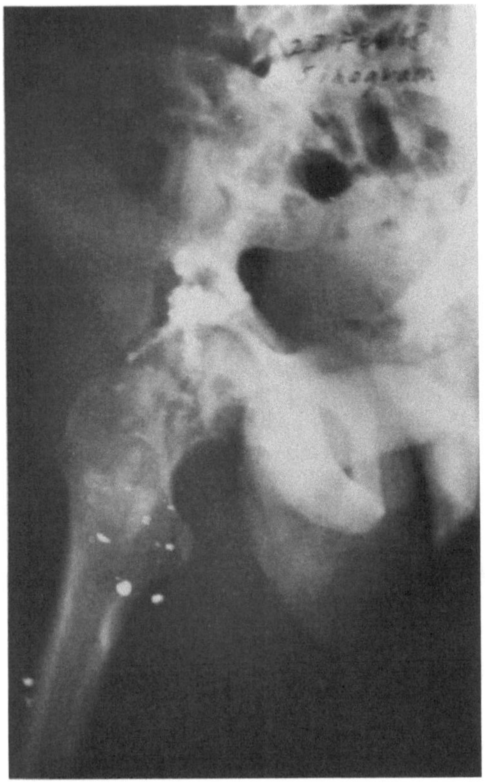

FIG. 6–32 Same patient as in Fig. 6–31. Artery repair initially successful, no formal arthrotomy; joint sepsis, arterial repair breakdown with sepsis and eventual above-knee amputation.

Management of Nerve Damage

Sciatic nerve injury occurred in about one-third of the joint injuries from combat missile wounds seen at Brooke General Hospital (9 in 29 injured, 1965–70). The principal factor governing the prognosis for neurological recovery is the exact anatomical state of injury to the nerve. The anatomical state of the nerve in a large contused missile wound in a badly injured patient are often not adequately determined and documented. An anatomically incomplete lesion—contusion or partial laceration—has a favorable prognosis for spontaneous, although incomplete, recovery of useful nerve function (Table 6–3). Only precise, correlated, concise documentation of the level of motor and sensory loss immediately following injury, the anatomical description of the nerve at wound débridement, and periodic documented motor and sensory testing during the months following injury can make this differentiation. Complete anatomical transection of the sciatic nerve at the level of the hip joint carries with it an extremely poor prognosis for recovery of useful neurological function even after the most meticulous elective delayed suture repair.[3] Certainly, routine exploration of the nerve at an early date in the postwound course, 4 to 6 weeks, without precise documented knowledge of the anatomical state of the nerve can lead only to surgical devascularization and further injury to some anatomically incomplete lesions. The nerve in apparent continuity embedded in extensive immature scar tissue at this time following missile wounding is easily devascularized in dissection. Attempts to resect the cicatrix within the nerve and perform reanastomosis may serve only to convert some anatomically incomplete lesions to complete lesions, with dismal prospects of any return of true useful neurological function. It is far more important at this time to restore joint mobility of the hip, knee, and ankle and to maintain flexibility and plantigrade position of the ankle and foot through continuous, appropriate, protective splinting and dynamic bracing.

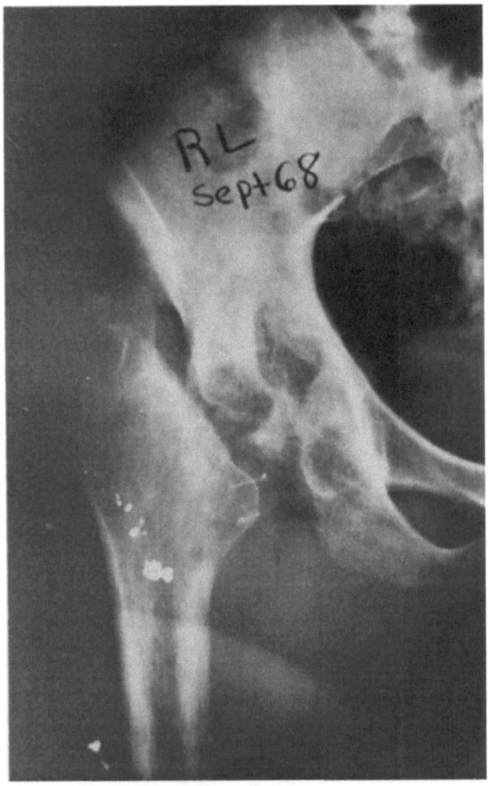

FIG. 6–33 Same patient as in preceding two figures. Femoral head and neck resection in treatment of extensive joint sepsis.

TABLE 6–3 Sciatic Nerve Injuries in Wounds of the Hip Joint: Brooke General Hospital 1965–70

Functional Severity of Nerve Deficit	Wounding Agent	Recovery Pattern	Time Period (months)
COMPLETE—two cases (no hamstring function)	Gunshot	1—Hamstring from 0 to good; tibial division from 0 to good; ankle plantar flexors with dyesthetic foot	11
		1—No return 10 months; exploration; nerve repair; no evidence of distal return 8 months postoperatively	18
INCOMPLETE—seven cases			
Peroneal division, 5 cases	Gunshot	4—Increased function from 0 to fair 1—No return	Av. 9.5
Tibial division, 0 cases			
Mixed division, 2 cases	Multiple fragment wounds	1—Increased function in tibial division; trace to good ankle plantar flexion with no peroneal return 1—Increased function from poor to good–minus, both divisions	12

When all of the documented evidence over a 6- to 8-month period points to a complete lesion with no evidence of spontaneous return of function distal to the level of injury, then and only then can an elective exploration and repair be performed on an extremity with mature wound scar, optimally mobile joints, and the sure knowledge that reconstitution of the anatomically disrupted nerve offers the only hope for recovery of any useful nerve function.[18] Resection of a neuroma to

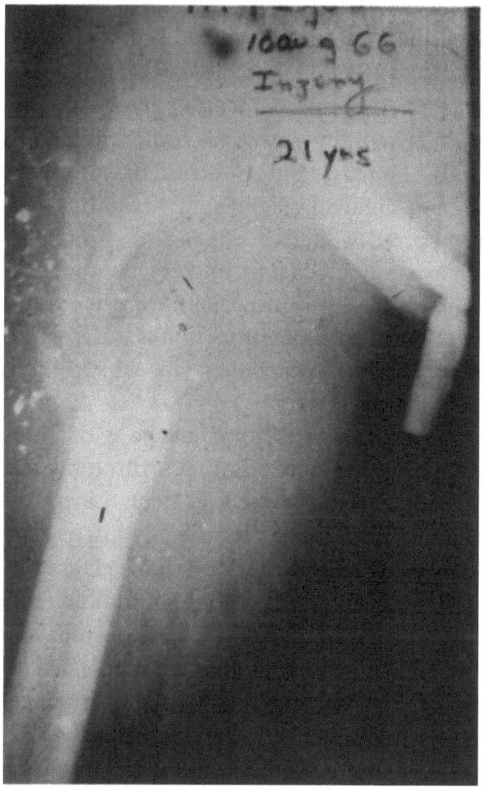

FIG. 6–34 High-velocity gunshot wound with involvement of the hip joint by missile fragments and extension from trochanteric fracture.

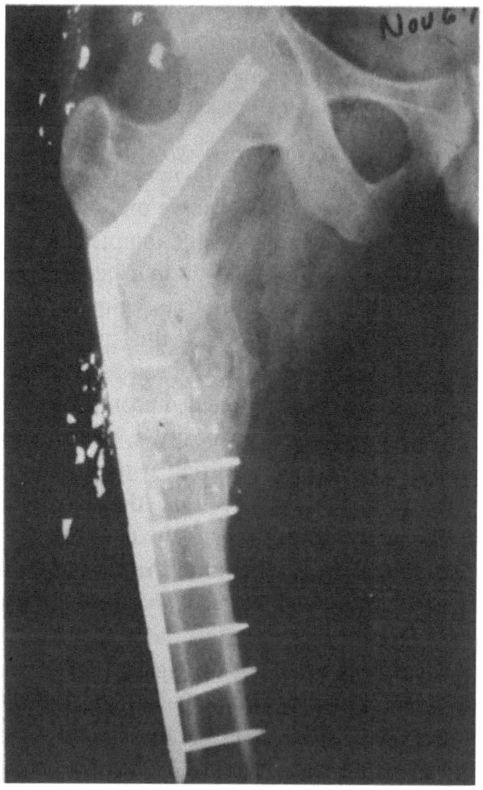

FIG. 6–35 Same patient as in Fig. 6–34. Uneventful healing after débridement and arthrotomy.

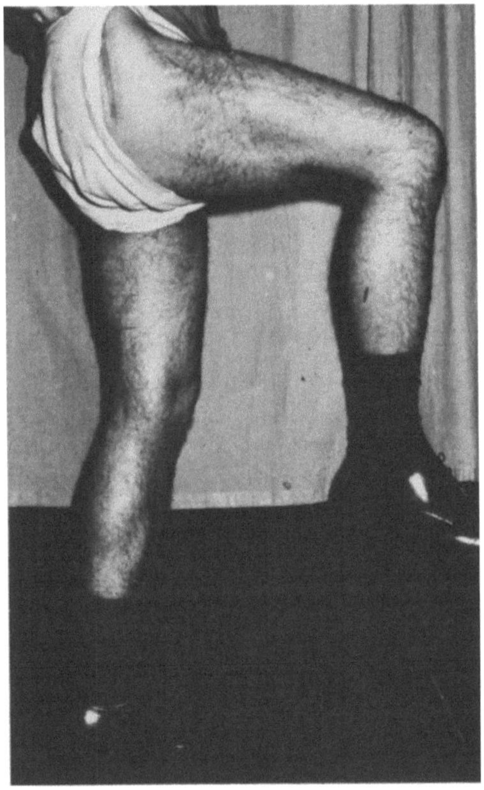

FIG. 6–36 Same patient as in preceding two figures. Good hip function following valgus osteotomy and bone grafting after wound maturation.

a level of normal-appearing nerve fascicles and end-to-end repair, gaining nerve mobility by knee flexion to 90° but resisting the temptation to dissect it extensively from its vascular bed, offers the best hope for success. If a large segment of nerve is anatomically disrupted, the prognosis is dismal.[3,22] Nerve grafts have been attempted but as yet have clinically not yielded promising results. Staged nerve pedicle transposition, sacrificing the peroneal division and suturing it as a pedicle to the proximal limb of the tibial division, with a delayed second-stage transfer in 6 weeks of this pedicle to the distal segment of the disrupted tibial division, has yielded occasional return of useful tibial division nerve function.

All surgical attempts to regain useful sciatic nerve function by repair are accompanied by periods of prolonged joint immobilization. The morbidity incurred from sciatic neuropathy is chiefly the loss of function below the knee. The insidious development of a rigid equinovarus deformity of the foot inevitably leads to trophic ulceration of the foot and ankle and eventual loss by amputation at some level below the knee. Both surgeon and patient must pay diligent and scrupulous attention to maintaining the plantigrade position of the foot and the flexibility of the joints of the foot and ankle as well as to protecting the skin. In the overall management of sciatic nerve injury, continuous appropriate foot care determines the morbidity regardless of the results of nerve repair. Syme's amputation, before ulceration of the heel pad or malleoli occurs, is an appropriate approach to rehabilitate a patient who cannot or will not engage in this prolonged, tedious care of the foot and ankle.

Antibiotics as Adjunctive Management in Hip Wounds

Joint sepsis indicates failure in the management of the hip wound. The basic principles of arthrotomy, colostomy, and delayed wound closure are requisites for success. Antibiotics certainly strengthen the effectiveness of these principles. Preoperative, intraoperative, and postoperative parenteral use of antibiotics has been proved to lessen the incidence of wound sepsis in major orthopedic surgery.[7] The choice of antibiotics depends on the environment in which the wound was incurred. Soil-borne bacteria such as *Pseudomonas, Proteus,* and *Clostridium* are the most common clinically significant organisms in combat-incurred wounds.[9] The use of effective agents such as aminoglycogides and cephalosporin is recommended. Cephalosporins are the agents of choice when soil contamination is not a significant factor in the environment in which the joint wounding occurred.

The advantage of joint lavage with antibiotic solutions at the time of initial arthrotomy and débridement are not clearly evident. Liberal use of large amounts of saline is probably just as effective. However, when 6 to 8 hours have elapsed before initial surgical care is instituted, antibiotic lavage with a polymyxin B/bacitracin/neomycin solution is recommended. It is also recommended at the time of the "second-look" after débridement to diffuse antibiotics with the same ones which will be given parenterally. The use of a continuous antibiotic suction-irrigation system in the treatment of the acute hip wound has not proved superior to the basic principles of arthrotomy and delayed wound closure, and is recommended only when

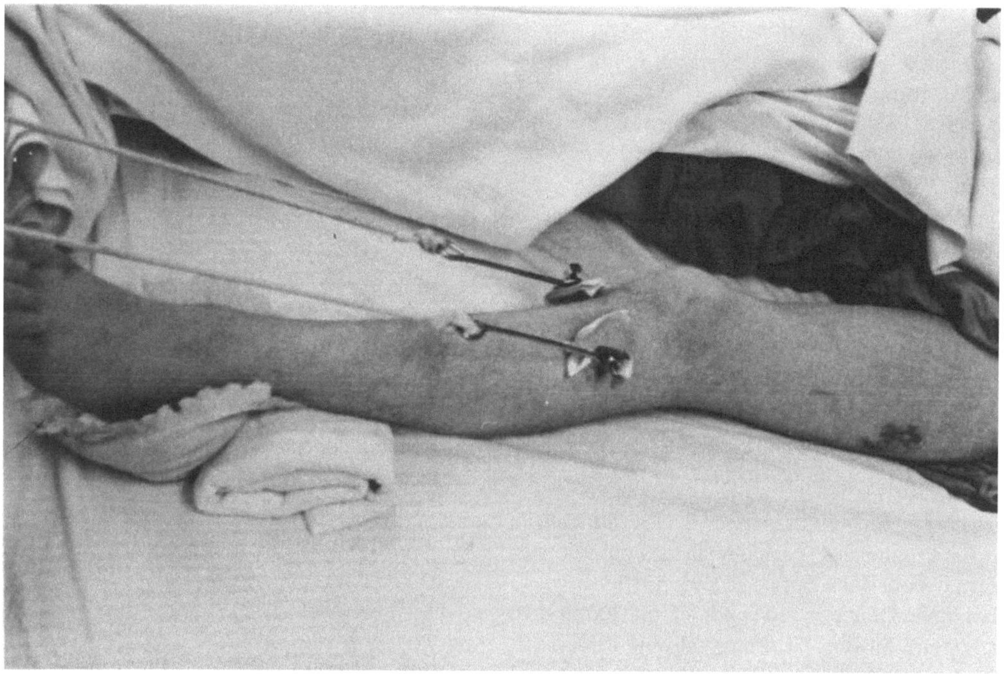

FIG. 6–37 Skeletal traction arrangement utilized after the acute phase of hip wounding (second or third week). Extremity freedom allows full assistive and active progressive range of motion to the ankle, knee, and hip.

treating established joint sepsis. Suction drainage can be employed during the immediate postoperative period.

Postoperative Management of Hip Joint Wounds

Wounds of the hip joint following arthrotomy and débridement are, in effect, traumatic arthroplasties and should be managed as such. Skeletal traction is applied to the extremity to maintain fracture reduction and allow early institution of supervised assistive and active joint motion. In cases of sciatic nerve injury, it is essential that the foot be maintained in a plantigrade position by appropriate well-padded splinting. A paralyzed ankle and foot should be gently mobilized several times daily through a full range of passive motion and the skin carefully cleansed and massaged. Extremity traction should be balanced and free from encumbering frames to allow comfort and maximum freedom of motion[14] (Fig. 6–37).

In the case of wounds incurred in combat or in instances where transportation of the patient over substantial distances is necessary, a one and a half hip spica affords the best method of immobilization. However, plaster immobilization time should be kept to a minimum. A spica can be applied a day or two before transport and carefully trimmed and relieved for safety and comfort. Patients with hip joint wounds preferably stay at the initial surgical treatment facility for several weeks until early wound healing is occurring and then are transported as expeditiously as possible to the final hospital destination; this measure minimizes plaster time and joint immobilization. Weight-bearing should be delayed for 3 months or until maximum controlled active hip motion has been obtained. Supervised progressive crutch-supported weight-bearing is then instituted, and ambulation progresses as dictated by the capability of the hip to increase walking time without pain. Periods of complete rest and light traction may be necessary during this phase of convalescence. Crutch- or cane-protected weight-bearing should be prolonged to a year or more so long as function is returning. Progress may be slow but in general continues for a year to 18 months.

References

1. Bateman, J. E.: *Trauma to Nerves in Limbs.* Philadelphia, Saunders, 1962.
2. Carney, P. W., Fitts, W. T., Jr., Kirby, C. K.: Gunshot wounds of major joints. J. Bone Joint Surg., 28A:607, 1946.
3. Clawson, K., Seddon, H. J.: Results of sciatic nerve repair. J. Bone Surg., 42B:205, 1960.
4. Deffer, P. A., Sellman, J. R.: Projectile wounds of joints. U.S. Med., Nov. 1, 1970.
5. DeMuth, W. E., Jr.: Bullet velocity as applied to military rifle wounding capacity. J. Trauma, 9:27, 1969.
6. Fischer, G.: Surgery one hundred years ago: a historical study (translated by C. H. von Klein). JAMA, 30:211, 1897.
7. Fogelberg, E. V., Zitzmann, E. K., Stinchfield, F. E.: Prophylactic penicillin in orthopaedic surgery. J. Bone Joint Surg., 52A:95, 1970.
8. Hampton, O. P., Jr.: *Wounds of the Extremities in Military Surgery.* St. Louis, Mosby, 1951.
9. Heggers, J. P., Barnes, S. T., Robson, M. C., et al.: Microbial flora of orthopaedic war wounds. Milit. Med., 134:602, 1969.
10. Hopkinson, D. A. W., Marshall, T. K.: Fire arm injuries. Br. J. Surg., 54:344, 1967.
11. Keggi, K. J., Southwick, W. O.: Early care of severe extremity wounds: a review of the Vietnam experience and its civilian application. Instructional Course Lectures, The American Academy of Orthopaedic Surgeons, Vol. 19; Chap. 12. St. Louis, Mosby, 1970.
12. Lucas, G. L.: Missile wounds of the bony pelvis. J. Trauma, 10:624, 1970.
13. *Medical Department, United States Army in the World War,* Vol. XI, Part One. Washington, D.C., Government Printing Office, 1927.
14. Perkins, G.: Rest and movement. J. Bone Joint Surg., 35B:521, 1953.
15. Pulmonary Effects of Nonthoracic Trauma. J. Trauma, special issue, 1968.
16. Rich, N. M., Baugh, J. H., Hughes, C. W.: Acute arterial injuries in Vietnam: 1,000 cases. J. Trauma, 10:359, 1970.
17. Seddon, H. J.: Three types of nerve injury. Brain, 66:238, 1943.
18. Sunderland, S.: Observations on the treatment of traumatic injuries of peripheral nerves. Br. J. Surg., 35:36, 1935.
19. Thompson, M. S., Omer, G. E.: Gunshot wounds of the hip joint. Surg. Gynecol. Obstet., 98:237, 1954.
20. Trueta, J.: *The Principles and Practice of War Surgery.* St. Louis, Mosby, 1943.
21. Urist, M. R.: *Battle Incurred Fractures About the Hip Joint.* Medical Department of the United States Army in World War II. Washington, D.C., Office of the Surgeon General, Department of The Army, 1956.
22. Woodhall, B., Beebe, G. W.: *Peripheral Nerve Regeneration Follow-up Study of 3,656 World War II Injuries.* Veterans Administration Medical Monographs. Washington, D.C., Government Printing Office, 1956.

CHAPTER 7

Soft-Tissue Lesions Affecting the Hip Joint

PAUL A. LOTKE

There are numerous problems about the hip which are confined to the soft-tissue structures about the joint and surrounding muscles. This chapter reviews the most common of these problems.

Transient Synovitis of the Hip

The most common cause of painful hip in children is transient synovitis. It is assumed to be a benign self-limiting condition afflicting children usually younger than 10 years. It is characterized by the abrupt onset of pain, limp, and limitation of motion unassociated with structural changes within the joint. It is important chiefly because it must be differentiated from more serious lesions such as Legg-Perthes' disease, tuberculous arthritis, pyogenic arthritis, rheumatoid arthritis, and other organic abnormalities of the hip.

Historical Background

Bradford and Lovett[3] in 1912 first described 25 cases of what they called "transient arthritis." They stated that the diagnosis was not tenable unless symptoms subsided within a few weeks and recovery was permanent. Since then, numerous reports have described this entity under various names: transient coxitis, coxitis serosa seu simplex, observation hip, acute transient epiphysitis, transitory synovitis, and toxic synovitis.[5,6,36,37] There were several older reviews on the subject by Rauch,[39] Lucas,[34] and others.[1,9,11,15,17,34,41,43] Drey in 1953 described the roentgenological features,[10] and more recently Jacobs[27] described his experiences with this problem.

Many etiological factors have been proposed for this entity.[4,5,11,13,15,35,37,41,42,44] They may generally be classified as traumatic, infective, allergic, and secondary to antecendent upper respiratory infection. All, in fact, may be causative, but to date, after several extensive reports of bacterial, viral, epidemiological, and immune studies, no one has been able to establish a definite etiology for the disease.[21,43]

Clinical Features

Transient synovitis mainly affects children under the age of 10 years, with an average age of 6 years. It is more commonly seen in male children with a male:female ratio of approximately 1.5:1. The true incidence of this problem cannot be estimated, as innumerable cases never come under a physician's care. Of the patients seen, only the more severely affected are hospitalized, and these are those most likely to be included in published articles. The onset of symptoms in most children is abrupt, and the presenting complaint is a limp, pain, or both. Pain is present in 85% of the patients. It is located in the hip in 75% and in the thigh or knee in the others. Night cries have been noted in many patients. Almost all the patients demonstrate an antalgic limp, and most show limitation of motion, usually in extension and internal rotation. In approximately half the patients, the hip assumes the position of flexion, external rotation, and slight abduction when the patient is lying down. These same patients have an abnormal stance characteristic of hip flexion contraction. A few demonstrate thigh atrophy. Occasionally there is tenderness over Scarpa's triangle.

Laboratory data have been included in most reports of synovitis of the hip. Routine blood tests, urinalysis, erythrocyte sedimentation rates, tuberculin skin tests, throat cultures, and miscellaneous agglutination tests and viral studies have been reported. Occasionally there is mild leukocytosis (to 12,000/mm^3) and a low-grade fever (to 38°C). In general, the laboratory studies are within normal limits and are mainly useful to help rule out other conditions.

Roentgenographic Findings

A two-view x-ray study, including the normal side, must be obtained for all patients. The main purpose is to exclude conditions such as Legg-Perthes' disease from the diagnosis. By definition, there should be no bony abnormalities. In 60% of the patients there are abnormal soft-tissue shadows, indicating inflammation about the hip.[22,23] Drey[10] showed that the gluteus minimus, the obturator internus, and the iliopsoas muscles were thickened, with disappearance or blurring of the adjacent intermuscular septa and increased haziness and density of the muscles. He noted a radiolucent streak along the inferior capsule (positive iliopsoas sign) in most of his cases. Another common x-ray finding is a widening of the medial joint space[49] (Waldenström's sign) believed to be caused by synovial thickening with lateral displacement of the femoral head. In addition, capsular swelling can be noted on the lateral aspect of the joint. It is important to realize that the soft-tissue abnormalities vary with the quality of the film and that the appearance of the abnormality can be altered by a slight change in the position of the involved extremity.

Clinical Course and Treatment

By definition, the symptoms are transient, usually subsiding within 3 to 21 days. Treatment is directed toward prevention of weight-bearing and restriction of activity. Traction is avoided, especially Buck's traction, as internal rotation and extension may increase the intracapsular pressures and compromise blood flow to the head. In the few instances when traction is utilized to assist in controlling an active child, it is applied lightly in the line of his deformity. Patients should not resume weight-bearing until they become asymptomatic, demonstrate a normal gait, and show no limitation of motion. Although complete prevention of weight-bearing is often difficult to achieve, it appears to have definite therapeutic value. Jacobs[27] demonstrated a prolongation of clinical course in those patients who failed to abstain from weight-bearing.

Follow-up roentgenograms are obtained to rule out the development of Legg-Perthes' disease.[12,14,29,31,49] It has been shown that 6% of patients with transient synovitis of the hip develop this problem. Those patients with recurrent or persistent synovitis especially should be closely followed, and all patients should have follow-up examinations for at least 18 months, as Legg-Perthes' disease may develop at any time within that interval.[38]

Differential Diagnosis

An early correct diagnosis is important to ensure optimal treatment and exclude other, more serious entities that might require specialized therapy. The differential diagnosis includes Legg-Perthes' disease, tuberculous arthritis, osteomyelitis, septic arthritis, rheumatoid arthritis, rheumatic fever, osteoid osteoma, syphilis, and slipped capital femoral epiphysis.

The roentgenographic findings are paramount in differentiating between Legg-Perthes' disease and transient synovitis. The earliest x-ray findings in Legg-Perthes' disease are flattening of the lateral side of the upper femoral epiphysis,[48] Waldenström's sign (Fig. 7–1), and narrowing of the transverse diameter of the obturator foramina on the affected side. Later findings include sclerotic changes in the capital epiphysis, possibly progressing to mottling and fragmentation. Some authorities believe that transient synovitis is an initiating factor in the development of Legg-Perthes' disease. The possible etiological relation between the two diseases is based on the facts that at the onset the diseases have similar clinical pictures and, occasionally, transient synovitis precedes Legg-Perthes' disease. However, it is difficult to ascribe a definite etiological relation to these two entities.

When differentiating tuberculous arthritis, it is important to obtain a history of exposure to the disease. The tuberculin test is positive, and the x-ray findings may show early bone atrophy or destructive areas in marginal lesions adjacent to the epiphyseal line.

Osteomyelitis and septic arthritis can be differentiated by the persistence of signs and symptoms

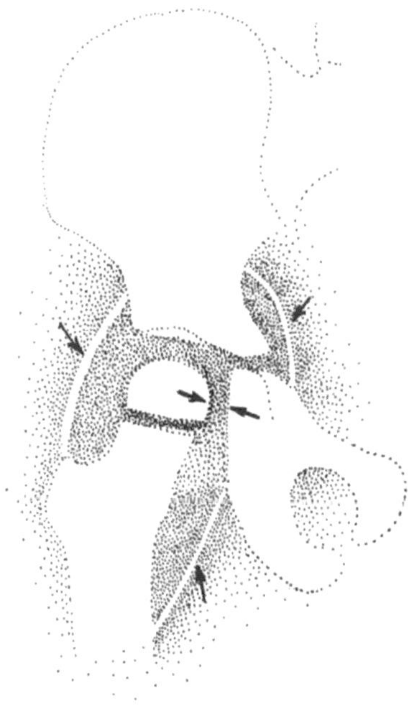

FIG. 7–1 Transient synovitis of the hip may show subtle x-ray changes (*arrows*) including widening of the medial joint space (Waldenström's sign), thickening of the obturator internus muscle shadow, and bulging of radiolucent streaks along the inferior and lateral aspects of the capsule.

of infection, both locally and systematically. The pain is usually more severe, with tenderness over Scarpa's triangle; fever and leukocytosis are usually apparent. X-ray films may show hyperemic deossification of the bone and later destructive changes.

Juvenile rheumatoid arthritis and rheumatic fever may be difficult to differentiate from each other, but they can be distinguished from transient synovitis. There is usually a history of previous upper respiratory infection or prior joint involvement, and fever, rash, and multiple joint involvement are frequently seen. Symptoms usually last more than 12 weeks in juvenile rheumatoid arthritis. The monoarticular presentation of juvenile rheumatoid arthritis is difficult to rule out during the first episode; however, the monoarticular disease most commonly appears in the knee and rarely in the hip.

Syphilis is rare; it can be excluded by searching for other stigmata, including serology. The x-ray findings of the luetic bone include metaphyseal periostitis and juxtaepiphyseal osteochondritis or erosions; these findings are usually diagnostic.

In slipped capital femoral epiphysis the x-ray findings are diagnostic. Good lateral x-ray studies are important, as the slip may not be apparent in one view. Statistically, there is a tendency for slipped capital epiphysis to occur in older children.

Miscellaneous Soft-Tissue Lesions

Numerous soft-tissue lesions affect the hip and frequently cause pain and disability. It is important to be able to recognize and differentiate these lesions from potential surgical lesions. They may be separated into inflammatory and posttraumatic conditions. The inflammatory lesions include inflammation of the bursae, snapping hip, meralgia paresthetica, and intraabdominal inflammations. The posttraumatic conditions include myositis ossificans, avulsions, and rupture of muscles.

Bursitis

At least 13 bursae are constantly present in the region of the hip, and a rather large number of other bursae are both small and inconsistent.[24] These are small pouches of connective tissue lined with a synovial-like membrane which may or may not connect with the joint. They are found between tendons and muscles or over bony prominences about the hip. Their function is believed to be a means of reducing friction and protecting sensitive structures from pressure. They are subject to all the inflammatory conditions: rheumatoid arthritis, gout, infections, and nonspecific inflammations.

Treatment of bursitis is determined primarily by the etiology. Conservative therapy is successful in most instances, but surgery is required for some conditions. The localized nonspecific idiopathic bursitis, which is the type most commonly seen, may be treated with a combination of systemic nonsteroidal antiinflammatory medicine (salicylates, indomethacin, or piroxicam etc.) and local measures (heat and rest). Frequently, injection of 10 to 20 mg hydrocortisone into the bursa affords rapid and long-lasting relief of symptoms. A source of local trauma or irritation to the bursa, i.e., occupational habit or wallet, should be sought and eliminated. Occasionally, if conservative treatment has not been satisfactory and the bursa is thickened and chronically inflamed, surgical excision is indicated. If the bursa is infected, the usual principles for treating infection are employed: The organism is identified and the infection treated with the appropriate systemic antibiotics. The bursa is aspirated, and warm soaks are applied to the area. Occasionally surgical drainage is required.

Systemic causes such as gout and rheumatoid arthritis are treated with appropriate medical regimens. Local injections of hydrocortisone can be effective.

The three largest and most constant bursae about the hip are the trochanteric, iliopectineal, and ischiogluteal, and they are most commonly involved in inflammatory conditions.

Trochanteric Bursa The trochanteric bursa is a large bursa between the tendon of the gluteus maximus and the posterolateral surface of the greater trochanter. Inflammation causes pain and tenderness over the trochanter or just posterior to the prominence[8] (Fig. 7–2). The pain of the trochanteric bursitis can be so diffuse that this misinterpretation of symptoms is understandable. A distinction can be made, however, by careful palpation around the posterior aspect of the greater trochanter where pain can become concentrated. However, tenderness in the sciatic notch is frequently found in disc disease. The diagnosis of a trochanteric bursitis can be confused with the diagnosis of a herniated disc with the pain referred down the posterior aspect of the leg.[46] Furthermore, there is pain in and around the trochanter on rotation of the hip joint. Both of these findings are absent with a herniated disc lesion.

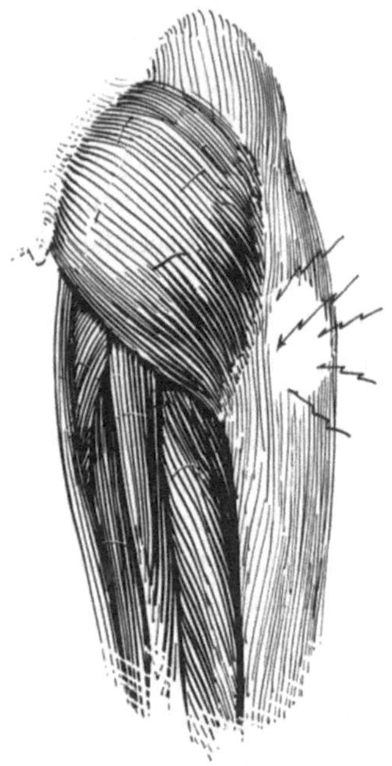

FIG. 7–2 Trochanteric bursitis. Inflammation in this bursa causes pain and tenderness over the posterior lateral aspect of the trochanter. It must be differentiated from other causes of hip pain, such as sciatica, stress fractures, and arthritis.

Pain is increased with pressure or when the hip is flexed and internally rotated. Occasionally the bursa is affected by an acute pyogenic or tuberculous infection. When acute infection is not clearly apparent, the possibility of tuberculosis should be considered. It has been reported that the bursa may be involved from a small tuberculous focus in the trochanter. Calcification about the trochanter bursa is not uncommon and is similar to that seen about the shoulder.[20,30] It is usually located in the adjacent tendons.

It has been observed that infected or loose total hip prostheses may cause pain in the trochanteric region.[47] Other intrinsic hip abnormalities may also result in trochanteric pain and must be differentiated from the bursitis.

Trochanteric bursitis is treated medically with antiinflammatory agents. When the pain is intense and very well localized, an injection of a cortisone preparation mixed with a local anesthetic can be extremely effective. My preference is to use 5 cc xylocaine and 1 cc triamcinolone injected directly into the site of maximal tenderness. The large volume allows coverage of a broad area, and the anesthetic agent gives some indication whether the right area has been injected. There is also some evidence to indicate that xylocaine itself has some antiinflammatory effects on crystalline-induced inflammations, i.e., from chondrocalcinosis, hydroxyapatite, or urate crystals. If the pain is not well localized, systemic nonsteroidal antiinflammatory medicine should be initiated, as mentioned previously.

Iliopectineal Bursa The iliopectineal bursa is deep to the iliopsoas tendon over the front of the hip joint[7] and is believed to be the largest synovial-line bursa in the body. It communicates with the joint in about 15% of adults. When inflamed, the pain and tenderness are in the lateral aspect of Scarpa's triangle.[25] Occasionally irritation of the adjacent femoral nerve and vessel causes referred pain along the anterior thigh and into the knee. Pain is elicited with tensing of the iliopsoas muscle during hip extension or forced flexion. Because this bursa may communicate with the joint, both spaces may be simultaneously involved. Extension into the bursa of proliferative synovium may be seen in rheumatoid arthritis or in patients with pigmented villonodular synovitis.

Ischiogluteal Bursa The ischiogluteal bursa lies between the tuberosity of the ischium and the gluteus maximus. It most commonly becomes inflamed in patients with occupations demanding prolonged sitting and therefore is called "tailor's" or "weaver's bottom." Appropriate chair padding and positioning may prevent recurrence. Occasionally the bursa is involved by acute suppurative infections which usually respond to conservative therapy.

Snapping Hip

Some patients are capable of producing an audible, palpable, but invisible snap on a lateral aspect of the hip as a tight fascia band slips over the prominence of the greater trochanter. Usually this gives rise to little inconvenience unless the underlying trochanteric bursa becomes inflamed or the patient is unable to tolerate the sensation, which is caused by the anterior edge of the gluteal aponeurosis snapping backward over the trochanter. Frequently the examiner cannot produce the snap, but the patient does so by flexing and internally rotating the thigh.

This entity, although not common, has been noted most frequently in adolescent and young women. Occasionally it is associated with a tic or leg-rotating nervous habit in which the patient unconsciously continues to snap the hip, a habit analogous to leg-bouncing. Recognizing this as a cause of the symptoms may be therapeutic.

Treatment is as with the other forms of bursitis. Surgical treatment is considered only if symptoms persist. Under local anesthesia the gluteal aponeurosis may be split longitudinally, its undersurface scarified, and the two edges kept apart by suturing the edges to the fascia that covers the vastus lateralis.

Other less common causes of snapping must be differentiated from the snapping hip. Occasionally osteochondromatosis manifests in this manner, or a clicking sound similar to that produced by cracking fingers may be noted in joints with severe degenerative changes or after osteochondral fractures.

Meralgia Paresthetica

A sensory mononeuritis of the lateral cutaneous nerve of the thigh is called meralgia paresthetica. The nerve is formed by fibers of the second and third lumbar roots. It courses across the anterior surface of the iliacus muscle and enters the thigh between the lateral border of the iliacus and below the upper end of the inguinal ligament. It pierces the fascia lata commonly just below and medial to the anterior superior iliac spine. It may, however, course through the fascia obliquely and attain a subcutaneous position several inches below the spine. In the thigh it divides into two branches: The posterior branch passes obliquely backward through the fascia lata and transmits cutaneous sensation from the superior lateral part of the buttock, and the anterior branch, which is the more important clinically, pierces the fascia lata through a small canal and transmits sensations from the lateral surface of the thigh as far distal as the knee.

This nerve is associated with dysesthesias such as tingling, burning, prickling, or "pins and needles" sensations. Occasionally there is hypesthesia. Its long, superficial course exposes it to various forms of injury, but in most cases there is no history of direct trauma. Various factors can irritate the nerve: tight belts or corsets, possibly prolonged walking, or long periods of acute hip flexion. The involvement is usually unilateral and seems to affect men three times as frequently as women.

The clinical course of meralgia paresthetica is variable, and the treatment depends on the etiology. Efforts are directed toward identifying an offending factor and eliminating its continued irritation. Local injections of an anesthetic agent can confirm the diagnosis. A local cortisone preparation may also be tried. However, if symptoms are arising from traction on the nerve as it courses about the iliac spine or as it emerges through the fascia, it may be necessary to split the fascia lata surgically or to correct the angulation of the nerve at the spine.

Occasionally the nerve is involved in a surgical scar secondary to an anterior approach of the hip or to obtaining a bone graft from the iliac crest. The resulting postsurgical neuroma may be excised with good relief of symptoms. Other problems such as tumors or inflammation proximal to the iliac spine must be considered and ruled out.

Intraabdominal Inflammations

Pain and spasm about the hip may be the presenting signs and symptoms of intraabdominal inflammation. The psoas muscle is affected in some cases of appendicitis. The hip is held in flexion and external rotation from the contraction and reflex spasm of this muscle. Any motion which stretches the muscle causes pain and increased spasm.[2] The obturator internus muscle, although covered by a relatively dense fascia, is also occasionally irritated by pelvic inflammation. If there is a pelvic abscess, i.e., one caused by a ruptured appendix, spasm of the obturator internus causes pain on internal rotation. Frequently this pain is referred to the hypogastrium; this referred pain is the "obturator sign" and is a useful test for pelvic pathology. It should be remembered that pain during examination of the hip may be related to problems above the inguinal ligaments.

Myositis Ossificans

Myositis ossificans has long been known to occur after surgery or trauma about the hip. The term encompasses all types of heterotopic bone formation, although there are various clinical patterns and initiating circumstances. In general, heterotopic bone forms in those areas where there has been a combination of hematoma and continued inflammatory reaction.

The condition may present in three patterns: (1) It may appear as a mass of bone lying within the muscle and separated from the bone by a layer of muscle. This is the classic presentation of myositis ossificans and usually occurs after severe repetitive soft-tissue trauma. (2) Heterotopic ossification may appear as a broad-based mass of bone contiguous with the underlying bone and periosteum, sometimes extending into and displacing the overlying muscle. This type may be the result of ossification in a subperiosteal hematoma and is seen after surgery or trauma; it might be better termed posttraumatic periostitis. (3) The heterotopic bone forms around the joint after fracture or surgery, appearing in the capsule and along the fascial planes. One or all of these patterns may be present in the hip, and all represent significant hazards to rehabilitation after surgery or injury.

The etiology of the heterotopic osseous formation is unknown. Several theories have been proposed in attempts to explain this phenomenon.[19,26,33] One concept is that during muscle strain or injury particles of periosteum are avulsed from the bony insertion of the muscle; the particles of periosteum, in turn, lodge in the muscle fiber and initiate osseous growth. Another theory postulates that bone formation stems from cell metaplasia as a result of muscle, tendon, or soft-tissue injury.[28] It is thought that osteoblastic function could be assumed by cells from any part of the body. Calcium salts, oxygen tensions, and enzymes also have been postulated to be directly related to heterotopic ossification.[32,47] As yet, however, no mechanisms for this process have been definitely established.

Pathologically, gross and microscopic appearances vary considerably with location and maturity. In general, disorganized cortical bone with active marrow cavities is apparent. Ossification and maturity are always greater in the periphery than centrally. In the early stage the periphery is poorly circumscribed, but laterally the lesion becomes well demarcated. As the lesion matures, the bony mass becomes smaller, the peripheral zones become differentiated, and the central areas continue to show highly cellular areas with atypical mitotic figures resembling sarcoma. The condition may be differentiated from a juxtacortical osteogenic sarcoma by a complete history, which includes trauma or surgery, and the microscopic appearance of the entire lesion.

Clinically, this heterotopic osseous tissue may become an important consideration with hip surgery and a difficult management problem. Small areas of ossification are frequently noted after reconstructive hip surgery. However, in some patients they become so massive they prevent hip motion and lead to fusion or failure of the reconstructive procedure.

The overall incidence of this problem is difficult to determine accurately because of the varying severity. However, if all grades of the heterotopic ossification are included, approximately 60% of patients after surgery to the hip have some evidence of heterotopic ossification.[16,27a,34a,40,42a,50] This process may be graded from mild to very severe. Fortunately, only about 0.5% of the patients have very severe ossification, and the remaining incidence is scattered along a broad spectrum of severity.

If one looks at the patients who are at the highest risk of developing ossification, several groups of patients are clearly defined (Table 7–1). The highest-risk patients are those with ankylosing spondylitis, followed by those who have had a previous episode of heterotopic ossification. This may include patients who had ipsilateral hip surgery and are returning for a secondary surgical procedure or those who have had a contralateral hip operated and have developed heterotopic ossification in that hip. Other groups include patients with DISH (diffuse idiopathic skeletal hyperostosis, or Forrestier's disease) and elderly men who have severe proliferative osteoarthritis in both hips. Persons who appear to be at low risk of developing heterotopic ossification include those with rheumatoid arthritis or osteonecrosis about the hip.

Although high-risk groups may be identified, the individuals within those groups who will develop heterotopic ossification cannot be determined. There was some evidence that the alkaline phosphatase level may be of predictive value in paraplegics, but this value may be elevated in all the postoperative patients and therefore does not appear to be a useful guide after hip surgery. Clinically, heterotopic ossification may be recognized by the onset of a sense of tightness which develops approximately 3 weeks after surgery. Many times the patients have been discharged from hospital on a satisfactory course only to be noted by the physical therapist to have a diminishing range of motion and increased inflammation about the hip. These patients are suspected of developing myositis ossificans, and so x-ray studies are performed (Fig. 7–3). The x-ray findings may become positive as early as 3 weeks, and clearly the ossification should be seen by 6 weeks. If one follows the clinical course of the development of heterotopic ossification, it is noted that by 3 months most of the ossification has been present and is beginning to mature. The maturation process takes 12 to 18 months before the activity begins to subside within the entire ossification mass.

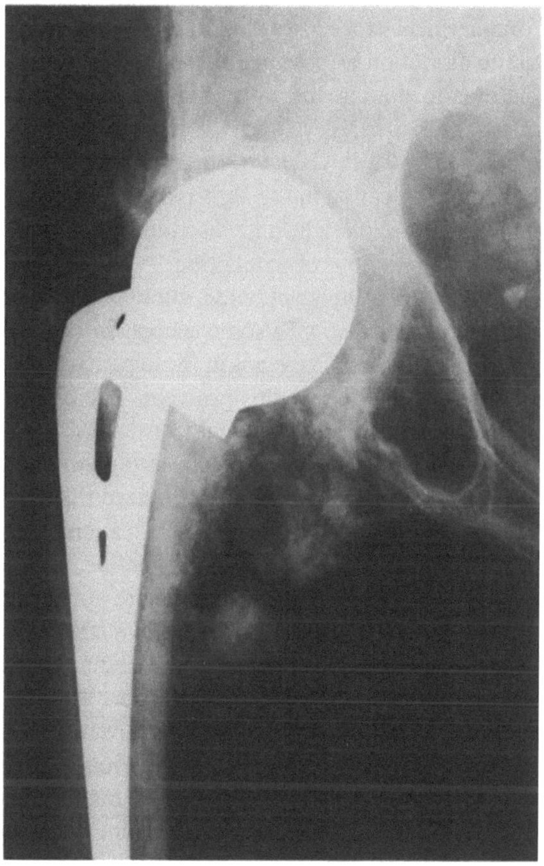

Fig. 7–3 Myositis ossificans. Note the marked formation of heterotopic bone around this prosthesis. If a secondary procedure is considered, preoperative EHDP or irradiation should be considered to prevent recurrence (see text).

Table 7–1 Heterotopic Ossification: High-Risk Patients

Ankylosing spondylitics
Patients with Forrestier's disease (DISH)
Male osteoarthritics with osteophyte formation
Patients undergoing revision surgery
Patients with ectopic bone formation in a contralateral hip
Patients undergoing surface replacement

If the heterotopic bone is so massive that it limits motion, excision of the bone may be considered, but not before the bone has fully matured. Bone scans are the most useful method to determine the activity of heterotopic ossification. Moreover, once this problem has been recognized, serial bone scans are evaluated to determine activity. When appropriate, surgical intervention is considered.

The best treatment for this problem is directed along the lines of prevention. It is important to recognize patients in high-risk groups and to consider prophylactic therapy. It is important to perform surgical procedures with as little trauma and tissue dissection as possible in order to reduce hematoma formation and muscle injury. Two treatments have been developed which appear to be quite successful in reducing the incidence of heterotopic ossification in the high-risk groups. These include the use of etidronate disodiumdiphosphate (EHDP) or the use of irradiation.

The use of a diphosphonate, such as disodium etidronate, has met with some success in the prevention of myositis ossificans in those patients with a history of developing this problem. The diphosphonates are simple chemical compounds with properties similar to naturally occurring inorganic pyrophosphate. It has been hypothesized that they are the regulators of biological calcification. They may be absorbed intact from the intestine. Unlike pyrophosphate, the diphosphonates are almost totally stable to chemical enzymatic degradation. Although the exact mechanism of action is still unknown, EHDP should be considered when reoperating patients with a history of severe myositis or those from other high-risk groups. The EHDP is administered at doses of 20 mg/kg/day for 1 month preoperatively and is continued for at least 3 months after surgery at the same dosage level. Lesser amounts have been shown to be ineffective, and with this dose it has been shown that there is a significant reduction in both the incidence of recurrent heterotopic ossification and in the quantity of bone which is present in those few patients who have had recurrences.

Another modality which has recently been used to prevent myositis ossificans is treatment with low-dose high-voltage radiation therapy [7a] (E. McC. Evarts, personal communication). It has been thought that the precursor to the heterotopic process, the osteoblast from the primitive mesenchymal cell, begins to proliferate shortly after surgery, and if radiation is applied as soon as possible after surgery the heterotopic ossification process may be arrested. It has been shown that a course of 2000 rads delivered over a 10-day period significantly reduces the incidence of the ossification. This low-dose irradiation appears to be relatively safe, with very few side effects. The only major contraindication is if the patient is a young, childbearing-age woman, but this specific contraindication is rare for high-risk ossification. There is some evidence to indicate that the combination of diphosphonate and high-voltage radiation therapy may be better than either one alone, and clinical trials continue in this regard.

It must again be emphasized that those patients in the high-risk group should be considered for a prophylactic treatment. In addition, if myositis is becoming a major postoperative problem, reoperation and excision of the myositis ossificans should await maturation of the bone; under no circumstances should this surgery be contemplated prior to 12 months from surgery and/or until the bone scan becomes cold.

Avulsions and Muscle Ruptures

Occasionally after a violent contraction or contusion, as during athletics, sudden pain and swelling about the hip or thigh can be secondary to avulsion or rupture of a muscle. The muscles most likely to be ruptured are the rectus femoris, adductor longus, and psoas.[18]

The rectus femoris is the muscle about the hip most commonly ruptured. It extends from the hip to below the knee and is susceptible to forcible blows in the thigh while firmly fixed. It may be torn from its attachments or at the musculotendinous junction at the level of the lesser trochanter, and it may appear as a firm tumor mass on the anterior thigh. Ordinarily the diagnosis is contusion or hematoma. If the fresh injury is recognized, it may be repaired surgically; otherwise, the ends cannot be sutured into opposition, and surgery should be avoided.

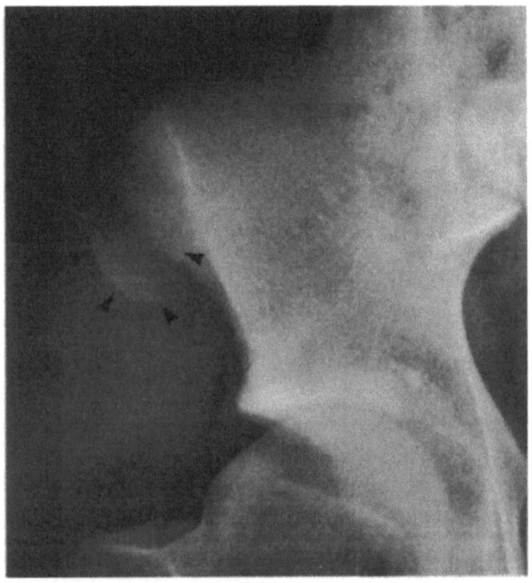

Fig. 7–4 Avulsion of the anterior superior spine of the ileum (*arrowheads*) after violent muscle contracture.

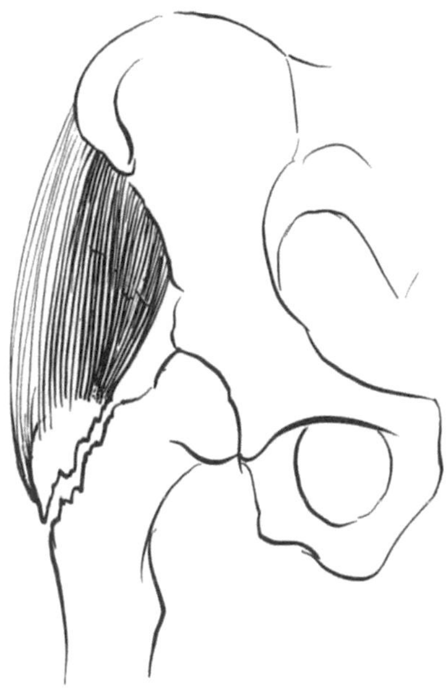

FIG. 7–5 Avulsion of the greater trochanter as occasionally seen after blunt trauma.

The same situation occurs with the adductor and psoas muscles. Formerly avulsion of the adductor muscle was an occupational hazard of horsemen and was called "rider's sprain." Nowadays this lesion is rare. If the lesion is massive and recognized early, the rupture is repaired. Partial rupture of the adductor can be painful over a period of 3 to 4 weeks.

Avulsions may occur from any of the several muscle origins and bony prominences about the hip. Most commonly these avulsions occur at the anterior superior spine of the ilium and the lesser trochanter, and occasionally at the greater trochanter and the ischium prior to fusion of the epiphyses (Figs. 7–4 and 7–5). The history is of unusual muscular violence. Examination reveals localized pain and tenderness. The injury can be distinguished from a contusion, as function of the involved muscle attachments is painful and active motion against resistance causes pain directly in the area of the avulsion. X-ray studies should be done and usually show the injury. Depending on the age and occupation of the patient and the extent of the separation, treatment is primarily conservative. In the young and athletic patient, if wide separation has occurred, treatment is prompt, accurate reduction and firm fixation.

References

1. Adams, J. A.: Transient synovitis of the hip joint in children. J. Bone Joint Surg., 45B:471, 1963.
2. Blair, W.: Psoas myositis or fibrositis in the differential diagnosis of lower abdominal disease. Am. J. Surg., 22:505, 1956.
3. Bradford, E. H., Lovett, R. W.: Treatment of hip disease. Am. J. Orthop. Surg., 9:354, 1911–12.
4. Burger, H.: Intermittent hydrarthrosis with allergic basis. JAMA, 112:2402, 1939.
5. Butler, R. W.: Transitory arthritis of hip joint in children: an investigation of arthritis of the hip in ninety-seven children. Br. Med. J., 1:951, 1933.
6. Caravias, D. E.: The significance of so-called "irritable hips" in children. Arch. Dis. Child., 31:415, 1956.
7. Chandler, S. B.: The iliopsoas bursa in man. Anat. Rec., 52:235, 1933.

7a. Coventry, M. B., Scanlon, P. W.: The use of radiation to discourage ectopic bone: A nine-year study in surgery about the hip. J. Bone Joint Surg., 63A:201, 1981.

8. Cozen, L.: Trochanter bursitis. Am. J. Orthop., 7:10, 1965.
9. Donaldson, W. F.: Transient synovitis of the hip joint. Pediatr. Clin. North Am., 2:1073, 1955.
10. Drey, L.: A roentgenographic study of transient synovitis of the hip. Radiology, 60:588, 1953.
11. Edwards, E. G.: Transient synovitis of hip joint in children. JAMA, 148:30, 1962.
12. Evans, D. L.: Legg-Calve-Perthes disease: a study of late results. J. Bone Joint Surg., 40B:168, 1958.
13. Fairbank, H. A. T.: Non-tuberculous coxitis in the young. Br. Med. J., 2:828, 1926.
14. Ferguson, A. B., Jr.: Synovitis of hip in Legg-Perthes disease. Clin. Orthop., 4:180, 1954.
15. Finder, J. G.: Transitory synovitis of hip joint in children. JAMA, 107:3, 1936.
16. Finerman, G. A. M.: Heterotopic ossification following total hip replacement. Symp. Contemp. Orthop., 5:95, 1982.
17. Fox, K. W., Griffin, L. L.: Transient synovitis of hip joint in children. Texas J. Med., 52:15, 1956.
18. Gaston, E. A., Wigglesworth, W. C.: Traumatic rupture of body of psoas muscle. Arch. Surg., 64:119, 1952.
19. Gerlach, U., Hohling, J. H., Themann, H.: Metabolism and structure of connective tissue during extraosseous calcification. Clin. Orthop., 69:118, 1970.
20. Goldenberg, R. R., Leventhal, G. S.: Supratrochanteric calcification, J. Bone Joint Surg., 18:205, 1936.
21. Hardinge, K.: The etiology of transient synovitis of the hip in children. J. Bone Joint Surg., 52B:100, 1970.

22. Hermel, M. B., Albert, S. M.: Transient synovitis of the hip. Clin. Orthop., 22:21, 1962.
23. Hermel, M. B., Sklaroff, D. M.: Roentgen changes in transient synovitis of hip joint. Arch. Surg., 68:364, 1954.
24. Hollingshead, W. H.: *Anatomy for Surgeons,* Vol. 3, 2nd ed. New York, Hoeber, 1969.
25. Hucherson, B. C., Freeman, G. E.: Iliopectineal bursitis. Am. J. Orthop., 4:220, 1962.
26. Huggins, C. B.: Experimental osteogenesis. Proc. Soc. Exp. Biol. Med., 27:349, 1930.
27. Jacobs, B. W.: Synovitis of the hip in children and its significance. Pediatrics, 47:349, 1930.
27a. Jowsey, J., Coventry, M. B., Robins, P. R.: Heterotopic ossification: theoretical consideration, possible etiologic factors, and a clinical review of total hip arthroplasty patients exhibiting this phenomenon. In: *The Hip. Proceedings of the 5th Open Scientific Meeting of the Hip Society.* St. Louis, Mosby, 1977, pp. 210–221.
28. Keith, A.: Concerning the origin and nature of osteoblast. Proc. R. Soc. Med., 21:301, 1927.
29. Kemp, M. B. S.: Some observations of Perthes disease. J. Bone Joint Surg., 47B:193, 1965.
30. King, J. W., Vanderpool, D. W.: Calcific tendinitis of rectus femoris. Am. J. Orthop., 9:110, 1967.
31. Kite, J. H., French, G. O.: Early diagnosis of flat headed femur. South. Med. J., 45:581, 1952.
32. Leonard, F., Scullin, R. I.: New mechanism for calcification of skeletal tissues. Nature, 224:1113, 1969.
33. Lewis, D.: Myositis ossificans. JAMA, 86:1281, 1923.
34. Lucas, L. S.: Painful hips in children. Am. Acad. Orthop. Surg., 5:144, 1948.
34a. Matos, M., Amstutz, H., Finerman, G.: Myositis ossificans following total hip replacement. J. Bone Joint Surg., 57A:13, 1975.
35. McMurray, B.: A report of six cases of coxa magna following synovitis of the hip joint. Br. J. Radiol., 20:477, 1947.
36. Miller, O. L.: Acute transient epiphysitis of hip joint. JAMA, 96:575, 1931.
37. Monty, C. P.: Prognosis of observation hip in children. Arch. Dis. Child., 37:539, 1962.
38. Ralston, E. L.: Legg-Calve-Perthes disease factors in healing. J. Bone Joint Surg., 43A:249, 1961.
39. Rauch, S.: Transitory synovitis of hip joint in children. Am. J. Dis. Child., 59:1245, 1940.
40. Ritter, M. A., Vaughan, R. B.: Ectopic ossification after total hip arthroplasty. J. Bone Joint Surg., 59A:245, 1977.
41. Rosenberg, N. J., Smith, E. E.: Transient synovitis of hip joint. J. Pediatr., 48:776, 1956.
42. Salter, R. B.: Experimental and clinical aspects of Perthes disease. J. Bone Joint Surg., 48B:393, 1966.
42a. Salvati, E. A., Wilson, P. D., Jolley, M. N., et al.: A ten-year followup study of our first 100 consecutive Charnley total hip replacements. J. Bone Joint Surg., 62A:753, 1981.
43. Spock, A.: Transient synovitis of hip joint. Pediatrics, 24:1042, 1959.
44. Stamp, W. H., Canales, G., Odell, O. T.: Late results of osteochondrosis of capital epiphysis of femur. JAMA, 169:1443, 1959.
45. Stover, S., Hahn, H. R., Miller, J. M.: Disodium etidronate in the prevention of heterotopic ossification following spinal cord injury. Paraplegia, 14:146, 1976.
46. Tronzo, R.: Trochanteric bursitis confused with referred pain from herniated lumbar disc lesions. Presented to the Philadelphia Orthopedic Soceity, 1969.
47. Vaes, G. M., Nichols, G.: Oxygen tension and the control of bone cell metabolism. Nature, 193:379, 1962.
48. Waldenström, H.: The first stages of coxa plana. J. Bone Joint Surg., 20A:559, 1938.
49. Wilke, L. H.: Juvenile osteochondrosis of the hip. JAMA, 192:393, 1965.
50. Wilson, P. D., Amstutz, H., Czerniecki, A., et al.: Total hip replacement with fixation by acrylic cement. J. Bone Joint Surg., 54A:207, 1972.

CHAPTER 8

Fractures of the Hip in Adults

RAYMOND G. TRONZO

Social Impact

Statistics gathered during the mid-1980s are quite different from those gathered previously because of three factors. (1) The commonplace use of the image intensifier roentgenogram with its updated memory bank has made surgical treatment of these injuries much more sophisticated with very accurate reductions and near-perfect placement of the internal fixator. (2) Stronger implants for more reliable fixation with low failure rates contributed greatly to a more favorable outcome. (3) A more optimistic attitude from the nursing sector has significantly reduced the mortality rate during the immediate postoperative period. Data collected before the late 1970s and early 1980s cannot be compared with the quality of survival in the present time frame.

Fracture of the upper end of the femur is one of the most common fractures in the body, especially in the elderly population. The *average age* at which these fractures occur is 76 (for men 74 and for women 79). The fracture patient's age reported in the literature is rarely below 40, and there is a distinct gap between age 17 and 30. Children's fractures are unique and were discussed in Volume I, Chapter 9. Women generally have a longer life span and therefore comprise most (75%) of the fractured hip population. Oddly enough, black women seldom break their hips.[1] In southern Florida, where there is a large elderly population, it is the single most frequent orthopedic admission in the hospitals. It is therefore an endemic disease within a retiree community.

Another interesting fact has come from Johnell et al.[7] in Sweden. They concluded that the *incidence* of hip fractures among the elderly population is increasing much faster than the increase in numbers would lead one to expect. The study showed that, although still lingering considerably behind women, the incidence among men has increased at an alarming rate. The authors cited similar trends from reports of other Scandinavian and British cities.

In yet another related Swedish study, Bauer et al.[8] presented interesting *cost figures*. In Sweden such figures are accurate and meaningful because of their tightly controlled national health plan. There, hip fractures now consume more hospital days than all of the noncancer abdominal surgery. It is a condition which is more expensive to individuals and society than any other "surgical" diagnosis. Bauer et al. found that improved surgical techniques with stronger implants and better reduction plus more accurate internal fixation with the use of the image intensifier allowed earlier weight-bearing, resulting in earlier discharge from the acute care facility. Their goal was to rehabilitate the patient maximally to a reliable gait with a walker so that they could go directly home rather than to an intermediary nursing home, or "geriatric center." With this program three-fourths of the patients returned home after 2 or 3 weeks in the acute care hospital. One year later 9 of 10 surviving patients were at home with no functional loss compared to what their functional status was at the 4-month mark. Their decrease in hospital stay has saved 1.25 million dollars in hospital days annually, or twice the hospital days used for all cancer surgery in Sweden. Bauer et al. further concluded that hospital convalescence is physically and mentally detrimental. It is 10 to 40 times more expensive than rehabilitation at home for patients who were relatively independent before they fractured their hip. Ceder et al., also from Sweden, found that one of the most significant factors in predicting the patient's prognosis was whether the patient was walking after 2 weeks.[9]

Mortality/Morbidity

Until the 1980s the *mortality rate* was devastating, ranging as high as 45%. The estimated annual U.S. mortality rate from all causes for 1977 showed that hip fractures had an overall mortality rate, including all ages, of 2%.[2] Coronary artery disease is the most frequent cause of death and is also the most frequent complicating disease in elderly patients who suffer a fractured hip. Mortality is a complex statistic. The time span is the most significant parameter to evaluate.

Miller[1] studied patients with fractured hips for a minimum of 8 months and found a yearly mortality rate, from whatever cause, of 27%. He suggested that this fracture should be viewed as a disease with a predictable rate and pattern of mortality: Those patients who survive 1 year may be considered cured, as their subsequent survival is similar to that of the population at large.

Knowelden et al,[3] calculated that 19% of patients with hip fractures die within a year after the injury. Kofoed and Alberts found that 3% died during the first month, 13% during the first 6 months, and 29% within the first 2 years.[4] The postoperative mortality is also considered the "hospital mortality rate." In St. Mary's Hospital in West Palm Beach, which represents a typical community hospital in southern Florida, the average hospital stay in 1985 was 11 days and the mortality rate was 3%.

A comprehensive study conducted by Kenzora et al.[5] on the mortality associated with hip fractures as related to age, treatment, preoperative illnesses, time of surgery, and complications from 1971 to 1977 is a valuable review. A total of 406 patients were followed until death or for at least 1 year. Their overall mortality rate was 14%. Sex, treatment of subcapital fracture by either internal fixation or arthroplasty, and the level of postoperative ambulation did not influence mortality. The number of preexisting medical conditions and the time of surgery following admission were highly significant, however. The recommendation is for any serious medical condition that may be present to be the treatment priority for at least the first 24 hours before taking the patient to surgery and that pulmonary therapy should be instituted before any surgery is performed.

An elderly group of institutionalized "captive" patients were thoroughly studied by Crane and Kernek.[6] These authors presented a 10-year review of 159 patients with 163 hip fractures (four were bilateral) in a single geriatric hospital and residential health facility (139 women and 20 men with an average age of 84.5 years). There were 65 femoral neck, 90 intertrochanteric, and 5 subtrochanteric fractures. Three cases had lost charts. Except for two cases all patients were treated surgically and had an average hospital stay of 14 days. Those who had an endoprosthesis stayed 3 days longer. Hospital mortality was 10.5%: 8% for neck fractures, 8% for intertrochanteric fractures, and 20% for subtrochanteric fractures. Causes of death were the many medical problems associated with this age group. At the 10-year follow-up, 51 patients were still alive. During the first 6 months these patients had the same life expectancy as their peers. Patients who were nonambulatory had a significantly higher death rate. The institution's daily census was 427, 13% of whom had hip fractures. Death from hip fracture accounted for 15% of all deaths during this period.

Although it was a select group of people, these results emphasize the increased likelihood of death following hip fracture in the very elderly as well as the fact that the more debilitated patients are at higher risk for such injuries. More than three-fourths of the patients who died within 2 months of discharge had been nonambulatory after surgery, whereas more than three-fourths of the survivors had been functionally ambulatory before surgery. The study also pointed out the great preponderance of women as the population approaches the upper age limits. The study showed that women carry a higher burden for sustaining hip fractures but seem to have a longer survival than do elderly men. One must realize that hip fractures in the elderly continue to be a major problem in terms of costs to both patients and society.

One of the most fascinating studies was reported by Mullen. It was a prospective study of 200 hip fracture patients older than 60 years. They undertook the study between 1981 and 1983 to assess the relation of patients' mental status at the time of admission, hospital confusion, complications, and death. Among the patients who became confused the death rate was 41%, but among those whose mental condition did not deteriorate, mortality was only 7%. Patients with normal mental status at admission had the lowest risk of death (2%). As mental status deteriorated during hospitalization, the death rate rose until it was at the 30% level for the most confused population. They also concluded: "Multifactorial analysis indicates admission mental status to be a reliable indicator of general health and survival. Hospital confusion is statistically independent of admission mental status."[10] Their paper clearly defined the responsibilities of the physician in regard to the total care of these delicate people. Such patients require close monitoring by a thorough team of medical experts as well as improved nutrition and vigorous physical activity. Just as they require good surgical care, so also do they deserve comprehensive medical care of the highest order administered with the same enthusiasm as that afforded the younger patient.

One can generalize from these data as they relate to *survival* that if an elderly patient fractures a hip while in good health, alert, and walking well she has a good chance of surviving the surgical treatment and living with the same life expectancy as her peers. If she is feeble, in ill health, and in her eighth decade, she may not have the reserve to survive the surgical treatment or may not be able to regain strength to ambulate well enough to return to the preoperative quality of living. Surgical care, however, offers the best gamble for any kind of meaningful existence.

It is difficult to predict whether an elderly patient is likely to sustain a second fracture on the opposite side if she survives the first one. Work done by Milton et al.[11] at the Mayo Clinic has shed some light on this subject. Their study spanned a 50-year period, which makes their data significant. A second fracture appeared in 1% of patients at 1 year, in 8% at 5 years, in 16% at 10 years, and in 20% at 20 years after the first fracture. They thus concluded that there was a definite risk of experiencing a second fracture to the opposite side. Moreover, the second fracture was often of the same variety as the first, and many times it was almost identical.

Nutritional Status of the Elderly Fracture Patient

It has always been assumed that the catabolic state of poor health in elderly patients is due to their poor dietary habits, which is true of the wealthy as well as the impoverished. Investigations by nutritional experts have now produced data to confirm this assumption. The British study by Older, Edwards, et al.[12] is noteworthy. They studied the nutritional value of voluntary food intake of elderly female patients who had undergone surgery for a fractured hip. Only vitamin A and calcium were found adequate. Their intake of protein, vitamin D, riboflavin, vitamin C, thiamine, and niacin fell short of recommended levels for healthy people. Inadequate thiamine levels were also found within the first 48 hours after surgery.

Calcium, an essential element for bone mineralization, was adequate. However, the intake of vitamin D was not; consequently the absorption and integration of the element into protein matrix was poor. This lack not only promotes osteoporosis but discourages bone healing.

Another interesting parameter was the nurse's estimate of the quality of the patient's food intake. Most often their estimate was as poor as the patient's. These patients obviously have a fickle appetite which must be changed with encouragement and awareness on the part of the nursing staff.

Posttraumatic confusion is often related to blood loss with its consequent decreased cerebral oxygenation combined with slow detoxification of the anesthetics used. Because of this deficit, one must not be too quick to pronounce the patient senile preoperatively and even more senile postoperatively.

Osteoporosis and Hip Fractures

Aging and bone quality (degree of osteopenia) as it relates to hip fractures is a very important parameter. Elabdien et al.[13] studied this problem. A series of 127 intertrochanteric fractures were analyzed with respect to fracture type, age, and bone quality. There was a continuous decrease in bone quality when measured by the "femoral score.'' These authors proved a direct relation between age and the severity of the fracture. The aging process starts earlier in women but accelerates in men after the age of 85. Consequently, the risk of sustaining a trochanteric fracture is more likely in men in their mid-eighties. Hence the increasing age of our population will produce more comminuted fractures in the upper femur with a greater demand to improve the surgical care if the quality of their survival is to be improved.

Singh et al.[14] developed an ''index,'' measuring the trabecular pattern of the upper end of the femur and using it as an indication of the degree of osteoporosis. They based their reasoning on the postulate that the amount of comminution of the fracture is directly related to the degree of osteoporosis. The validity of this index as a practical clinical tool has been seriously challenged.[15,16]

Three fracture sites are common in osteoporotic bone. In order of frequency, they are the vertebral bodies, the distal end of the radius, and the upper end of the femur. Freeman et al. investigated the possibility that hip fractures result from fatigue (stress) on the femoral neck.[17] A study by Garrett and Vernon-Roberts took exception to this concept.[18] A clinical, radiological, and histopathological study of femoral heads from 125 patients with fracture of the neck of the femur and from 30 cadavers was carried out to identify various risk factors. The findings showed that (1) the Singh index was unreliable as a radiological indicator of the bone content of the femoral heads; (2) the bone content of the femoral head in patients sustaining a fracture of the femoral neck did not differ from that of the controls; (3) osteomalacia was not found in any of the heads examined; and (4) the distribution of trabecular microfractures did not support the hypothesis that fracture of the neck was the result of progressive fatigue. It was concluded that the single most important factor leading to fracture in this Australian population was injury caused by falls, and that such injury was frequently associated with other disease processes.

Lips et al.[19] also studied parameters for screening people at risk. Reproducibility of the Singh index was poor. The patients with femoral neck fractures had a higher vertebral index, more vertebral crush fractures, and a lower Singh index (when measurable) than the control group. There was no difference in these radiological indices between cervical and intertrochanteric fractures. The radiological indices correlated poorly with each other and with histomorphometric data from bone biopsies of the patients. The authors concluded that there is need for a more accurate technique for local assessment of the bone mass in the femoral neck.

The newest equipment for studying osteoporosis is the quantitative computed tomography (CT) scan.[20] CT has been used for noninvasive quantitative bone mineral determination. The technique's usefulness in this area lies in its ability to give a quantitative image. It can be used to measure trabecular, cortical, or integral bone centrally or peripherally. Advances in CT technology, especially in external localization capabilities, point the way for advanced scanners to be modified for quantitative CT measurements at minimal cost. A reduction in patient scanning exposure makes this an attractive technique for noninvasive, accurate measurement of bone mass. It may become the tool of the future for predicting which femoral neck fracture is too osteoporotic to expect a reasonably good result if a pinning procedure were performed.

It is not within the scope of this text to go into the voluminous metabolic details of osteoporosis. The U.S. government has been holding hearings on the need to treat osteoporosis earlier and on how such studies may be conducted through their agencies. A subcommittee hearing unfolded some surprising statistics. The disease with its complications costs 3.8 billion dollars per year in the United States and kills 40,000 victims a year. It affects some 20 million Americans, mostly women after the age 30 (the point at which estrogen levels begin to decline). Their interest in hip fractures focused on the fact that 18% of all fractured hip patients die within their first year after injury. In addition to hormone depletion, poorly balanced diets contribute to the osteoporotic phenomenon. Through such studies it is finally being recognized that more education on nutrition is needed in our medical schools.

''Transient Osteoporosis'' of the Hip

Transient osteoporosis of the hip is an obscure syndrome, although it has been well documented in the literature.[21] Because it is so seldom recognized, it has been misdiagnosed as tuberculosis, avascular necrosis, stress fracture, malignancy, synovial chondromatosis, and villonodular synovitis. However, its true diagnosis is easy if there is a high level of awareness and suspicion. There is no need for aggressive procedures because the disease runs a purely benign course; it is self-limiting and ends with no disability. All laboratory tests are normal except for the x-ray films. The hallmark of the syndrome is pain in the groin, buttock, or the hip itself. The pain may be sudden and severe, or it may be insidious and mild. In 30% of the reported cases the opposite hip is affected as well. Its course runs 2 to 6 months.

X-ray patterns characteristic of this disease do not develop until 3 to 6 weeks after the onset of pain. Bone scans are positive earlier, showing increased uptake in an intense homogeneous pattern that affects the entire femoral head. This pattern spreads into the diaphysis in about half of the patients. The routine x-ray picture shows a demineralized femoral head.

Treatment is nonspecific. Steroids, nonsteroids, bed rest, traction, heat, physiotherapy, sympathetic blocks, and protected weight-bearing have been tried. None seems to alter the ultimate outcome, which is benign.

Related Trauma

Trauma associated with these fractures is usually minor. A slip on the rug or a slick floor is the usual cause. The patient may simply twist her leg and fracture her hip without actually falling. The author had one patient who fractured her hip as she raised herself from a low chair. The old adage that an elderly patient fractures her hip first and then falls is difficult to prove. Such an event is called a "drop fall." It was recorded in only 2% of a large series.[22] More severe trauma is substantiated in younger patients, below 60, as in car accidents or industrial mishaps. Curiously, the left hip is fractured more frequently than the right.[2]

A group in England[23] sought to identify preventable factors which cause these fractures. They reviewed 384 femoral neck fractures and 226 comparable controls during a 1-year period. In the fracture group one-third had had a previous fracture after age 60. The younger patients could identify a definite fall or loss of consciousness.

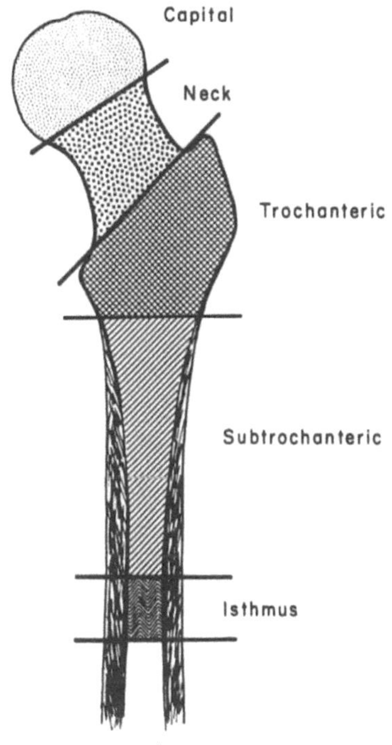

FIG. 8–1 Regions of various fractures of the upper femur.

The elderly fracture group simply found themselves on the floor—a "drop attack." Neurological disease was present in 43% of the fracture patients. Chronic brain syndrome was also more common at all ages in the fracture group. Loss of balance was associated with a cerebrovascular accident, which was more common in patients under age 75 in the fracture group. Visual impairment was equally common and was the usual cause for imbalance. The most striking difference between the fracture group and the controls was the patients' general physical state, which was poorer in the fracture patients.

Fracture Regions

It is important to determine the anatomical region of the hip fracture because each region has distinct characteristics of healing, reduction parameters, and postoperative behavior. Fracture regions are depicted in Fig. 8–1. Fractures within the femoral head are the rarest and are called *capital* fractures. They usually occur in association with dislocations of the hip joint (Fig. 8–2). Isolated fractures of the *greater trochanter* are uncommon.

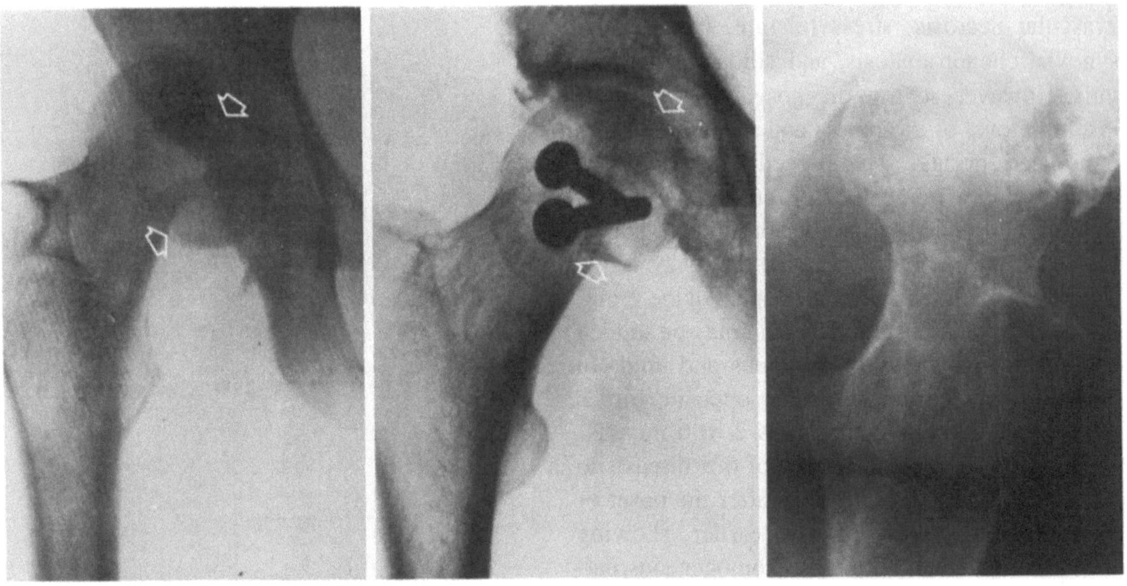

A B C

FIG. 8–2 Capital fracture **(A)** fixed by embedding the screws **(B)** into the articular cartilage. Arrows indicate the plane of the fracture. (From DuQuennon, A., et al.: Rev. Chir. Orthop., 61:209, 1975.) **(C)** Capital fracture as part of a fracture dislocation of the hip joint. It was missed on routine films. Typically it is an anterior fragment which is broken off when it strikes the posterior edge of the acetabulum as the head dislocates posteriorly. The new double-threaded screw should be used instead of the conventional screws with heads as seen here (Herbert screws).

(Fig. 8–3). They can disguise intertrochanteric fractures. Usually avulsion fractures, they can also be the result of a direct blow, in which case one should be careful to look for an obscure intertrochanteric component. A laminogram is essential. Isolated fractures of the *lesser trochanter,* also uncommon, are avulsion fractures usually seen in younger patients. The iliopsoas, when suddenly and forcefully contracted, pulls the fragment upward (Fig. 8–4).

The two major fracture regions are in the neck and between the two trochanters. Fractures within the *femoral neck* are referred to as medial fractures, cervical, transcervical, or intracapsular. Basi-cervical, or basilar neck, fractures are not included here, as traditionally done in the past, but are included under trochanteric fractures. Any fracture occurring within the area between the lesser and greater trochanters is called an *intertrochanteric fracture.* Pertrochanteric and trochanteric fractures are other labels given to them. Fractures which split off between the lesser trochanter and the femoral isthmus are called *subtrochanteric* fractures. There is often a crossover of the latter two areas. The fracture then derives its label from the region where the most of the fracture fragments reside.

Classification

There are three reasons why it is important to have a classification for fractures: (1) It becomes a research tool for properly comparing one set

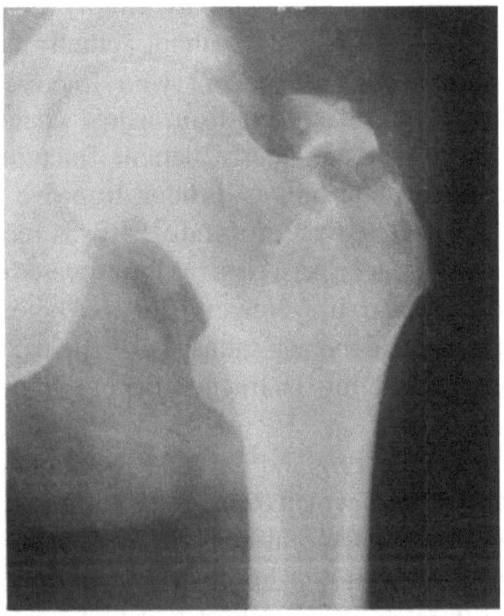

FIG. 8–3 Fracture of the greater trochanter: an avulsion injury within the insertion of the gluteal muscle tendon.

of data with others. (2) It is a means of prognosticating the outcome of one type over another. (3) It allows mapping out a treatment scheme for achieving a favorable outcome. Unfortunately, no one classification has yet to serve any of these needs completely.

X-ray studies are crucial for any fracture analysis. Garden[24] noted: "Much of the blame for long, continued failure to understand and resolve the problems of intracapsular fracture of the femoral neck must be attributed to the deplorable quality of hip joint radiology in those early days. The evil reputation of subcapital fractures and the misleading assumption made from misinterpretations of the slipshod radiographs that were then presented continued to affect our thinking about this fracture at the present time." This was stated 10 years ago and holds true today. The early writers looked at the anatomical site of the fracture[25,26] and categorized the fractures as subcapital and transcervical types. These labels have stuck and are loosely used. Subcapital refers to those fractures just below the head, and transcervical refers to fractures of the midportion of the neck. Other phrases are "high neck" and "low neck" and have simple labeling value only. In reality, the exact location cannot be accurately determined by preoperative x-ray studies unless there is some universal method of obtaining the x-ray films and of positioning the patient while in pain with a severely deformed leg.[24,27] Askin and Bryan thought that there was no difference between the two types, and if there appeared to be, it was due to x-ray artifacts.[28] Garden pointed out that the fracture line is an x-ray projection which varies in obliquity with any rotation of the distal fragment and not the fracture line per se because the femoral neck is spiral in shape.[29] The femoral neck must be placed parallel to the film, which would require sedation and careful reduction by an attending orthopedic surgeon, a very impractical situation. Linton proposed that most femoral neck fractures were at angles of 45° to 60° and that the low-angled ones were the early stage of the same fracture mechanism which would cause all of them to eventually become vertical.[30]

Pauwels, in a never-to-be-forgotten paper, classified these fractures by the obliquity of the fracture across the neck in the anteroposterior (AP) x-ray film.[31] Type I was fairly horizontal at 30°, type II at 50°, and type III at 70°. The more vertical type at 70° was supposedly at the mercy of severe shear forces and consequently held the worst prognosis. Pauwels completely ignored the coronal plane of the fracture, which may be more important than the sagittal plane. Furthermore, it had no value for preoperative planning, as only the postreduction x-ray films can give any clue to where the fracture line is really located. Subsequent investigators failed to find any validity to this method.[32,33] Finally Pauwels' classification has been abandoned as a serious means of typing femoral neck fractures.

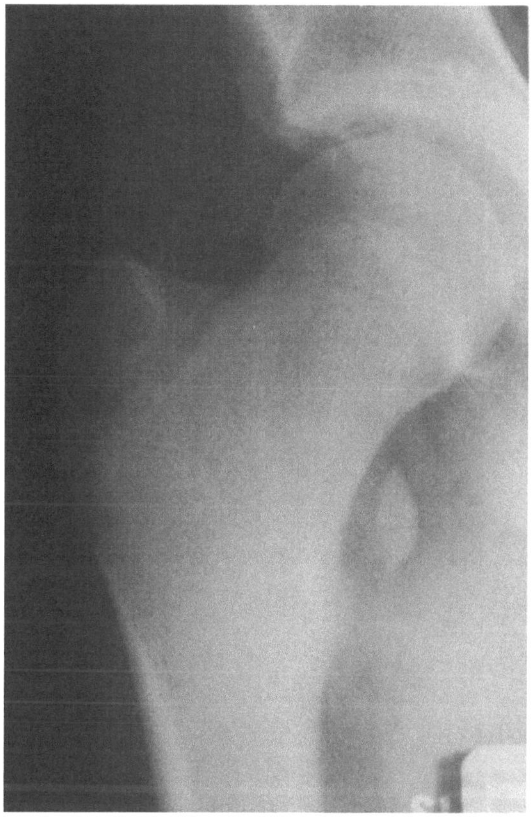

FIG. 8–4 Fracture of the lesser trochanter: an avulsion injury of the epiphysis which usually separates away with contracture of the iliopsoas tendon.

The most quoted classification has been that used by Garden.[24,34] He used the degree of displacement as a measure of typing femoral neck fractures. He based it on prereduction x-ray films *in the AP view only* (Fig. 8–5). The criteria are as follows:

Type I: Slight valgus displacement which has been called an impacted fracture.
Type II: No displacement.
Type III: Partial displacement with an intact reti-

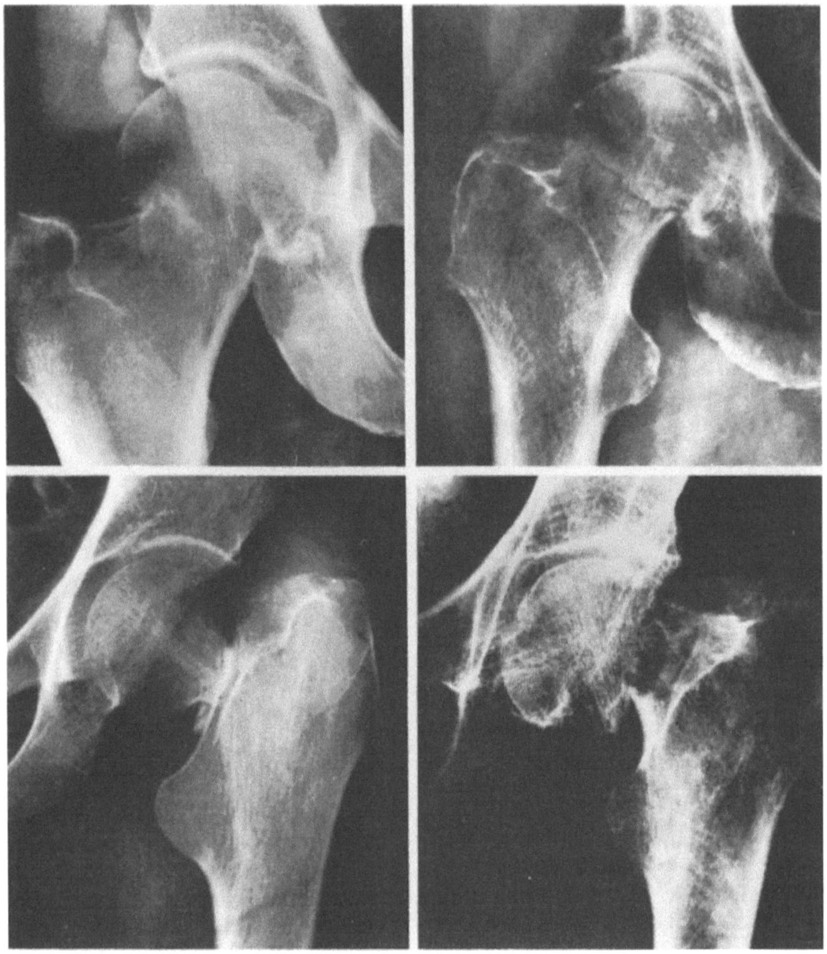

FIG. 8–5 Classification of subcapital fractures. Stage 1 (**A**): Incomplete subcapital fracture commonly known as the "abducted" or "impacted" fracture. The medial trabeculae at the junction of the head and neck sometimes appear to be bent rather than broken in the manner of a greenstick fracture. The appearance of abduction is the result of a posterolateral rotation of the proximal on the distal fragment. Stage II (**B**): Complete subcapital fraction without displacement. The alignment of the medial trabeculae in the two fragments is undisturbed. Stage III (**C**): Complete subcapital fracture with partial displacement. The direction of the medial trabeculae in the capital fragment shows that this fragment is rotated in a medial direction. Stage IV (**D**): Complete subcapital fracture with full displacement. Intimate contact between the two fragments has been lost, and the capital fragment is free to return to its normal position in the acetabulum as shown by the direction of its medial trabeculae, which now lie in alignment with their counterparts in the pelvis. (From Garden, R. S.: Stability and union in subcapital fractures of the femur. J. Bone Joint Surg., *46B:* 630. 1961.)

naculum which should be detected by looking at the trabecular pattern of the femoral head. The trabeculation of the neck does not line up with the trabecular pattern of the acetabulum. This is supposedly due to the fact that the retinacular fibers are intact and act as a tether which causes the head to rotate back to its normal anatomical orientation.

Type IV: The head is completely separated from the neck with complete laceration of the retinaculum and its blood vessels. Therefore the head rotates back into position so that its trabecular pattern lines up with the acetabulum.

In practice, few people have been able to distinguish between types III and IV. London[35] was the first to admit to this difficulty as a preoperative evaluation, and even after reduction and pinning the distinction remained esoteric. Therefore investigators simplify the classification into "displaced" and "undisplaced" (relatively speaking) neck fractures.[36–40]

Stable and Unstable Typing

Femoral neck fractures can be categorized into stable and unstable groups. *Stability* implies the presence of inherent characteristics which render any reduction needed relatively easy and the form of fixation reliable and predictable. *Instability* refers to those fractures whose reduction is quite difficult to achieve and internal fixation equally difficult to maintain.

A classification is proposed here by the author which has helped prognosticate a favorable outcome. It also aids in planning a treatment program. Unlike the Garden classification, which does not utilize lateral x-ray films, this one depends heavily on the analysis of lateral x-ray studies. Much of the fracture's behavior can be predicted by viewing the *lateral position* of the fragments and estimating the extent of the posterior comminution. CT scans are now available to help evaluate this aspect of the fracture (Fig. 8–6). The second parameter used to arrive at this classification is the appearance of the fracture line as it winds around the femoral neck as seen on the A/P x-ray film.

It must be noted that the x-ray studies used here are not special views in any way because it is impractical to request special studies when the patient is rushed to the radiology department and x-rayed with the leg positioned in whatever way that is comfortable at the time. This may in fact be a more realistic approach to the problem because the fragments seem to stabilize themselves in their own individual fashion. Furthermore, the fragments rarely change unless anesthesia is given and/or the leg is forcefully maneuvered.

The fractures are grouped into various characteristic *patterns*. It is not the intent to burden the reader with more types to be committed to memory. The patterns presented here serve as an atlas which can be referred to when trying to decide on a plan of treatment:

Unstable: complete separation in the lateral view
Stable: displaced but not separated
Impacted: an old term newly defined—no surgical treatment needed

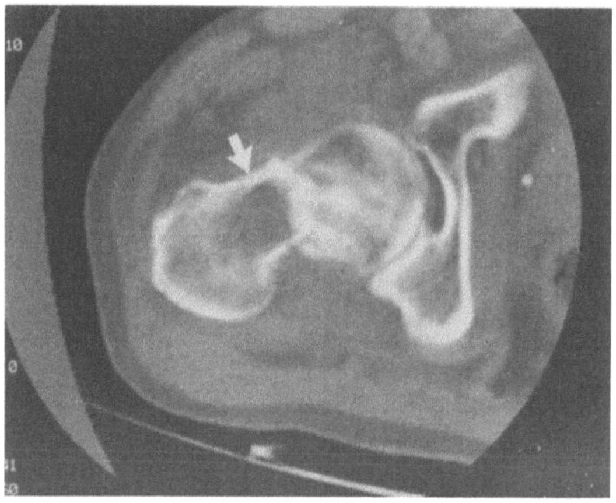

FIG. 8–6 CT scan of a displaced, unstable, femoral neck fracture. Note the magnitude of osteoporosis in the femoral neck, which is the single most important reason for fixation failure and collapse of the fracture. The arrow points to the hollowed neck.

Unstable Fractures

Unstable fractures of the femoral neck are distinctly displaced in both planes, either varus or valgus. In the lateral view the fragments are completely separated from one another. There is little or no continuity between the head and the neck. Marked comminution of the fragments posteriorly is the hallmark (Fig. 8–7). Most are almost impossible to reduce anatomically or near-anatomically. Consequently, they are difficult to hold reduced. One must decide whether a closed reduction, open reduction, or arthroplasty is preferred.

Unstable Pattern I The neck is fractured high, almost transversely (Fig. 8–8), and there is complete separation of the fragments. The comminution occurs in the posterior portion of the head fragment (Fig. 8–9). In the AP view one can see the sharp extension on the inferior part of the neck (Fig. 8–10). If the head is in less external rotation, more of the intact neck can be appreciated (Fig. 8–11). Frequently the patient's leg is severely rotated outwardly causing the AP radiograph to appear more like a lateral view (Fig. 8–12).

The unstable pattern I is the most common type of neck fracture seen in the elderly female patient. It comes closest to being a true subcapital

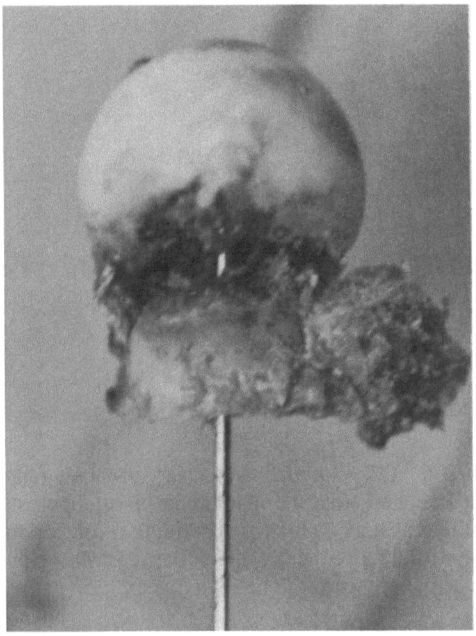

FIG. 8–7 Unstable fracture. Marked comminution of the fragments posteriorly is the hallmark. A gap has been created in the compression side of the femoral neck when the fracture collapses posteriorly.

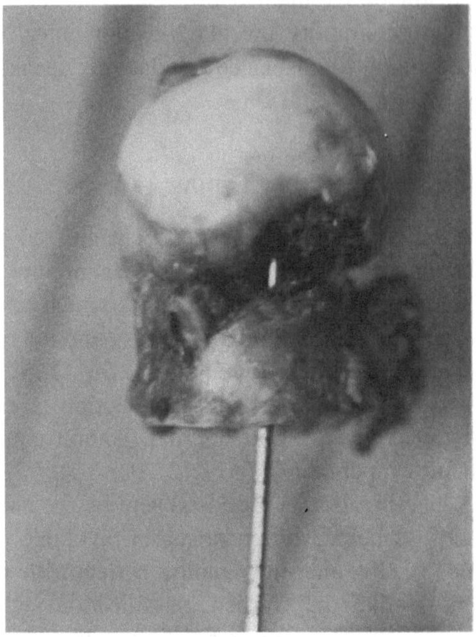

FIG. 8–9 Once the fracture is reduced, *if* it reduces, there remains a significant gap in the posterior portion of the head–neck junction. Comminution occurs mainly in the neck fragment, but some of the comminution also occurs in the head itself where a butterfly fragment is frequently seen which is here shown as a flap. This is the same fracture as in Fig. 8–7.

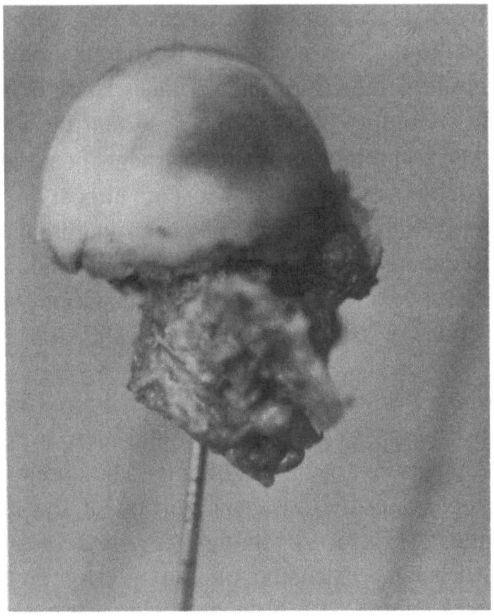

FIG. 8–8 The unstable pattern typically seen in the *elderly* patient shows a squared-off neck and a very comminuted posterior head segment. The fracture is at the junction of the edge of the head. The head is not only rotated onto the neck for an angular deformity, but the neck is shifted as it points anteriorly and the head shifts posteriorly. Note the bruising of the articular cartilage from the impact.

fracture, as the osteoporosis is most severe at the head–neck junction. The femoral neck is a hollow shell (Fig. 8–6). Posteriorly it looks like an explosion took place.

Unstable Pattern II Less frequently the fracture is not as transverse. There is more of the neck on the head fragment; this ''beak'' appears as the inferior part of the head (Fig. 8–13). The beak has been mistaken as being in the AP plane and near vertical as proposed by Pauwels' type III. In reality, it is a short spiral fragment coming off the posterior neck. A small butterfly fragment may even be present as part of the comminution pattern (Fig. 8–14). It is an ominous sign, as it bespeaks of a fracture that will be difficult to reduce and just as difficult to hold reduced. The fragments are separated with some contact posteriorly at the site of the deformity or at the hinge, like an open book with the opening or gap anteriorly, as seen in the lateral view (Fig. 8–15). In the middle-aged population, this fracture takes

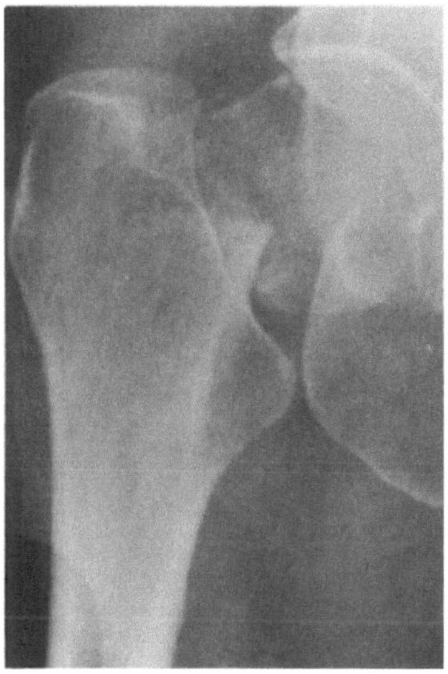

FIG. 8–10 In the AP x-ray one can see the sharp extension on the neck which gouges into the head. Note the prominent lesser trochanter indicative of the leg being externally rotated.

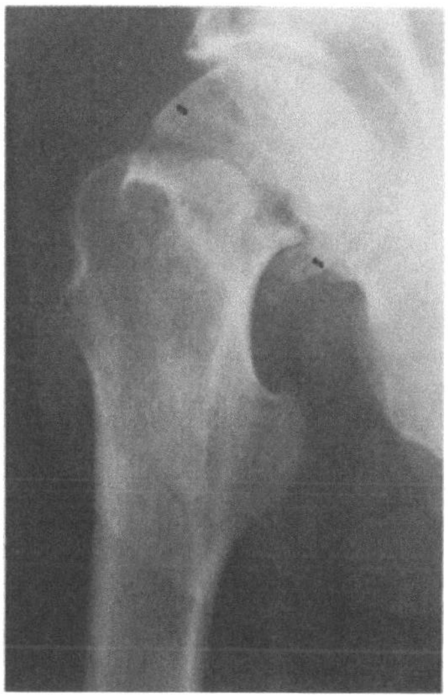

FIG. 8–12 Because of the severe rotation of the head, it is almost impossible to detect the trabeculations in the head that are essential for adhering to Garden's classification. For this reason, the Garden classification is often impractical.

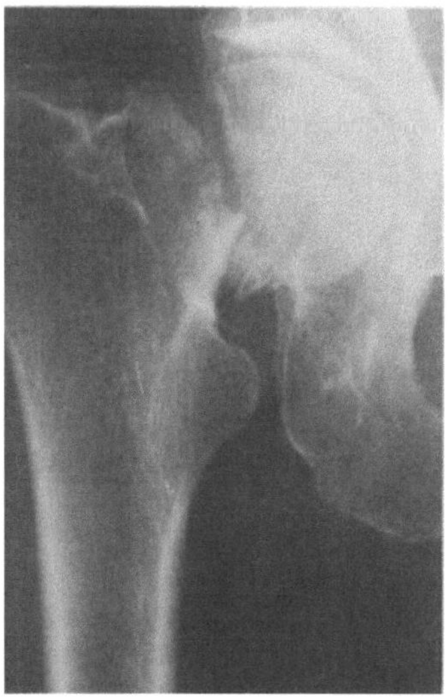

FIG. 8–11 The head is twisted in less external rotation so that less of the neck can be seen. This is a neck fracture.

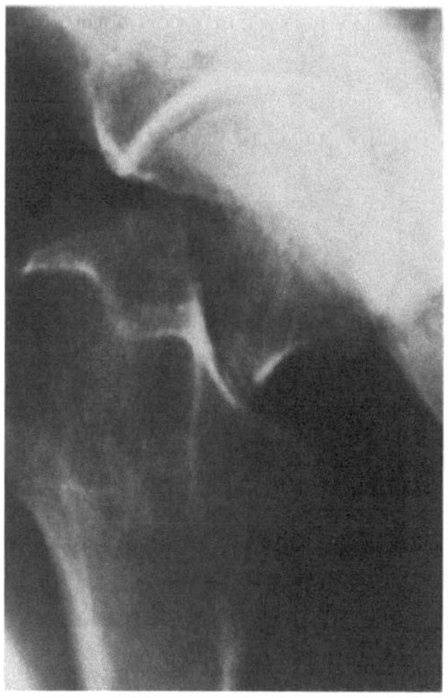

FIG. 8–13 X-ray of an Unstable type II with the head as a major fragment. Its inferior "beak" is obvious since the head does not rotate in the socket because the posterior retinaculum is completely severed leaving the fragments independent of one another.

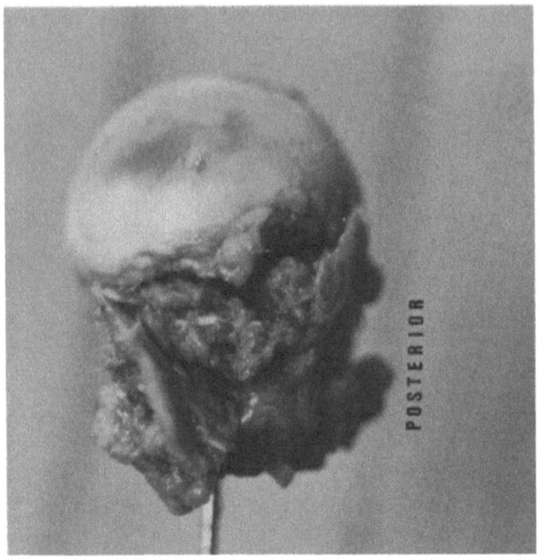

FIG. 8–14 Note the short spiral type of butterfly fragment coming off the posterior portion of the neck, which is the compression side.

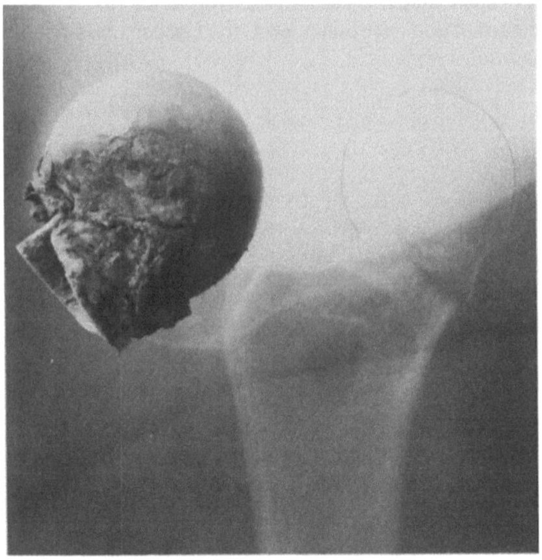

FIG. 8–15 Lateral view. The fragments are less separated, with some contact posteriorly at the apex of the deformity or at the hinge, similar to a book with the opening or gap posteriorly.

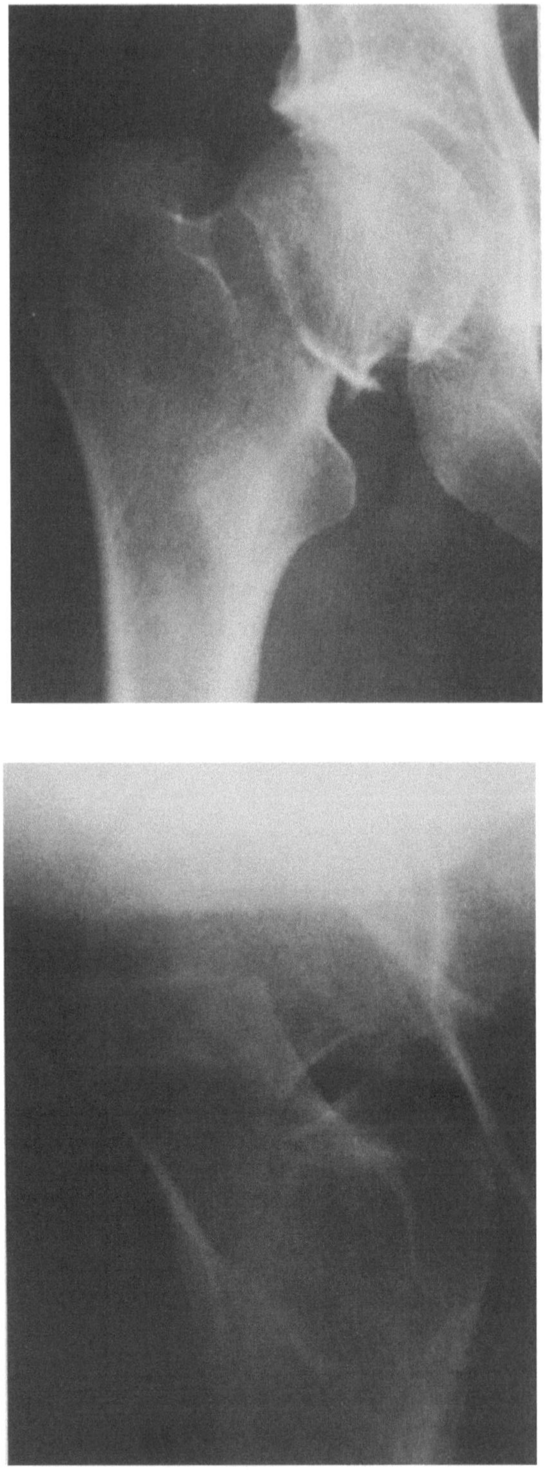

A

B

FIG. 8–16 **A** AP view. Fracture takes on a similar form in the middle-aged population with what seems to be minimal displacement. The white line is caused by the fracture edge as seen from a head-on view. **B** On closer look from a lateral x-ray, one can appreciate the "white" line across the fracture which indicates that the head fragment is severely angulated. The "white" line represents the turned-up edge of the head fragment as it is superimposed on the neck.

on a similar form in the AP view with what seems to be minimal displacement (Fig. 8–16A). On closer look one can appreciate the "white" line across the fracture which indicates that the head fragment is severely angulated (Fig. 8–16B) because the "white" line represents the turned-up edge of the head fragment. These fractures have a somewhat better chance of being adequately reduced. There is always a lateral shift of the fragments as well as a residual angular deformity (Fig. 8–17).

Unstable Pattern III Markedly displaced valgus fractures as seen in the AP view (Fig. 8–18A) are unstable and must be distinguished from the slightly displaced version, as discussed under Stable Fractures. These are also markedly displaced in the lateral x-ray view (Fig. 8–18B). They roll into valgus because there is comminution superiorly as well as posteriorly. *They are not truly impacted.* The valgus configuration cannot be improved without making them worse, whereas the lateral postion may be improved by careful manipulation. These fractures were formerly grouped together regardless of their displacement and were considered stable fracture situations, which is incorrect by this investigator's analysis because they can be almost impossible to properly reduce into a more acceptable varus postion. The slightly displaced valgus fractures are quite different and are not included here because they are true stable complexes.

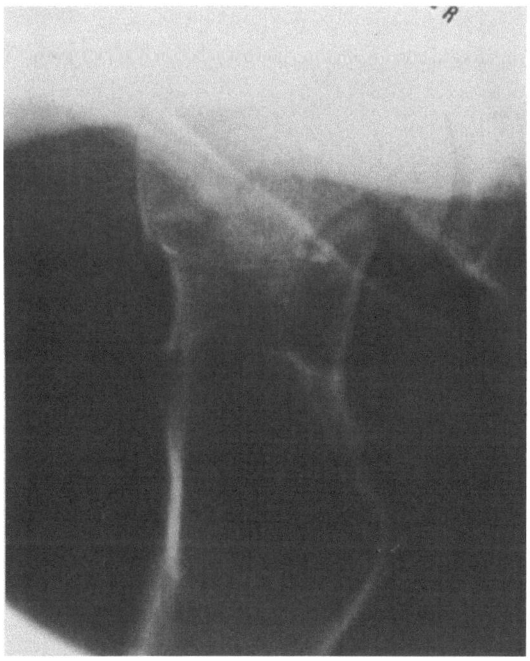

Fig. 8–17 The lateral x-ray is the most important tool for appraising both the characteristics as well as the quality of reduction of a neck fracture. Here the neck is well reduced but the head is still angulated posteriorly due to the comminution.

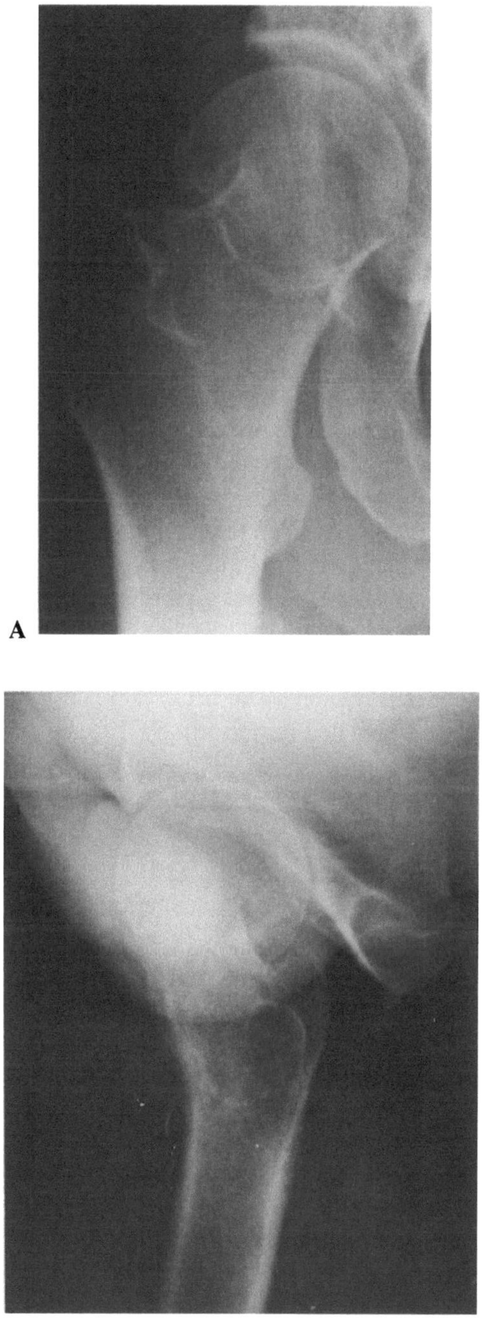

A

B

Fig. 8–18 **A** Unstable type III is the valgus fracture. This fracture is deceivingly unstable. **B** In the lateral x-ray the neck looks squared off. There is comminution all across the fracture line. Because the head is rolled off posteriorly there is a double fracture line on the AP x-ray (A) which is mistaken as impaction.

Unstable Pattern IV In young adults and adolescents the femoral neck is not osteoporotic; its cortex is strong and thick. The posterior neck does not become as comminuted, if at all. In patients in their forties and younger, the femoral neck fractures in a spiral manner with a short, oblique pattern (Fig. 8–19). These fractures are very difficult to reduce and pin[41] because of the spiral obliquity of the fracture line (Fig. 8–19B).

Stable Fractures

When there is less osteopenia, less posterior comminution, and consequently less displacement, the fracture is considered a stable one. Whatever displacement is present is easily reduced, and the hip is easy to pin. Open reduction is not a consideration. Healing is quick, nonunions are rare, and aseptic necrosis is seldom a complication.

Stable Pattern I This pattern represents a valgus or abducted fracture. The neck, jammed into the head, is angulated posteriorly by 10° and in the AP view sits abducted by 10° to 15° (Fig. 8–20). The head is is still perched precariously, so it must be pinned. Bentley[145] showed how it can roll off if not pinned (see Impacted Fracture, below). They must be destinguished from what the author has redefined as "undisplaced impacted" fractures, Fig. 8–28.

Stable Pattern II Short *oblique* fractures have little or no displacement in either plane (Fig. 8–21). They are not well impacted and can become easily displaced if treated casually. They must be pinned.

Stable Pattern III (*Stress Fractures*) Stress fractures are grouped in this category. Rare and peculiar, they are most commonly found in the younger population who are athletic. If one should appear in an older patient as a spontaneous fracture, it is likely associated with some osteogenic disorder.[42] An elderly patient can present with a fairly acute onset of pain in the hip or groin, and internal rotation of the leg produces consider-

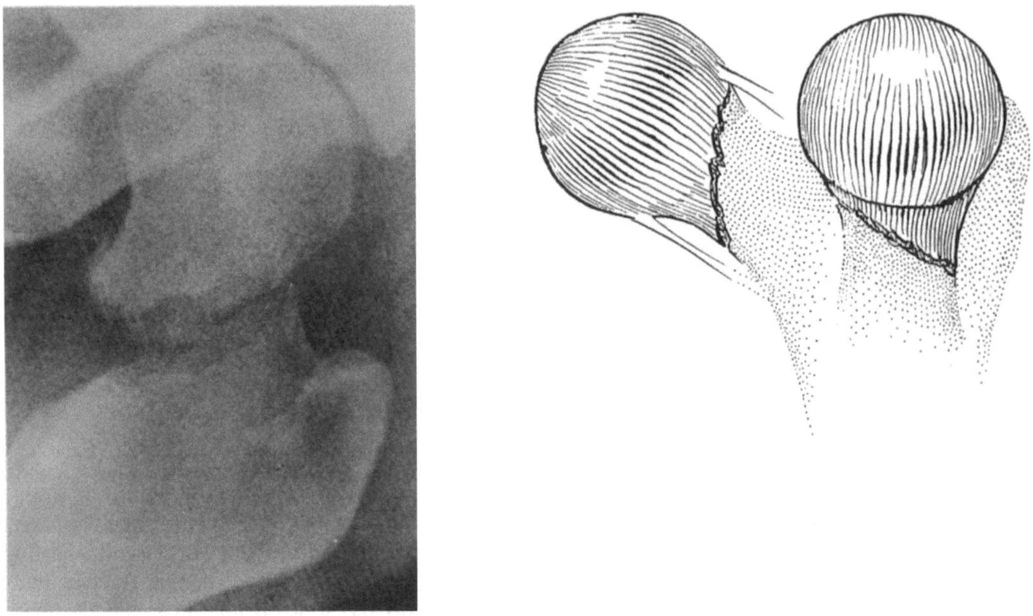

A

B

FIG. 8–19 **A** This is a very oblique, almost vertical fracture type seen in young adults and adolescents. What makes it so difficult to manage surgically is that it is a spiral fracture so that keeping the fragments together is virtually impossible without firm fixation. (Adapted from Swiontkowski, M. F., Umquist, R. A., Hanse, S. T.: Fractures of the femoral neck in patients between the age of twelve and forty-nine years. J. Bone Joint Surg., 66A:837, 1984.) **B** The manner in which the spiral fragment occupies two planes on the femoral neck at one time is demonstrated by the artist.

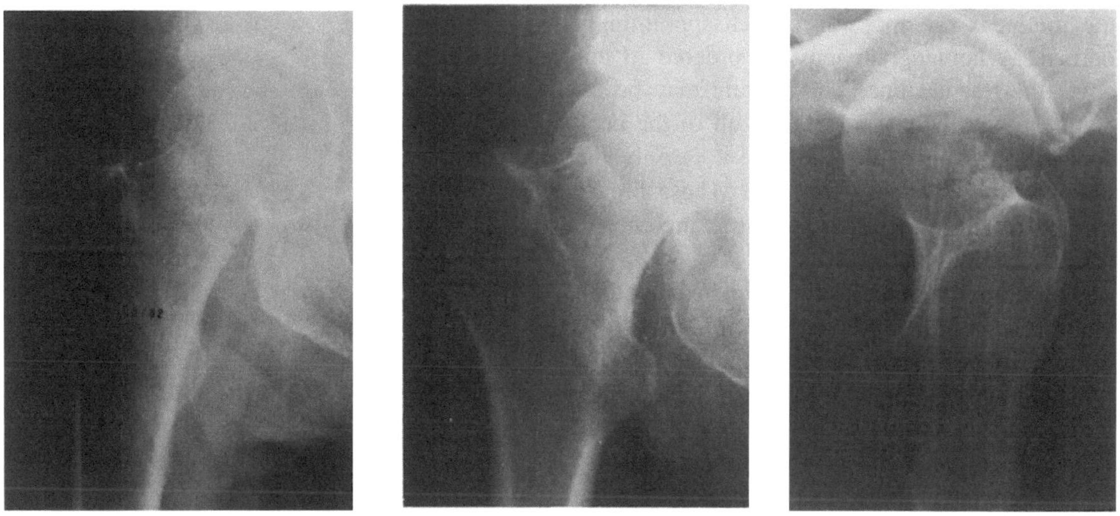

A B C

FIG. 8–20 **A** Stable type I fracture. The head fragment is only moderately abducted and only slightly rotated posteriorly. It is inherently stable and is impacted to some degree. **B** Another example of an abduction fracture showing the impacted nature of the squared-off neck being jammed into the head fragment. **C** The most important view to be used in determining stability is the lateral x-ray. Here there is only slight angulation which translates into a very stable fracture type.

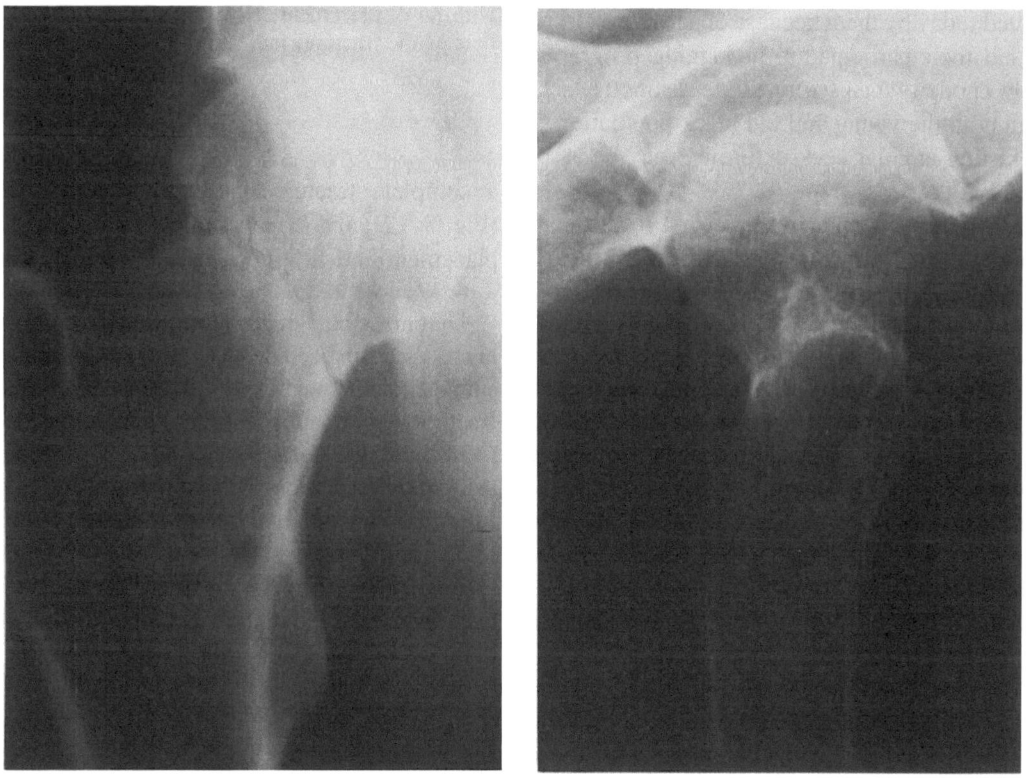

A B

FIG. 8–21 **A** Stable pattern II fracture. Note the short, oblique fracture line through the upper neck. The fracture is only slightly displaced, but that does not mean it is an impacted type of fracture. This fracture, along with stable fracture pattern I, can easily shift and migrate into varus as been shown by Linton. **B** There is slight displacement (10°) posteriorly in this lateral x-ray. (From Linton, P.: Types of displacement in fractures of the neck of the femur. J. Bone Joint Surg., 31B:184, 1949.)

able pain. The pain can be disabling even though the routine x-ray appearance is disappointingly normal. A laminogram must be ordered to uncover the fracture line. The fracture may be incomplete with only the superior half of the neck appearing fractured; occasionally it is only the inferior neck that looks fractured. These breaks can be treated in the older patient as incomplete fractures, but must be pinned.

The more common variety is seen in the young, vigorous athletic man who engages in some physical activity with short spurts of intensity, e.g., army recruit on a forced march.[43,44] Such a fracture occurs in otherwise normal bone. A male patient in his twenties may present with a history of experiencing progressive groin pain,[43–45] or the fracture can occur in a younger patient with an open epiphysis.[46] Bilateral cases have been reported.[47] These fractures may appear simultaneously with other stress fractures, e.g., in the metatarsals.[43] They have been called "spontaneous fractures[42] and fatigue fractures.[48] There have been reports of these fractures in increasing numbers among joggers.[49] Women are being plagued today by them because of aerobic exercising and their participation in jogging programs. Oddly enough, such fractures are distinctly lacking in both the young and old black population.[49] Preexisting angular neck deformity may be associated with a stress fracture.[36]

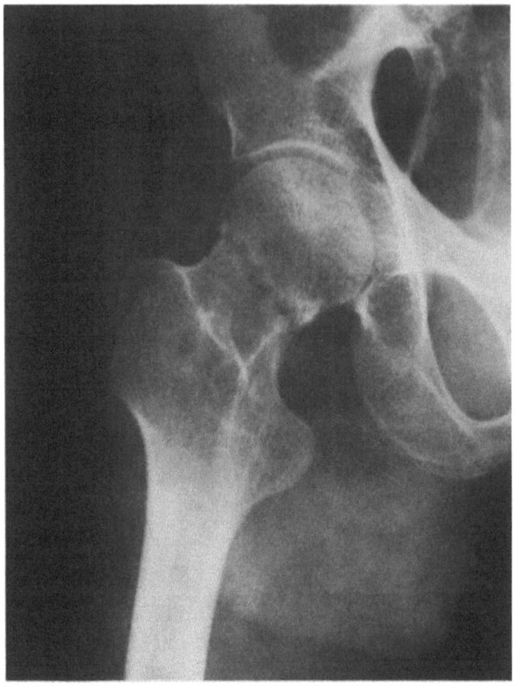

FIG. 8–22 Stable pattern III: stress fracture. There is little or no comminution, a complete fracture line with no displacement. Note the slightly sclerotic borders of the fracture, indicating its chronic nature.

Historically, Blecher was the first to draw attention to stress fractures as distinct entities.[50] Other major reports are by Morris and Blickenstaff[51] and Devas.[43] Ernst's report emphasized the high incidence of complications when these fractures are allowed to become displaced.[52] They typically require more time for healing than that needed for other neck fractures.[43,50] There is little or no comminution (Fig. 8–22), and there is usually sclerosis on either side of the fracture line (Fig. 8–22), indicating the chronic nature of the situation.

Devas[43] defined two forms: (1) a transverse "distraction" or oblique fracture seen in the superior neck perpendicular to the femoral neck; and (2) a type of "compression" fracture with a more horizontal line seen in the inferior neck. There is typically sclerosis on either side of the fracture which Devas suggested is evidence that these are fatigue fractures. Morris and Bleckenstaff[51] defined three types: (1) an incomplete fracture in the neck with sclerotic borders (Fig. 8–23); (2) a complete fracture line with no displacement (Fig. 8–22); and (3) a complete fracture with displacement and little to no sclerosis indicative of a more acute process (Fig. 8–24).

Diagnosis may be difficult. Such fractures must always be suspected, even though initial x-ray studies may be negative. If the problem is a stress fracture, the x-ray films may become positive 10 to 14 days later because of endosteal or subperiosteal callus formation.[50] Bone scans are very helpful as they are positive before routine x-rays films reveal a fracture.[52] "The subtlety of symptoms associated with impending stress fractures is often responsible for the diagnosis being missed. A patient in one of the groups, young or old, who demonstrates pain in the hip or knee with exertion, limitation of hip motion, or localized anterior tenderness, in spite of negative x-rays, *has a stress fracture of the femoral neck until proven otherwise.*"[36] Tenderness may be minimal because of the heavy musculature over the hip area. Stressing the joint in extreme internal rotation usually elicits pain.

The incidence of nonunions and avascular necrosis has not been accurately measured because of the rarity of the fracture, the inconsistency of early diagnosis, and the various modes of treatment.[50]

These fractures can be difficult to manage because they are deceivingly treacherous. Treating them in traction is more of a gamble than one may realize, because they can displace while the patient lies in bed.[50] It is recommended that these fractures be pinned as early as possible or as soon as the diagnosis is established, regardless of age.[53] Pinning them is not easy. If the fracture is in a young muscular athlete, the bone is hard so that predrilling may be necessary before pins can be properly placed across the fracture. Nor can they be allowed to bear weight early because the fracture can displace. Since they are slow to heal, they must be monitored carefully before the patient is given free use of the leg. Morris and Blickenstaff[51] reported nine displaced fractures, four of which never united and three of which required two operations to achieve union. Walsh recommended bone grafting in displaced versions.[54] DeLee thought that a hemiarthroplasty

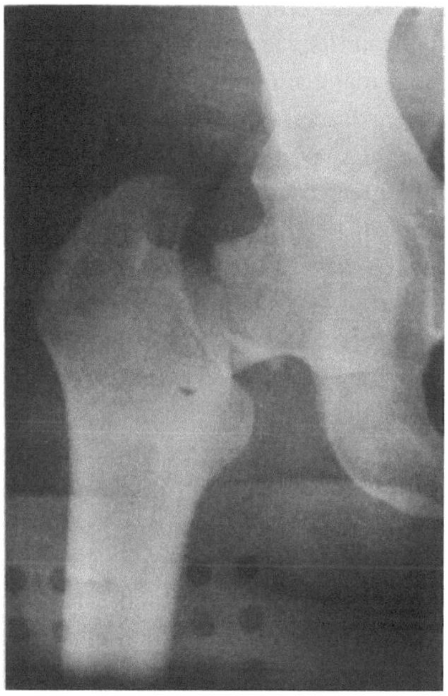

FIG. 8–24 Stress fracture. Note the complete fracture with displacement in this young athlete with no sclerosis, indicating the acute nature of the fracture. The edges are sharp. There is very little posterior comminution. The fracture plane is not so oblique as in other traumatic femoral neck fractures.

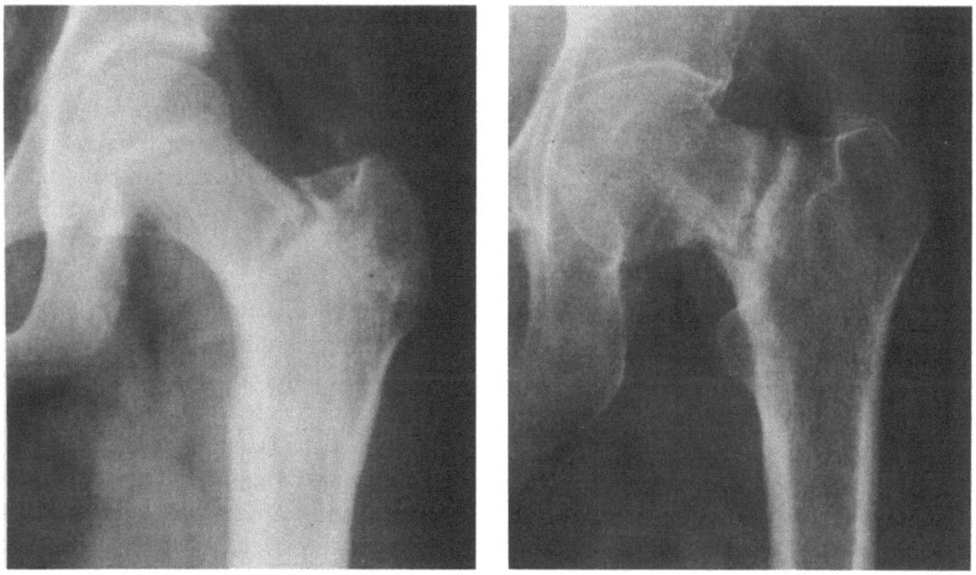

A B

FIG. 8–23 **A** Stress fracture with an incomplete fracture line typically seen at the base of the superior portion of the neck. **B** Stress fracture with varus deformity and a complete fracture line.

was justified as primary treatment in the older patient with a displaced stress fracture.[36]

Surgical management comprises closed reduction of these fractures if they are displaced, after which they are pinned. When treated early the displacement is usually not severe, and a good reduction can be expected. However, if the displacement is severe, one must be ready for an open reduction. Proceeding directly to a hemiarthroplasty is justified in the elderly patient,[36] but in the younger patient everything should be done to preserve the natural femoral head. A sliding compression screw is not recommended because it is too difficult to screw across the thick femoral neck. The head can easily rotate with such a device, which may compromise the vital arterial blood supply. Furthermore, such a large implant in and of itself may cause enough destruction inside the femoral head to destroy the blood supply to it. Any of the new heavier pins is a better choice, when at least three are inserted.

Stress Fracture After Pinning Tronzo first described a unique type of stress fracture.[55] If an intertrochanteric fracture is fixed with a device which penetrates only to the head–neck junction, a stress riser is created which can produce a fracture (Fig. 8–25). Such fractures have been confirmed to exist by others.[56–58] The second fracture usually occurs after the original fracture is healed, when the stress riser effect eventually comes into play. It is best treated by a total hip replacement because the acetabulum will have undergone enough degeneration to make a hemiarthroplasty unsuccessful. Hopefully this fracture will become extinct when surgeons realize that the implant must penetrate well into the head past the head–neck junction.

"Impacted" Fracture Redefined

Traditionally, impacted fractures have been considered together as one type of neck fracture. Even though they are recognized as distinctly different from undisplaced fractures, they are still grouped with them. Collectively they are "Garden I" fractures, and all supposedly have "inherent stability."[59] It has been reported that the impacted fracture assumes a valgus or abducted posture because the cortex of the femoral neck has been driven into the cancellous femoral neck[96] and thus there is assumed to be a built-in stability.[57,60,61]

Because of this assumption their treatment is controversial. Must they be pinned? Can they be left unpinned? Could they be disimpacted if abducted too severely? Crawford[62] described a variety which clinically produces little pain; indeed the patients came to medical attention several days after their falls and after they had been bearing weight on the leg. So why not let them continue?[59,63,64]

Although varus impacted fractures have been reported, there is some doubt that they actually exist, and some say they may be a misinterpretation of AP x-ray studies only. Lowell found that such fractures became displaced after conservative treatment, indicating that there is no inherent stability. He believed that all fractures showing any degree of varus or valgus, or any posterior angulation greater than 30°, require internal fixation.[65] MacAusland and colleagues recommended that *all* impacted fractures be treated the same as other femoral neck fractures and pinned to prevent further displacement and nonunion.[66] This has long been advised by Fielding[67] and Pankovich.[59] Yet there is still confusion as to when one should be treated surgically.[67,68] The incidence of lost reduction varies from 8 to 20% and that of aseptic necrosis from 13 to 40%.[36]

This author has made a concerted effort to study these relatively undisplaced fractures in order to sort out the variables responsible for such reportedly inconsistent behavior. Perhaps a more careful look at them would uncover some specific pattern that would help formulate a more reliable treatment plan. These fractures were studied using a posterior approach and were treated via a hemiarthroplasty. From these clinical observations three distinct types of fracture evolved.

When the head displaces in both directions to a significant degree, it not only angulates but *shifts* off the femoral neck (Fig. 8–18). The most significant feature is the extreme posture of the head seen on the lateral x-ray film. These fractures have been reclassified as *unstable pattern III*. This extreme deformity must be corrected for several reasons. If left, the joint will have a large amount of necrosis and nonunion, and the patient will ultimately have a knock-knee deformity (Fig. 8–26). Aufranc[69] recognized the true nature of this fracture when he wrote in 1958: "There are favorable and unfavorable impacted fractures. . . . The angle of the valgus postion should not be greater than an angle in which the general

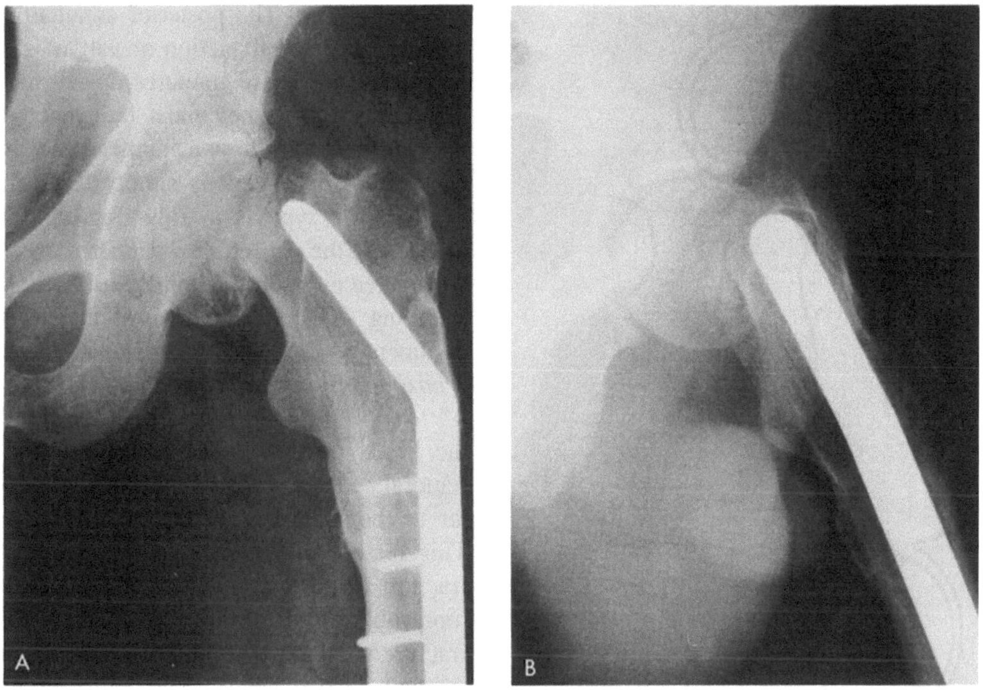

Fig. 8–25 A unique stress fracture occurred when a nail was too short to cross the point of stress at the neck–head junction created by the tip of the nail. This was first described by Tronzo in 1973 and has since been referred to as the "Tronzo fracture"; it is an avoidable phenomenon if the fixation device were to extend deep into the head past the femoral neck junction.

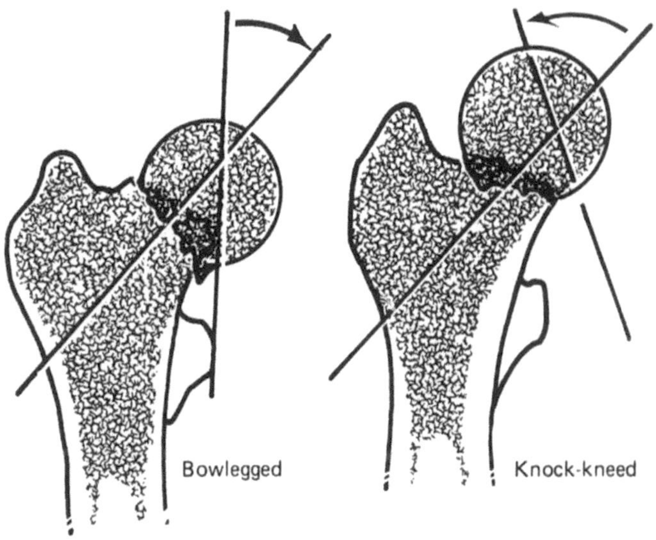

Fig. 8–26 When the head fragment is shifted in severe valgus, the patient can be expected to walk with a knock-knee deformity. Should it be left in varus, the patient becomes bowlegged.

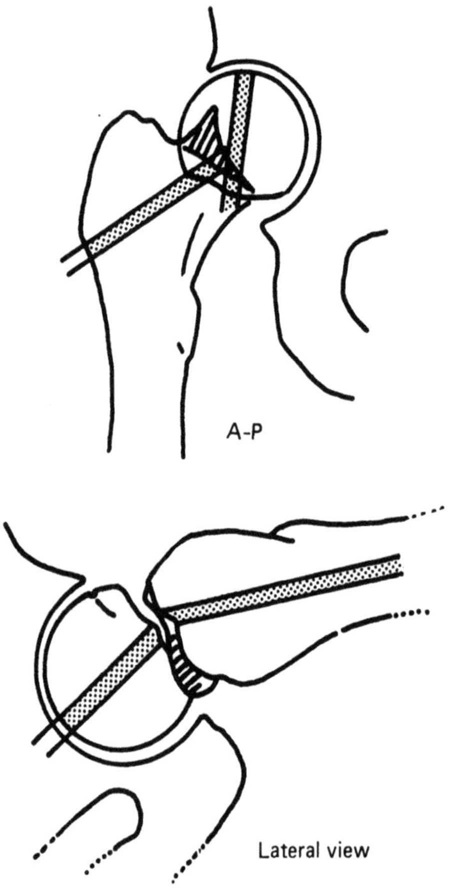

FIG. 8–27 Garden's classification of fractures, which depends on observing the trabecular pattern in both head and neck, was first conceived by Aufranc. These drawings demonstrate the very unstable nature of the so-called valgus or impacted fracture. Aufranc stated, "The head is so severely displaced that it will surely go to either nonunion or aseptic necrosis." Time and observation have proved him correct with regard to this fracture. (From Aufranc, O. E.: In: *Fractures and Dislocations of the Hip.* Edited by E. F. Cave. Chicago, Year Book 1958, Chap. 25.)

trabecular pattern of the head fragment is less than perpendicular. A valgus position forming an angle greater than this may result in aseptic necrosis or nonunion" and loss of reduction. (Fig. 8–27). Furthermore, at surgical exposure they can easily be rolled off the neck completely. Aufranc acknowledged that his views were not shared by all of his colleagues at the Massachusetts General Hospital. "Some members of the Fracture Clinic do not believe that an increased valgus position is necessarily a hazard."[69] In this author's opinion Aufranc was astute as well as correct. Yet few people heard him.

A second group of fractures have been called *stable pattern I.* The fragments here are driven into each other. The posterior angulation is less than 15° and the abduction or valgus is likewise less than 15°. These fractures do not have to be manipulated, but they must be pinned because they are well fixed to one another and may disimpact when the patient is simply lying in bed.[68]

The third type is a truly impacted fracture, called here the *undisplaced impacted* fracture and considered as a separate entity. It is distinguished by being so jammed into itself that no surgical treatment is needed. *The critical point is that there is no angulation seen in the lateral view, (although 2° to 5° may be tolerated).* In the lateral view the head is seen to sit squarely on top of the femoral neck, and the fracture line is perpendicular to the long axis of the neck (Fig. 8–28A). This feature distinguishes it from the stable II fracture (Fig. 8–21), where the fracture line is more oblique to the long axis which makes the fracture vulnerable to rotational stresses and subsequent displacement. The impacted head is perched in abduction or in valgus in the AP view by no more than a few degrees (Fig. 8–28B) (10° is acceptable *if* there is absolutely no angulation seen in the lateral view).

These truly impacted fractures are so stable that they can be treated conservatively by watchful waiting with no surgical stabilization needed. Clinically, they have other distinguishing features. All patients with undisplaced impacted fractures were younger, between 55 and 72 years of age, the average age being 66. There was no deformity of the affected leg, and the patient usually walked in to be checked using no external support. There was little or no pain, but there was a bothersome ache in the groin or the knee for several days. A minor traumatic episode could be faintly remembered. A trial of passive motion was painless, although any forceful internal rotation to the extreme can cause pain. The patients could raise and rotate their legs easily without more than an achy feeling.

Tronzo and Penner have collected data from 42 of these fractures over a 4-year period. All of the patients were managed with 1 to 3 days of bed rest either at home or in the hospital (if they had been admitted by the referring physician). They were instructed on crutch walking or ambulation with a walker, and they practiced nonweight-bearing, progressing to partial weight-bearing and finally to full weight-bearing as the

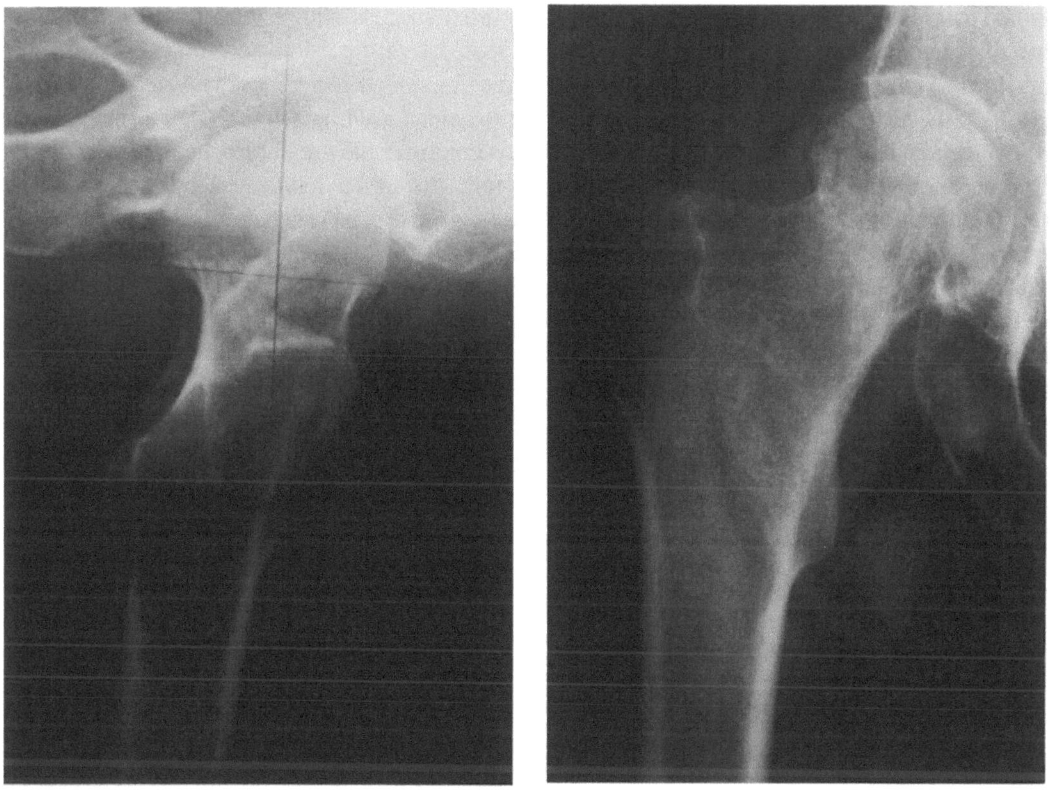

A B

Fig. 8–28 **A** Undisplaced, truly impacted fracture. The head is precisely impacted into the neck at a near-perfect perpendicular angle as seen in both views. The displacement is only a few degrees in either direction (no more than 5°). **B** The most important view is the lateral, where only a few degrees can be tolerated if this fracture is to be treated without pinning. This fracture is distinct from the undisplaced fracture seen in Fig. 8–21.

pain disappeared. They were told generally to restrict their activities considerably. They were judiciously warned that the fracture might ''fall apart,'' which would then require surgical pinning. They were further warned to come into the office immediately should they experience sudden or progressive groin pain. All of the patients chosen for such treatment were estimated to be alert and able to fully understand the instructions so that complete cooperation was anticipated. In one patient the fracture slipped slightly into varus 4 weeks later after she was walking with full weight-bearing despite pain. She declined surgical treatment, and the fracture healed without further migration and to her satisfaction. So far there have been no nonunions or necrotic heads. Healing time, as measured by the complete absence of pain, was 10 weeks maximum.

Bentley[68] reviewed a series of 73 ''impacted'' fractures. In effect, he collected together so-called impacted fractures, some of which were slightly displaced and some of which were undisplaced.[68] Four fractures in his patients (5.5%) disimpacted during the first 2 weeks. Two others fell into varus and healed, and a seventh ''rotated externally somewhat.'' That gave a 9.5% rate of slips. He did not attempt to distinguish which fractures slipped and which did not. If he had categorized them as outlined here, his data would possibly have matched ours.

Management of Fractures by Region

Femoral Head Fractures

Fractures confined only to the femoral head are rare injuries (Fig. 8–2). They can be isolated, as in gunshot wounds, but usually are part of the hip fracture/dislocation complex. Thompson and Epstein classified dislocations of the hip into five groups.[70] It was their fifth grouping which contained associated femoral head fractures when the hip dislocated posteriorly. Pipkin, in a classic paper, further divided these fractures into four types.[71] The head fragment may be either above or below the fovea, and it may be associated with an additional neck fracture or with a major fracture complex of the acetabulum. The size of the fragment is an important dimension. The fragment is typically anterior and superior. CT scans are crucial to mapping out the surgical approach to the injury. It is well to be suspicious of head fragments in any fracture/dislocation of the hip joint.

There are guidelines to follow: Closed reductions should always be tried, *but be aware of the possibility that one can create a femoral neck fracture while forcefully reducing the femoral head.* An open reduction is needed if the fragment fails to fall into a nearly anatomical position or if the attempt fails altogether. If the fragment is less than 25% of the volume of the head, is inferior, and is non-weight-bearing, it can be excised. When the fragment approaches one-third the volume of the head, it should be fixed with some form of internal pin or screw (Fig. 8–3). Associated neck fractures are difficult and take priority, being fixed first; the head fragment is then separately pinned. Total hip arthroplasty must be considered when both sides of the joint remain distorted.

Bipolar devices have no place here, where there is always some degree of damage to the acetabular surfaces. Acetabular fractures are fixed, and then the head fragment is treated by following the routine guidelines for a femoral neck fracture. The ligamentum teres is kept intact if possible; however, it may have to be sacrificed if the entire fragment must be delivered in order to attain an anatomical reduction, which is important for a good functional result. Total hip arthroplasty may have to be considered, especially for the older patient who would be a candidate for the procedure because of age alone.

There are two approaches to internal fixation. One is to pin the fragment by threading thin Steinmann pins up from the femoral neck, thereby piercing the fragment. The other is to screw the fragment into place directly with AO malleolar screws, which can be countersunk below the articular cartilage.[72–76]

Dowd and Johnston, on the other hand, reported success with a nonoperative regimen.[77]

A lateral incision formulated by Tronzo is recommended for comprehensive exposure to the hip joint (Volume I, p. 100). Do not hesitate to osteotomize the greater trochanter for better exposure; it can be reattached by two crossed AO screws and washers. Refer to Mears and Rubash, Chapter 5, for a detailed description of the star-shaped incision for yet another comprehensive exposure to these complicated acetabular fractures. Surgical management of these fractures belongs to the seasoned hip surgeon with appropriate skills and experience.

Femoral Neck Fractures

Fractures through the femoral neck are variously described as transcervical, cervical, or subcapital. They cover an area from the base of the caput to (not through) the intertrochanteric line. Women are more often affected than men and within an age range that is climbing. In 1975 at St. Mary's Hospital in West Palm Beach, Florida, the average age of women with these fractures was 77. In 1985 the average age was 81. At the time of this writing, August 1985, there were four women on one orthopedic floor with fractured hips whose ages ranged from 90 to 96. It was once thought that patients with femoral neck fractures were about 3 years younger than those with intertrochanteric fractures. It is not true in our series. Their age paralled intertrochanteric fractures. (The "basicervical" fracture is not included here but is discussed in detail under intertrochanteric fractures.)

In a classic treatise on femoral neck fractures, Speed attributed notoriety to them by branding them "the unsolved fracture."[78] Dickson tried to dilute the label's impact.[79] Barnes added another note of pessimism by calling them "the unsolvable fracture."[80] The only uncontrolled complication is the development of avascular necrosis, and even that problem is being lessened by more accurate reductions and more efficient internal fixation. Arthroplasties using improved designed implants have become more successful with a much better functional outcome. These fractures are no more mysterious or unsolvable than any other major fracture and maybe less so than many.

Anatomy of the Femoral Neck

The general anatomy of the femoral neck can be reviewed by referring to Volume I, Chapter 3. There are several unique features of the upper end of the femur which must be appreciated to understand the behavior of these fractures.

The most important of these is the vascular supply to the femoral head. Figure 8–29 depicts a special complex of vessels. This blood supply is discussed in detail by Crock and Dickens in Volume I. For the first time anywhere the venous drainage of the upper femur has been described by them, and the main arterial supply was considered in three areas: (1) the arterial ring outside the capsule which is located at the base of the femoral neck; (2) the ascending cervical arteries closely attached to the femoral neck as they emerge from the extracapsular ring; and (3) the arteries of the round ligmament. The parent blood supply comes from the obturator artery to the round ligament; and the medial and lateral femoral circumflex arteries converge to make up the extracapsular arterial ring. The most important arterial complex is located posteriorly in a synovial fold as a collection of the ascending cervical arteries. They are called the *retinacular arteries of Weitbrecht.* [81,82] These critical vessels are vulnerable when the neck fractures. It has been assumed that this complex is completely disrupted by markedly displaced fractures, partially lacerated by mildly displaced ones, and unharmed by undisplaced fractures. The sequence parallels the incidence of nonunion and/or avascular necrosis in the femoral head for three variations of femoral neck fractures.

As the ascending cervical arteries cross the surface of the neck, they send several smaller branches into the metaphysis of the upper femoral area. The luxuriant vascular supply to the metaphysis and neck explains the absence of avascular changes in here as distinguished from what occurs in the femoral head. The vessels can be divided into four subgroups: anterior, medial, posterior, and lateral, as they are oriented to the femoral neck. At the margin of the articular cartilage a second, smaller ring is formed which was first described by Chung as the *subsynovial intraarticular arterial ring.* [83] Important vessels arise from this ring and are called the *epiphyseal arteries.* Claffey demonstrated that aseptic necrosis occurred in those neck fractures which disrupted this ring at their lateral entry.[84] Trueta and Harrison believed that the epiphyseal blood supply in

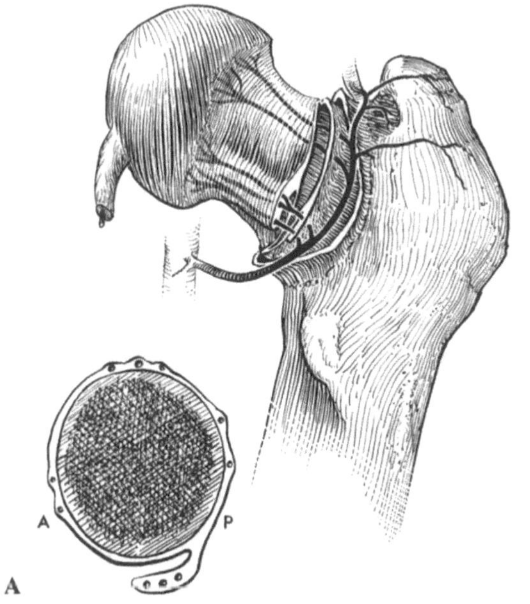

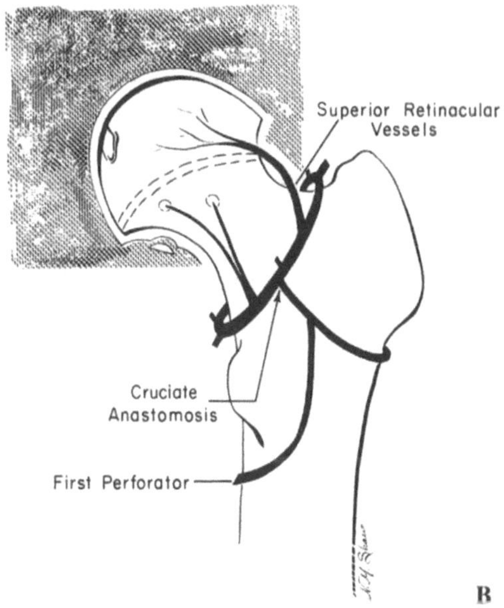

FIG. 8–29 **A** Retinacula on femoral neck. Inset shows them concentrated superiorly and inferiorly. **B** Isolated femoral head at the end of the cervical pedicle. Basal anastomosis sending superior and inferior retinacular vessels to the head, posterior aspect illustrated.

the adult, distinguished from that in the child, arises largely from the lateral epiphyseal arteries, which enter the head posterosuperiorly and secondarily from the medial epiphyseal artery entering through the ligamentum teres.[85]

The artery passing through the round ligament from the obturator artery has been ascribed various levels of importance. It occasionally branches off the median femoral circumflex. Claffey observed that its presence per se did not make it capable of supplying the femoral head well enough to keep it alive should all other sources of blood become shut off.[84] Wertheimer and Fernandes Lopes found that it was large enough to supply sufficient blood to the head in only one-third of the patients studies.[86] The artery may have anatomical variations; thus in some individuals it may be large enough to keep the head alive in the presence of ruptured retinacular vessels, whereas in others it may be quite inadequate. This could explain why some femoral heads survive despite displacement at the time of fracture.

After the insult to the femoral head, there may be two sources of revascularization: The residual uninjured vascular supply may be sufficient to sustain the femoral head, and vessels from the neck and surrounding tissue may repair themselves before damage ensues.

That portion of the femoral neck which is intracapsular—all of the anterior and the posterior two-thirds—has no cambium layer in its periosteum that could participate in peripheral callus formation.[87,88] Healing of the fracture must depend on endosteal callus formation alone.[89–91] Furthermore, the fragments must be impacted; otherwise the synovial fluid lyses any clots that form.[92]

The external and internal geometry of the femur and femoral head have been studied extensively. Ward's triangle is described in Volume I, Chapter III, with the compressive and tensile trabeculations illustrated. The head is not a true sphere, nor is the acetabulum a true hemisphere. Such an anatomical configuration may be necessary for improving spread of the synovial fluid over the articular surfaces.[93–96] One must be mindful of the fact that the femoral neck in reality is a tube with an intermedullary cavity, as in the longer femoral shaft. This tube becomes hollowed to varying degrees directly relative to age. The forces demonstrated by Rydell[97,98] are important factors contributing to the progressive weakness of this cylinder of bone as it becomes fatigued.[17]

Rydell used a strain gauge on a femoral prosthesis to study the forces which play on the femoral head and neck. When standing on one leg a force was developed that was 2.5 times the body weight. With one leg support, holding a cane in the opposite hand, the force across the hip joint may be reduced to that of the person's body weight. This is important for rehabilitation. At rest in a two-legged stance, there is a force one-half of the body weight across the hip joint.

Rydell also observed that by lifting the leg from a supine position with the knee straight, such as getting out of bed, a force 1.5 times that of the patient's body weight is produced.[99] One must appreciate the presence of these powerful forces when getting an elderly patient out of bed, especially in situations where the fracture repair was less than ideal.

Biomechanics of Neck Fractures

DeLee extensively reviewed the various theories on the mechanism of how these fractures are produced.[36] Kocker, as far back as 1896, expounded on two possible modes: (1) a direct blow to the greater trochanter; and (2) lateral rotation of the leg causing the neck to be twisted off (Fig. 8–30). The head is firmly fixed by the anterior capsule and the iliofemoral ligament while the neck rotates posteriorly. The posterior cortex impinges on the edge of the acetabulum and buckles under the forces generated. Scheck pointed this out in early publications, and most other authors agree.[100–102] What is at issue is whether all neck fractures are comminuted. After exposing hundreds of these fractures for hemiarthroplasties, this writer has yet to see one that was not comminuted; it is just a matter of degree. This fact explains why the head is so typically twisted backward.[103–104]

A third mechanism was proposed by Urovitz et al., who favored the idea that these are fatigue fractures.[105] Freeman's group studied the relation between osteoporosis and fatigue forces.[106,107] The mechanism they suggested is one of cyclical loading which causes micro- and macrofractures in the femoral neck, especially posteriorly, as observed by this writer so many times at arthroplasty. A stress fracture of this type becomes complete even after such minor trauma as is typical with these elderly patients. The torsional forces which produce the fracture precede the fall by mere seconds as the muscles contract to axially load the femoral neck along its longitudinal axis. The patient, however, can identify only with the inevitable fall to the floor.[94]

The biomechanical explanations which emerge from these accumulated data are as follows. The patient falls on the affected leg with the foot firmly planted and the hip positioned in slight flexion as the body is thrown backward and is externally rotated (Fig. 8–30). Two major fragments are produced which move in two planes simultaneously. The head must roll backward because of the pull of the iliopsoas tendon (Fig. 8–30) as it tightens over the head anteriorly, thereby causing the posterior cortex to buckle. The most common position is varus with backward angulation of the head, the apex of which points anteriorly, and some degree of rotation which is difficult to appreciate. The final AP position is most likely due to the manner in which the greater trochanter is struck at the time the person makes contact with the floor, either adducted or abducted. Linton, however, thought that the head shifts from valgus to varus as a normal sequence of events.[108,109]

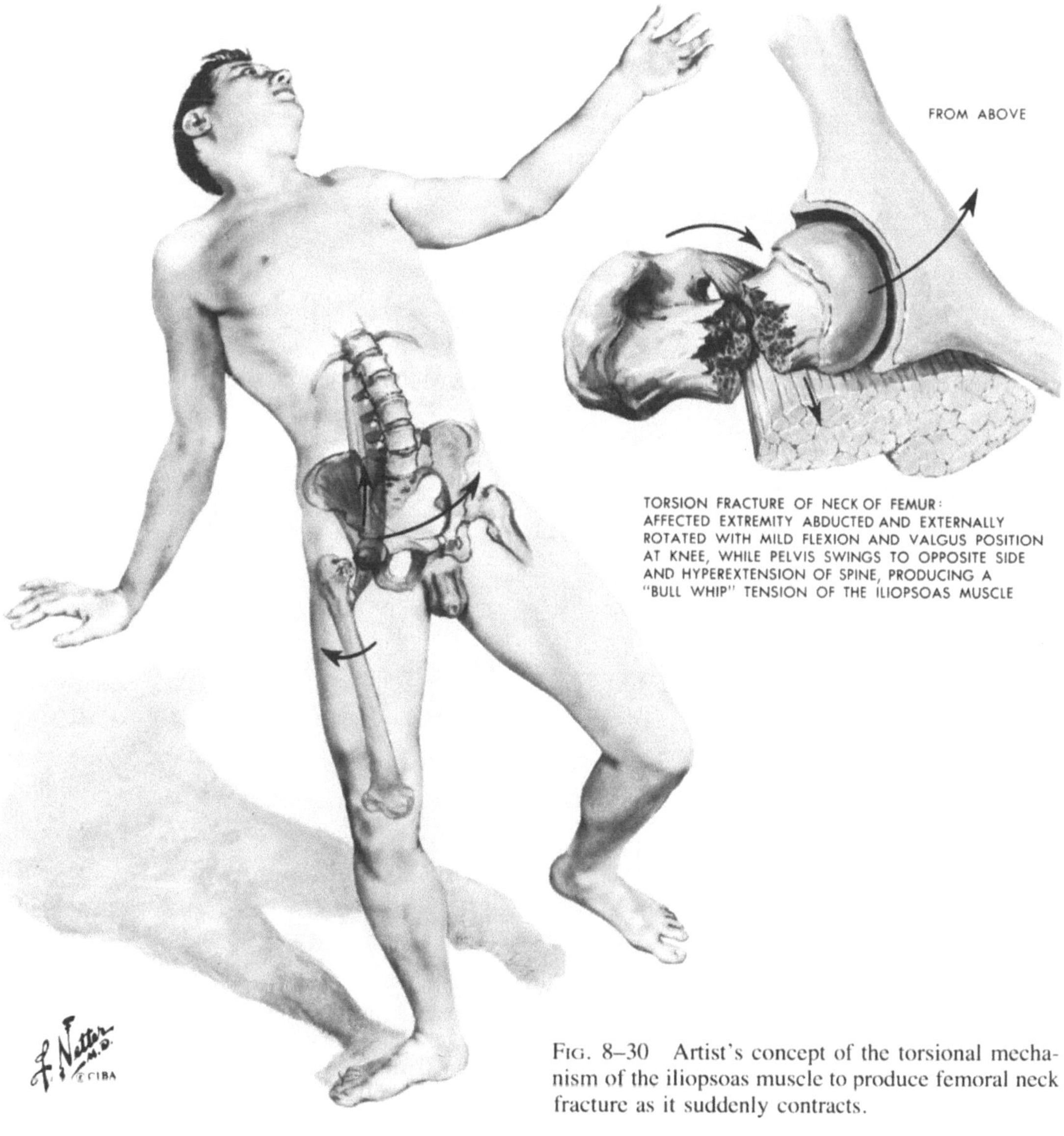

FIG. 8–30 Artist's concept of the torsional mechanism of the iliopsoas muscle to produce femoral neck fracture as it suddenly contracts.

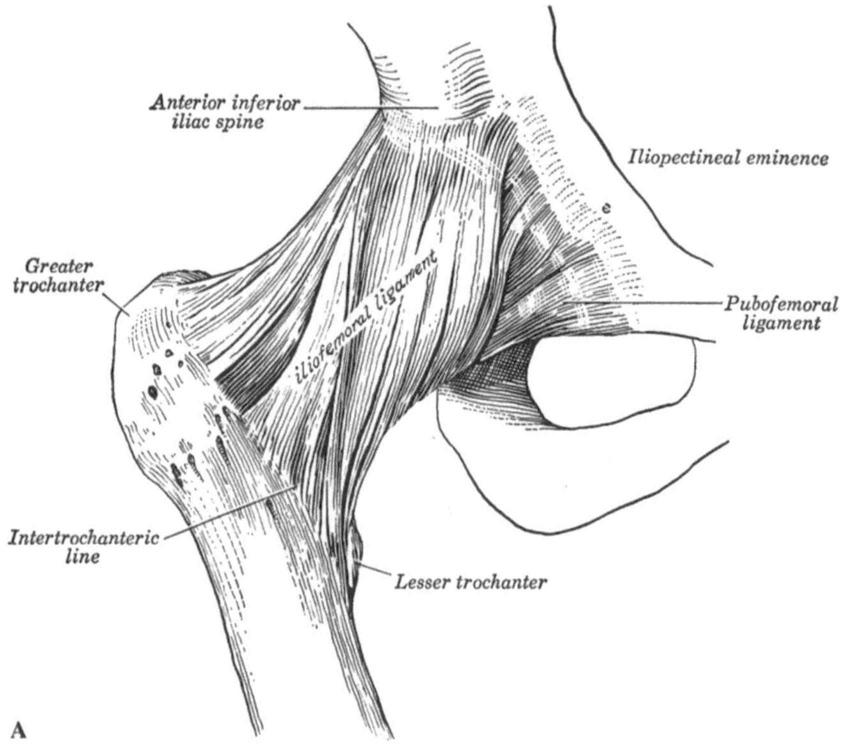

A

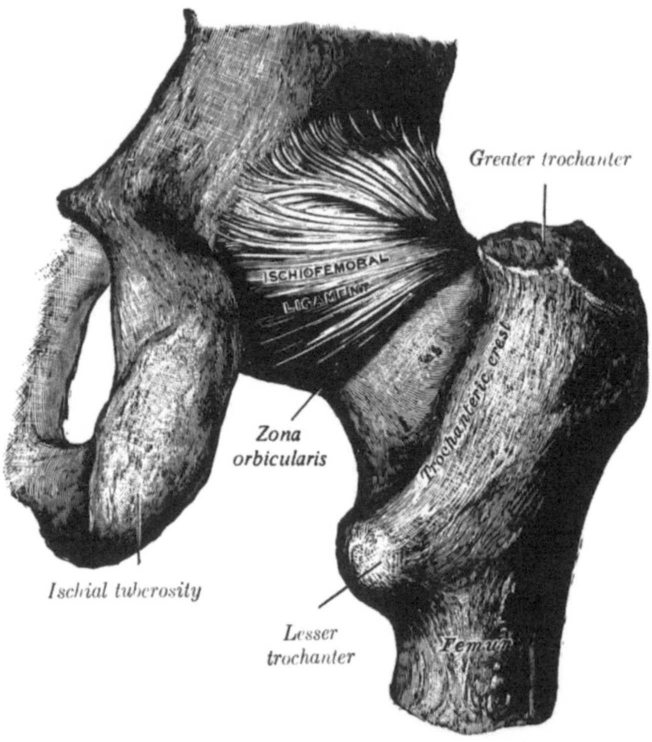

B

FIG. 8–31 **A** The iliofemoral ligament is a very strong wall of fibers that spirals covering the entire head and neck. It firmly attaches anteriorly along the intertrochanteric line. **B** The ischial femoral ligament continues to spiral around the neck posteriorly but leaves its base uncovered. Instead of attaching to bone, it rolls up into a thick band called the zona orbicularis. (From *Gray's Anatomy*, 29th ed. Philadelphia, Lea & Febinger, 1973.)

The magnitude of the force coupled with the individual progression of osteoporosis determines the degree of displacement.

The influence of the capsule on the fracture mechanics of the femoral neck has been given little attention. It is this author's opinion that the capsule with its iliofemoral ligament is very important to the uniqueness of femoral neck fractures. The twisting fiber network comprising the iliofemoral ligament creates the strongest and largest ligament in the body. It can reach tremendous size. The author measured one in a 40-year-old man who had had an open reduction for a fresh fracture–dislocation. It was 0.75 inch thick. The anterior portion is a solid wall which strongly resists forces playing through the long axis of the femoral neck (Fig. 8–31A). Therefore the neck can only bow backward. The posterior portion acts like a sling around the femoral neck because it does not attach to any bone (Fig. 8–31B). Anteriorly it attaches to the acetabulum above and to the base of the neck (Fig. 8–31A). There is a distinct ridge, or groove, around the head–neck junction posteriorly (Fig. 8–32). The ligament thickens sharply on its posterior side into what is called the zona orbicularis (Fig. 8–31B). This part of the ligament can snag the head into a grip as it twists around this bony groove. Remembering that the femoral head is not perfectly spherical (nor is the acetabulum), it can become mechanically locked into the cartilagenous socket.[24] When the twisting fibers of the ligament contract, this portion grips the head, like a powerful hook, jamming it into the incongruent acetabulum and producing bending moments along the posterior femoral neck.

The bony architecture also contributes to the unique characteristics of femoral neck fractures.

A 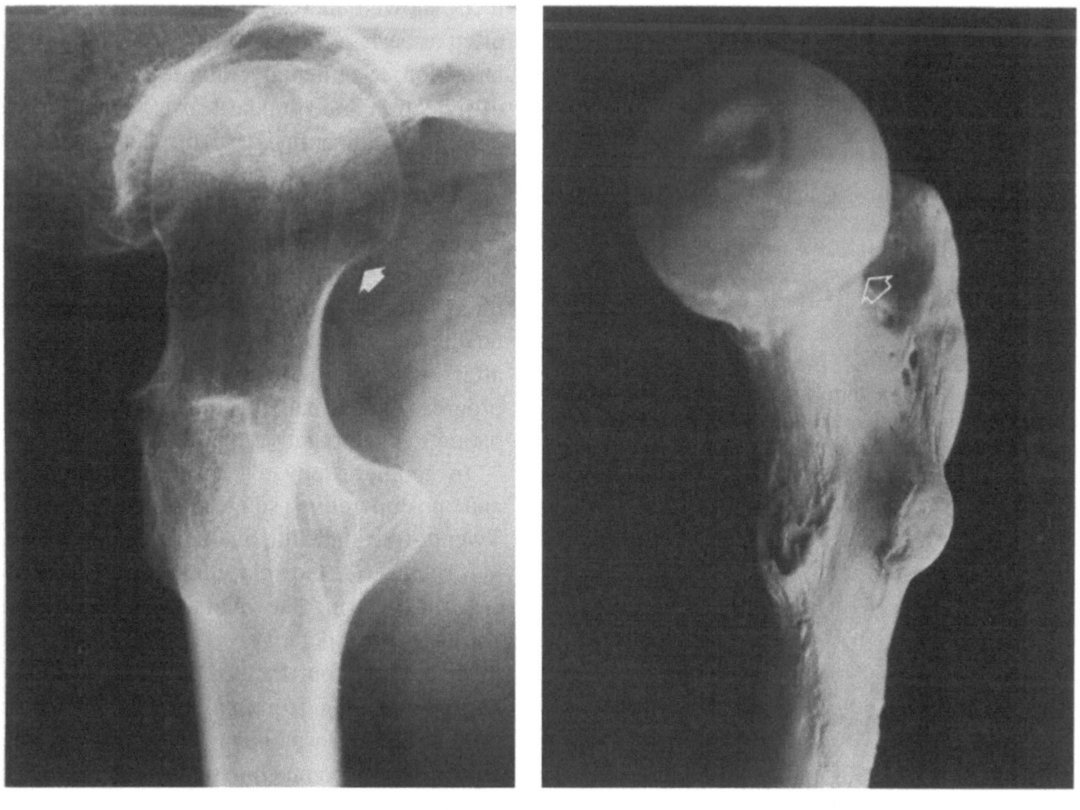 B

FIG. 8–32 **A** X-ray view of the coronal characteristics of the bony architecture. The neck sits well anterior to the trochanter, especially the lesser trochanter, which is entirely displaced posteriorly. The posterior edge of the femoral neck is grooved deeply (arrows) for the rope-like zona orbicularis fibers, which are stoutest posteriorly. The bone of the neck is thinnest posteriorly, mostly at the posterior base of the neck as it blends into the lesser trochanter. **B** Cadaver specimen mirroring the x-ray picture seen in **A.**

Both trochanters are offset to the posterior side of the neck, especially the lesser trochanter. The latter is entirely posterior, not medial, which is an illusion when viewing an AP x-ray film (Fig. 8–32). The short external rotators are also attached between the two trochanters, all of which produce traction on the bone. Tension forces cause the cortex to become thin, especially the posterior cortex. This fact can be confirmed at primary arthroplasty. The comminuted fragments are typically multiple thin particles which fold into themselves (Fig. 8–33).

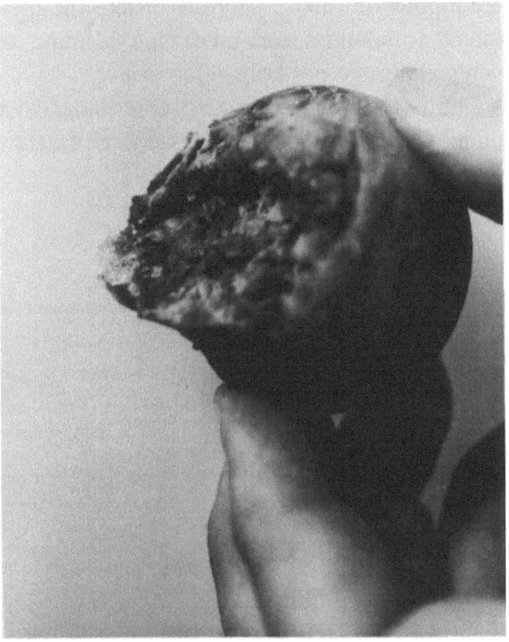

FIG. 8–33 Multiple thin fragments of bone constitute posterior comminution on the head fragment. They typically fold onto themselves, which is a feature not easily recognized on the routine x-ray film. Because of this feature, neck fractures can be slow to heal.

Management of Femoral Neck Fractures

Role of Scintimetry

Since the early 1960s radioactive isotopes have been used to help prognosticate the outcome of femoral neck fractures. Both nonunions and segmental collapse after these fractures are thought to be caused by injury to the blood supply of the femoral head; scintigraphic findings of deficient vascularity have regularly been associated with complications.

The leaders of these ongoing investigative studies are in Sweden, headed by Stromqvist et al.[110] They studied 39 patients with femoral neck fractures, following them clinically and radiographically by technetium-99m methylenediphosphonate (^{99m}Tc-MDP) scintimetry 2 to 29 days and 4, 8, 12, 24, and 36 months after surgery or until redisplacement, pseudarthrosis, or segmental collapse occurred. The scintimetric data were calculated by selecting regions of interest on the fractured and intact sides over the femoral head, neck, greater trochanter, and shaft; ratios of fractured side/intact side were obtained for each region. Bone metabolism after femoral neck fracture was expressed and analyzed numerically.

Prognosis regarding the course of healing could be predicted with precision by studying femoral head uptake; normal uptake was associated with healing, whereas defective uptake was observed in conjunction with subsequent complications. However, femoral heads with primary uptake defects showed increased uptake after 4 months, often as early as 6 to 8 weeks, indicating revascularization. Segmental collapse, as well as loss of reduction and pseudarthrosis, appear to be related to vascular injury to the head. The uptake in the femoral neck, trochanter, and shaft areas was increased in all patients with femoral neck fractures. Subsequent normalization was considerably slower in patients with complications. That there was any significant difference from normal healing was not apparent until 12 to 24 months after operation, indicating that healing was not progressing normally from the beginning of the patients' postoperative phase.

In another study by Stromqvist et al.[111] pre- and postoperative scintimetry was compared. Twenty-four patients, average age 73, were studied. Eighteen had displaced fractures. Scintimetry was done during the operation and within 5 to 15 days postoperatively. Fixation was accomplished with a four-flanged nail with an anchoring hook protruding from its tip (the Rydell nail). Weight-bearing was begun from the first postoperative day. Seventeen patients were followed for 4 months after injury. Six with increased uptake and eight with decreased uptake preoperatively had comparable results during the postoperative follow-up. Those with an intermediate uptake before operation had decreased uptake after surgery.

This finding meant there was further injury to the blood supply of the femoral head as time passed.

Fitzgerald[112] summarized the role of scintimetry at this time:

> All surgeons who treat patients with femoral neck fracture would like to be able to identify those preoperative patients with irreversible damage to the vascular supply of the the femoral head. Scintigraphy has demonstrated that damage to vascularity of the femoral head is rarely an all or nothing phenomenon but rather it is a gradient. We have yet to identify the degree of damage to the femoral head which will lead to irreversible changes.
>
> This interesting study is an attempt to identify the degree of vascular insult which precludes normal healing. The use of dedicated computer systems and regions of interest allows the nuclear radiologist to be more specific than was previously possible. The data generated . . . indicate: (1) certain patients have significant damage to the vascular supply to the femoral head at the time of injury, and (2) further damage to the vascular supply of the femoral head does indeed occur at the time internal fixation devices are implanted.
>
> Before widespread use of these techniques can be advocated . . . investigators must show stronger correlation between the abnormal scintigraphic findings and the ultimate clinical result, that is, a direct correlation between decreased uptake of ^{99m}Tc-methylene diphosphonate and the development of osteonecrosis or femoral neck nonunion.

A similar study using the same technique was reported by Holmberg and Thorngren.[113] In a series of 152 patients, they found the qualitative evaluation to be less accurate than the numerical method. They concluded that ^{99m}Tc-MDP scintimetry is a powerful tool for evaluating the vascular status in the femoral head after femoral neck fractures. The authors did not, however, discuss the cost of the computer hardware or software necessary for the processing of such quantitative analysis. Although this method is a distinct improvement in predicting the outcome of femoral neck fractures, the lack of appropriate equipment may limit its practical application.

Preoperative scintimetry is still not a practical tool when planning treatment for femoral neck fractures. Accuracy is not yet high enough to make the technique meaningful in any preoperative plan. From a practical standpoint, one cannot depend entirely on the preoperative scan. Even if the scan shows a poor uptake no surgeon would remove a femoral head in a stable fracture, e.g., undisplaced or impacted fracture, or in a displaced fracture in a young patient, as there is a fair chance that the study is giving a false reading. There is also a chance that the head will revascularize, thereby saving a good serviceable head. On the other hand, if the scintimetry procedure were extremely accurate and could reveal the extent of vascular damage, e.g., indicating that there is no possibility of the damage being repaired, the technique would become a valuable diagnostic tool.

For preoperative analysis of the status of femoral head blood flow, then, scintimetry remains a research tool. Postoperative studies, on the other hand, are another matter. Scintimetry can help greatly in pointing out impending nonunions and necrotic heads before they become more of a problem in management than they need be.

Nonsurgical Management

Prior to the 1980s there was a place for nonsurgical management of femoral neck fractures in bedridden, senile patients and/or demented institutionalized people. Sherk et al.[114] reviewed this issue and concluded that there was justification for "skillful neglect" as there was an appreciable number of surgical complications in the surgically treated group in whom the quality of life did not improve all that much.

In another study Lyons and Nevins advocated what they called "nontreatment" of fractured hips in senile patients.[115] They claimed that their patient population was composed exclusively of those with "severe organic mental syndromes." Their reasons for nontreatment were partly humanitarian, partly pragmatic, and partly economic. Such a policy requires certain essential conditions. The most important is that the prognosis of the patients' chances of mobilization must be made with great caution and be based on sufficient hard data; otherwise that patient may be doomed unnecessarily to the sad confinement of bed or chair for the remainder of her life.

Hyams[116] took issue with this philosophy of managing such patients: "I would deplore the use of the word senility to mean brain failure. It implies an advanced and irreversible situation without hope and without everything, and it encourages woolly thinking and a pessimistic attitude. The latter may sometimes be justified; the former, never."

In our locale neglecting these people skillfully

or not skillfully is intolerable. There are some emotional reasons for this attitude as well as some factual reasons. Why should a demented or a senile bedridden patient be asked to suffer the pain of a broken hip? They perceive pain as well as the mentally competent person. Why should their leg be left deformed? Nursing care of a patient left in bed with a broken hip deteriorates rapidly because the nurse becomes intimidated by it and tends to leave that patient alone rather than move her for fear of hurting her further. Nurses may also take the unspoken attitude that the patient must be a terminal case if the doctors do not want to treat her. Furthermore, what happens to these same people if they are passed off to the most junior resident to manage or if a second-rate job is done on the basis that "anything is better than nothing" because it does not matter anyway? Such an attitude compounds the problem. A couple of pins stuck into the hip "percutaneously"[117] as expediently as possible or a prosthesis casually jammed into place as fast as possible does not help the situation either. These already handicapped people need the best, not the worst, care. They should all be treated with optimism.[118] This author is repeatedly gratified to see these people walk into the office with a walker, alert and happy again, after having been in the hospital, confused and with what appeared to be little hope for recovery. With good nursing care and a good diet that reverses their preoperative starvation diets, they seem to have a new lease on life. Such situations are seen in members of wealthy families as well as in the average retiree.

Patients with severe flexion contractures and bedsores are another matter; they really are terminal with insurmountable surgical and medical problems. They should be left alone. The only femoral neck fracture per se which may be treated nonsurgically is the truly impacted fracture as redefined by this author (see as discussed earlier in the chapter).

Surgical Management

Closed Reduction

Reducing a displaced femoral neck fracture can be a tedious process. Fracture tables were not available during the early part of this century, and so a regular operating table was used, the patient's leg being draped over the edge of the table and various manuevers pursued. With the Leadbetter technique the hip was flexed to 90° and traction applied with the leg adducted. Internal rotation was then applied and the leg pulled down into extension with slight abduction. The "heel/palm" test is a valid measure of a good reduction: When the heel is rested on the palm of the surgeon's hand, it should sit up without falling back into external rotation.[119] The Whitman manuever is done in the opposite direction. Traction is applied with the leg in extension. As strong traction is applied, the knee is internally rotated.[120]

Despite the use today of fracture tables or image intensifiers, femoral neck fractures of the unstable pattern are almost impossible to reduce anatomically. One must be patient and carefully watch the x-ray monitor. Massie[121] used forceful internal rotation, whereas Garden[24] made a strong case for gentle manipulation. Flynn has been a modern-day advocate of manipulating the fracture outside a fracture table.[122] He gently flexes the hip beyond 90° in slight abduction and neutral rotation. An assistant steadies the foot while the surgeon applies traction in line with the femoral neck, then internally rotating it slowly as the leg is extended. X-ray studies help to decide if more or less abduction or adduction is needed. If successful, the leg is then tied into the fracture table. Compton[123] confirmed the usefulness of this method.

Another approach was reported by Deyerle.[124] With his method the fractured leg is internally rotated until the femoral neck is seen on x-ray film to be parallel to the floor. The position is verified by a clear lateral view. The leg is tied into the fracture table, and gentle traction is applied by an assistant. The surgeon simultaneously pushes in forcefully on the greater trochanter while at the same time levering out on the knee (Fig. 8–34). At this point the fracture should be well reduced with possibly some slight residual valgus. If the angulation persists (apex pointing anteriorly), as seen in the lateral view, an additional step may be tried: The surgeon pushes hard on the anterior aspect of the hip with both hands while an assistant stabilizes the opposite iliac crest (Fig. 8–35). If it works, an audible "crunch" is heard.

At no time should strong traction be used on the leg because this position creates a "Japanese finger trap,'' either keeping the fragments distracted or holding them so tightly they cannot be properly pushed together. Furthermore, such traction may pull the distal fragment into an unacceptable valgus position.

One final maneuver may be tried. If the operating room light is in a room with a central base, a crutch can be placed upside down with the arm pad against the patient's anterior hip joint (the tip wedged up against the light base) (Fig. 8–36). The operating table can be moved upward, with the the crutch pressing down on the fracture, thereby reducing the anterior angulation. The image intensifier can still be placed in a position to obtain a lateral view of the hip to verify the reduction. It should look like the case illustrated in Figure 8–37. Once reduction is complete, the crutch is removed to make way for the image intensifier to check the AP position. If the fracture resumes its old position of varus, it must be opened or replaced with a prosthesis. If it goes into severe valgus, an attempt must be made to improve it. A rolled-up sheet wrapped around the inner thigh may be used, pulling laterally. This maneuver should make the fragments go into adduction. Valgus positions, when marked, result in more femoral head necrosis than varus postures. They also cause knock-knee deformities (Fig. 8–26).

Open Reduction

An open reduction requires a preoperative master plan. Most cases can be fairly well anticipated depending on the protocol employed by the group or in the department, or by one's own set of rules. Although Arnold approached all femoral neck fractures as candidates for closed pinning, he was prepared for an alternate operative plan. The operative permits were so prepared that the patient was ready for an arthroplasty if the closed reduction should fail in an older patient, and for an open reduction should it fail in a younger patient. He, however, did not define the age limits for

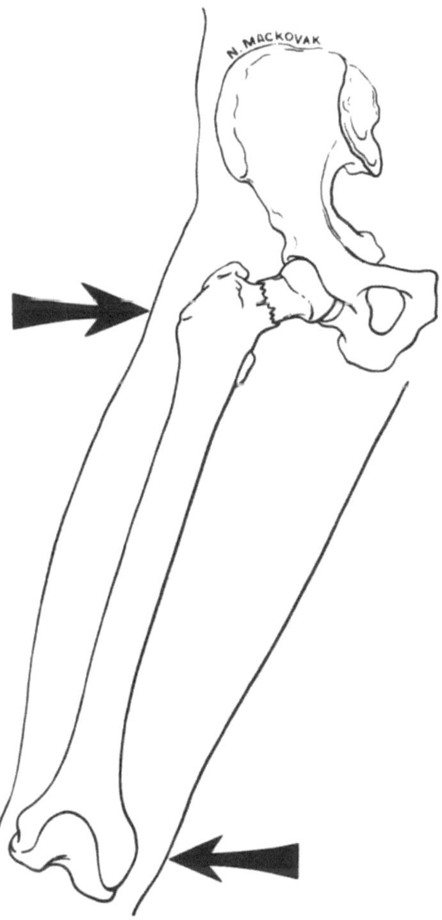

Fig. 8–34 With the leg parallel with the fracture table under strong traction, the hand and shoulder exert heavy pressure over the lateral side of the trochanter. The opposite hand pulls against the medial side of the knee, rotating the neck under the head and producing a slight overreduction in the anterior posterior plane.

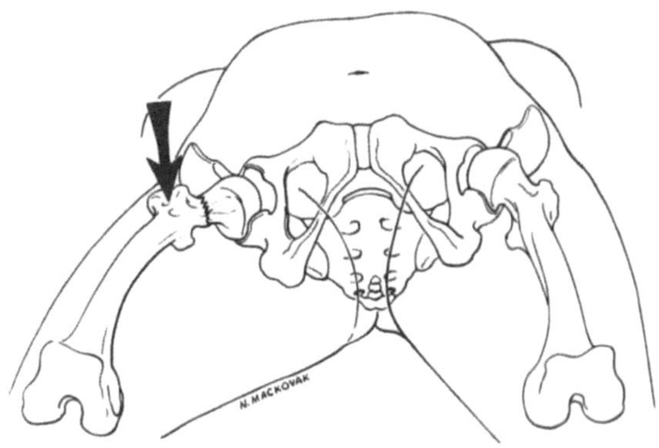

Fig. 8–35 With the patient on the fracture table, strong downward pressure is exerted over the trochanter with two hands (*arrow*). An assistant holds counterpressure over the opposite iliac crest to prevent the pelvis rotating on the sacral crest. This produces a crunch and places the ''ice cream back on the cone'' in anatomical or slightly overreduced position in the lateral plane.

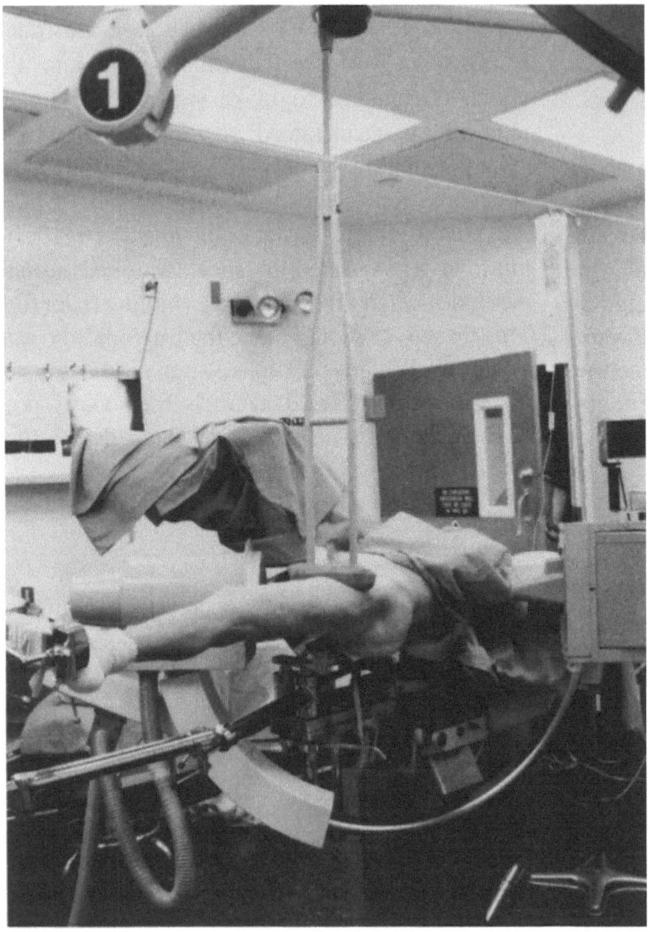

Fig. 8–36 When the neck fragments remain angulated in the lateral view after routine maneuvers have failed, a crutch can be used to force them into alignment by wedging it up against the OR light base. With the rubber handle held against the anterior hip, the OR table is pumped upward until the fragments reduce themselves. Do not use strong traction here. The crutch is then removed and the area prepared for surgery. *Marked internal rotation is usually necessary in most reductions of displaced femoral neck fractures.* With the modern use of image magnification, the reduction can be dynamically viewed as the best maneuver is tried. Sometimes, a second crutch under the knee flexes the hip enough to improve the reduction.

each of these two groups. This is the grayest area in orthopedics.[125] The question may never be clearly settled because of several factors that determine such decisions. For the sake of preventing repetition, these are discussed in the section on arthroplasties (see later in the chapter).

One point is clear when it comes to treating the young patient with a fractured femoral neck; an open reduction is necessary when a stable, near-anatomical reduction cannot be achieved by any of the closed methods. Swiontkowski et al. defined "young adults" as patients between 12 and 49.[126] These entities are usually unstable fractures with obliquity and separation (Fig. 8–38) that chances for a successful closed reduction are slim. Moreover, one is reminded that these fractures must be reduced anatomically, otherwise redisplacement, nonunion, and femoral head necrosis will surely ensue. Therefore these displaced fractures are best managed with an open reduction, Swiontkowski's Seattle group[126] recommended drilling a lag screw perpendicular to the fracture line to compress the fragments together and further help maintain stability of the reduction (Fig. 8–39). These are difficult surgical cases. They should be attempted only by an experienced surgeon. The AO malleolar screws are ideal implants for fixation (Fig. 8–40).

Surgical Approach The choice of a surgical plan is a personalized one because it depends on the skills of the individual surgeon and his or her past experiences. What one can do best is what one should have as his preference. The usual surgical approach is a Watson-Jones incision, or a variation of an anterolateral incision (Fig. 8–41) with the patient in a prone position. The head and neck can be seen, and there is

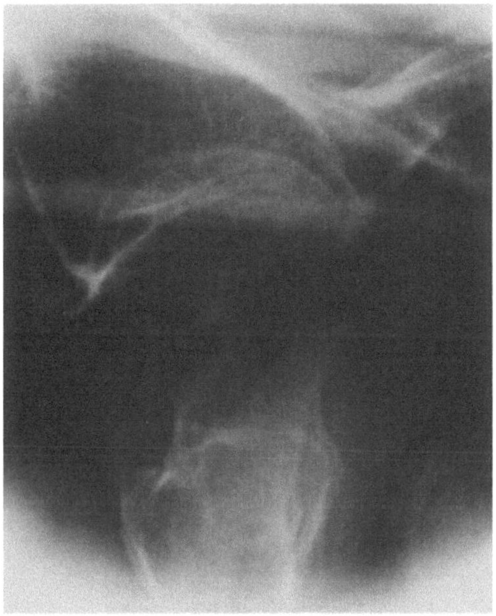

FIG. 8–37 Fracture reduction that can be achieved by wedging a crutch against the anterior portion of the patient. This is the same unstable fracture that is seen in Figs. 8–8 and 8–9. Note the posterior comminution and gap after reduction has been achieved.

sufficient exposure for introducing the pins into the lateral cortex just distal to the greater trochanter. It is usually necessary to fix the head fragment to the socket with two thin Steinmann pins in order to prevent the head from rotating around as the fragments are being reduced.

The author prefers the antero-lateral exposure with the patient on her side as previously reported[55] and has been updated (Fig. 8–64). Because the comminution is posterior, with the head folded back on itself, such an exposure is needed to visualize this area and to be prepared for a supplementary bone graft. This lateral approach affords excellent exposure posteriorly as well as anteriorly when the patient is placed directly on her side. X-ray films are likewise easily obtained in this position for both AP and frogleg lateral

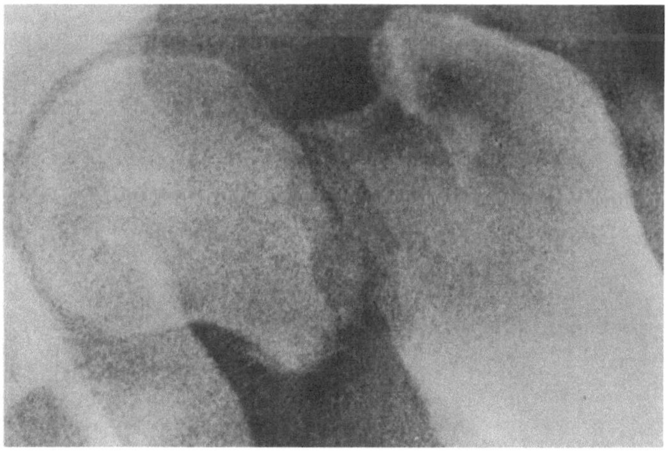

FIG. 8–38 Fracture of the femoral neck unique to young adults with marked obliquity and separation. It must be treated with an open reduction in order to achieve anatomical stability. (From Swiontkowski, M. F., Umquist, R. A., Hansen, S. T.: Fractures of the femoral neck in patients between the age of twelve and forty-nine years. J. Bone Joint Surg., 66A:837, 1984.)

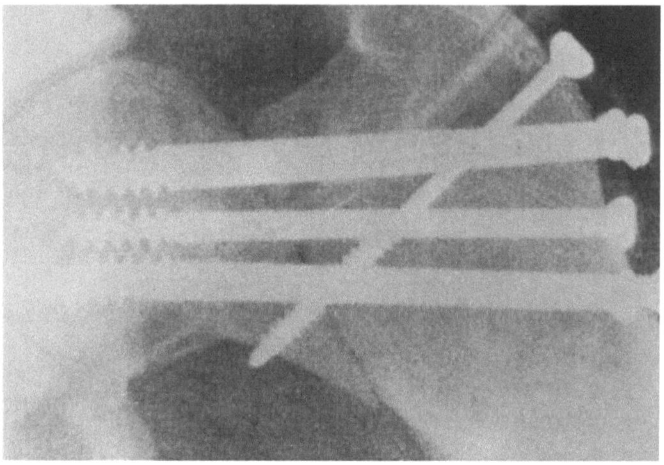

FIG. 8–39 Technique of stabilizing this spiral oblique fracture by placing an AO screw perpendicular to the fracture line as recommended by Swiontkowski et al. (From Swiontkowski, M. F., et al.: Fractures of the femoral neck in patients between the age of twelve and forty-nine years. J. Bone Joint Surg., 66A:837, 1984.)

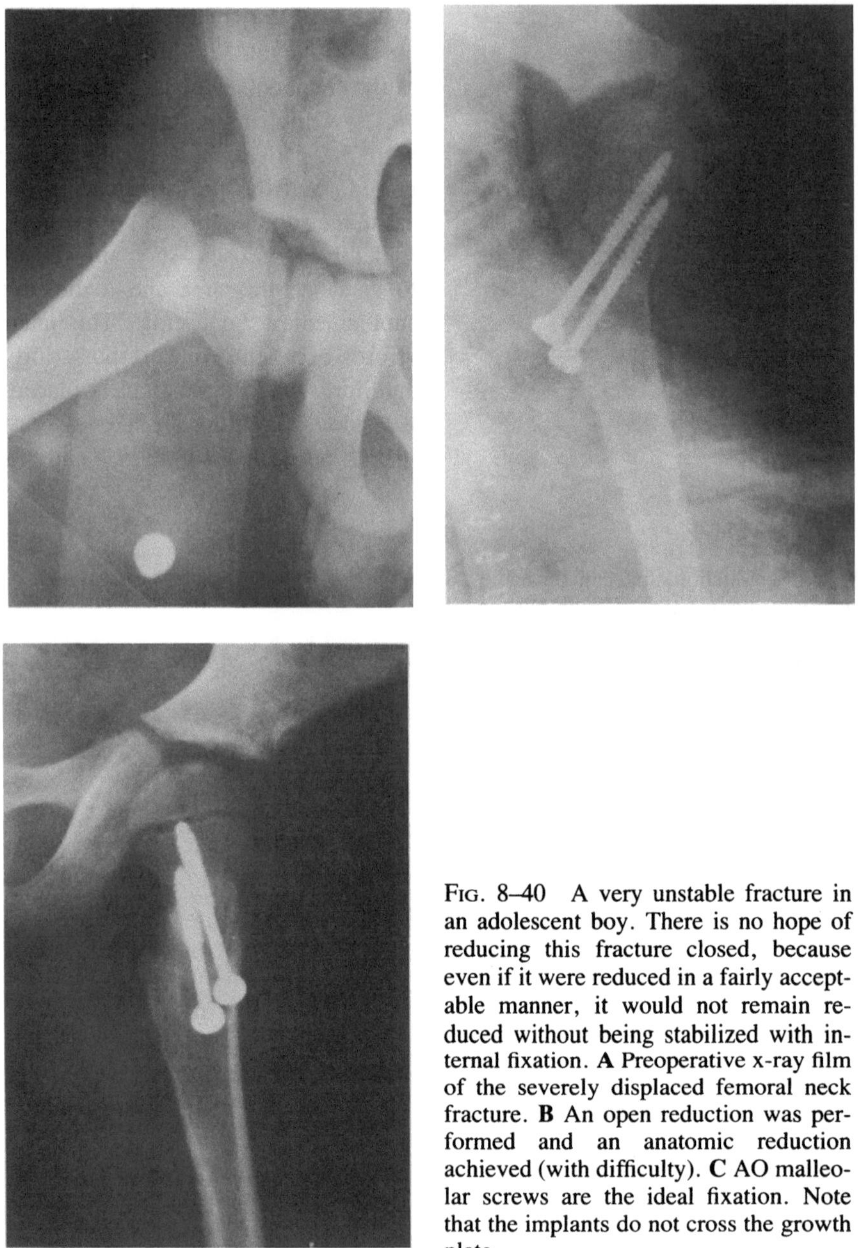

A B C

FIG. 8–40 A very unstable fracture in an adolescent boy. There is no hope of reducing this fracture closed, because even if it were reduced in a fairly acceptable manner, it would not remain reduced without being stabilized with internal fixation. **A** Preoperative x-ray film of the severely displaced femoral neck fracture. **B** An open reduction was performed and an anatomic reduction achieved (with difficulty). **C** AO malleolar screws are the ideal fixation. Note that the implants do not cross the growth plate.

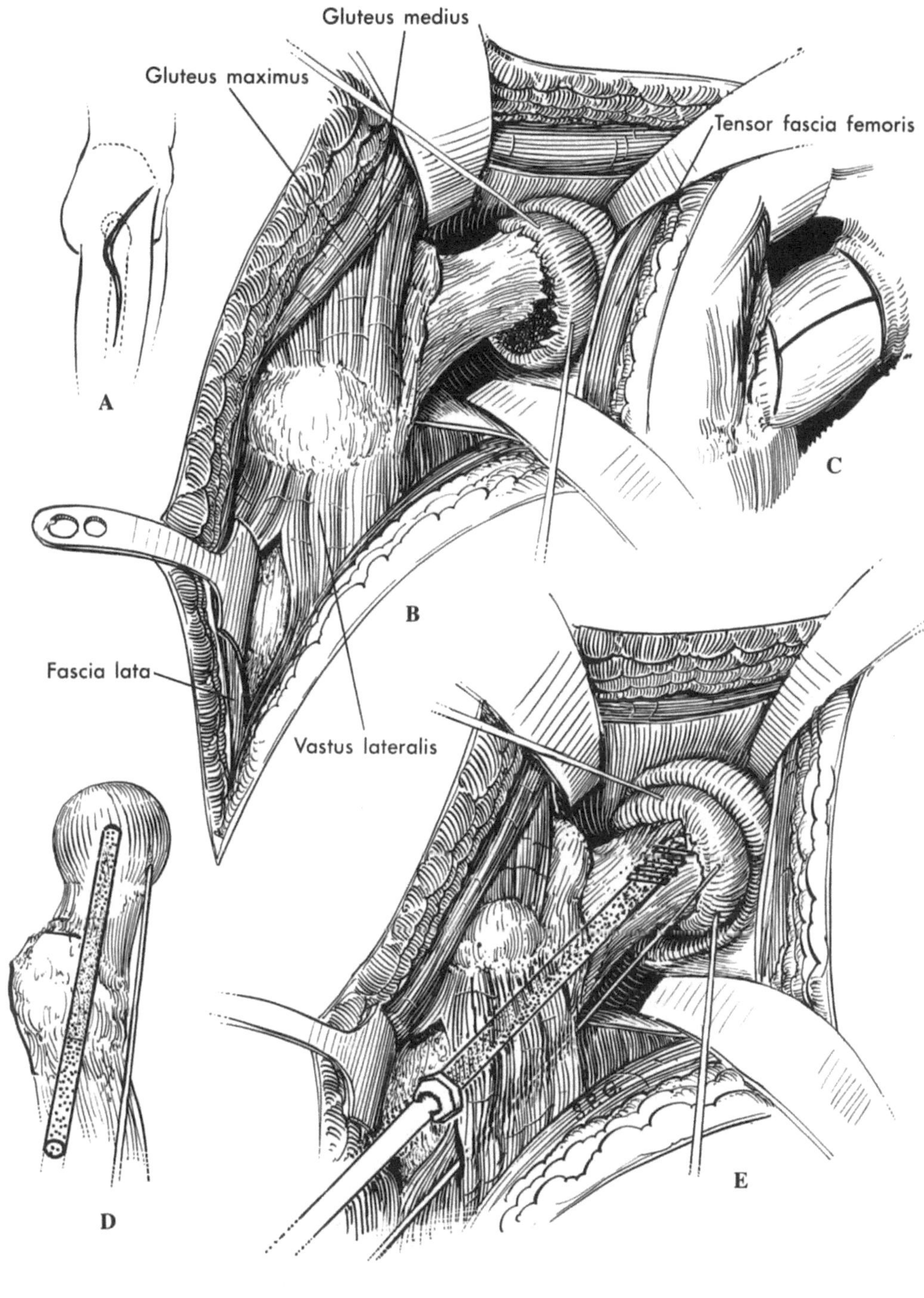

FIG. 8–41 Surgical technique of open reduction for cervical fractures. **A** Modified Watson-Jones incision curves posterior to the greater trochanter. **B** Access to the anterior capsule is gained by splitting the fascial interval between the tensor fascia femoris and gluteus maximus. At this level the gluteus medius is found and can be retracted laterally. The tensor fascia femoris muscle is retracted upward and medially. **C** The capsule is opened with a vertical incision and then across at the edge of the acetabulum and base of the neck so that there is maximum exposure. **D** A pin placed across the neck of the femur gives the operator a perfect lateral path to the center of the head. **E** The head is fixed to the acetabulum by piercing it with two Steinmann pins. After the shaft is reduced to the head by abduction and slight internal rotation, the surgeon drills a screw of his choice (Haggie, Asnis, Ace, etc.) from the exposed lateral cortex into the head. A minimum of three such screws are used. An x-ray should be obtained at this point to check their position into the head and whether they have been screwed reasonably parallel. Whatever adjustments are needed can be done as a final step before closure (see Figs. 8–44, 8–47, and 8–48).

views. If there is too much loss of bone and/or if the fracture line is too much of a spiral oblique configuration to allow good stabilization of the fragments, a femoral neck osteotomy is performed. This step is best done with an ossilating saw rather than with an osteotome, which may not cut the bone smoothly, sometimes fragmenting it even more. Once the osteotomy is completed, the beak of the head fragment may fit down into the neck or sit more squarely on the neck. Proceeding posteriorly may raise some concern about damaging the blood supply going through the retinaculum, although Meyers et al. have shown this not to be the case.[127,128]

Quality of Reduction

The lateral x-ray view is the most important one when evaluating femoral neck fractures pre- and postoperatively, yet its importance is commonly understated. Garden's words in 1974 emphasize their importance[24]:

> In the assessment of reduction after subcapital fractures it is customary to rely more on the anteroposterior than the lateral radiograph; this especially applies to those who still think in terms of valgus/varus displacement . . . with more informative radiographs, however, the immediate postoperative lateral radiograph has been found to be of greater importance than any other radiographic evidence in the treatment of subcapital fractures. I have come to rely on the appearance of the fragments on the lateral radiographs as the best mirror of reduction and the best guide to prognosis.

He used two parameters to compute his ''alignment index'' (Fig. 8–42). (Oddly enough he ignored the lateral x-ray in arriving at his classification.) The first, measured on the AP view, is called the frontal alignment. The medial trabeculations or the compressive stream can be used as a constant landmark to measure the varus/valgus tilt. If the central beam is used, it measures 160° in the average patient (Figs. 8–42 and 8–43A). If there is any question about this measurement, the opposite hip is measured. The second parameter is found in the lateral x-ray film or the coronal plane. The central axis of the head and neck should be perpendicular to one another at 180° (Fig. 8–42 and 8–43B). Therefore an ideal alignment index is 160°/180°. The reduced and pinned fracture seen in Fig. 8–44 is about as close to that ideal as possible.

Garden's group found that an alignment index which ranged between 150° to 180° in either plane was acceptable and correlated well with a lower union rate and lower necrosis of the femoral head.[129] He and his colleagues studied 1503 femoral neck fractures over a 36-month period. It is impressive to note that all of them were treated by a closed reduction. The implants used for internal fixation are unknown to U.S. physicians: the Tulloch Brown sliding nail, Garden's big cross screws, and the Smyth triangular screws.

The results of Garden et al.'s analysis of such a massive number of fracture cases are worthy of review: The shearing angle of Pauwels did not affect the union rate or the incidence of femoral head necrosis. When there was a residual varus deformity in displaced fractures, only 50% healed. When the alignment index came within 155° to 180°, 75% healed. When the residual lateral angulation exceeded 20°, only half united. A ''marked'' valgus reduction carried the highest rate of femoral head necrosis. Few failures of fixation occurred when the implant was seated within 0.5 cm of the articular surface and in the center of the head in both views. When there was a frankly poor reduction, 85% developed femoral head necrosis. Sixty-six percent of the displaced fractures united. In women only 17% of stage III fractures and 12% of stage IV fractures healed before 6 months. Seventy-four percent united when weight-bearing was resumed within 2 weeks. The incidence of union increased by 2% when walking began between the second and sixth weeks, by a further 3% when weight-bearing was delayed until 7 to 12 weeks, and by an additional 4% in a small group who were not allowed to bear weight until 3 months postoperatively. Sixty percent of the displaced fractures were healed within 6 months.

Internal Fixation The choice of apparatus for internal fixation of a femoral nick fracture is between a single large device and several smaller threaded pins. Fielding[67] championed the Pugh sliding nail, whereas others have preferred the sliding hip screw.[130] There is some recent evidence, however, to suggest that a single large nail or screw may do more damage to the vascularity of the femoral head than realized. Bauer and associates,[200] using ^{99m}Tc-MDP imaging, noted that two hips fixed with a large triflanged nail had good vascularity before pinning but no

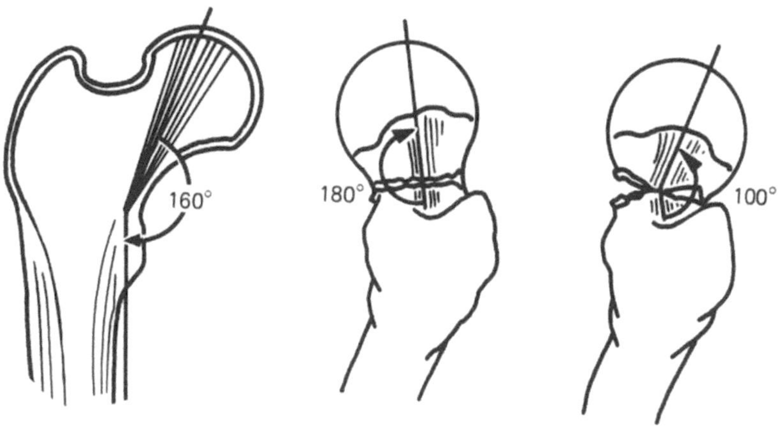

FIG. 8–42 Garden's alignment index utilizing the trabecular pattern which occupies the tension trabeculae seen in the head and neck. The index can be used to estimate the quality of reduction. In the AP view the trabeculations usually go from 150° to 160°. Garden accepted 160° as the ideal figure. In the lateral view it should be parallel and 180°. If the head should shift and angulate posteriorly, as seen in Fig. 8–3, it would be measured at 150°.

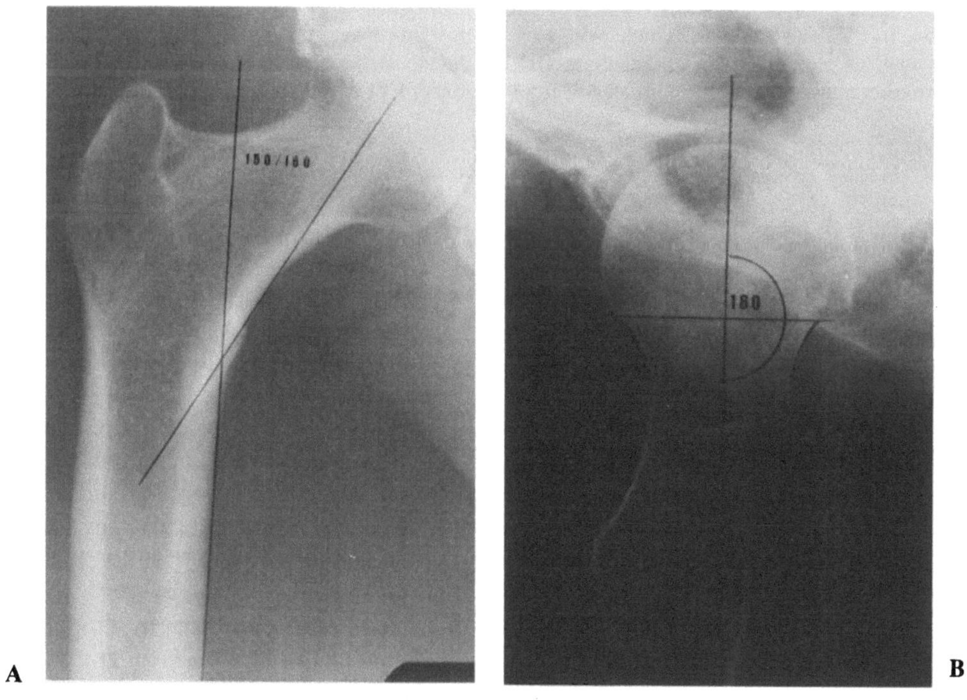

FIG. 8–43 X-ray views illustrating the Garden index concept. **A** The AP view with a 150° to 160° range. **B** The 180° degree range seen in the lateral x-ray film.

vascularity shortly after pinning. They concluded that this "should focus interest on the effect of the shape of the nail and the accompanying operative technique . . . perhaps multiple thin nails and a less traumatic technique should be preferred."[131] These Swedish surgeons have gone from the larger Rydell three-flanged pin to two smaller cylinder pins, both with retractable hooks at their tip to snag the femoral head (Fig. 8–45). There is a further objection to a large implant

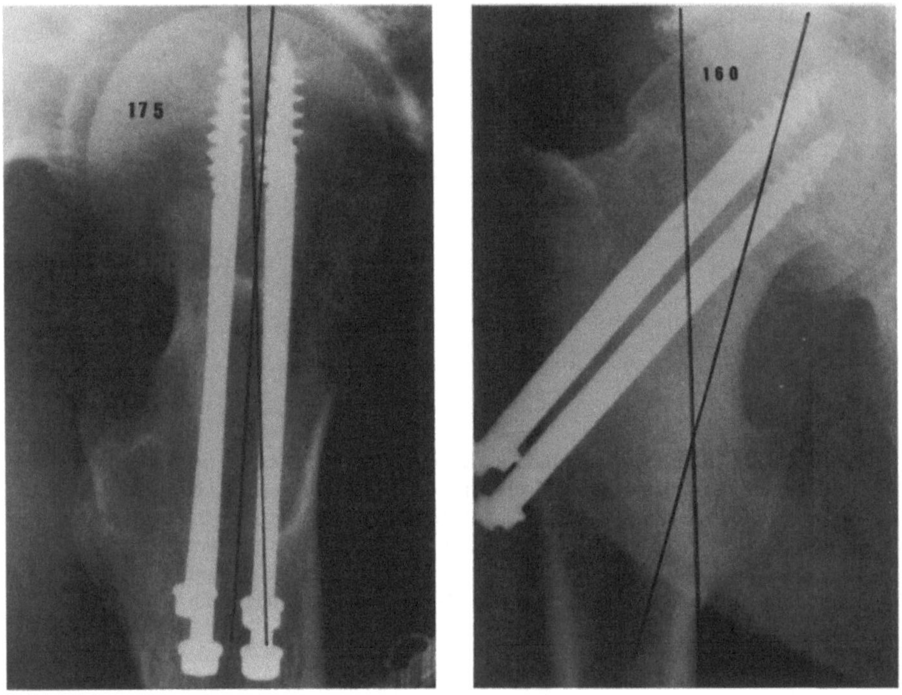

A B

FIG. 8–44 The fracture, which would be an unstable fracture type II or III, was reduced as well as possible, with an excellent Garden index. This fracture went on to heal without complications, which substantiates Garden's concept of what can be expected when the index is close to ideal.

such as a Pugh nail: It can distract the fragments, and the head can tilt away, losing an otherwise good reduction. A single screw causes rotation of the head as it approaches the hard subchondral surface, and supplementary pins must be used.[132] There is also experimental evidence that multiple pins into the femoral neck are stronger than a single sliding compression screw.[133]

The implant preferred by American surgeons is a small threaded pin used in multiples of three to six. The first to advocate the use of these pins was Austin-Moore.[134,135] These thin pins are placed in a quadrilateral pattern parallel to one another so that the fragments can more easily impact. Today, pins are heavier and stronger with lag-like threads for better anchorage in the head, e.g., Haggie, Knowles, and Guffon pins. Swiss surgeons have used AO screws instead of threaded pins.[136] The newest device, promoted by Asnis (Fig. 8–46), is cannulated and is a modification of the Howse screw. It is stouter than the ever-popular Knowles device. There are other versions by Ace, Richards, and Mecron. The Asnis type of screw (Howmedica) is becoming popular because of its refined instrumentation and seemingly extra purchasing power: In one research paper it was shown that the Asnis screw had significantly more holding power than did Knowles pins.[137] It promises to facilitate parallel pinning of the fragments. This author has found the system too cumbersome, and Asnis himself showed a case in which the pins were not parallel.[138] With better instrumentation the idea has a bright future.

This author prefers the Guffon pin because the tips are sharp and can be quickly started into the lateral cortex. Moreover, this pin is strong, and it has larger lag threads for grasping the femoral head well.

There are laboratory data on the strength of pins fixing the femoral neck. The work by van Auderkercke et al. is timely.[139] They concluded that there is no significant difference in strength when three, five, or seven Knowles pins are used, and that the strength of a sliding nail plate is not superior to the strength of multiple pinning. The different failure mode of five or seven pins

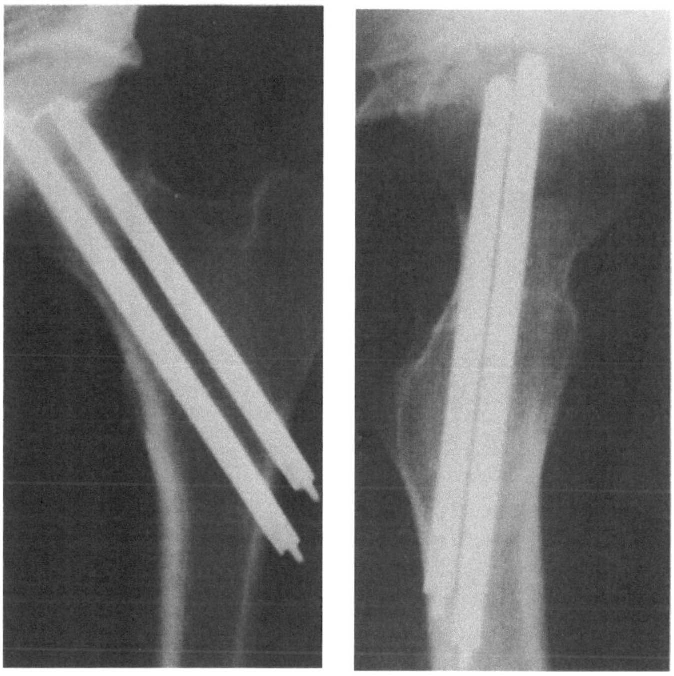

FIG. 8–45 Hansson nails, used in Sweden, are heavy stainless steel pins with a central screw that causes a sharp blade to extrude at the tip, thereby locking the pin into the head, thus locking into the femoral head. Although these pins are available from European suppliers, they are not used much in the United States, so there is little experience and data from American sources.

compared with a three-pin fixation can be explained by the damage to the trabecular structure by too many pins and the central placement of some of the pins in the weaker area of the cross-section of the femoral neck. The trabecular bone in the central area represents only a thin porous network. Pinning in this area results in failure of the supporting cancellous bone rather than a plastic deformation of the pins. Thus it is the ultimate property of bone that is the limiting factor.

Another study by Ruben et al.[133] confirmed the efficiency of multiple pinning. This experimental study demonstrated the rigidity and durability of Knowles pin fixation of femoral neck fractures. A fracture was created by an osteotomy, then reduced and fixed with Knowles pins. Four groups of reduction and pin configurations were created: optimal reduction and pinning, poor reduction, poor pinning, and comminution. Three months of walking by a patient with a neck fracture were simulated with the materials testing machine. The results showed that Knowles pinning of a femoral neck fracture can provide adequate support for immediate full weight-bearing until healing has been reached. Stability and durability of the fixation were compromised by loss of cortical bone support, comminution of the posterior cortex, short pins not engaged into subchondral bone, nonparallel pins, and osteoporosis. The pin placement was parallel to the long axis of the femoral neck, which is 130°, not the radical 150° proposed by some.[129]

From a practical standpoint, placing four pins in a rectangular pattern appears to satisfy all criteria for good pin placement. Occassionally the neck is small, so three pins in a diamond pattern do just as well. The position of the pins in the femoral head is critical. The superolateral portion of the femoral head is vulnerable to vascular damage by implants, as pointed out long ago by Claffey[84] and Brodetti.[140] A more inferior place-

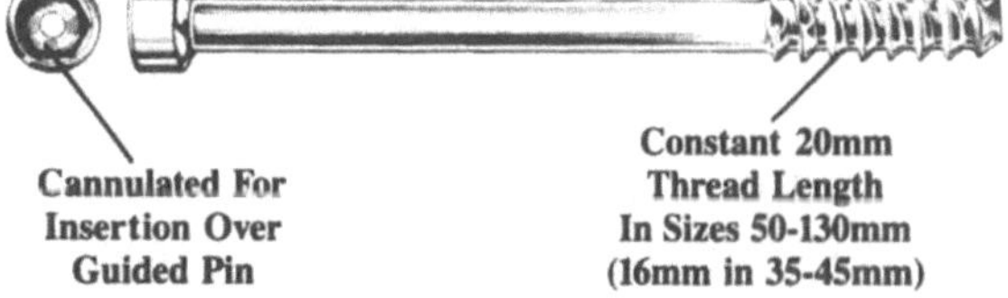

FIG. 8–46 A Cannulated screw designed by Asnis.

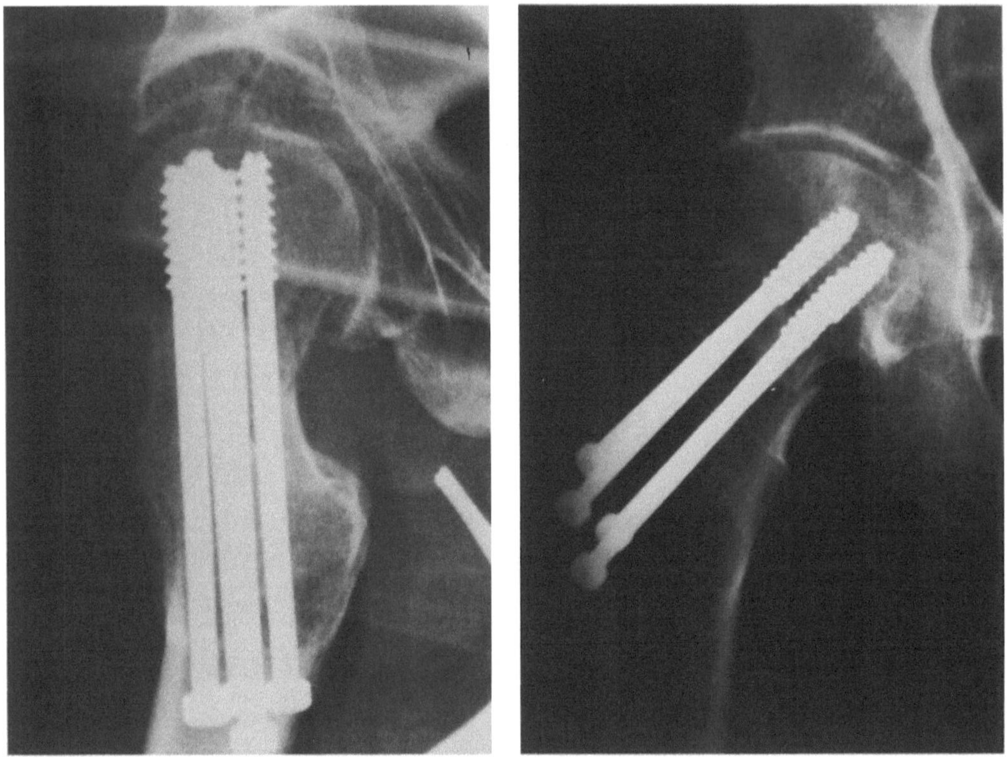

B C

FIG. 8–46 **B, C** X-ray films, AP and lateral, showing a femoral neck fracture fixed by Asnis screws. In this system, guide pins are first inserted through a gig in order to assure a more precise parallel placement of the screws.

ment in the sagittal plane and a central location in the coronal plane is ideal. This positioning, however, has been challenged by Crowell et al.[137] They concluded that "Although the Asnis device showed increased holding power over Knowles pins, fixation with either device is severely compromised in osteoporotic bone. Traditional recommendation has been to place four pins in the posteromedial location for optimal fixation, but our findings suggest that there is increased trabecular densities in the central and two lateral locations where the pullout forces were also the greatest."

This study and its results must be put into perspective in that the vital blood supply to the femoral head can be damaged by pins drilled into the superolateral area of the femoral head. It once was thought that a more posterior position in the lateral x-ray view would be favorable in preventing further posterior collapse of the head on the neck by propping up that part of the head. This does not actually happen. A more balanced placement of the pins is theoretically better because rotation and impaction would be better controlled. After the pins have been placed properly, the fracture can be impacted by the lag effect of the pins. Attempting to impact the fragments before pinning can cause the fracture to go into extreme valgus or occasionally into varus. The fragments invariably collapse, one on the other, postoperatively with compression from the muscle contractures and with early weight-bearing if the pins had been placed reasonably parallel. Finally, the tip of each pin is screwed into the head as far as possible. Ideally it should go to the subchondral bone (Fig. 8–46).

Guide Pin Placement Placement of the guide pin has been facilitated immensely by use of the image intensifier and, even more so, the newest memory screens. Critical positioning of the guide pin in the lateral view can consume considerable exposure time. Tronzo found a simple, reliable method for accurately placing a master guide pin for near-perfect lateral positioning and reported it in 1974 as an extramedullary guide pin.[141] It has since been recommended by DeLee,[36] Pankovich,[142] and Zickel[227] in their texts on technique for hip nailings. It can be very reliable if the technique is followed precisely.

After a short lateral incision is made just below the greater trochanter; the cortex is exposed by dividing first the tensor fascia and then the vastus lateralis. A ⅛ inch Steinmann pin or one of the stouter guide pins (anything less bows and bends too much to be useful) is used to pierce the remnants of the vastus lateralis and into the base of the capsule. This step is critical. The pin must pass *along the anterior femoral neck* and stop as it goes into the *edge* of the femoral head (Fig. 8–47). It should be so placed that a mallet must be used to tap it into the head. By placing a finger over the capsule, one can follow the pin's path as it passes along the neck. If it should not do so, it will pass over the head into the pelvis or catch the dome of the head, causing the pin to fall into an oblique alignment. This "intracapsular," or "extramedullary," pin can now be used as a guide for final drilling of the four pins (Figs. 8–48 and 8–49). The same pin should have been placed in the AP plane at about 135° to the shaft and aimed either at the center of the head or into its inferior two-thirds (Fig. 8–50).

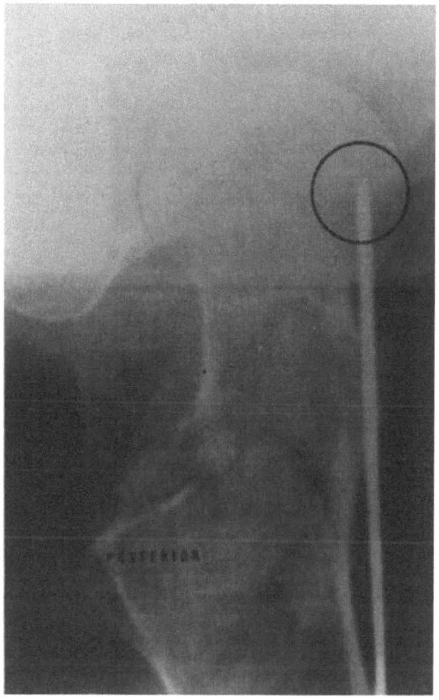

Fig. 8–47 Tronzo's technique of placing a guide pin along the neck of the femur into the "edge" of the head. This site is just beneath the capsule and outside the medullary canal. Thus the technique has been called extramedullary guide pin placement or intracapsular guide pin placement. The pin can be kept in place and used as a guide for accurate placement of the pins, using the lateral view of the hip.

Open Pinning Versus Percutaneous Pinning

In addition to an open reduction of the fracture site itself, there are two methods of pinning a femoral neck fracture. One is to expose the lateral cortex just below the greater trochanter and insert the pins directly into the femoral neck. This is called the open technique. (Although the fracture itself is not exposed it is still a major surgical procedure exposing bone—thus the common label, "open pinning" as being distinguished from an "open reduction.") This method is mandatory for the Asnis type of system whereby parallelism is controlled by a special guide instrument placed up against lateral cortex. This technique is the author's preferred method because it is more direct and seems more reliable in obtaining precise placement of the pins. However, unlike percutaneous pinning, it can be complicated by deep wound infections, which rarely occur with percutaneous pinning.

Pinning a femoral neck fracture percutaneously is an alternate procedure. It took Arnold to produce a collection of data to give the technique credibility.[144] The procedure, the details of which

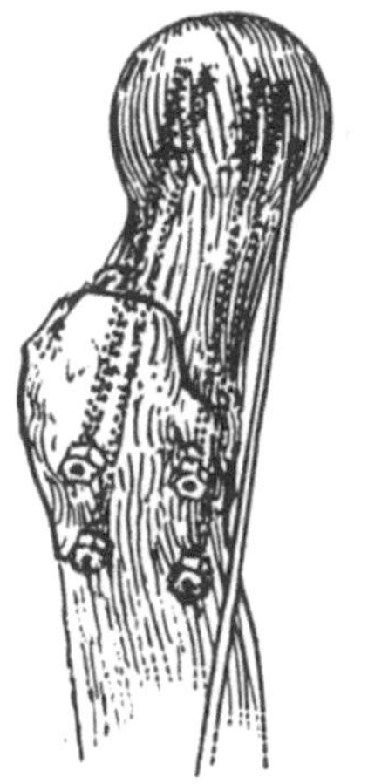

Fig. 8–48 Keep the extramedullary guide pin in place for it can be very helpful when aligning the pins in the all-important lateral view.

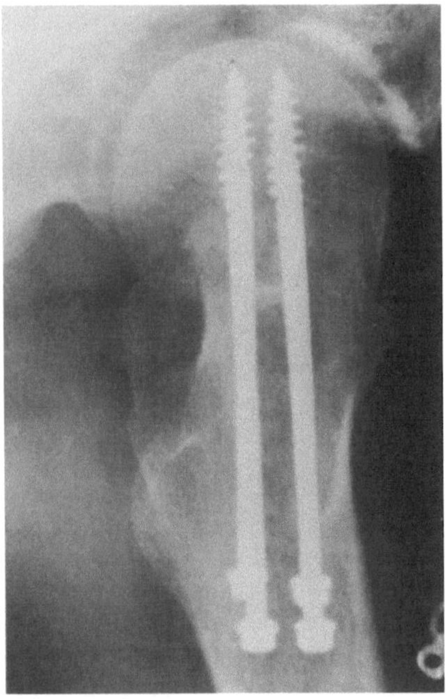

FIG. 8–49 An ideal parallel placement of the four pins quadrilaterally in the center of the head in the lateral view.

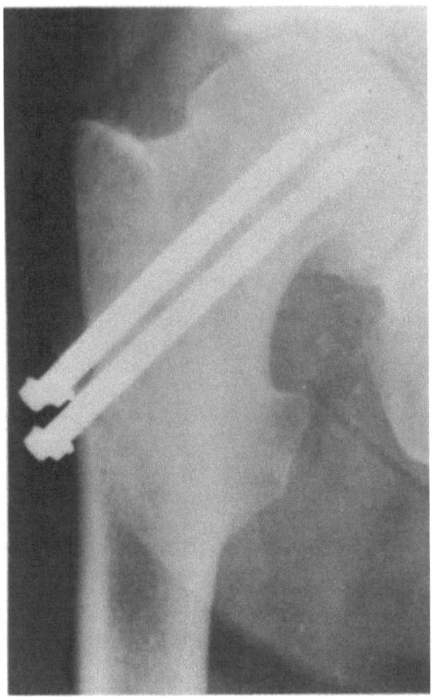

FIG. 8–50 In the AP view the pins are also parallel, placed in the lower inferior medial portion of the head, thereby avoiding damage to the vascular supply of the head.

can be found in Arnold's paper, may be more demanding than it first appears, but as with other procedures precision comes with practice. Arnold's statistics from nearly 1000 cases of displaced femoral neck fractures are impressive: no infections and an 85% healing rate (in "well reduced, well pinned cases"). He used percutaneous pinning with few exceptions, the latter being "fractures of the elderly," fractures in patients with parkinsonism, and fractures with evidence of posterior comminution. If varus displacement occurred during the first 1 to 3 months, a secondary arthroplasty was done, either hemiarthroplasty or total hip replacement. Young adults who did not have a good closed reduction were treated with an open reduction whereas older patients underwent a primary arthroplasty if the fracture did not reduce satisfactorily.

Pin Complications Complications can occur operatively or in the early postoperative period. This author knows of a guide pin that was inserted too far into the pelvis which penetrated the internal iliac artery, resulting in a postoperative death when the cause of the patient's shock went unrecognized. Knowles pins can migrate into the pelvis causing damage to the external iliac vein,[145] into the left ureter,[146] into the bladder,[147] and into the abdominal cavity in a case of parkinsonism reported by Arnold.[207] In the latter instance the pin migration was supposedly due to the patient's tremors. Altner reported a case in which the guide pin was advanced into the pelvis and lost there. The patient expired from peritonitis.[148] Shaw formulated a scheme to prevent pin penetration into the hip joint from going unrecognized,[149] based on the use of a cannulated screw, e.g., the Asnis device, and the injection of contrast material through the cannulation.

Prevention of Pin Migration Certain precautions should be followed to prevent migration of guide pins and Knowles pins. Guide pins should never go across the hip joint. It is important that they be monitored as they enter the head so that their final resting place is well established.

If the hilt of a Knowles pin passes beyond the cortex of the lateral shaft, it will have also gone past the head into the joint, thereby leaving a path for the pin to migrate easily into the pelvis. If there is no further room for another path, either do without the pin or use some bone cement poured into the hole around the pin which has been backed out and then drilled into its proper place. If a cannulated screw is used, liquid cement can be injected through the nail into the head, assuming that the guide pin had not gone into the hip joint, otherwise a ''cement arthrogram'' will follow. A package with its syringe and cement is being readied for marketing with a new fenestrated screw system.[150]

Bone Grafts

Bone grafting has been reserved for nonunion of the femoral neck. Judet[151] used a muscle pedicle graft for this purpose (Fig. 8–51). Meyers et al. refined the concept and promoted its use for nonunions and as a primary procedure for displaced femoral neck fractures in young patients (Fig. 8–52).[127,128,152–154] It seems reasonable that a vascularized pedicle bone graft would be proper treatment as a primary procedure in young patients with a displaced femoral neck fracture. Such a situation carries with it a nonunion rate of 20% and a 30% rate of segmental collapse. Meyers claimed that his procedure reduces both rates to 5% each.[152] The procedure seems straightforward (Fig. 8–52),[155] but it was challenged by

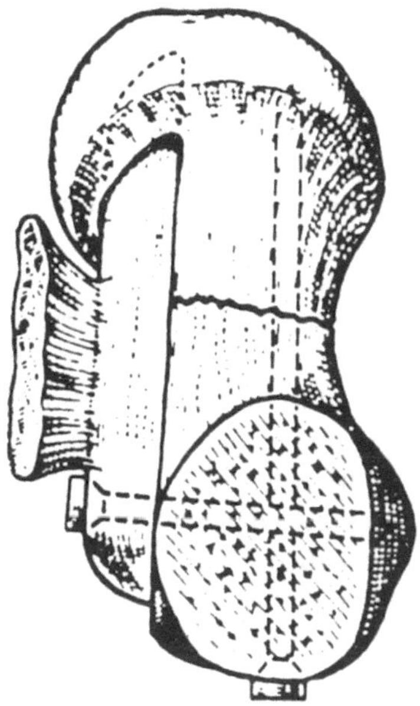

FIG. 8–51 The pedicle graft first devised by Judet is inserted into the compression side of the femoral neck (posterior cortex). It is used to fill in the posterior comminution as well as aid in supporting the fractured femoral neck. It may or may not be a true vascular graft. (Adapted from Judet, R.: Traitement des fractures du col de femur por graffe pediculae. Acta Orthop. Scand., 32:421, 1962.

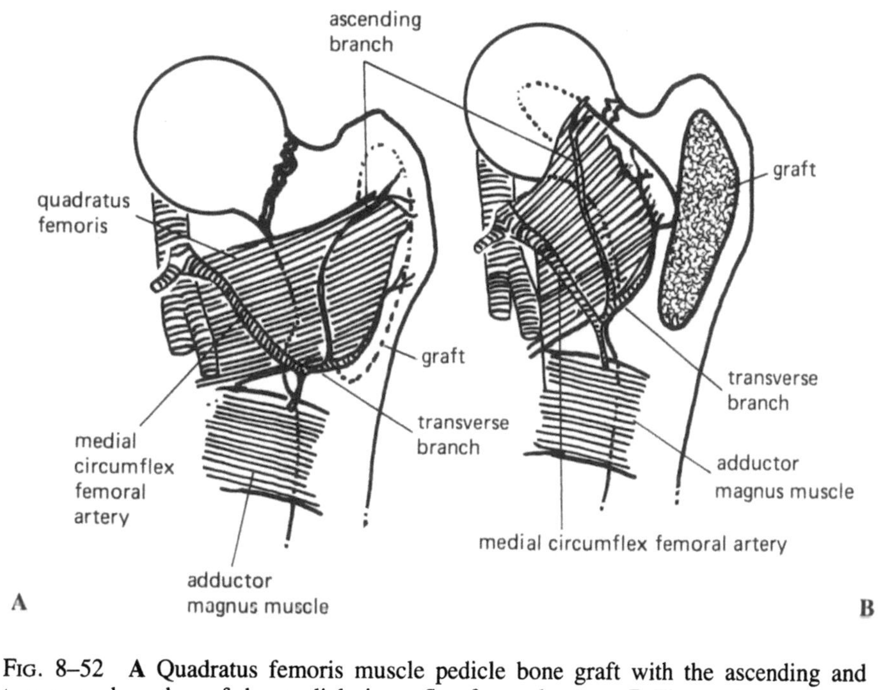

FIG. 8–52 **A** Quadratus femoris muscle pedicle bone graft with the ascending and transverse branches of the medial circumflex femoral artery. **B** The graft rotated and inserted into the femoral head. (Adapted from Chacka, P. B.: Vascularised pedicular bone grafts. Mt. Orthop., 8:127, 1984.)

Ferguson: "Since the beginning of recorded orthopedics there have been operations to improve blood supply by transplanting muscle. However, there are few tissues less suited than muscle to accomplish this result, since muscle has end-artery circulation. The various muscle transplants for vascular improvement operations have not survived the test of time."[128] A study by Morwessel and Evarts[156] also challenged Meyers' enthusiasm and cast doubt on his technique as a primary procedure. As outlined by Meyers, it accomplishes the following: (1) fills in the gap left by the comminution in the posterior neck: (2) provides additional mechanical support to the fracture; and (3) provides the latticework for revascularization of a potentially avascular head.

The surgical technique is not easy, and it must not be attempted by a novice. Meyers recommended putting the patient prone on the fracture table with the leg free so that it can be manipulated. He used a Gibson incision (Fig. 8–53). The principle is to mobilize the quadratus muscle with a generous block of bone which lies between the two trochanters and then insert it into the posterior femoral neck, across the fracture site and parallel to the neck (Fig. 8–53B). This author prefers to put the patient on her side and utilize his modified lateral incision (Fig. 8–64).

The fat overlaying the quadratus muscle is carefully stripped medially to clearly define its attachment to the posterior surface of the greater trochanter up to the intertrochanteric line. The ascending and transverse branches of the medial circumflex femoral artery run along the superior and inferior margins of the muscle, and the muscle must be handled carefully to avoid damaging these important vessels. A rectangular block of bone as outlined in Fig. 8–53B is cut out by first marking its boundaries with a drill and then using an osteotome. The graft is extended by about 1 cm beyond the superior edge of the muscle so it can be pushed up under the head. The inferior end of the graft is close to the lesser trochanter and calcar where the cortex is thicker; hence this part must be well predrilled in order not to fracture it (which is the single most common technical error in the procedure). This step also avoids creating a stress point, which can in turn produce a

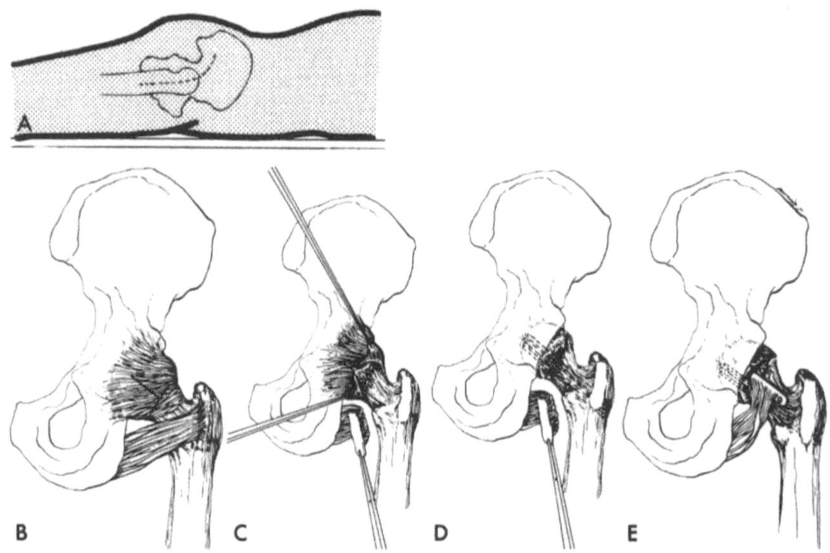

Fig. 8–53 Steps in the surgical procedure. **A** Skin incision. **B** Outline of pedicle graft, which includes the trochanteric crest and the insertion of the quadratus femoris muscle. The capsular incision is drawn in as an inverted T. **C** The capsule is cut and retracted, and the pedicle graft is elevated and retracted to expose the fracture line. **D** Four Hagie pins have been inserted. The tip of each pin should reach the subchondral area of the head. **E** The pedicle graft is inserted into the prepared opening in the head and fixed with one screw in the neck of the femur. (From Meyers, M. H., Harvey, P., Jr., Moore, T.: The muscle pedicle bone graft in the treatment of displaced fractures of the femoral neck: Indications, operative technique, and results. Orthop. Clin. North Am., 5:779, 1974.)

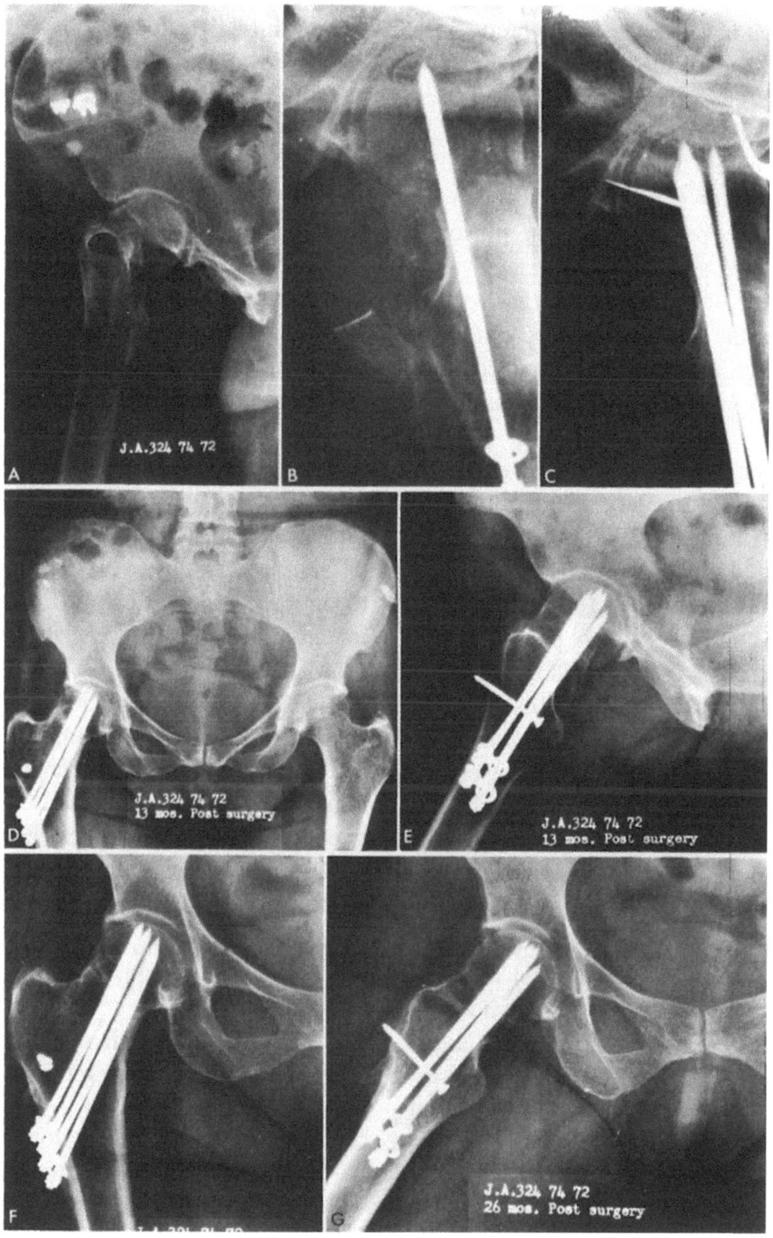

FIG. 8–54 **A** Subcapital fracture, 1 day after injury. **B** Fracture reduced and fixed with one Hagie pin. This photograph reveals a large defect in the posterior cortex of the neck. The pin placement is good. **C** All the Hagie pins have been inserted. Pin placement is good. **D** Anteroposterior view 13 months after surgery, showing union of the fracture. **E** Lateral view 13 months after surgery showing union of the fracture. **F** AP view 26 months after surgery, showing osseous union. **G** Lateral view 26 months after surgery, showing osseous union. The pedicle graft appears viable at the fracture site. (From Meyers, M. H., Harvey, P., Jr., Moore, T.: The muscle pedicle bone graft in the treatment of displaced fractures of the femoral neck: Indications, operative technique, and results. Orthop. Clin. North Am., 5:779, 1974.)

subtrochanteric fracture. The medial part of the graft is not drilled because the drill would necessarily penetrate the muscle, causing damage to the vessels. The graft is approximately 0.5 cm thick and 1 cm wide. As the graft is lifted out of its bed, the muscle is peeled away from the underlying capsule as far as possible to freely mobilize the muscle–pedicle unit. The muscle is wrapped in a saline sponge and retracted away medially. The rest of the short external rotators is detached from the back of the trochanter and retracted medially. The capsule is opened, or if it is already torn it is opened further parallel with the neck.

The fracture is now exposed, and the necessary maneuvers are done to reduce the fracture. An assistant applies traction while holding the leg internally rotated, abducted, and flexed. The lateral shift is the most difficult deformity to correct and may require the assistant to push the knee outwardly as he pushes the upper femor inwardly or vice versa. The pins are drilled across the fracture in a quadralateral fashion. The cannulated screw system has an advantage here because guide pins can be used and the pin placements checked by x-ray studies. This step avoids tearing up good bone tissue in repeated attempts to gain ideal pin placement.

Once reduced and pinned, a slot is made in the neck at the edge of the head, and a path is dug out of the head for the graft to slide into place on the surface of the femoral neck. Cancellous bone can be curetted out of the greater trochanter to fill any defect at the site of comminution before the graft is put into place, or iliac crest bone can be harvested for this purpose. The pedicular graft is then rotated so that its proximal end is passed through the prepared slot in the head. The graft is affixed in place by a malleolar screw. An example of one of Meyers' cases is shown in Figure 8–54. It is not possible to close the capsule, but the rotator tendons can be reattached to the greater trochanter.

Weight-bearing is not permitted for at least 6 to 8 months depending on the healing process followed by scans and laminograms. Before discharge a bone scan is done as a base study to be used later for comparison. Meyers found that most patients showed good vascularity by 6 months. Among his 233 patients the average time to union was 3 to 4 months in 132, and 6 months in the others with a union rate of 93%; no consistent pattern could be found in the 23 cases of nonunion, except for the three patients with parkinsonism. Late segmental collapse occurred in 5.6% of the fractures that united.

Technical complications were not minor, which should alert one to the technical liabilities of the procedure. In Meyers et al.'s series[154]: "The pedicle was fractured in eight instances during the operative procedure. This was not serious and required innovations such as extra screws for fixation or wire fixation." There were three subtrochanteric fractures that resulted from overzealousness when obtaining the graft. Two pins broke. One pin migrated into the pelvis, requiring an intrapelvic, extraperitoneal approach to remove the metallic fragment. The lesser trochanteric fractured twice, but these fractures were of no significance. In two cases the graft appeared to have become dislodged from the head. Deep infection was troublesome in that it occurred in 6% of the cases.

Baksi of India grafted 56 patients with ununited femoral neck fractures. Union occurred in 75%, delayed union in seven patients, and only a repeat nonunion in five. Technical failures numbered two. He added multiple drill holes into any sclerotic area in the femoral head and used silk sutures to secure the graft into the head.[58]

Use of Endoprostheses

The use of endoprostheses in the treatment of fresh fractures of the femoral neck has become an established procedure, with certain reservations. Although it was first done during the 1950s its use is still embroiled in controversy. Originally, it was a viable alternative for salvaging a failed femoral neck fracture. When it became an alternative to cup arthroplasty, it became apparent that it was also a viable alternative to internal fixation of fresh fractures in the elderly patient. Now it appears to face extinction because of the success of total hip replacement. Or have progress and technical refinement given it renewed credibility via bipolar devices?

The exact place for an endoprosthetic replacement in the management of fresh fractures in an elderly patient remain confusing even after reviewing an up-to-date bibliography. There is no consensus in the literature, as most reports reflect personalized views with little objective evidence of controlling variables. Old style prostheses cannot be measured against new designs that provide improved fixation and improved articulation with the acetabulum.

A critical parameter which is impossible to control is the skill of the surgeon executing the operation. A surgeon practicing alone may be compelled to pin all fresh femoral neck fractures for the simple reason that department policy allows him to perform such a procedure alone, whereas he must have staff assistance if he were to choose an arthroplasty. A great deal of attention is broadly swept away by such a callous approach to an already handicapped patient. Another issue complicating the results is the question of whether to use a prosthesis with cement, without cement, or with a microporous coating. The situation is further clouded by the reappearance of bipolar (double-head) prostheses. Despite personal distortions and blind spots, there are honest divergent positions, expressed by the following deductions:

1. "After all, the best place for a prosthesis is in the instrument cupboard, just as the best place for a viable femoral head is on the neck of the femur" (stated by Nicoll in 1963[55]).
2. "Nailing a femoral fracture is nothing more than the first stage of a two-stage arthroplasty." (author unknown).
3. "The bad results of nailing are the results of bad nailings."[157]

Pinning Versus Endoprostheses in the Elderly Arnold[144] reviewed 1000 cases of femoral neck fractures treated percutaneously as primary treatment. He found a mortality rate of 1.5%, 89% union rate, 11% nonunion rate, symptomatic femoral head necrosis in 8%, and an infection rate of 0.5%.

Failures were treated with a bipolar prosthesis or a total hip replacement. Arnold considered that a prosthetic replacement should be done as a secondary procedure because it resulted in a lower mortality rate than if done as a primary operation. He would rather pin an unstable fracture initially and do the arthroplasty as a secondary procedure. He performed the hemiarthroplasty during the same initial hospitalization when it became apparent that the pinning would not result in a stable reduction. This was "an important factor in our choice of pinning as primary treatment."[144] Today because of "DRG's," such a policy could not be tolerated; it would have to be one or the other in favor of the procedure which had the shortest hospital stay.

Johnson et al.[158] followed 40 patients with a mean age of 73 (range 38 to 93) with ^{85}Sr scintimetry, x-ray studies, and clinical examinations for 5 years. Thirteen of the fractures healed without complications, 22 developed femoral head necrosis, and 5 showed clear evidence of nonunion. Increasing pain (although not always incapacitating) during weight-bearing was an early sign of necrosis and nonunion. These two developments were treated with secondary arthroplasties. Five patients with femoral head necrosis were asymptomatic. The patient's living situation proved important. Those who had partners chose not to undergo an arthroplasty operation. "It is concluded that a primary arthroplasty in femoral neck fractures should be avoided."[158]

Bray and Chapman made a strong case for pinning femoral neck fractures:[159]

1. Weight-bearing: Patients with adequately pinned hips can bear full weight immediately after surgery. There is less soft tissue dissection and therefore less pain. The patients with percutaneous pins need no drains and abduction pillows to curtail immediate ambulation. The sooner these patients are out of bed and ambulating, the less likely they are to develop associated medical complications of hospitalization.

2. Dislocation: The reported incidence of prosthetic dislocation after primary arthroplasty in the treatment of femoral neck fracture averages nearly 10%. [*Editors note:* The implications of immediate dislocation after primary arthroplasty suggest that the procedure may be more skill-sensitive than is practical, as there can be malalignment of the components, inappropriate component size, or poor patient selection.] There are no dislocations after a pinning.

3. Deep wound infection: Multiple reports in the literature suggest the incidence of deep wound infection in the treatment of femoral neck fractures averages 11% for hemiarthroplasties and only 0.5% for percutaneous pinnings. An infected hemiarthroplasty is an absolute catastrophic complication to the elderly patient.

4. Treatment failures: Late complications of a hemiarthroplasty include loosening, protrusio, component migration, calcar absorption, and heterotopic bone formation. These failures must then be treated by another major operation in the form of a revision arthroplasty with the same set of complications, but with a higher rate of morbidity.

On the other hand, open reduction and internal fixation [are] not without failure. Many reports over the last 10 years have suggested nonunion rates from 5% to 15% and late femoral head necrosis between 7% and 12%. These complications are undoubtedly related to the type of fracture, the acceptance of a poor reduction, and inadequate fixation.

However, if there are advantages to treating failures, the pinned group has several to mention. The major advantage of these treatment failures is that many patients are either free of pain or have symptoms so mild that they do not require a reconstructive procedure. We agree with Arnold that a secondary femoral head replacement for a failed percutaneous pinning have a substantially lower incidence of complications than do primary replacements. Any surgeon routinely caring for elderly patients with hip fractures would agree that surgical options are far greater approaching the patient with failed pinning than those patients with failed hemiarthroplasty.

Evidence Favoring Endoprosthetic Replacement Results with improved technique, more experienced surgeons, better designs, and better patient selection are reflected in the literature of the 1980s. The justification for using an endoprosthesis in fresh femoral neck fractures is that it hopefully will circumvent the complications associated with pinning such fractures. There is good reason to search for a solution to these complications that plague elderly patients, whose life span and quality of life are so tenuous anyway.

Nonunions have been reported to range from 10% to 33%.[38,39] In one study necrotic heads were frequently found when examined at primary arthroplasty.[160] Johnson et al.[158] reviewed nine contemporary reports of internal fixation of femoral neck fractures and found an average failure rate of 36% among 2647 fractures. This was compared to another nine reports which favored endoprosthetic replacement as the treatment of choice for displaced femoral neck fractures; in the latter they found an accumulated failure rate of 13% among 1247 such fractures.

Welch[161] reviewed 300 cemented hemiarthroplasties. His conclusion was "that hemiarthroplasty, cemented in place, in the treatment of displaced femoral neck fractures in elderly persons is a rational procedure. It carries no greater morbidity rate and may even decrease these parameters when modern technology is employed. In the long run it would appear that greater than 90% of the prostheses are serviceable for the duration of the patient's life."

Soreide et al.[162] conducted a prospective study by randomizing displaced fractures into two groups, those treated with internal fixation and those treated with a Christiansen endoprosthesis. Immediate weight-bearing was allowed in both groups as tolerated. The prosthetic group walked to full weight-bearing quicker. Mortality rates were the same: 20% after the first year. Morbidity was different in that blood transfusions were routinely needed for the prosthesis group. The pinned group were hospitalized a shorter time and had less exposure time in the operating room. Soreide et al. concluded that a hemiarthroplasty for the treatment of an acutely displaced femoral neck fracture provided the elderly patient with more definitive treatment because there were fewer reoperations and overall better results after the first year.

In another prospective study Sikorski and Barrington[163] compared internal fixation with primary endoprosthetic replacement in patients 70 years and older. They also compared the posterior approach (Moore) with an anterior approach (McKee). They concluded that internal fixation offered no advantage over hemiarthroplasty in the treatment of displaced femoral neck fractures. "The morbidity of internal fixation was awesome. They had a high rate of technical failures and over 30% had to be revised. Persistent pain and prolonged rehabilitation were major drawbacks to the group treated with internal fixation." These

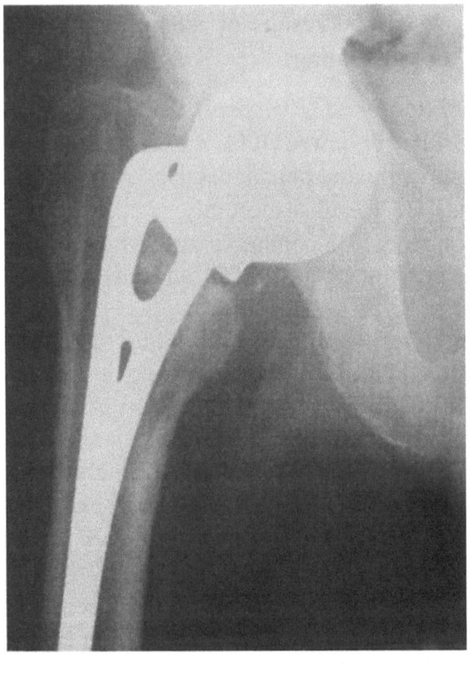

FIG. 8–55 There is erosion of the inferior neck or "sinking" of the implant. Note the early erosion of the acetabulum, evident from a loss of the joint line.

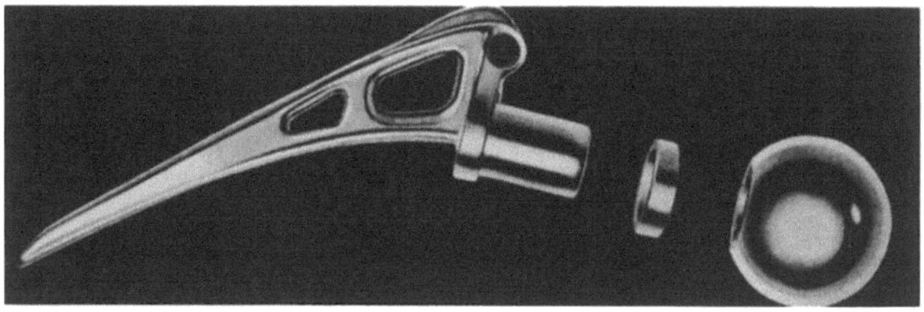

FIG. 8–56 Skuderi prosthesis was the first trunion-bearing device allowing motion to take place at the head and neck junction given "universal rotation" (two planes at once).

authors found better results in patients managed with posterior incisions. Dorr[164] reported similar findings in a comparative study: There was persistent pain in 50% of those treated with internal fixation and in only 10% of those with a cemented Bateman prosthesis. Moreover, 30% of the pinned group experienced failure of fixation.

Bipolar Prosthesis A two-part endoprosthesis has come into vogue. It has been called a universal head, a double-headed prosthesis, a double-interface, a bicentric, and a bipolar prosthesis. The latter name sounds more sophisticated and so has caught the imagination of the orthopedic public, but no one knows what the term really means. It means many dollars in Medicare payment to the surgeon if it is used as a "modified total hip arthroplasty."

A major problem with a conventional endoprosthesis is that over long usage the acetabulum is eroded, the stem loosens, and the prosthesis "sinks in" (Fig. 8–55). During the early 1950s Scuderi recognized this problem and tried to solve it by a design change. He put the head on a trunion and used washers or shims for varying the neck lengths (Fig. 8–56). It never gained much attention and so was lost on the shelf. During the 1970s Christiansen rediscovered the trunion idea and revised the prosthesis with a polyethylene bearing[165] (Fig. 8–57). According to Bowman et al.[166] the current rage was started by Bateman. Its design concept is to lock a spherical head into a socket so that the head swivels instead of just rotating on a simple trunion. The theoretical advantage is to keep the acetabular side quiet with as little motion as possible while the major motion takes place at the swivel. The stem was originally fenestrated similar to a Moore prosthesis. Another theoretical advantage is that the double action on the rotating head relieves some of the torque stresses being put on the stem and thus preserves the fixation of the stem in the femur (Fig. 8–58). The early Bateman design had the troublesome feature of drifting into varus and getting stuck there. The engineers at the Osteonic company solved that by placing the femoral ball into the socket in an eccentric position, making it self-centering. They then changed the stem design to be wedged in two dimensions and in different sizes for different canals thus achieving a better fit, a "canal-filling" concept. Each manu-

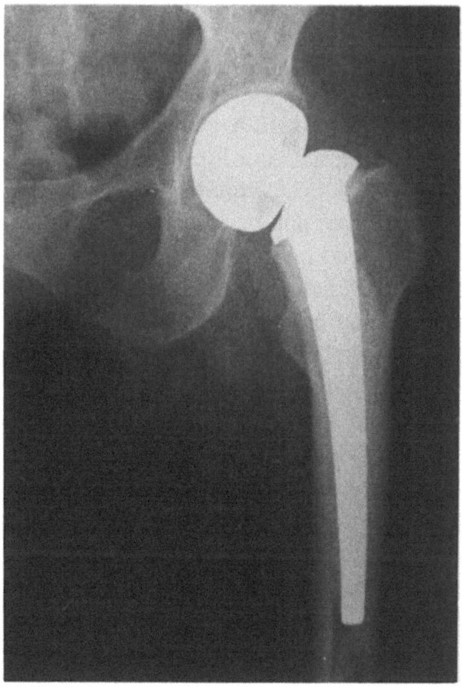

FIG. 8–57 Christiansen prosthesis has a unique trunion bearing for double-action motion which may allow less acetabular wear. It could be easily replaced later by a total hip device.

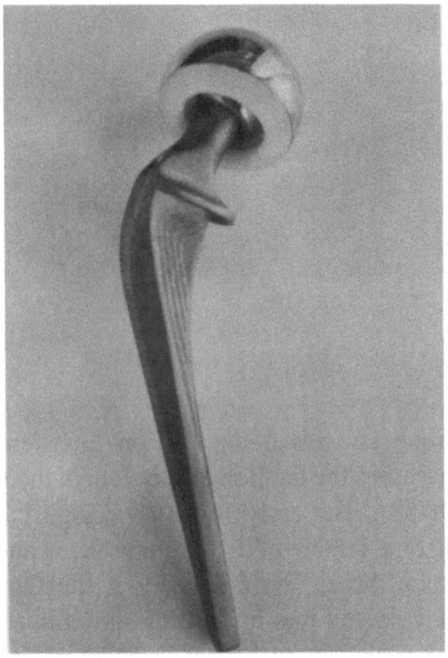

FIG. 8–58 The Osteonic prosthesis is a "canal filling" type of device used for a press-fit fixation. The center of the head is offset enough in the socket to make the head portion fall into valgus rather than into the less acceptable varus.

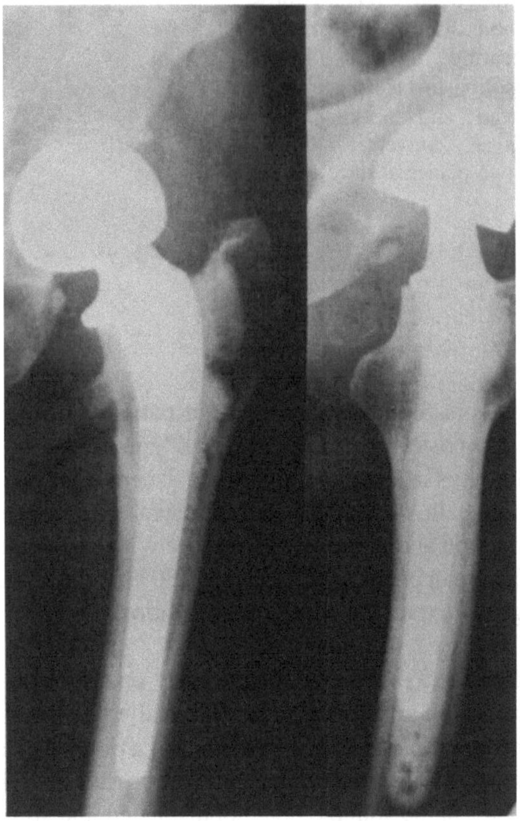

FIG. 8–59 Any of these bipolar prostheses, such as the Osteonic prosthesis, can be either press-fitted or cemented into position, as is the case here.

facturer has its own marketing version. The prostheses can be used with or without cement (Fig. 8–59).

There are few scientific data to support the idea in general and none to clearly support one design over the other. A cemented Müller endoprosthesis costs one-third less than the cemented bipolar system. The problem of erosion of the acetabulum has not been solved. Drinker and Murray[167] found measurable wear in the acetabulum in 53% of their cases. The problem of femoral stem loosening has not been solved either by the double action of the femoral head device. Figure 8–60 shows a displaced femoral neck fracture in a 52-year-old man who had been treated with an Osteonics device inserted 2 years prior to this picture. The stem became loose but not infected. Similar effects were demonstrated with a bipolar implant when used for femoral head necrosis in young patients.[168]

The use of cement remains another unsettled issue. Charnley proposed that if an endoprosthesis were cemented into place the system would be so rigid that wear on the acetabulum would be accelerated.[169] He thought that a slightly loose stem would piston just enough to act like a shock absorber, thereby helping to diminish acetabular wear. Some believe that the diminution is enhanced further by the bipolar device.[160]

Kwoh and Cruess[170] studied the effects of a unipolar prosthesis on the acetabulum in dogs when it was cemented into the femoral shaft. At 6 weeks focal surface changes were noted in the articular cartilage, and at 6 months there was extensive destruction of the entire cartilage.

Figure 8–61 shows the acetabulum of a patient who had been treated with an Osteonics device that was press-fitted into place.

Cabanela and Van Demark[171] found no difference between a cemented Thompson prosthesis and a cemented bipolar prosthesis in an elderly patient who had suffered a displaced femoral neck fracture. They did believe, however, that there may be an advantage in using a bipolar device in active elderly patients with displaced neck fractures. They also recommended it in elderly patients with nonunion of the femoral neck for reasons that are not clear, as they had only eight patients to refer to for analysis: three had excellent results, three good, and two fair!

Drinker and Murray[167] made several observations: Although the postoperative dislocation rate was the same for bipolar and unipolar devices, reduction of the bipolar prosthesis was more difficult. If the parts came apart, an open reduction became necessary. Conversion to a total hip arthroplasty usually required reconstruction of both components. These investigators were using the older solid head/neck designs, and so they could not make up for instability due to short necks.

The new replaceable modular heads may be of help. Inner bearing motion stopped after 4 years, thus throwing all of the wear back onto the acetabular floor. This author has revised cases where the opposite was true. In these cases the acetabulum was thin and fragile because there was stress shielding by the inner bearing taking all of the load and not distributing it over a larger area of the acetabulum. Despite some early failures, Murray[172] has remained enthusiastic about the bipolar prosthesis. He too recommended it for active elderly patients with a displaced femoral neck fracture because, like Drinker and Murray, the results with a cemented bipolar prosthesis was better in the active biologically younger person.

The only advantage that may be defensible is its potential ease of converting it to a total hip replacement. If a bipolar prosthesis fails by eroding the acetabulum, it can be revised by leaving the stem in place and installing a matching acetabular component. That may or may not be the case in the future when more data will have been collected. Cabanela and Van Demark found it difficult to revise, and three of four revisions had to have the femoral component revised as well as the acetabular reconstruction.[171] If it is realized that these stems also loosen with time, how can one know the exact status of the stem fixation at that moment when only the acetabular side had been revised? For instance, if the socket has been revised in April, why is it not possible for the stem to eventually become loose by May? It is possible that the stem had been loose at the April revision but was missed at a time when it too could have been revised. The true cause of pain in an arthroplastic joint can be elusive. A total revision may ultimately be needed. It is possible that those people who are planning on only an acetabular revision will be looking at a newly

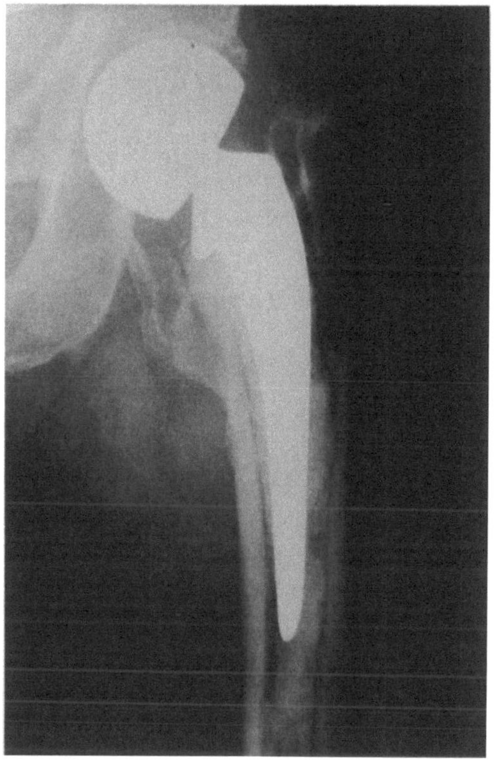

FIG. 8–60 Bateman-type prosthesis that has shown early migration into the acetabulum and loosening of the bone cement bond.

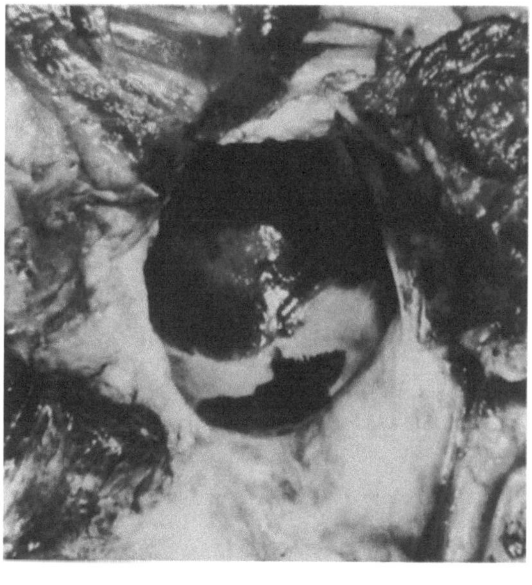

FIG. 8–61 Focal necrosis and intracartilaginous hemorrhaging or a collection of blood clots within the surface layer of the articular cartilage of the acetabulum can be seen 3 years after an endoprosthesis.

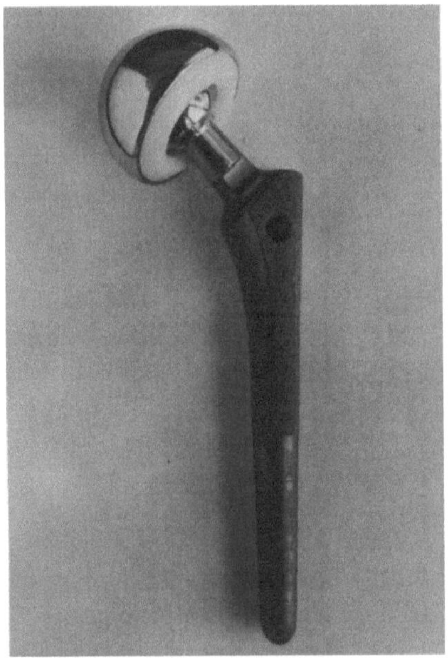

FIG. 8–62 The Tronzo BioBond prosthesis is the newest of the canal filling, straight stem implants made of titanium with a plasma sprayed coating. Its fenestration is also porous on its surface for long-term locking once a thick bar of bone matures which will in turn support the device. It can be used with or without cement, with or without a bipolar head.

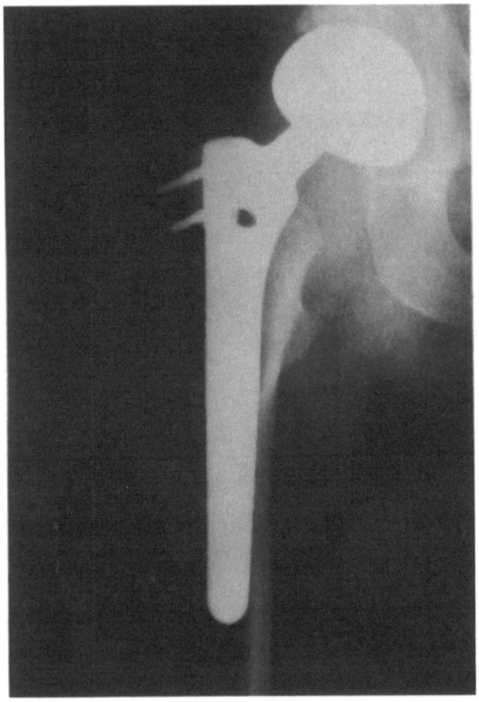

FIG. 8–63 Tronzo Bio-bond bipolar prosthesis with a microporous coating used as a bipolar replacement for a femoral neck fracture without cement.

created procedure to be known as a "two-staged revision."

There is one complication unique to this device. The head can pop out of its socket if the hip should dislocate. This author has had one patient with a Bateman device do this. The newest designs have better retention rings, so this complication may have been reduced. An additional problem unique to the device is the difficulty of reduction once dislocation has taken place. The swivel head can get caught on the edge of the acetabulum, making open reduction a necessity.[161,162]

Cement Versus No Cement Versus Microporous Fixation A cemented prosthesis clearly produces a better result than an uncemented prosthesis according to data from modern studies.[158,160,164,166,171–179] A cemented bipolar prosthesis functions better than a noncemented one.[173] Ordway et al. concluded: "The improvement with cement is so significant as to warrant a slight increase in the technical instrumentation for the extra step in the procedure."[175] It remains to be proved whether newer versions of the Austin-Moore prosthesis such as BioMet's Anatomical Press Fit (APF) will fare better than a cemented or a microporous system (BioBond system). It also remains to be proved whether a microporous system has any advantage over a cemented endoprosthesis. We are currently investigating the ramifications of employing a bipolar, microporous device in an elderly population (Figs. 8–62 and 8–63). There appears to be no difference between the two systems on a short-term basis except that the BioBond system can be inserted quickly by eliminating the cementing steps. However, there is more bleeding postoperatively with this system, as the intramedullary cavity continues to ooze because there is no coagulation effect from the hot cement against the bleeding trabeculations. So far this phenomenon has not been a problem. A long-term study is required, however, to prove the worthiness of the BioBond concept. Despite these convincing data, a number of surgeons have resumed use of the old (two-sized—narrow and broad) Austin-Moore prostheses.

Charnley made the monumental discovery of using methylmethacrylate when he borrowed it from his brother-in-law who was a dentist. Charnley, frustrated with the progressive looseness of Austin-Moore prostheses, poured his brother-in-law's dental acrylate into the femoral canal around the stem. It worked well, and a new era in orthopedic surgery was born.[180] He later compared uncemented prostheses with cemented ones.[181] There are now many more reports that favor cementing in a prosthesis than there are against its use.

Surgical Technique The technique for inserting an endoprosthesis is the same for a solid-head device as for a double-head device. The individual's preferred incision should be used and his favorite system installed. There are a few points that may increase the success rate of the arthroplasty. The fractured femoral head must be removed carefully from the acetabulum to avoid damage to the sensitive articular cartilage. Measuring the head is critical for attempting to reduce acetabular erosion. Head sizes come in millimeter increments, which are rather fine to measure grossly. Cabanela and Van Demark of the Mayo Clinic reported that they no longer relied on the suction test for assessing the fit of a trial head.[171] They recommended using a trial system with metal heads which can be x-rayed in the acetabulum while the patient is on the operating table. They aimed for concentricity of the metal cup with the subchondral bone image, which invariably resulted in selecting a prosthetic size slightly larger than the removed head. The neck should be anteverted by about 15° to 20°. The angle can be judged by placing the lower leg parallel to the wall (Fig. 8–64F).

Surgical Exposure for Inserting an Endoprosthesis This author prefers a lateral exposure with focus on the posterior aspect of the hip joint. Figure 8–64 is a series of illustrations depicting this surgical approach. By placing the patient directly on the side, a straight incision can be made which allows the leg to be maneuvered in any direction for access to either the anterior or the posterior side of the hip joint. For patients in whom the capsule is normal, e.g., those with fresh fractures of the femoral neck, only the posterior part needs to be approached. It is not a Gibson or a Moore incision, as they were executed with the patient prone for the purpose of exploring only the posterior area. By placing the patient laterally, the incision can be made more anteriorly with a straight cut, which keeps instrumentation away from the sciatic nerve. Damage to the sciatic nerve is avoided by not exposing it, but its location is constantly packed off (Fig. 8–64C). It is

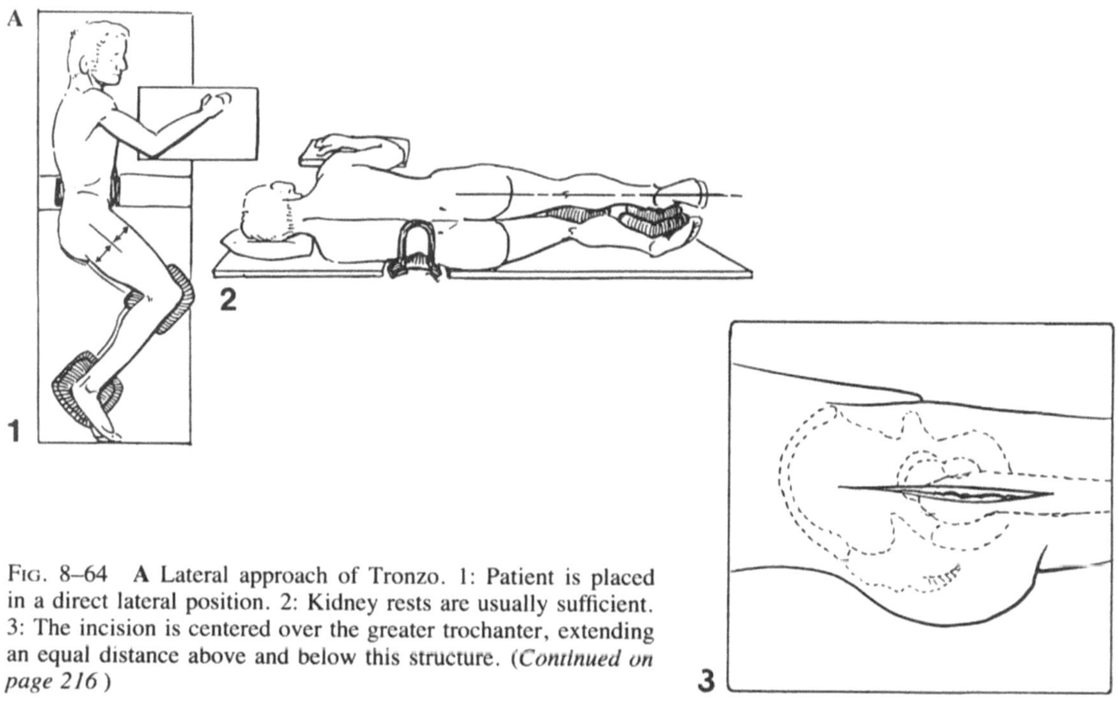

FIG. 8–64 **A** Lateral approach of Tronzo. 1: Patient is placed in a direct lateral position. 2: Kidney rests are usually sufficient. 3: The incision is centered over the greater trochanter, extending an equal distance above and below this structure. (*Continued on page 216*)

B

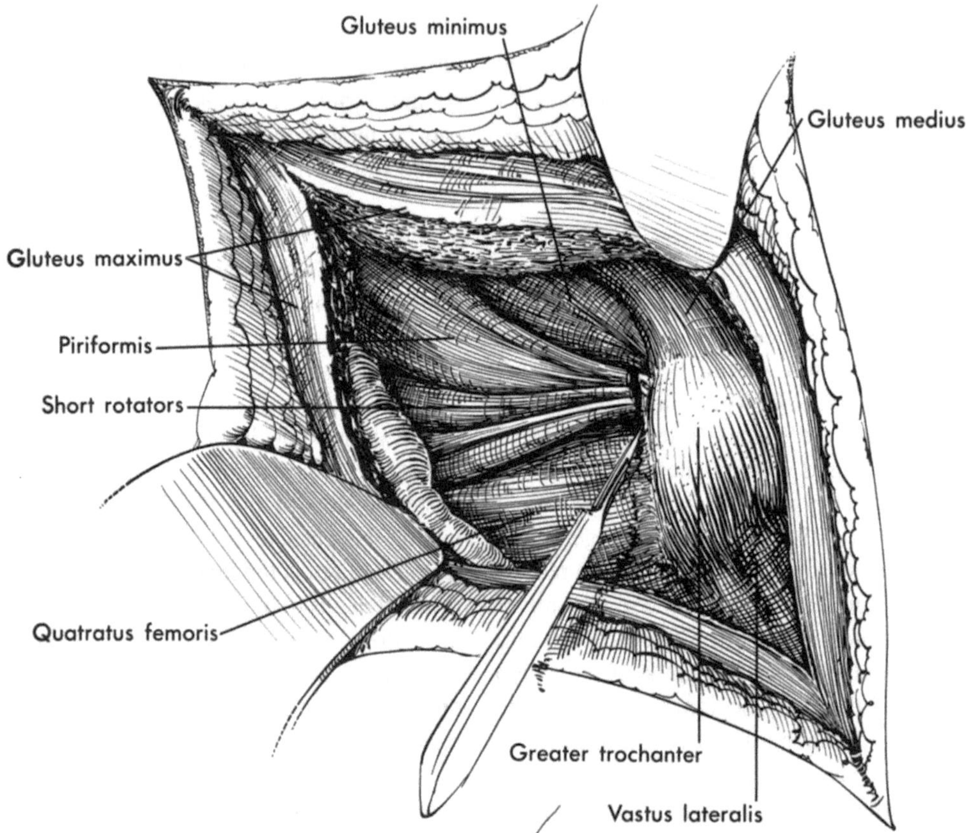
Gluteus minimus
Gluteus medius
Gluteus maximus
Piriformis
Short rotators
Quatratus femoris
Greater trochanter
Vastus lateralis

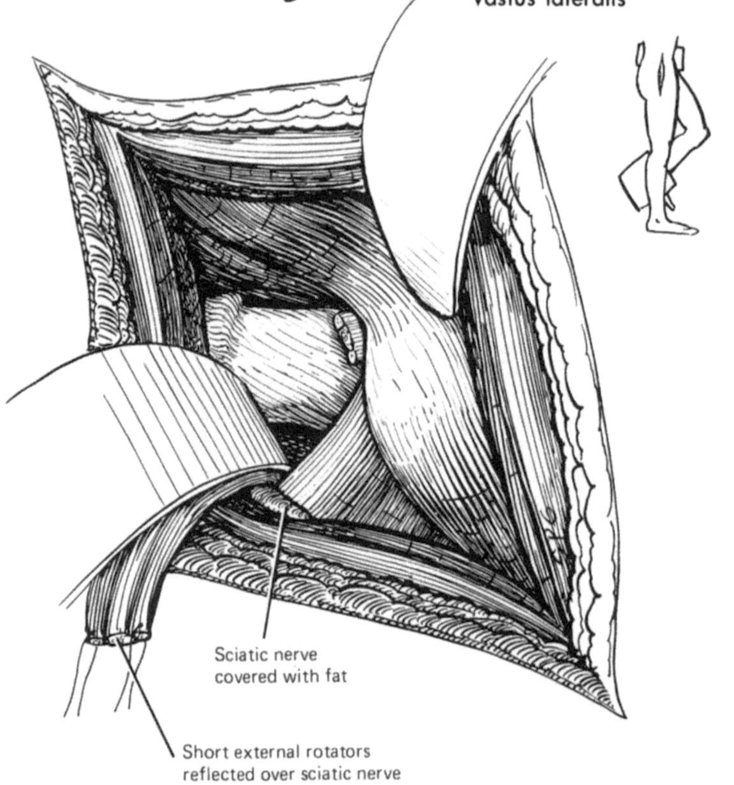
Sciatic nerve
covered with fat
Short external rotators
reflected over sciatic nerve

C

FIG 8–64 **B** After the fascia lata is cut, the gluteus maximus is then easily split with blunt dissection in a direct line with its fibers. The loose areolar tissue is cut sharply away to visualize the lower border of the gluteus medius and its neighboring mass of short external rotators. Cut up under the gluteus medius as far as possible into the insertion of the gluteus minimus and then sweep the knife downward across the piriformis, the internal obturator, the glemilli, and the external obturator muscles. Cut as close to the bony insertions as possible. Go only to the capsule. Reflect this mass of muscle down over the posterior lip of the acetabulum by scraping away from the capsule. **C** Abduct the leg and rest it on a padded Mayo stand in extension which relieves tension on the gluteal muscles for easier dissection. Throughout this procedure, the sciatic nerve is left embedded in its protective layer of fat and is not dissected out. One must keep the sciatic nerve in mind at all times, remembering where it should be anatomically. It is protected by a large moist sponge deep to a smooth, broad retractor (wide Richardson's or Deaver's). Additional protection is given to the sciatic nerve by stripping the short external rotators away from the capsule to form a muscular flap which can then be retracted over the sciatic nerve, again keeping a sponge between this mass and the retractor.

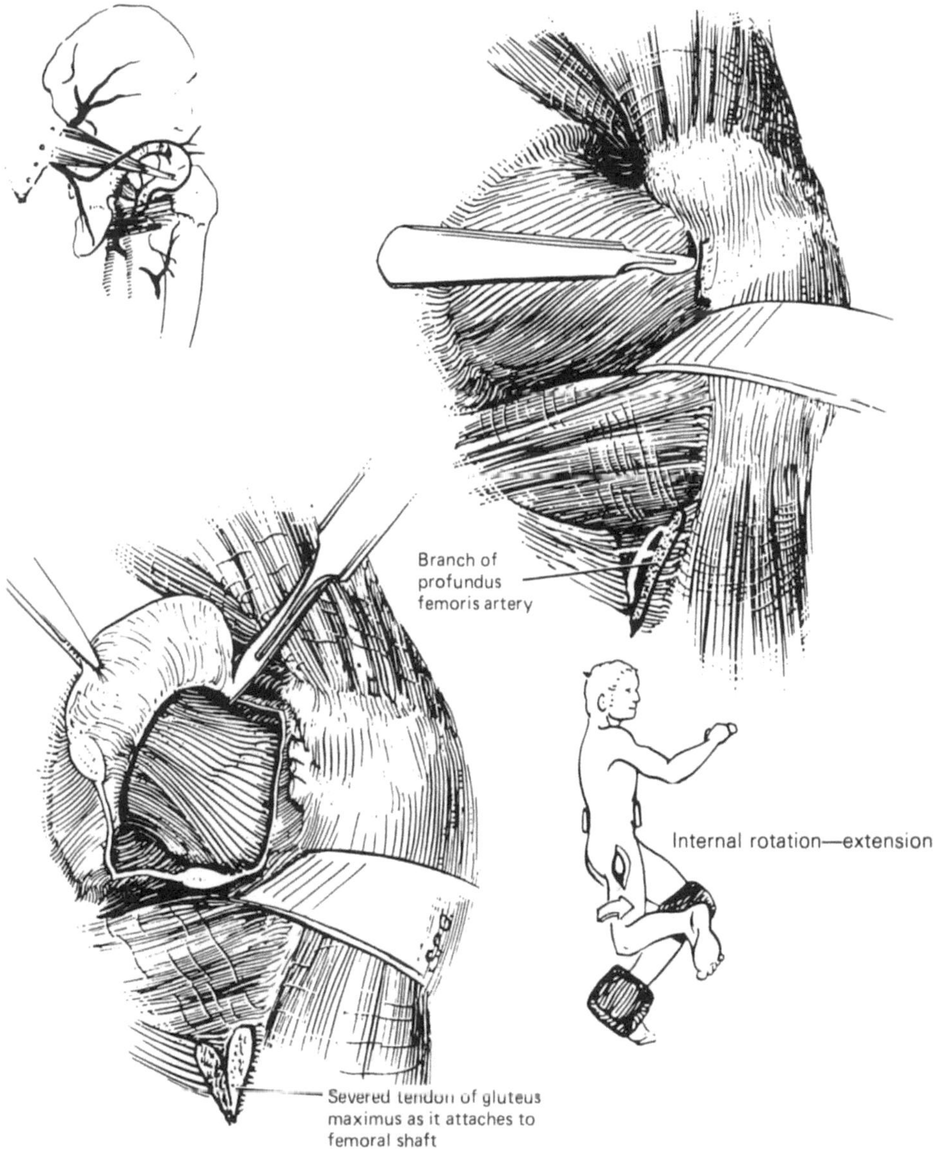

D

FIG. 8–64 **D** The vascular supply to the soft tissues is important to appreciate: the superior gluteal artery may be damaged by splitting the gluteus maximus too deeply, and bleeding can be extensive when the capsule

(*Continued on page 218*)

is excised, especially in rheumatoids and avascular necrosis. Excise the capsule well into the piriformis fossa (X) because it is at this point where the new straight stem prostheses will enter the greater trochanter. The quadratus femoris muscle is retracted aside as the inferior capsule is excised. It is usually best to release the broad tendon of the gluteus maximus as it inserts into the femoral shaft because it is usually contracted, which prevents full mobilization of the femur. Be wary of a branch of the profundus artery which resides immediately under the tendon; cut it about a quarter of an inch from the shaft, otherwise it will retract deeply making its ligation difficult and bloody.

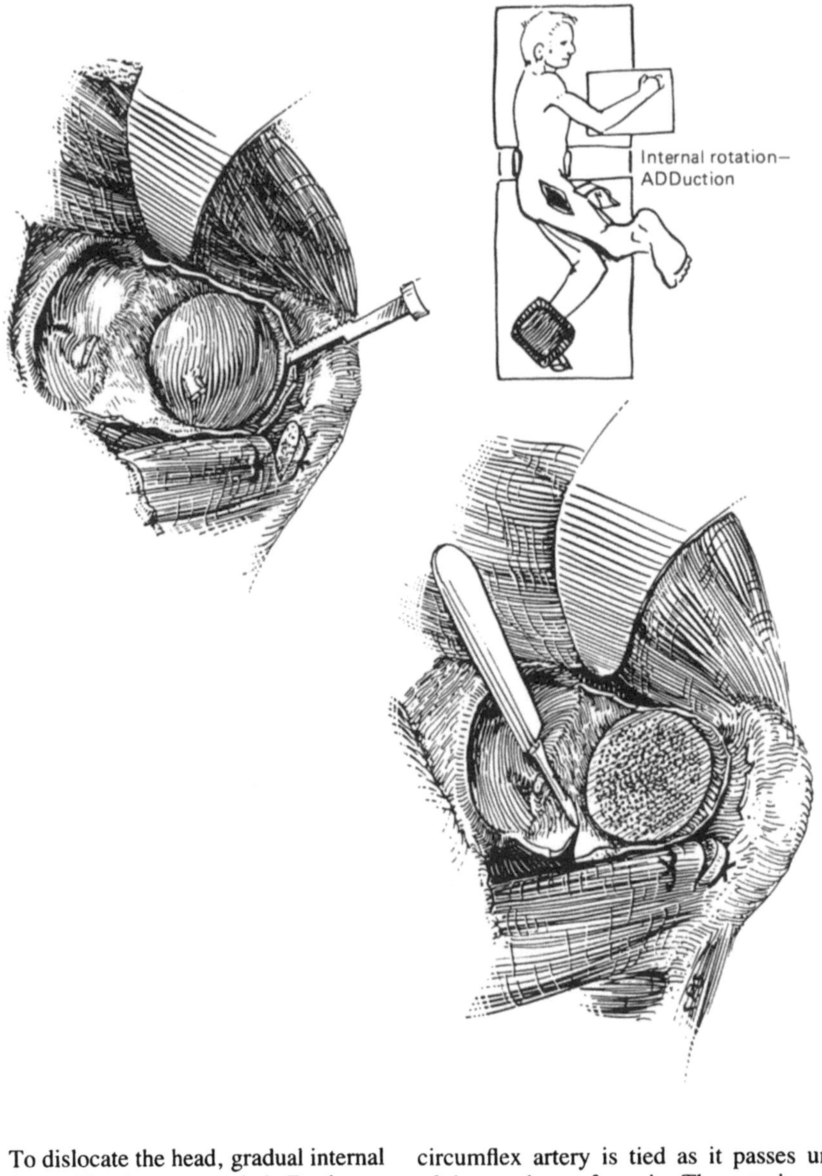

FIG. 8–64 **E** To dislocate the head, gradual internal rotation and marked adduction are needed. For better exposure of the inferior neck, cut through the quadratus femorus muscle. The branch of the medial femoral circumflex artery is tied as it passes under the edge of the quadratus femoris. The anterior capsule can be cut away or at least incised.

necessary to cut out a generous block of bone from the greater trochanter in order to have a straight path to the femoral canal for instrumentation, reamers and rasps, so as to accommodate straight stem prostheses (Fig. 8–64F).

Another "lateral" approach has been recently popularized by the "PCA" group of surgeons. They have given Hardinge[182] credit for it as the originator. He named it a "direct lateral" approach. Bauer and his colleagues must be given the credit for its conception since they published it in 1979.[183] Their name for it is the "transgluteal" approach which is a more accurate description since it is actually another antero-lateral inci-

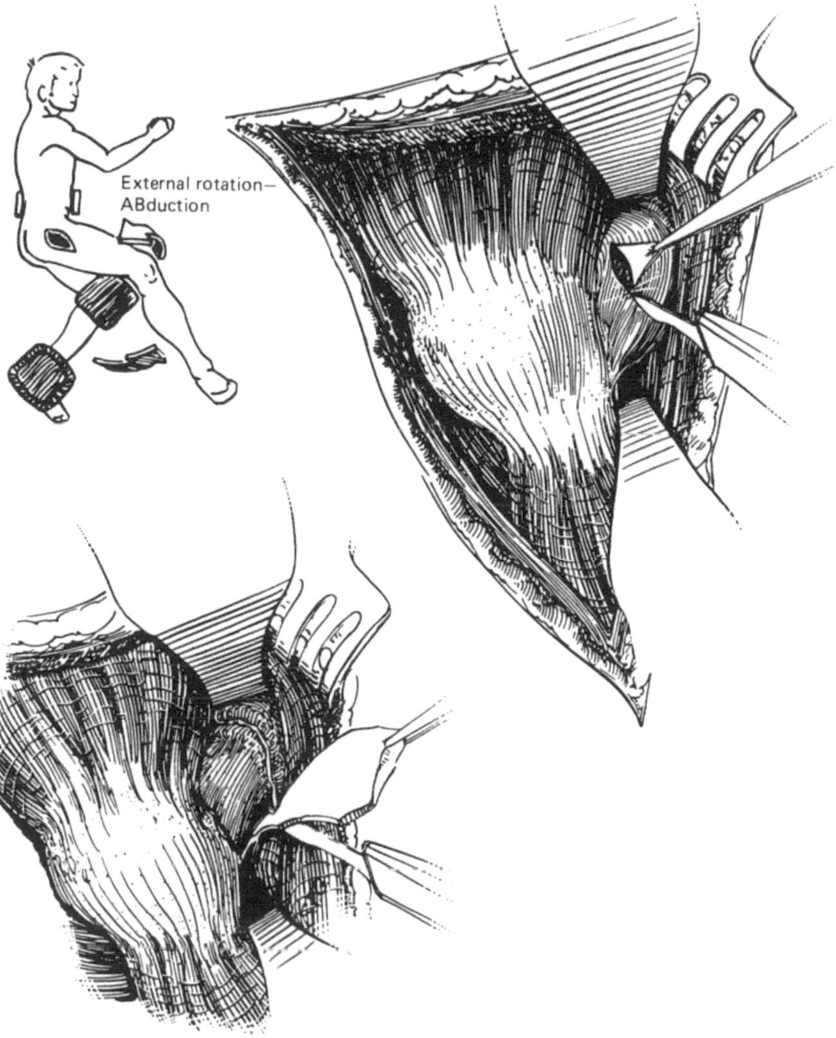

FIG. 8–64 **F** Anterior exposure is easily obtained by rotating the leg externally with abduction. The reflected tendons of the rectus femoris are cut and that muscle retracted while an anterior capsulectomy is performed. An alternate approach is to incise the capsule close along the intertrochanteric line thus releasing the tight capsule.

sion executed by going through the anterior quarter of the gluteus medius muscle and tendon to gain access to the anterior region of the hip joint (Fig. 8–65). The patient is positioned prone instead of in the true lateral position. It is especially useful for curved prostheses because of its wide anterior exposure, but it can be utilized for any of the prostheses (Fig. 8–66).

Preventing Prosthetic Dislocation Dislocation of the prosthesis has been cited as a major disadvantages of a hemiarthroplasty. The reported rate varies from 4.5%[184] to 12%.[185] When treating a failed (pinned) femoral neck fracture with a hemiarthroplasty, the dislocation rate is higher.[185] When it occurs, it can become a major complication and prolong the time to ambulation and recovery. Careful attention to the prevention of this potential problem must become almost a ritual with the nursing staff.

The patient must not leave the operating room table without an abduction pillow. Although am-

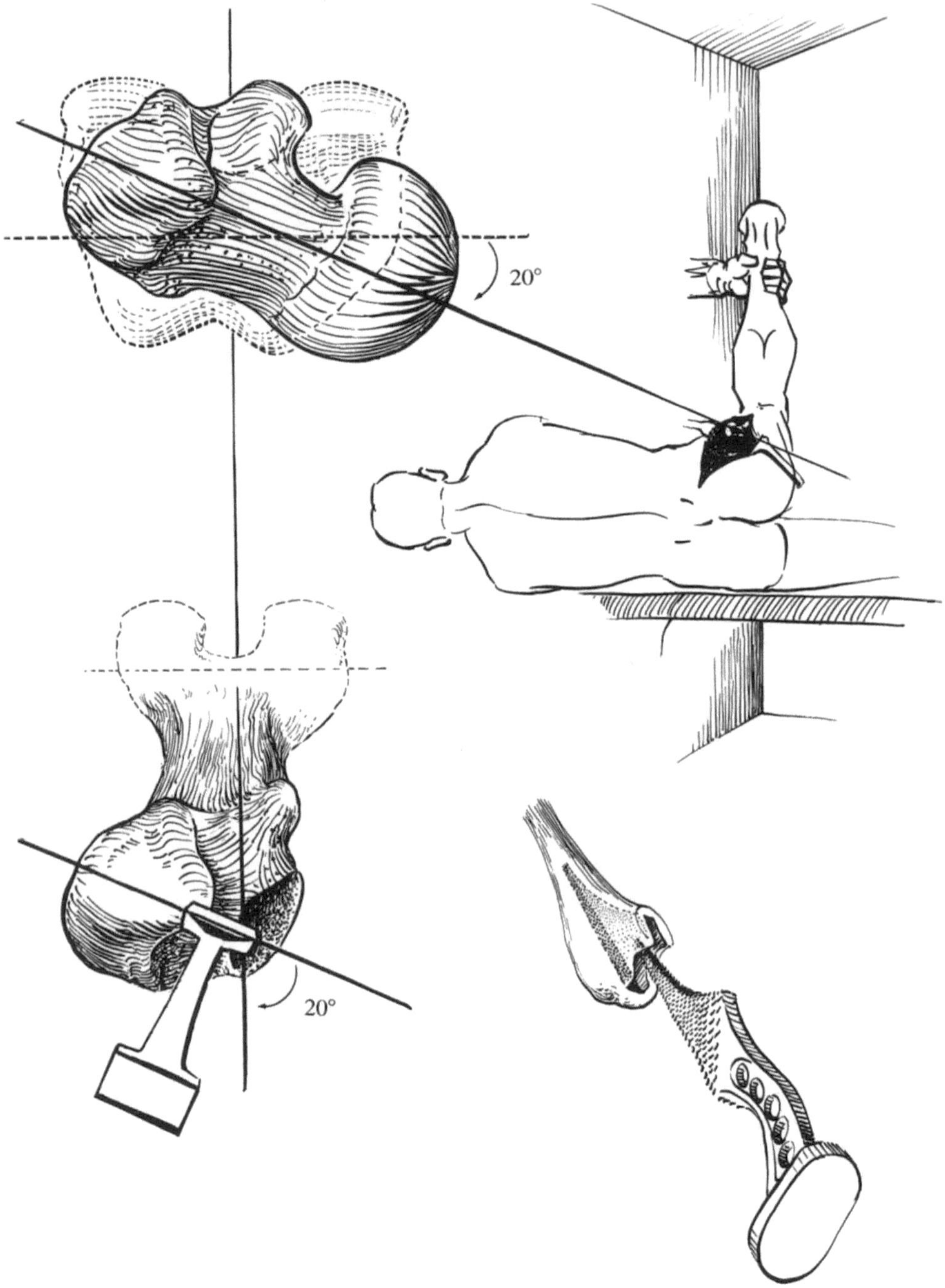

FIG. 8–64 **G** Anteversion is determined by turning the leg upward and making it parallel with the corner of the room. The box osteotome is set at about 15° to 20° to the axis of the femoral condyles at the knee or 90° to 100° to the perpendicular of the upright leg. The author has found this method superior to any that depends on landmarks on the upper femur itself because in cases of congenital dysplasia all structural characteristics are distorted. The new straight stem prostheses make it necessary to cut deeply into the *most* lateral aspect of the greater trochanter in order to accommodate the thick distal portion centered into the femoral isthmus. Rasp as far laterally as possible.

A

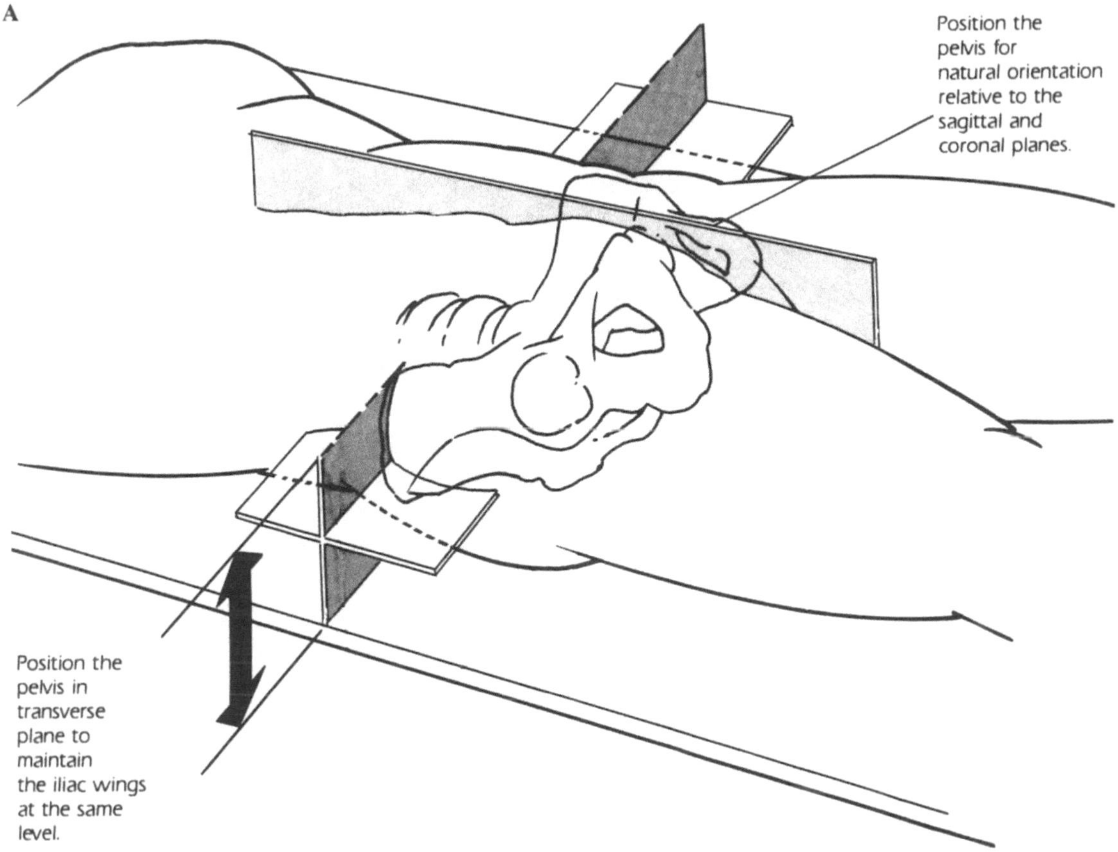

B

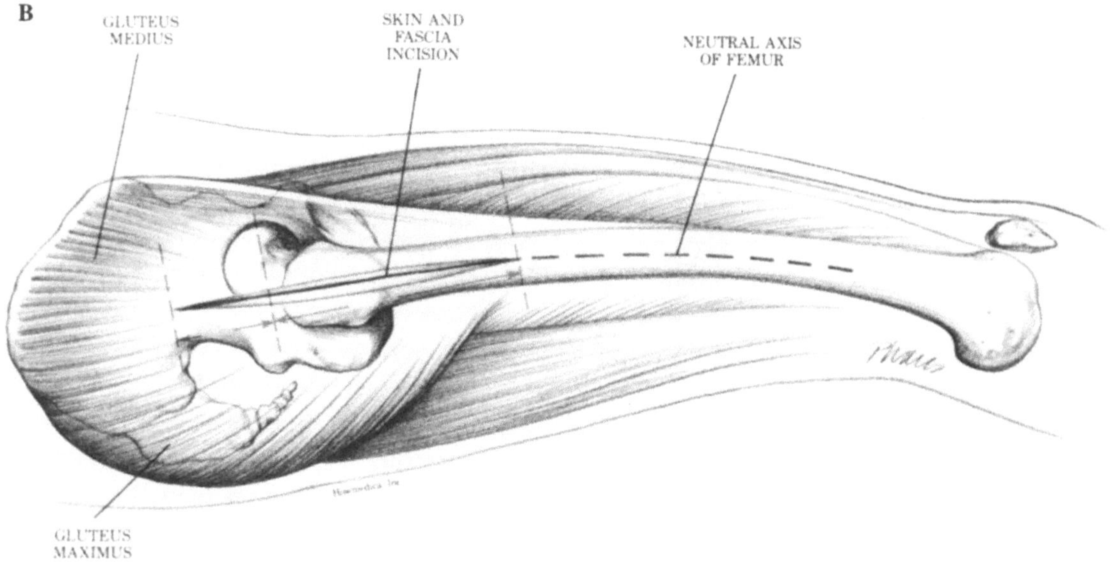

FIG. 8 65 Bauer's "transgluteal" approach or Hardinge's "direct lateral" approach: **A** Position the patient in a level prone posture for proper orientation of the acetabulum. **B** A lateral incision is made along the axis of the femur splitting the gluteus maximus and the tensor fascia. (*Continued on page 222*)

C

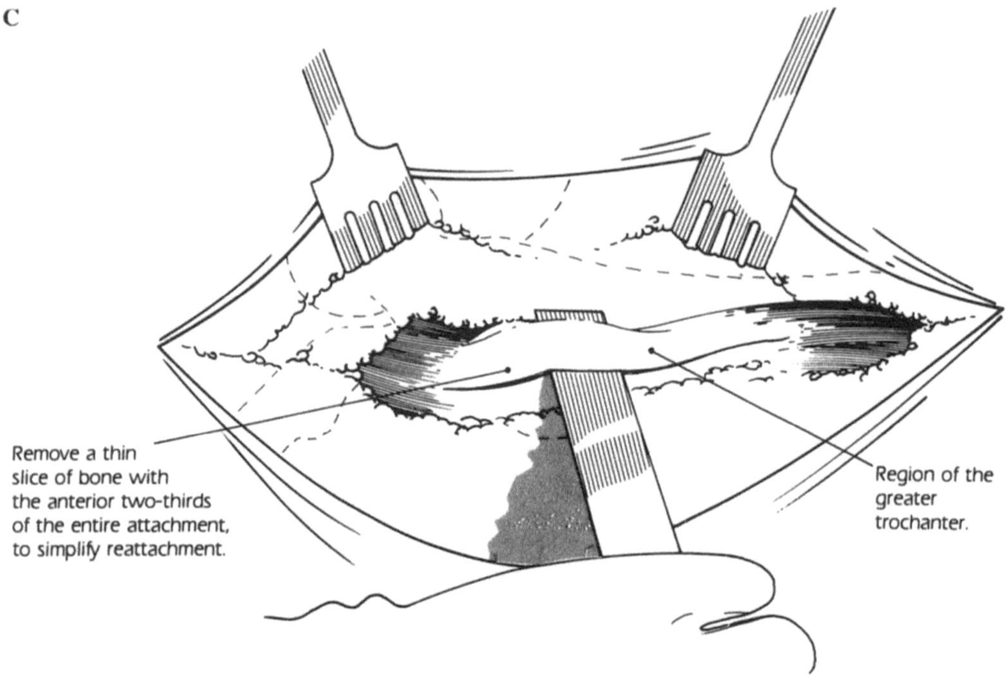

D

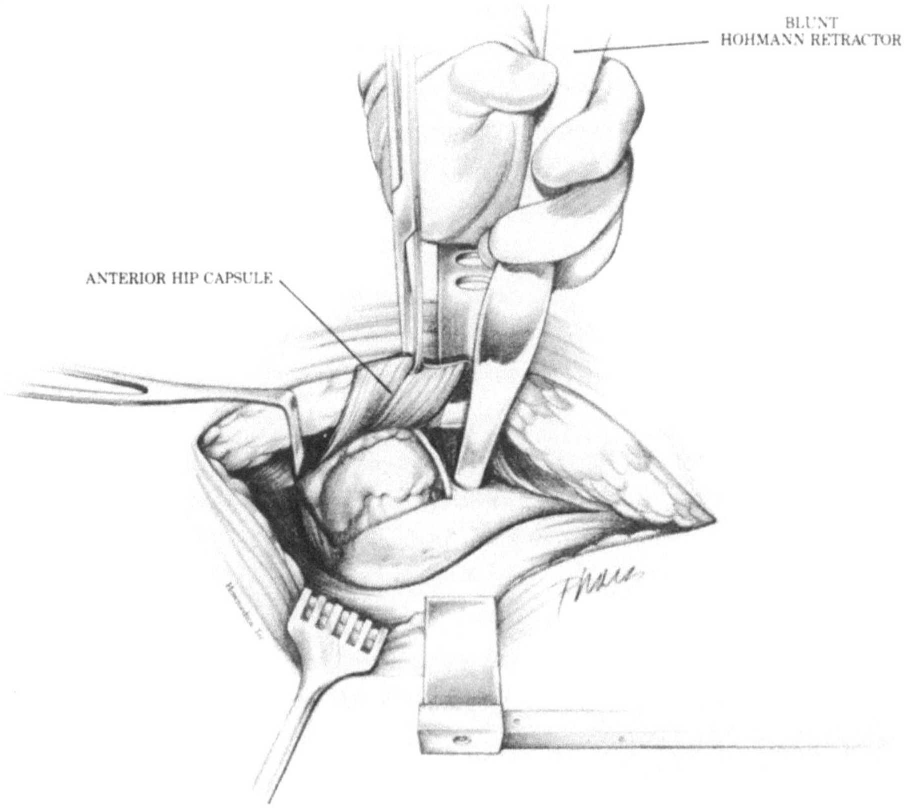

FIG. 8–65 **C** The unique feature of this incision comes at this point when the anterior part of the gluteus medius tendon is split and peeled off of the anterior surface of the greater trochanter with a sliver of bone (optional). **D** The gluteus medius flap is retracted medially as the anterior capsule is cleared away with a periosteal elevator and then a generous capsulectomy is performed.

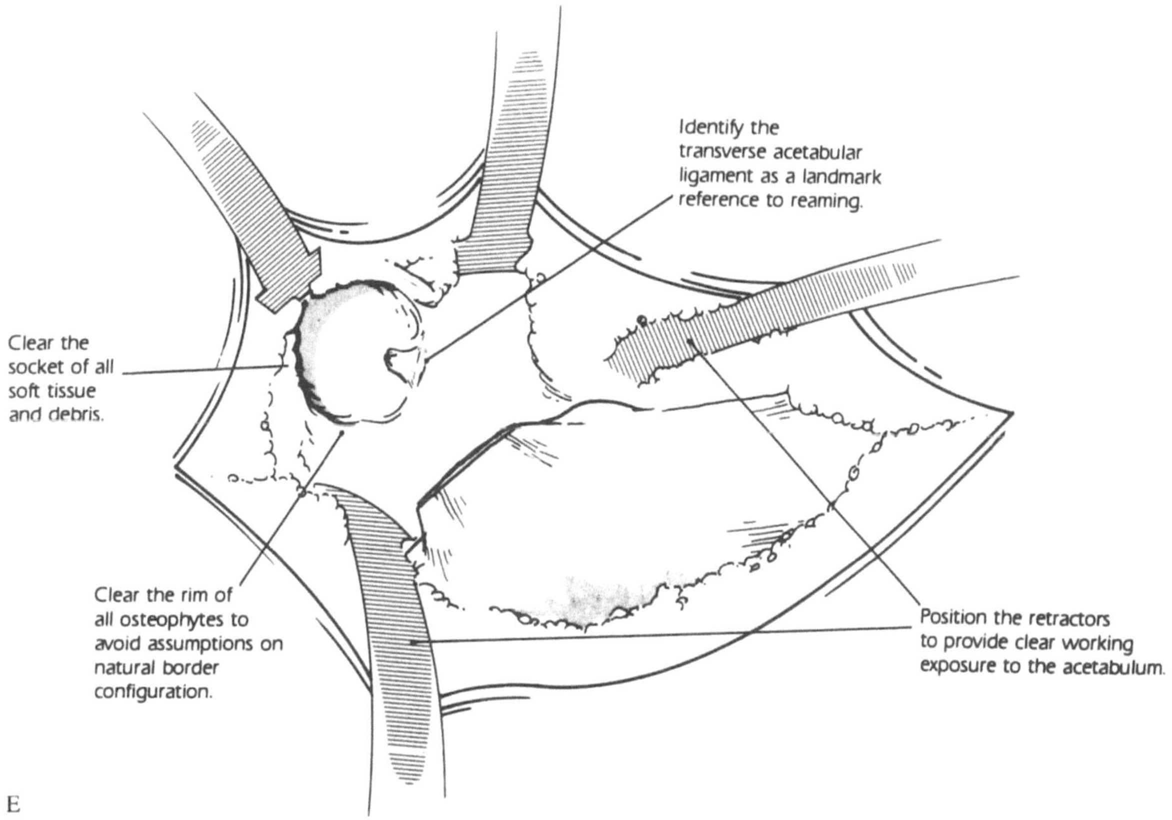

FIG. 8–65 **E** After the neck is amputated the acetabulum can be exposed for its reconstruction. A series of Hohmann retractors are the best instruments to use here.

bulation is started as soon as possible or as soon as the patient can physically and mentally cooperate, within the first 2 to 3 days, the patient must be rehabilitated carefully with legs abducted while sitting, walking, and in bed for at least 6 weeks. The 10-day period in the hospital is usually uneventful with an experienced staff, but the time at home or in a nursing home becomes critical.

Execution of the arthroplasty must be meticulous. The stem must be inserted with some type of firm fixation, with the head anteverted 15°–20°, and the head should fit precisely.

A new surgical approach for the arthroplasty can help to prevent dislocations. Until recently the posterolateral incision was a popular approach. It was postulated that by cutting loose the posterior structures the prosthesis becomes vulnerable to dislocation posteriorly. Dislocations are less likely with an anterior approach. Roberts et al.[186] studied this problem and found that patients with the posterior approach had less "perioperative" morbidity but a few more dislocations. Iyer[187] designed a method to prevent posterior dislocations: He took down the posterior curtain (capsule and tendons of the short external rotators) with a block of the greater trochanter and its attached gluteus medius en masse. When these structures were reattached, the posterior path to potential dislocation was blocked. This author tried the method and, after a period of learning the technique, modified it as shown in Fig. 8–66. Improvements include the use of AO screws, a special broad washer, and AO nuts to keep the bone compressed together (Fig. 8–69).

Wires, heavy ribbons, or sutures will not hold the friable piece of bone without breaking through it. The width of the cut into the trochanter is important. It should be about one-fourth of its entire width, or about 0.5 inch. If it is any wider, part of the femoral neck is also divided. That much bone makes reattachment a bit more tedious because it must be scooped out to accommodate

A

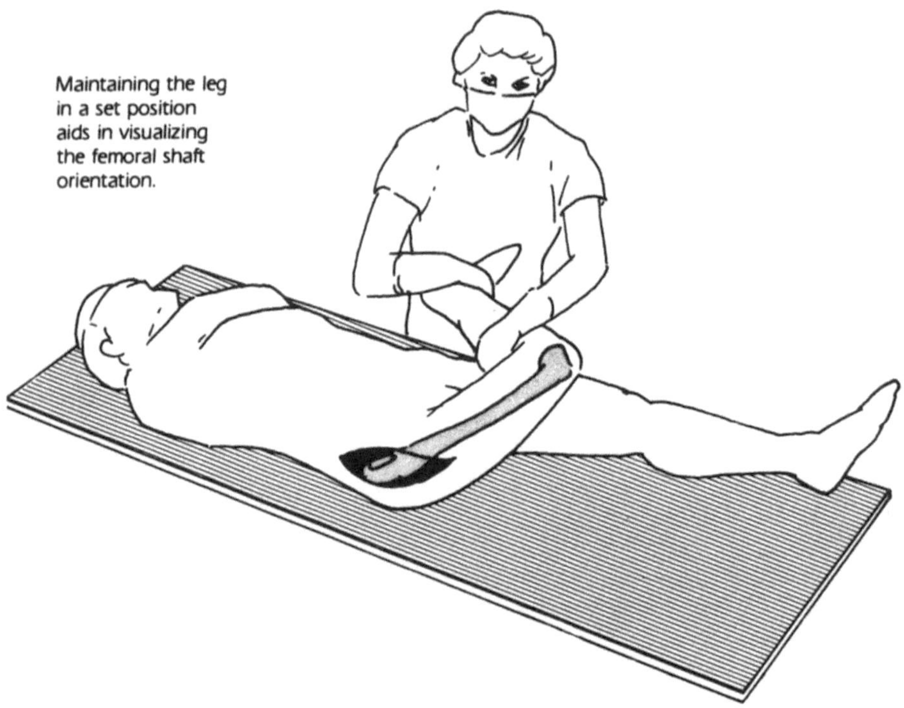

B

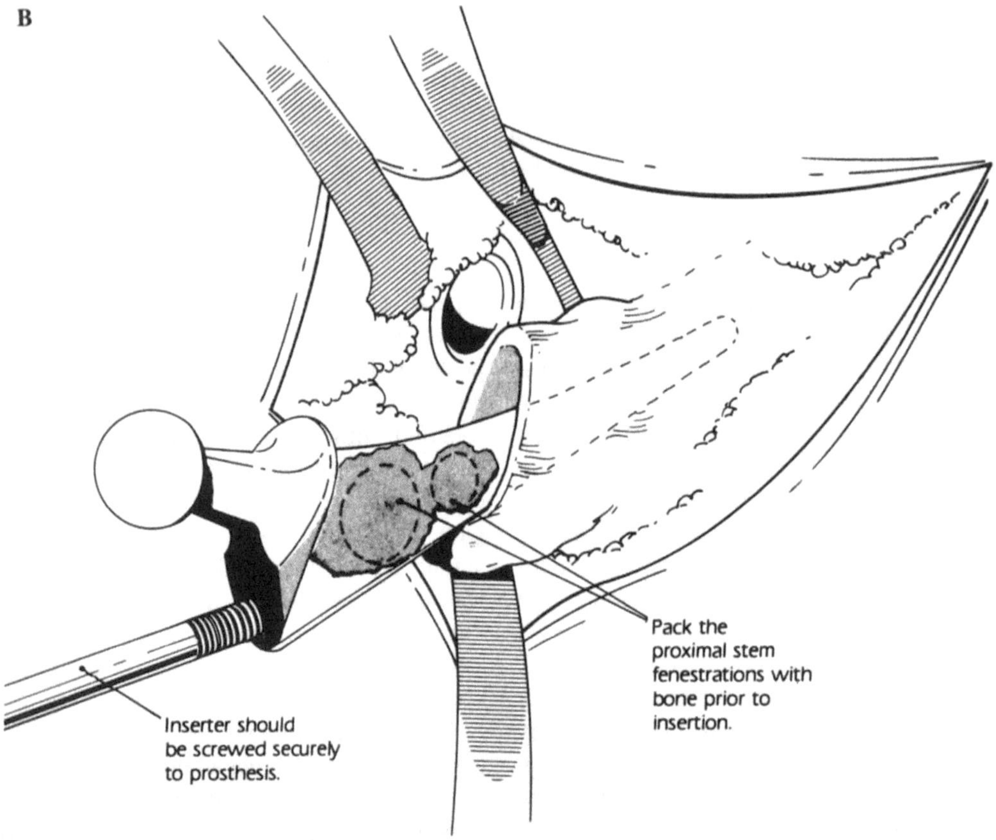

FIG. 8–66 Use of the Bauer incision for an arthroplasty: **A** If a hemiarthroplasty is in order, no further work need be done on the acetabulum. If a total hip is to executed, at this point the acetabulum is prepared with appropriate reamers and the leg is flexed in extreme external rotation. **B** Appropriate sized reamers and rasps

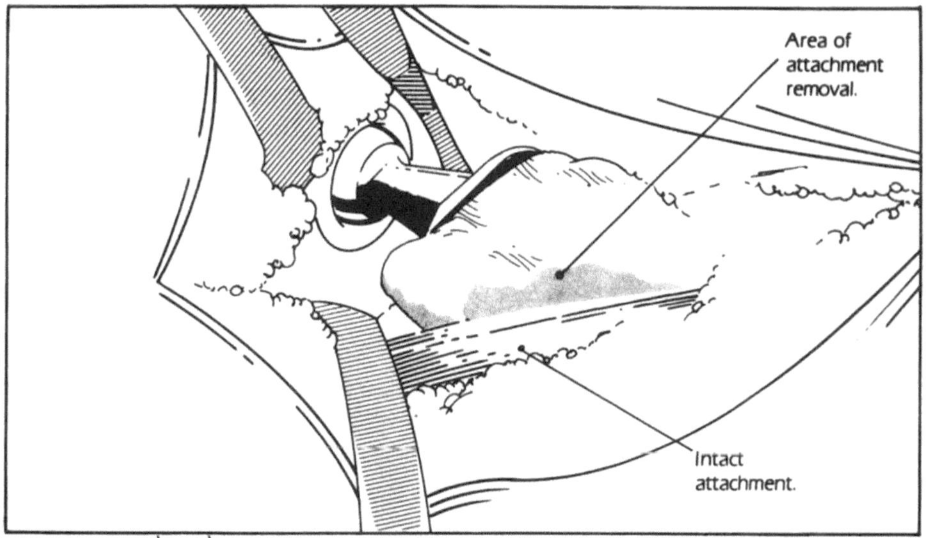

C

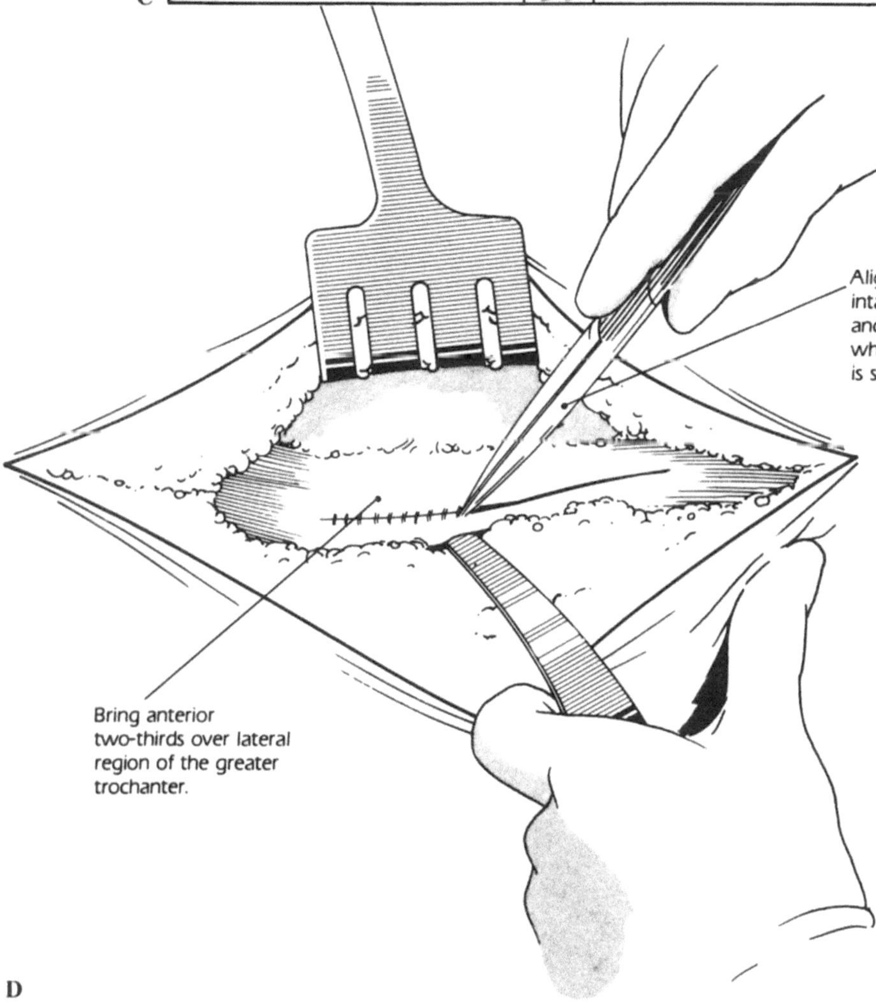

D

are used to prepare the femoral shaft and the femoral implant is driven in place with 15 degrees of anteversion. In this case a BioBond prosthesis is being bone grafted before insertion. **C** The prosthesis is reduced and the wound is closed by carefully approximating the gluteus medius tendon. **D** After the prosthesis has been reduced, the gluteus medius tendon is brought back together. (Artwork courtesy of the Biomet Corp. and Howmedica)

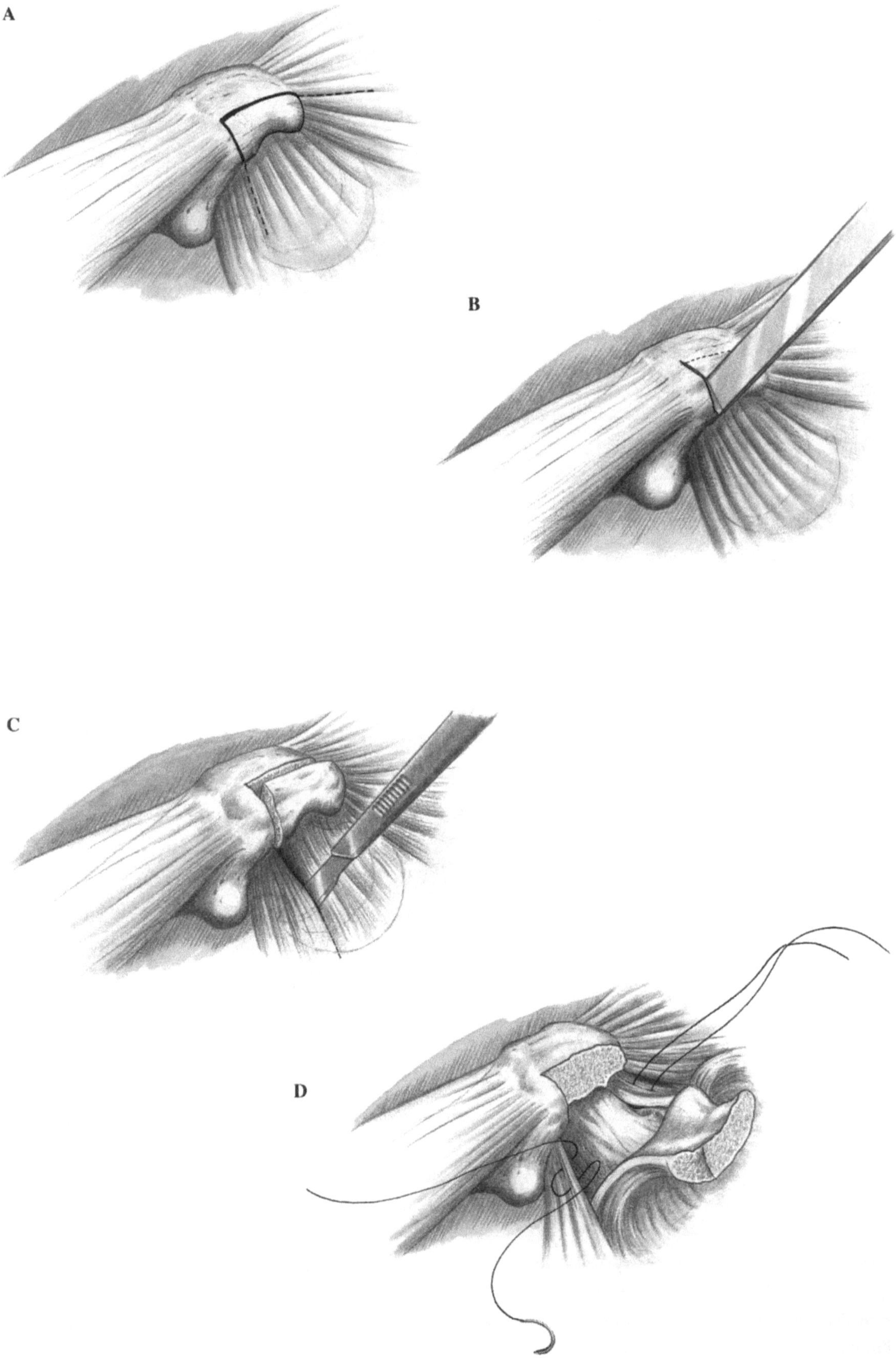
A
B
C
D

E

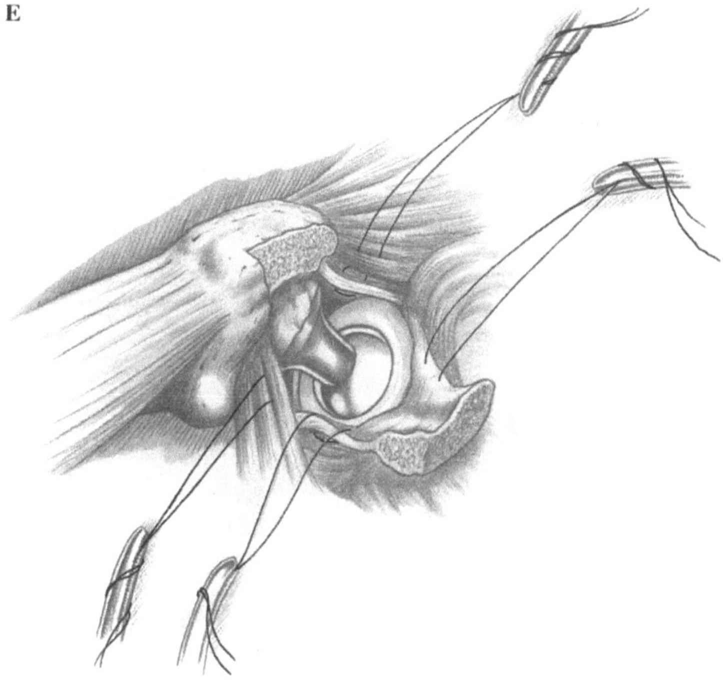

F

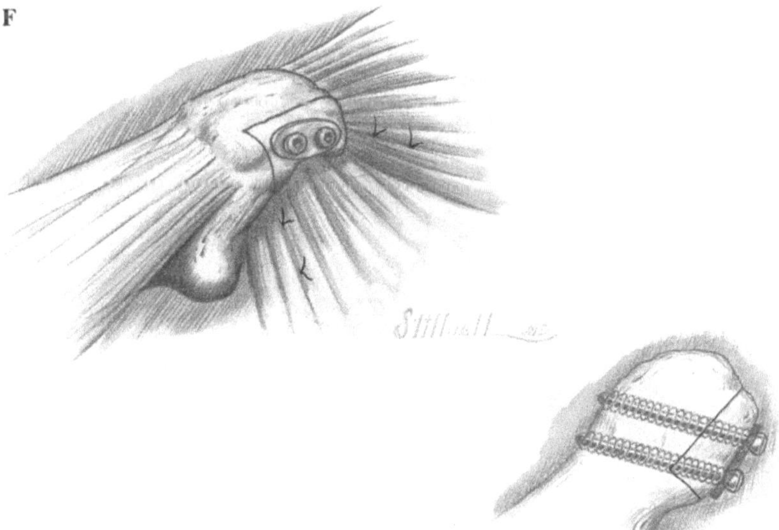

FIG. 8–67 Trochanteric splitting incision (a new posterior approach). Tronzo's Method: **A** One third to one quarter of the posterior portion of the greater trochanter is outlined. It will be separated as one unit with the gluteus medius, external rotators, and capsule. **B** A straight osteotome is used to split the trochanter down into the trochanteric crest. **C** The gluteus medius fibers and part of the quadratus muscle are cut through deep into the capsule with a single sweep of the scalpel. **D** Sutures are placed into either edge of the opening to be used later for a tight closure. It is easier to do this step now rather than later. **E** After the prosthesis has been inserted and reduced into the acetabulum, both sides of the flap are sutured close. The special two-holed curved washer (Biomet Corp.) are put against the trochanter and screwed into place. **F** Cancellous AO screws are used. Note they must pass through the opposite cortex to insure their proper purchase.

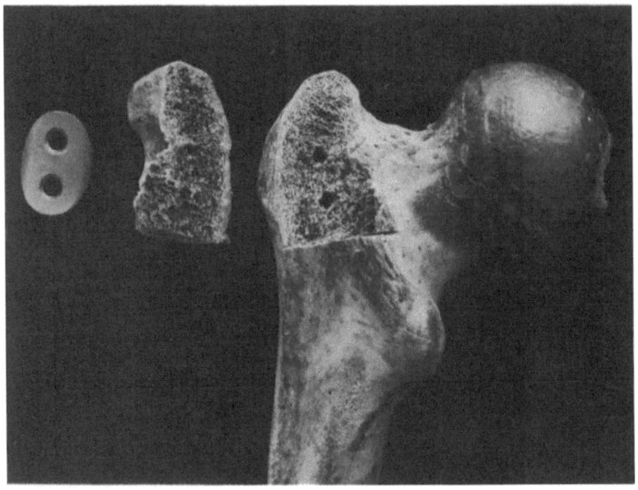

A

FIG. 8–68 **A** The essential ingredients of the new posterior approach are the special washer (Biomet Corp.) and a generous block of bone taken posteriorly with the capsule and short rotator tendons attached as a single flap.

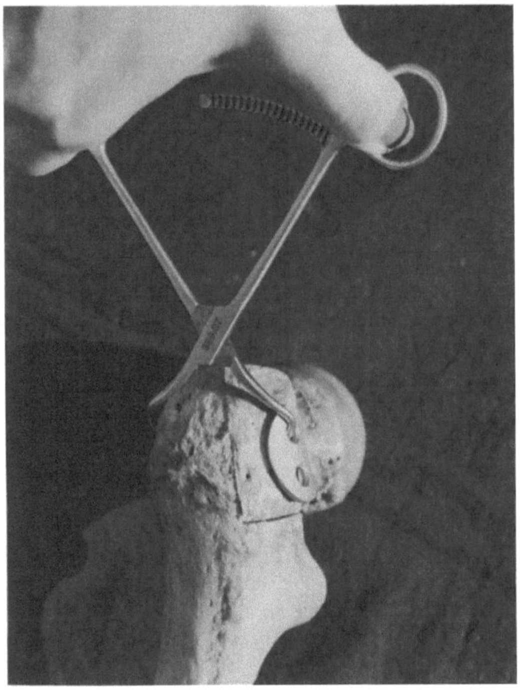

B

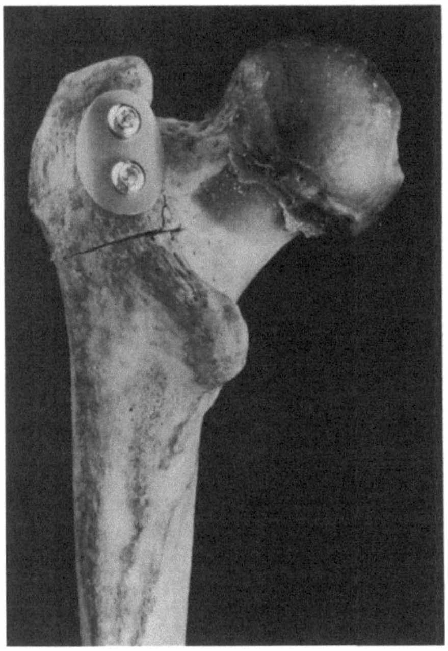

C

FIG. 8–68 **B** An AO bone clamp is required to hold the bone and washer in place while the first screw is inserted. **C** The special washer evenly compresses the bone back together. It is necessary—otherwise the screws would sink into the soft bone.

the prosthesis, making the whole procedure more cumbersome than need be. Anything smaller leaves only a sliver of bone to be screwed back into place. Therefore take time to calculate the initial cut. A special two-hole washer, made by the Biomet Corporation, is used with AO cancellous screws (Fig. 8–68C). Also be sure to make the screws go past the opposite cortex. When standard cortical screws are used, they must be bolted to the opposite side with the AO nut system (Fig. 8–69)—otherwise the screws will pull out.

These procedural refinements make reattachment easier and more secure. This very promising method is now used routinely by the author. As yet there have been no dislocations. The rehabilitation period for the patient is more vigorous and

FIG. 8–68 **D** The washer does not interfere with the soft tissues as it supports the reestablished posterior wall.

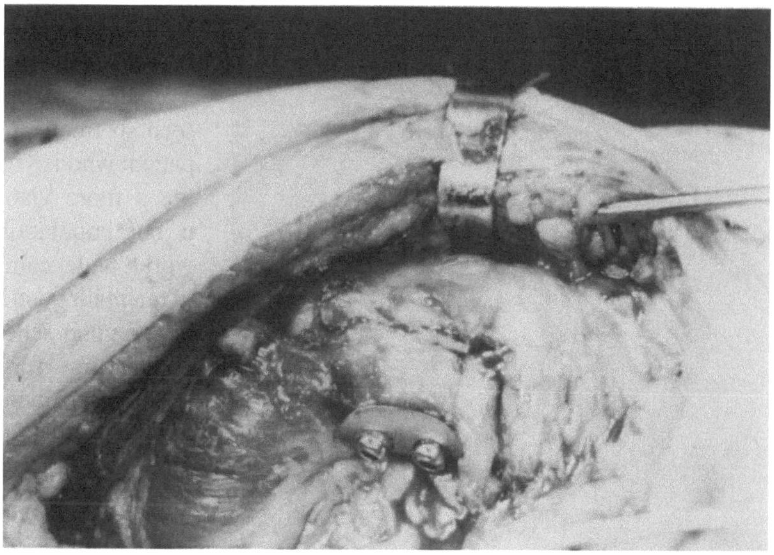

D

much less hazardous. Once mastered, the extra steps do not prolong the arthroplasty. In fact, there is a favorable trade-off. There is less bleeding because the osteotomy is cut through the upper third of the quadratus muscle, which avoids severing the ever-present branch of the medial femoral circumflex artery. An additional bonus is the exposure itself, which is quite good for viewing both posterior and superior areas of the femoral neck for direct access to the upper femur where the prosthesis is to be inserted.

Total Hip Replacement Total hip replacement is being used more frequently because of convincing data that it is one of the most successful arthroplasties ever devised for the hip joint. Just when it should be used in the treatment of fresh fractures of the femoral neck is still unsettled.[177,184,185–190] A clear indication for a total hip replacement is an unstable femoral neck fracture complicated by acetabular diseases, e.g., rheumatoid arthritis, osteoarthritis, traumatic arthritis, Paget's disease, or severe osteoporosis, associated arthritis (Figs. 8–70, 8–71). Patients who have had a failure from pinning benefit from a total joint replacement when there has been disturbance of the acetabulum by hip pins or by degenerative changes secondary to nonunion of the femoral neck.[184,190] Total hip replacement is an alternative only in older patients who, if younger, would be candidates for a bone grafting procedure.

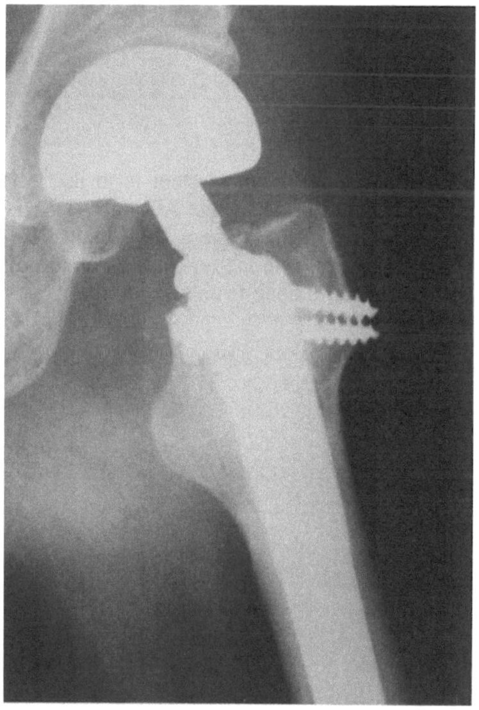

E

FIG. 8–68 **E** An x-ray showing the *cancellous* bone screws in place. Cortical bone screws used alone will not hold this soft bone together.

Total hip replacement is an excellent salvage operation for femoral head necrosis in the older patient. There is also growing encouragement for the use of total hip arthroplasties in the elderly patient who is active enough to be considered chronologically young.[177,184,188,189,191] If these patients fit the criteria for treatment of an unstable neck fracture with an endoprosthesis, they do

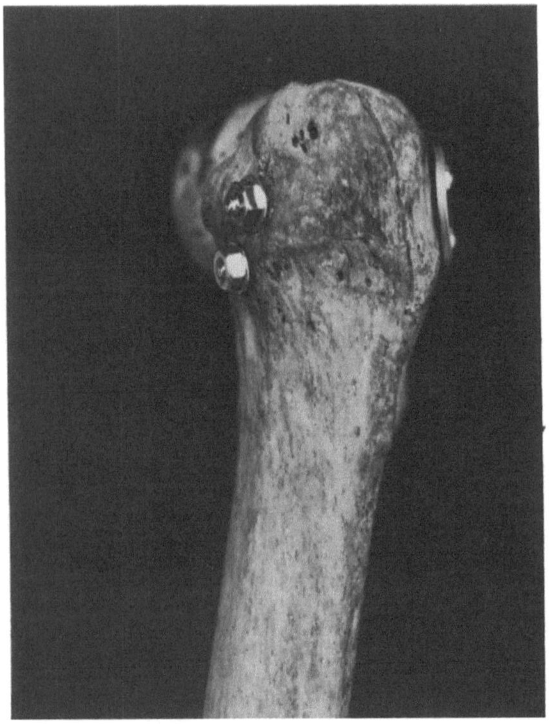

FIG. 8–69 A more secure system is to use cortical screws bolted into place by the AO nuts. This is the preferred method. It may take a few minutes longer, but it is the most reliable method of fixation to prevent the soft trochanteric bone from separating.

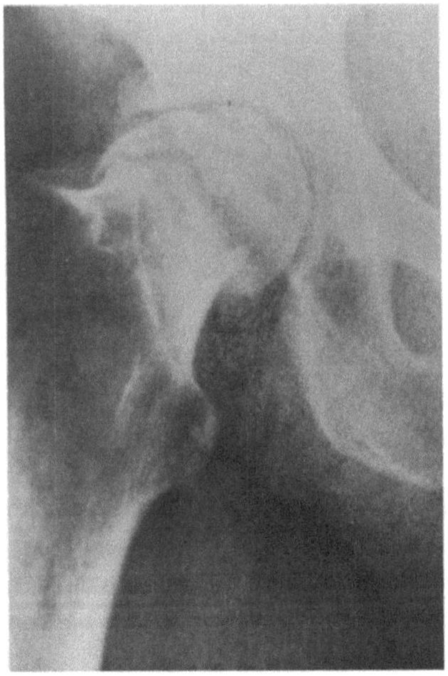

FIG. 8–70 Fractures in an osteoarthritic hip joint are typically high into the neck at the neck/head junction.

much better with reconstruction of the acetabulum by a total hip replacement.

Total hip replacement is an excellent, definitive, one-stage procedure. It avoids the erosion seen so frequently with an endoprosthesis in the patient who is vigorous. This indication is becoming a more viable alternative because not only is our population growing older but there is a world wide campaign to encourage the elderly to maintain good health by exercising and walking on a regular schedule. Bryan stated that "the operating time for a total hip replacement is not significantly increased. I prefer a total hip arthroplasty in the more vigorous patient because pain relief and function are usually better. I prefer to prescribe the operation based on the pathologic findings and physiologic capabilities rather than on chronologic age."[191]

Defining this patient category is tricky. Clearly someone like President Reagan—who chops wood, rides horses, and keeps a business schedule that would rival that of a 40-year-old executive—is such a person. He would certainly do poorly with an endoprosthesis but would regain his vigor in short order with a total hip replacement. Klein of Georgetown University School of Medicine puts the President in the "young-old" bracket, which is somewhere between 65 and 75. Beyond that is Klein's "old-old" group.[192] When President Reagan reaches 76 he may well extend the limits of the "young-old" category and still be an excellent candidate for a total hip replacement should he ever sustain an unstable fracture of the femoral neck.

Indications for Endoprosthesis An endoprosthesis is indicated in the following situations:

1. Unstable femoral neck fractures in an elderly, relatively inactive patient. It makes no difference if the fracture is reducible or irreducible by closed manipulation, so long as it falls into the unstable grouping.
2. Pathologic fractures or impending pathologic fractures of the femoral neck.
3. Associated illnesses: mental disorders, parkinsonism, hemiplegia, blindness.[174]

Bipolar Prosthesis According to Murray,[172] a bipolar prosthesis is indicated for:

1. Displaced femoral neck fractures in active elderly patients.
2. Possibly indicated where there is mild arthritis associated with the fracture.

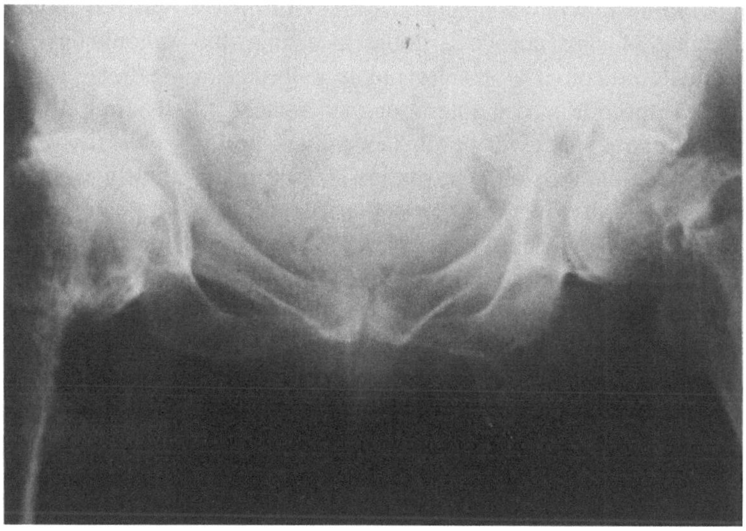

FIG. 8–71 Patient with bilateral degenerative joint disease with a fracture on the less involved side. These are uncommon fractures because the upper femur is hard from the osteoarthritis.

3. Femoral head osteonecrosis following a femoral neck fracture.

Total Hip Replacement Total hip replacement is indicated for:

1. Unstable femoral neck fractures associated with any arthritic process, e.g., rheumatoid arthritis, osteoarthritis (Figures 8–70 and 71), traumatic arthritis, or Paget's disease.[193]
2. Severe osteoporosis of the acetabular floor associated with unstable fractures.
3. Active, vigorous "young-old" patients with an unstable femoral neck fracture.
4. Salvage for failed femoral neck fractures such as nonunions and femoral head necrosis. It yields better functional results and has fewer postoperative dislocations than does a hemiarthroplasty.[185]
5. Salvage of a failed endoprosthesis.

Contraindications to Endoprosthesis Any infection that may threaten the deep tissues and joint which would not only worsen the infection but would seriously render the prosthetic replacement a failure contraindicates use of an endoprosthesis. However, bringing a deep infection under control is usually easier with an endoprosthesis than with total hip replacement.

Anyone under the age of 60, regardless of the type of fracture, should not be treated primarily with any type of prosthesis; a prosthesis should be reserved as the last resort. In this age group if all else fails, e.g., an irreducible fracture open or closed, a total hip replacement would yield the best overall results. In a young adult a prosthetic device is especially contraindicated, as there are other alternatives such as osteotomy, bone graft, and fusion. Only in the rare situation is use of a prosthesis justified in a young patient. The presence of a malignant tumor is an example.

Preoperative Preparation

It was once thought that femoral neck fractures were emergencies, and that any accompanying medical abnormalities must be secondary to an emergency operation. That concept no longer exists. The medical problems take priority over the fractured hip. Many elderly patients have congestive heart failure, electrolyte imbalance, dehydration, and anemia from being on their typical starvation diets. Moreover, their diabetes may need adjusting, and their pulmonary dysfunction may need careful monitoring. All of these medical abnormalities require careful correction and attention preoperatively as well as postoperatively. On the other hand, they must not be managed casually but with a sense of urgency. All efforts must be mobilized to maximize the patient's good health in order to take him or her to the operating room within 24 to 48 hours if possible. The operation should be considered an urgency, not an emergency.

The leg is splinted in Buck's traction with about 5 pounds of weight and the patient made comfortable. There is no evidence to support the contention that delay further harms the femoral neck. Whatever damage has been done to the femoral head was complete at the time of impact; nothing of consequence is going to change the ultimate outcome, as the fragments will stay in their respective places unless roughly treated.

Antibiotics are given prophylactically just prior to making the incision. The routine in widespread use is 1 g of a cephalosporin pushed and 1 g dripping in slowly during the operation. The same antibiotic is given in a dose of 1 g every 8 hours for at least 24 hours or until the Hemovac is removed and drainage from the Hemovac site has stopped.[194,195]

Postoperative Care

Pinned Fracture Early ambulation is the key to successfully avoiding much of the threatening medical complications. If alert enough, the patient is out of bed and into a chair the first day after surgery and ambulating on the second day. A well reduced, securely pinned fracture can be expected to allow full weight-bearing. These two factors reflect the difference between success and failure.

Laboratory studies have proved that well placed Knowles pins bear the patient's weight well.[133] A clinical study by Arnold's group[196] followed two groups of elderly patients with femoral neck fractures treated with Knowles pins. One group was kept from weight-bearing until the fracture was healed according to x-ray studies. The patients in the second group were encouraged to bear full weight as much as possible and as early as possible. Most of these patients were at their maximum weight tolerance by 4 weeks, using either a cane or a walker for a more comfortable and steady gait. "The results concerning stability of the fracture were comparable, indicating that early weight-bearing did not adversely affect the stability of a properly reduced and pinned displaced fracture of the femoral neck. Factors that did aversely affect stability following fixation with Knowles pins included the degree of initial displacement of the fracture (Garden type IV), failure to adequately reduce or fix the fracture, and severe demineralizing bone disease as measured in an iliac crest biopsy obtained at surgery."[196]

From a practical standpoint, patients can be divided into two groups. The first group contains those patients with stable fractures who had a good reduction to start with and even had an improved reduction at the time of surgery, which should have produced an excellent pinning. These patients can be asked to walk with full weight-bearing almost immediately after surgery. They typically become pain-free within a few days. Early weight-bearing enhances bone healing by its compressive forces. The pins control the impaction that takes place early, aiding the healing process.

The second group, those who sustained an unstable fracture, are more feeble and inherently slower to recover from their surgery. These patients experience some thigh spasm and groin pain. They must be ambulated more slowly and their fracture watched carefully because some of the best reduced and best pinned fractures collapse quickly and lose their reduction because of severe osteoporosis. These patients can become quite disabled. Early arthroplasty may be considered an early solution for their disability. Arnold performs it even during the immediate postoperative period,[144] as do European surgeons.[185,197] On the other hand, some of these unstable fractures go on to heal if weight-bearing is graduated on a careful schedule. Watchful waiting in this group is worthwhile.

Physical therapy is important. Abduction exercises and quadriceps drills improve gait and help smooth out the ambulation process as the patient regains control of the fractured leg. Any patient suffering spasms of the thigh should not undergo such a program until the pain and spasm subside with heat and rest. The patient is allowed to progress from a walker to a cane to no support as she regains her confidence. Some do not return to their preoperative mental state and must realistically stay on a program of a bed to chair existence.

Prevention of thromboembolic disease is a topic which could easily occupy all of the pages in this text. However, with early ambulation there has been a definite decrease in this complication. The prophylactic routine used most widely among orthopedic surgeons is aspirin in doses of 600 mg twice a day.[198–201] Such a regimen is not accompanied by the feared postoperative hematoma or drainage as are heparin, coumadin, low-molecular-weight dextran, or the newest is Embolex. There has been some evidence that aspirin's antiplatelet effect may be a sex-linked phenomenon in favor of men.[199] Snook and colleagues reported significant protection in both men and women suffering a fractured hip who received 1.2 g of aspirin per day. Repeated studies have shown that low-dose heparin is not effective in preventing thromboembolic disease in patients undergoing hip surgery [202,203]; in fact, it causes more problems than expected. Patients with a documented history of thrombosis require attention and should be anticoagulated with warfarin, low-molecular-weight dextran, or heparin. Antiembolic stockings should be used routinely, as they may help. The aspirin regimen is maintained for about 4 weeks or until the patient is ambulating to maximum capacity.

Intermittent pneumatic compression prevents thrombosis by improving blood flow in leg veins. It has been shown that it also increases fibrinolytic activity which may be an additional contribution to its antithrombotic properties. A combined thigh and calf device is now available which may be the most effective method of preventing deep venous thrombosis in hip surgery (Jobst Inc.).[340]

Postoperative Care for a Hemiarthroplasty

With a cemented hemiarthroplasty the patient becomes comfortable quite rapidly. Such patients are prompted to ambulate the day after surgery, bearing full weight on the leg as tolerated. During the first 6 weeks measures must be taken to prevent dislocation. Assuming that the prosthesis was inserted properly, a dislocation should not occur unless the patient becomes uncooperative or the nursing care becomes too casual. Some patients become so disoriented and irascible that it is almost impossible to convince them to follow preventive measures.

During ambulation they must be taught a wide-based gait. When sitting they must keep their knees abducted and neutrally rotated with an abduction pillow to remind them of their artificial joint. While in bed they must use an abduction pillow. The abduction pillow should be used for an arbitrary period of 6 weeks. By then enough capsular-like scar tissue should have developed to contain the prosthetic head in the socket. The position to be avoided is flexion to 90° and adduction past neutral. Patients with parkinsonism and spastic hemiplegics are especially vulnerable to this complication. They should be routinely placed in one of the stock abduction braces for 6 to 8 weeks (Fig. 8–72). Abduction strengthening exercises are important to the prevention of a dislocation. The patient may proceed from a walker to a cane as rapidly as tolerated, using the cane on the side opposite the arthroplasty.

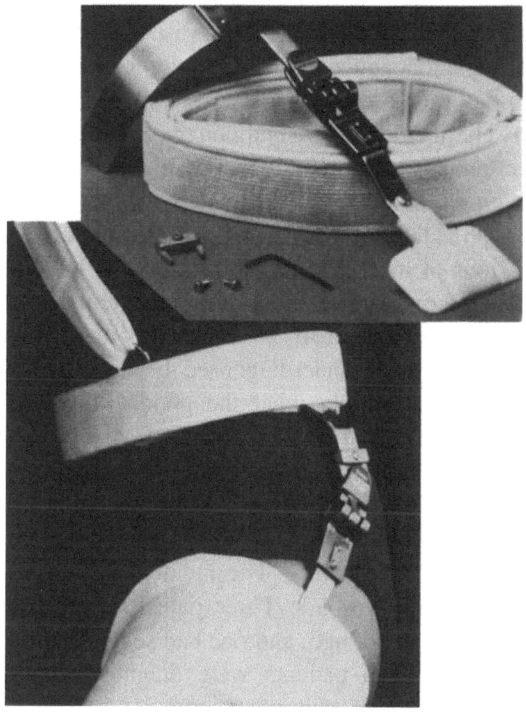

FIG. 8–72 Abduction braces are available as stock items. They hold the leg abducted while allowing flexion in varying degrees, adjusted by a wrench supplied with the device. The abduction brace can be applied to the thigh with plastic casting material.

Patients with an uncemented, press-fit prosthesis experience some thigh pain and groin discomfort. Their ambulation must be more gradual and prolonged than that for the patient with a cemented prosthesis. The more precise the fit or the tighter the fit, the less is the postoperative discomfort.

Medical Complications

Medical complications associated with surgical care of femoral neck fractures include all of the usual problems that result from any major operation and mirror the patient's preoperative medical status. Of major importance is the phenomenon of thromboembolic disease. Early vigorous ambulation has reduced this complication considerably. Once diagnosed, the patient must be actively anticoagulated. Elderly patients can be difficult to manage because of their delicate metabolic balance. Not uncommonly they respond erratically to the anticoagulant and so require a careful day-to-day monitoring.

The incidence of a pulmonary embolus is uncertain as autopsy studies report a wide variation, from 6% to 64%.[204] Prophylaxis for this complication is tedious and carries considerable complications of its own. The autopsy reports have uncovered more evidence of pulmonary emboli than is recognized clinically.[204] This entity may or may not be grossly underdiagnosed because autopsy studies relate only what the patient died *with,* not necessarily *from.*

Day[202] reported autopsy findings from the San Francisco General Hospital. There was an in-hospital mortality rate of 6.2% (35 of 565) among fractured hip patients. The incidence of pulmonary emboli was 1%. Three patients were more than 80 years of age, and one had severe multiple sclerosis. Two patients were diagnosed before death as having pulmonary emboli, a diagnosis which could not be confirmed at autopsy.

Leg vein thrombosis is usually of minor consequence when unassociated with pulmonary embolus, but it must be treated, and prolongs hospitalization. The question is whether it really is a significant antecedent to the development of a pulmonary embolus. There is evidence to suggest that it does not pose a major threat in this regard.[205–208] Day stated: "Detection of deep venous thrombosis is only an intermediate step, and although it has been assumed to be true, there is no proof that decreasing the incidence of deep venous thrombosis necessarily decreases the number of deaths from this disease. In fact, studies which have used this diagnosis as the principal end point have reported a remarkably low incidence of deep venous thrombosis. There is no scientific justification for continuing to highlight deep venous thrombosis to the extent that has been done in the past . . . as a leading cause of death in fractured hip patients."[202]

Complications of Hemiarthroplasty

Dislocation The overall dislocation rate reported during the 1970s was 10%.[209] With more experience gained the rate has dropped to below 3%.[210–212] A postoperative dislocation (Fig. 8–73) is the single disadvantage unique to this operation compared to any hip pinning. Patients treated with a hemiarthroplasty have been hospitalized longer in order to prevent dislocations. Likewise, postoperative rehabilitation must follow a more cautious course with careful supervision, all of which increases hospital costs. For this reason the Scandinavian countries are encouraged to pin hips rather than perform an arthroplasty. Soreide et al.[213] published an analysis of a prospective analysis of the comparative costs and the consumption of hospital resources in a Norwegian setting:

> As regards the initial stay in the hospital, prosthetic replacement was found to be associated with higher costs by a factor of 2.4. This difference was reduced by a more expensive follow-up and frequent readmissions and reoperations in the patients who had undergone a hip pinning. Considering the total costs, prosthetic replacement was found to be 1.6 times more expensive than internal fixation.

Sikorski and Barrington[210] characterized a prosthetic dislocation as "rare," as they had only one in their series of 57 patients with prostheses. These problems are not rare but uncommon, with an incidence of 4 to 10%. Sharma and Sankaran more correctly labeled dislocations as a serious complication. They had dislocations in 4 of 145 cases, but 3 of those had to be converted to Girdlestone arthroplasties.[211]

Causes of Dislocation

1. Neuromuscular diseases such as a hemiparesis following a stroke, Parkinson's disease, cerebral palsy, or similar disease can cause such a muscular imbalance that the hip joint is at risk. Should a prosthesis be inserted in such a patient, the patient's hip must be carefully protected for a minimum of 6 weeks. A diligent program is instituted of constant gait training and use of an abduction pillow at night for another 6 weeks. A stock abduction brace (Fig. 8–72), is a good prophylactic measure to be used over a prolonged period of time. At surgery it may be prudent to perform an adductor tenotomy to ensure that the leg is held in sufficient abduction. Many demented, bedridden, cachectic patients have such generalized atonia that they have a "loose hip joint" and easily dislocate their prosthesis if allowed to lie in bed with their hips flexed and adducted. If such a patient has flexion-adduction contractures at the outset, a prosthetic replacement is contraindicated. A hip joint at risk should be protected in one of the new abduction braces (Fig. 8–72) set at 45–60° of flexion.

2. Inaccurate fit of the prosthetic head into

the acetabulum is a common cause of dislocation. A too-large head dislocates more easily than one too small. Today most manufacturers offer head sizes in 1-mm increments, which is an improvement over the old 1/16-inch increments. Cutting too much neck off can render the joint excessively loose. Leaving too much neck on can make the prosthesis too tightly fitted into the joint, causing an adduction contracture and a late dislocation. A head with too much anteversion leads to an anterior dislocation, and one seated with too much retroversion results in a posterior dislocation. About 20° of anteversion is proper. Particles of cement or a particle of bone can fall into the acetabulum, creating a blockage that causes a dislocation, as the head may not become fully seated. Before the head is reduced one must be certain that the socket is completely cleared of all debris.

3. Deep infections can cause a late dislocation (Fig. 8–74). The joint capsule becomes so attenuated by the infection that it no longer can contain the head in its socket or the pus builds up under so much pressure that it crowds out the prosthesis. Widened joint spaces must be looked for, as they are ominous. In Salvati and Wilson's series deep infections accounted for one-third of the dislocations.[214]

4. Noncompliance by the patient is a frequent cause of dislocation. Be careful of the disoriented patient, who may not cooperate during the early postoperative period. Such patients should be restrained with a well fitted abduction pillow in place until they are alert enough to understand the principles of their new gait. The nursing staff must be trained to keep the patient sitting with no more than 80° of flexion, abduction of at least 30 to 40°, and held in neutral rotation.

5. The type of incision may contribute to the vulnerability of the hip joint. True posterior incisions such as the Southern exposure cut loose all of the posterior structures that ordinarily block a posterior exit of the prosthesis. In a prospective study by Sikorski and Barrington, no difference was found between anterior and posterior incisions.[210] In another prospecitve study on total hip arthroplasties there was a significantly higher incidence of dislocations in posterior incisions. The use of a new incision described by Tronzo (page 244; Fig. 8–66), may prevent this problem.

A hip dislocation is usually diagnosed easily enough. The hallmark to look for is shortening of the patient's leg, which is typically adducted,

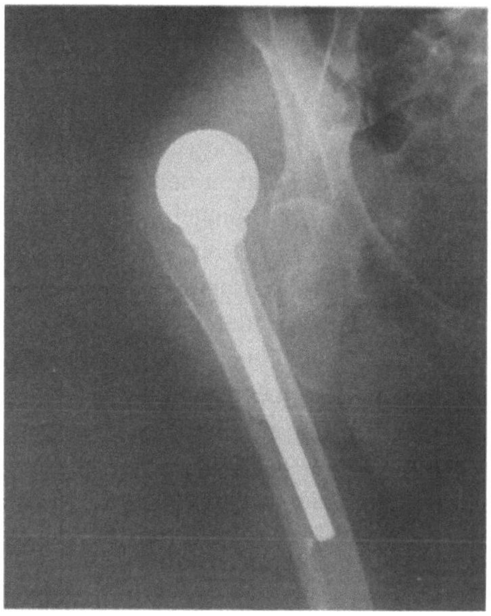

FIG. 8–73 Dislocated prosthesis postoperatively, usually superior and posterior.

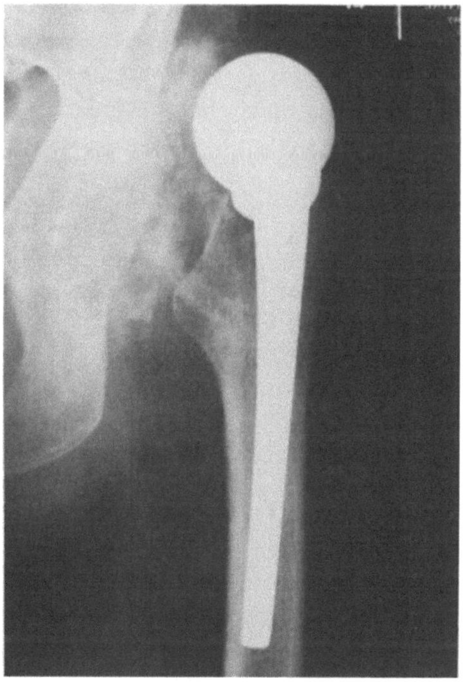

FIG. 8–74 Deep joint infection can be a cause of a dislocation from distension and edema within the capsular substance which becomes attenuated and weakened.

flexed and internally rotated. The hip either feels different with minimal discomfort or is acutely painful.

Treatment of a Dislocation If any of the mechanical causes can be identified, an open reduction is obligatory. Unfortunately, it is not an easy feat. When it becomes obvious that the dislocation will not respond to conservative measures, the problems may become identified only at an open reduction. Most first dislocations respond to a closed reduction in the patient's room with intravenous diazepam (Valium) and meperidine (Demerol). If three such attempts fail, general anesthesia becomes necessary. The reduction should always be scheduled for a "closed reduction, possible open reduction."

There are three maneuvers for a closed reduction. The most common one is the Bigelow, followed by the Allis, and then the Stimson. In the Bigelow maneuver the patient is on his back. The leg is flexed, adducted, internally rotated, externally rotated and extended simultaneously, and finally abducted. Strong traction is applied to the leg during the procedure, almost lifting the patient off the bed, while an assistant pushes down on the iliac crests (Fig. 8–75).

The Allis maneuver is similar. Here the patient is flat on his back in bed. The leg and thigh are strongly pulled in the line of the deformity (adducted) while an assistant pushes down on both iliac crests; with gradual forced flexion the leg is rotated inwardly and outwardly until a click is felt or heard. The leg is then abducted and extended (Fig. 8–76).

The patient is laid prone on top of a table or

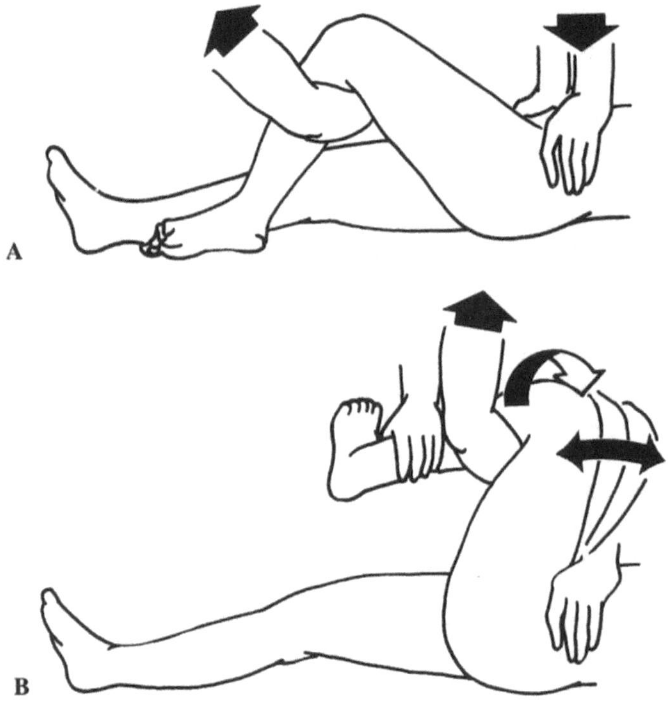

Fig. 8–75 Bigelow method of reducting a posterior hip dislocation is accomplished by: **A** holding the patient firmly supine on the floor or bed with countertraction by an assistant over the iliac crests. **B** The leg is pulled gradually in flexion and severe adduction while held in internal rotation. **C** When motion is felt as the head begins to slip over the acetabular edge, the leg is externally rotated and abducted. At this point a thud is felt and heard as the head pops back into place. **D** The leg is returned to extension and abduction. **E** Bigelow also described a method of reducing anterior dislocations which are very uncommon. The leg is pulled in the line of the deformity while in its typically abducted position. It is externally rotated and then gradually abducted and internally rotated as it gets eased over the acetabular rim and reduced. It is then held in neutral position and abducted while healing takes place. Reduction of anterior dislocations is accomplished by a reverse maneuver.

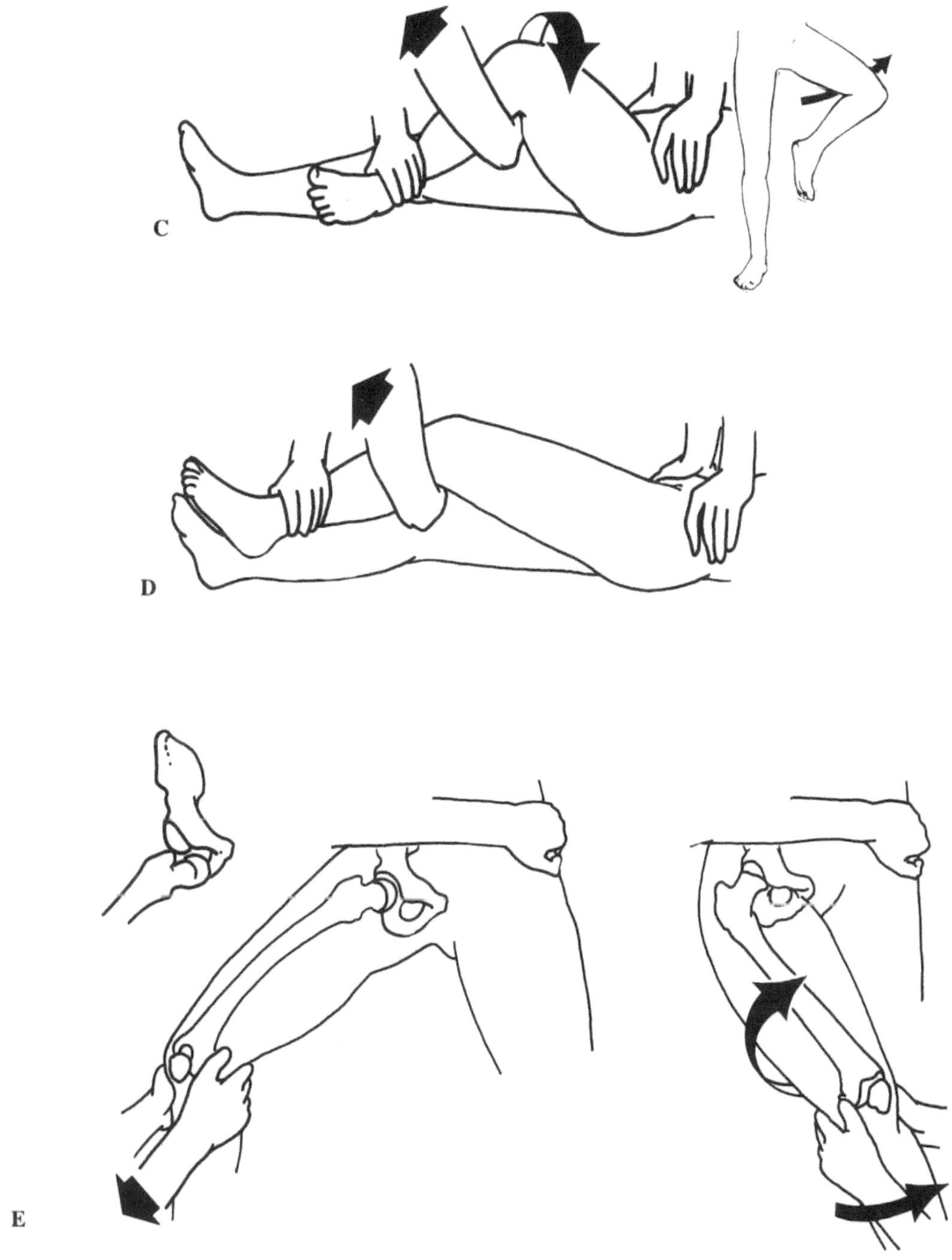

FIG. 8–75 *Continued*

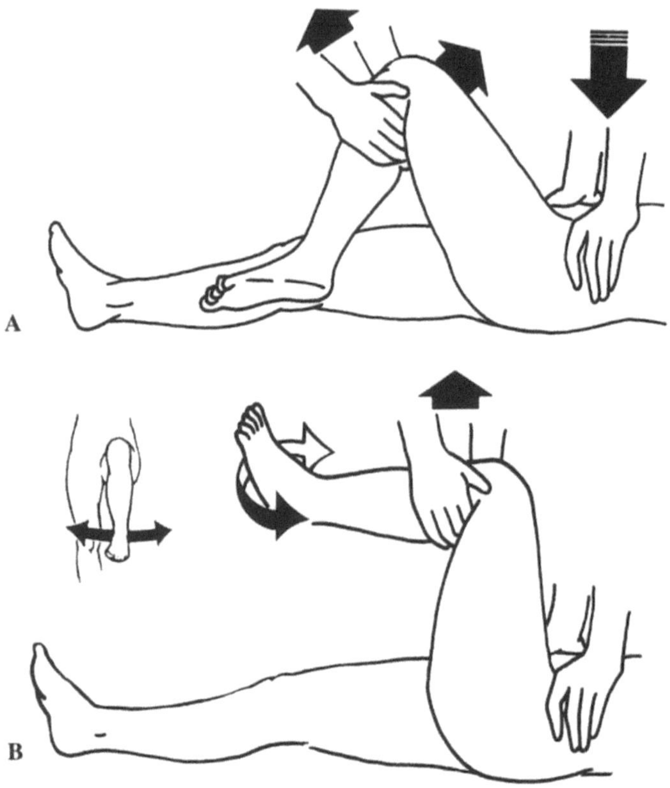

Fig. 8–76 The Allis maneuver is carried out with the patient supine. **A** The leg is pulled in the line of the deformity while the leg is flexed and adducted. **B** Wiggle the flexed leg externally and internally. When the posteriorly placed femoral head is pulled upward, it pops into place. The leg is extended and abducted and protected with an abducted pillow.

a high examining table, with his hip flexed over the edge of the table for the Stimson method. While an assistant holds the patient down on the table, the surgeon forces both hip and knee into flexion. The leg is rotated inwardly and outwardly, with forceful traction being steadily applied (Fig. 8–77).

"Bipolar" prostheses pose a special problem in the reductions of their peculiar dislocations. The sharp edge of the ball may snag on the edge of the acetabulum and become lodged there, requiring an open reduction to dislodge it. Another problem can arise with some of the older models when the head pops off completely. The Norwegians call this phenomenon a "delerin luxation."[212] It certainly requires an open reduction.

Should the dislocation occur a second time, serious thought should be given to an open reduction to pinpoint its true cause. There is the possibility that the acetabulum has been so damaged as to render it incapable of containing the head any longer. A total hip arthroplasty is performed at this point.

Management after a closed reduction is to put the patient in an abduction brace for at least 6 weeks with partial weight-bearing in abduction. Management after an open reduction is dictated by what is found at surgery. Usually an abduction brace for 6 weeks is sufficient to allow scar tissue to form well enough to stabilize the joint.

Occasionally an improperly sized prosthesis is chosen and the stem gets stuck in the femoral canal, usually about one-third to one-half way down the length of the prosthesis. It will move no further, nor can it be pulled out. Trying to remove it with an extractor can be futile. The author offers his approach to the problem (Fig. 8–78). Saw through the lateral cortex along the anterior border of the stem. The split cortex allows the femoral shaft to expand enough to permit its removal with the extractor.

If the dislocation is due to the prosthesis being too anteverted or too retroverted, the prosthesis must be removed and reinserted with a proper orientation, otherwise the dislocation will only get worse as the lip of the acetabulum becomes progressively more deformed. Such a procedure is formidable if the prosthesis is biologically bonded inside the canal. Two saw cuts can be made along the broad sides of the prosthesis (Fig.

FIG. 8–77 The Stimson method takes advantage of gravity. One or two pillows are placed on an examining table. The patient is placed prone over the edge of the table while the legs are left to dangle. The dislocated leg is pushed toward the floor while internally and externally rotated. It is an effective method and should be tried if either the Allis or Bigelow maneuvers fail. Do not try to rush the reduction. Steady traction is applied while rotating the leg inwardly and outwardly until the head goes back into its socket.

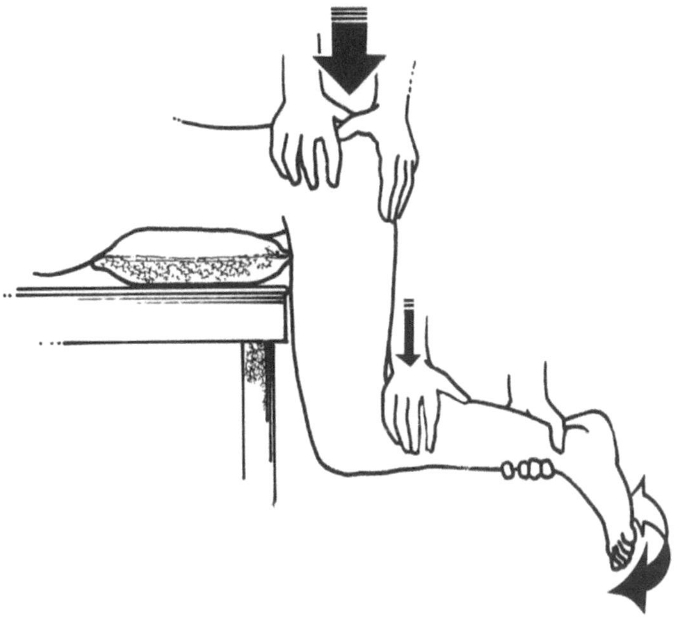

8–79). The major part of the bony ingrowth can be swept away with the saw and the stem extracted in the usual manner.

Nerve Damage Partial paralysis or complete paralysis to the sciatic nerve is the most common nerve injury. Next in order are the femoral, peroneal, and obturator nerves.[174] The head pushes against the anterior surface of the sciatic nerve, stretching the posterior fibers where the components making up the peroneal nerve reside (Fig. 8–80). A footdrop ensues. Before any reduction, examine for the neurological status of the leg. Once discovered, an electromyogram (EMG) is obtained to record the nerve's progress. Some recovery can be expected over a 6- to 12-month period. There is little recovery after this time, and seldom is it a complete recovery. If the paralysis follows an open reduction, surgical severance versus stretching becomes a diagnostic challenge. An EMG helps decide if and when the nerve should be explored for repair.

The femoral nerve can become damaged from stretching by Hohmann retractors when they are placed around the edge of the acetabulum.[215] These patients usually recover fairly well.

Femoral Stem Loosening A prosthesis left uncemented in the femoral shaft of an osteoporotic patient can be expected to loosen within

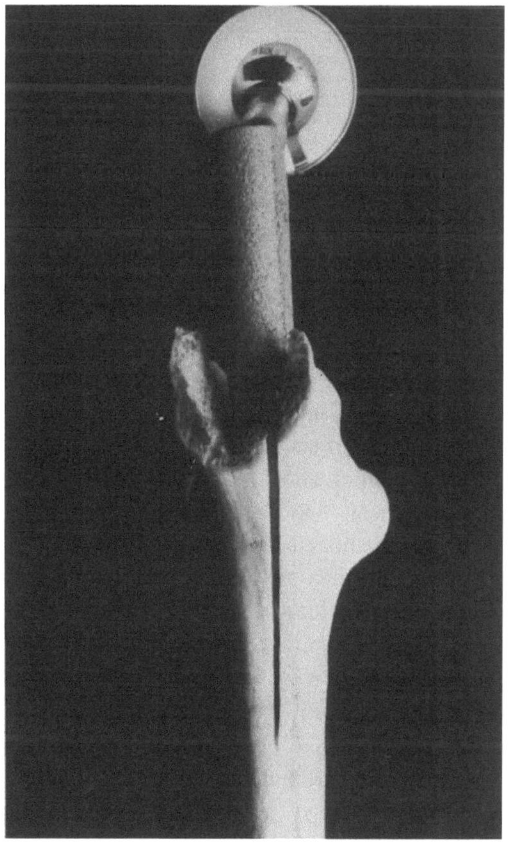

FIG. 8–78 Tronzo's method of releasing a stuck prosthesis. Cut into the lateral cortex along a siting parallel to broad side of the prosthesis, which allows the cortical tube to expand enough to allow withdrawal of the stem.

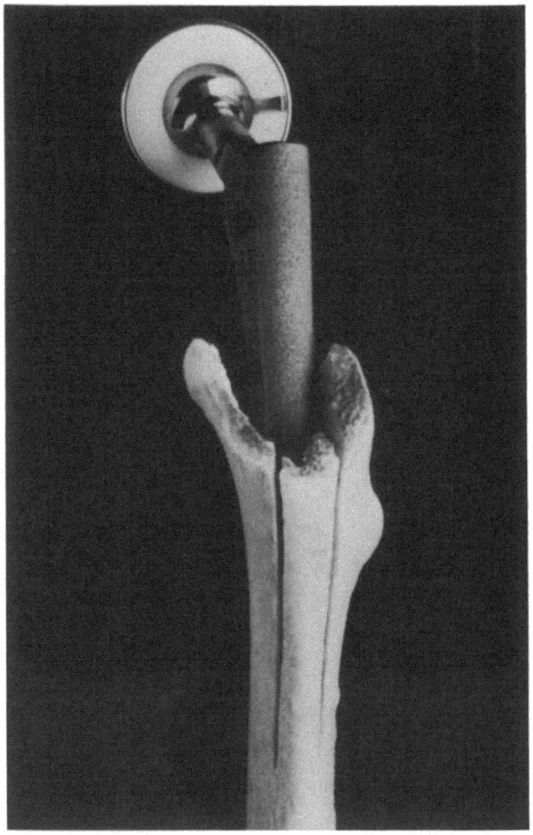

FIG. 8–79 Tronzo's method of removing a biobonded stem. By cutting the lateral cortex on either side of the flat surfaces, enough prosthesis is released from bony ingrowth to make it possible to extract the stem.

weeks or days of its insertion. A carefully fitted one that comes in seven sizes, or more, may be a different phenomenon. A tightly fitted, porous, coated prosthesis may be an even different situation. Both prosthetic types are being widely used, but not enough data have accumulated to furnish any hard information.

Loosening is typified by pain in the thigh on weight-bearing. Percussing the thigh produces pain. Deep infection around the prosthesis is a dreaded possibility. A characteristic x-ray finding is a sclerotic line around the stem with condensed bone around the tip. In chronic cases there is a "window-wiper" effect seen in the lower part where the tip has swept back and forth causing erosion in a window-wiper pattern. In general the x-ray film shows a halo where the eroded bone is around the prosthesis. The prosthesis may begin to sink as the inferior femoral neck becomes eroded mechanically by the metal or by slow destruction from a deep infection (Fig. 8–81). It may eventually drift into a varus position. Should the prosthesis be placed into varus initially, it is at risk for developing loosening.[174] Sikorski and Barrington followed their patients for only 2 years, and 12% of the uncemented prosthesis were definitely loose by the end of that period.

Acetabular Erosion Erosion and protrusio of the acetabulum is a major late complication of a hemiarthroplasty. Its cause and solution remain unsettled. Some of the more obvious causes are a prosthesis too tightly fitted into its socket, a head too small causing uneven wear, technical abuse of the articular cartilage at surgery for its insertion, a loose stem, and deep infection (Fig. 8–88B).

A controversial issue is whether cemented prostheses cause accelerated wear of the acetabulum. This concept was promulgated by Charnley when he said that the prosthesis needs to be able to piston within its femoral bed so as to act like a shock absorber. He made this statement despite the fact that he turned the world of international orthopedics upside down when he reported dramatic successes with Austin-Moore prostheses by cementing them into place.[181] He later rested his

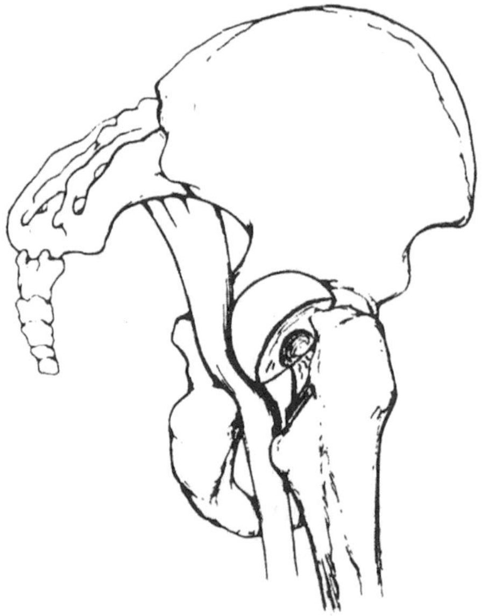

FIG. 8–80 The posterior fibers of the sciatic nerve become stretched by the prosthesis, causing peroneal nerve paralysis.

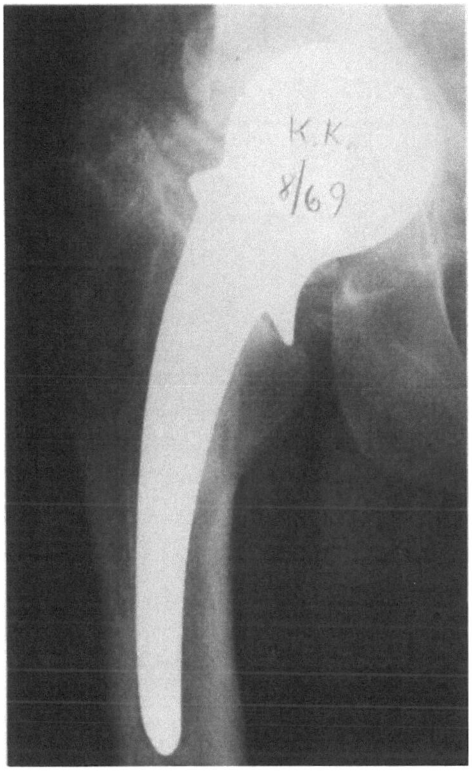

FIG. 8–81 Femoral prosthesis may "sink" in the canal as the calcar becomes eroded either from a deep infection or from mechanical wear secondary to the rotation of the stem. This parallels the patient's thigh pain and/or groin pain. Note also the acetabular erosion.

case on the findings of seven cases.[181] His words have been taken as gospel ever since their publication. At a meeting in Arizona sponsored by the Harrington Arthritis Foundation in 1984 no one on the panel could substantiate Charnley's seven cases. The use of a bipolar rotating head has been offered as a cure to the problems, but there are no convincing data as yet to prove its worthiness. The earlier version, e.g., Christiansen's trunion bearing device (Fig. 8–82), was thought to prevent acetabular erosion, but it too has produced poor results.[212]

The geometry of the femoral head and its mated acetabular partner may be the most significant factor in the development of acetabular erosion when such a foreign element as a metal prosthesis is introduced into the hip joint. One must be reminded that the human femoral head is not a perfect sphere (Fig. 8–83), although it is manufactured as such.[216] Nor is the acetabulum a true hemisphere[217] (Fig. 8–84). Both parts are "out of round" especially the femoral head. The deliberate mismatch is thought to exist as an elaborate scheme to massage the synovial nutrients into the hyaline cartilage. In a normally functioning hip joint, the force of compression widens the acetabulum as the femoral head flattens (Fig. 8–84). Cathcart[218] designed an oval ("out of round") head into an endoprosthesis to help restore this mechanism. It seemed to be a correct idea theoretically, but no long-term clinical proof has been made available to prove its worth. The idea has not caught on. Extensive studies have been done to measure these geometric parameters to better understand the effects of a prosthesis in a human socket.[219,220] From one's own intuition, it is difficult to expect the acetabulum to successfully remodel itself to accommodate a steel hemisphere without pain, cartilage damage, and eventual bony protrusio.

Ectopic Calcification Ectopic or heterotopic calcification is not as bothersome in a hemiarthroplasty as it is following a total hip arthroplasty. (See Chapter 7 for details of prevention and treatment.) Earlier authors have reported an incidence of 25%[221] and as much as 40%.[222] In neither of these studies did its presence cause any significant interference with joint function. Only occasionally (in about 6%) did it grow large enough in the abductor muscle or in the superior capsule that it had to be excised.[222]

Infection Postarthroplasty infection rate is a difficult complication to evaluate. Superficial infections are seldom an issue. The deep infection is the important one to consider. During the 1960s the rate was as high as 20%.[223] As the technique has become better understood and progressive skills were passed on to the house staff, the rate has fallen. It was once thought to be significantly higher than in Knowles pinning of the fracture. In our experience it has no more of a risk than a Knowles pinning, a 1% infection rate in either case. Superficial infections are easy enough to detect with redness, tenderness, and fever. Such infections are treated with local heat and aggressive antibiotics. If the infection does not respond in 2 to 3 days, a deep infection is likely. The wound must be drained of its infected hematoma. Removing a few sutures and opening a small hole with a hemostat on the floor is usually inadequate.

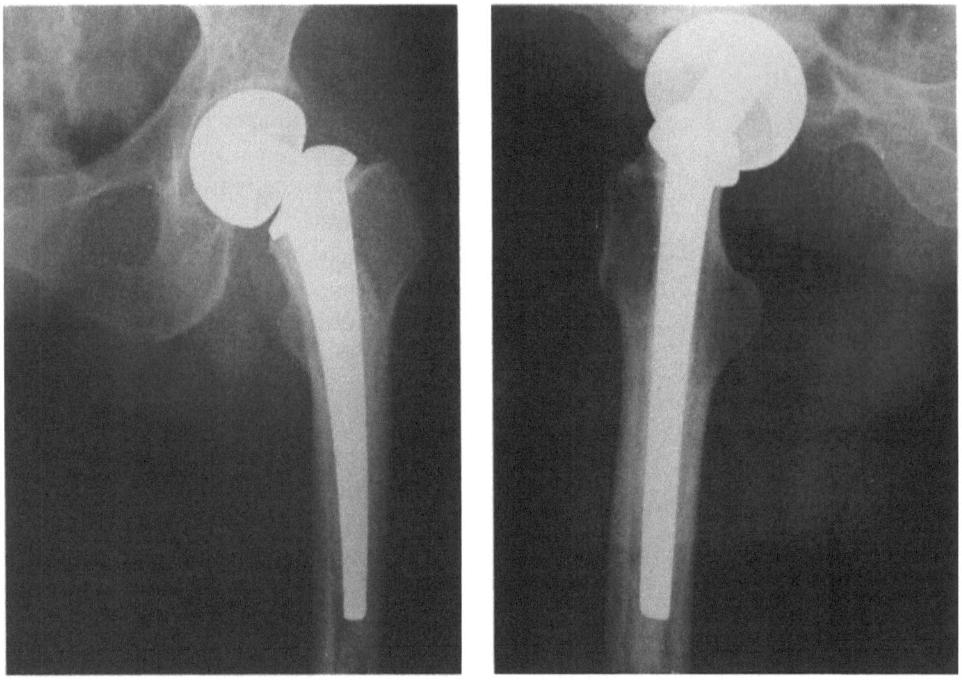

Fig. 8–82 Christiansen prosthesis has a unique trunnion bearing for double-action motion which may allow for less acetabular wear. It could be easily replaced later by a total hip device.

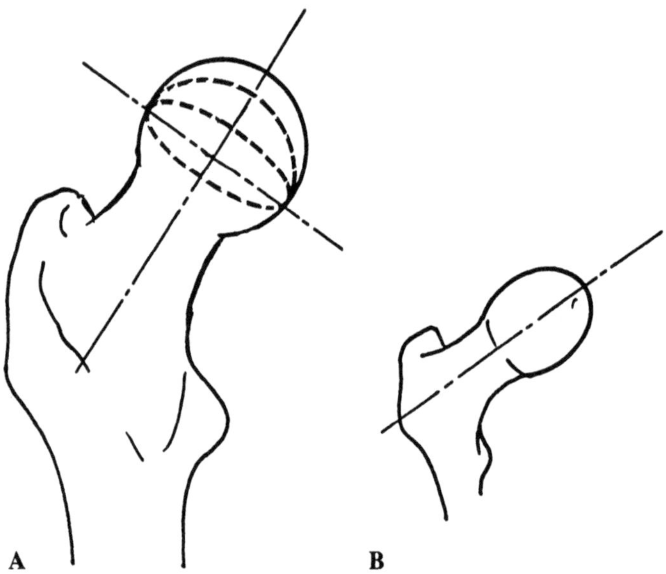

Fig. 8–83 The femoral head is not a true sphere as we envision it to be as depicted in **A.** In reality, it is egg-shaped and slightly "out-of-round" as illustrated in **B.**

More aggressive drainage in the operating suite is much safer and more definitive. The wound can be lavaged and closed over a new drain.

Deep, late infections are difficult to diagnose, as they are difficult to distinguish from mechanical loosening. There are two forms. One may be called "early late" and the other is called "late late." The former appears a few months to a year after surgery. The patient seldom has any obvious fever. The hallmark is a poorly defined never-ending ache in the thigh. There may also be a vague ache in the groin that gradually develops into a pain that persists even through the night and is aggravated by weight-bearing. Rehabilitation is unusually slow. The only laboratory study that may be helpful is an elevated sedimentation rate. X-ray films may show only subtle changes of demineralization around the prosthesis. As time progresses, a faint sclerotic border appears within the demineralized zone (Fig. 8–85). The joint space may be slightly narrowed, which would not occur so early if it were due to mechanical erosion. A bone scan helps, as does joint aspiration under x-ray control. If ignored, the process may cause more diffuse heterotopic bone, especially in the inferior capsule, which is not typical of aseptic bone condensation. The prosthesis may be seen as sinking into the neck of the femur (Fig. 8–86). The prosthesis may even dislocate without any obvious trauma because the capsule becomes attenuated and the joint fills with pus under pressure.

The "late late" infection develops more quietly, over a period of a year or longer. There are no systemic signs. Symptoms are more subtle, with the eventual development of pain that is located mostly in the groin or thigh. The ESR is high, and the bone scan is positive. The x-ray films show a border of sclerosis with no demineralization. At this point one faces a diagnostic dilemma because this set of circumstances may well represent a mechanically loose prosthesis. A joint tap may yield a positive culture. *Staphylococcus epidermidis* is usually the offending organism, which can be difficult to eradicate by antibiotics alone. In other cases appropriate antibiotics first and then removal of the prosthesis may be a logical sequence. Most of the time the prosthesis must be removed along with thorough débridement and a long course of antibiotics. (See Chapter 12 for more details of a Girdlestone arthroplasty.) Closed suction irrigation has not

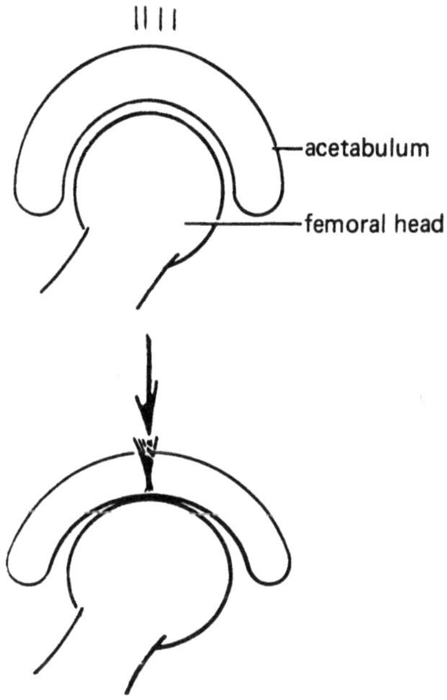

Fig. 8–84 The acetabulum expands under compressive loads generated against it by the femoral head.

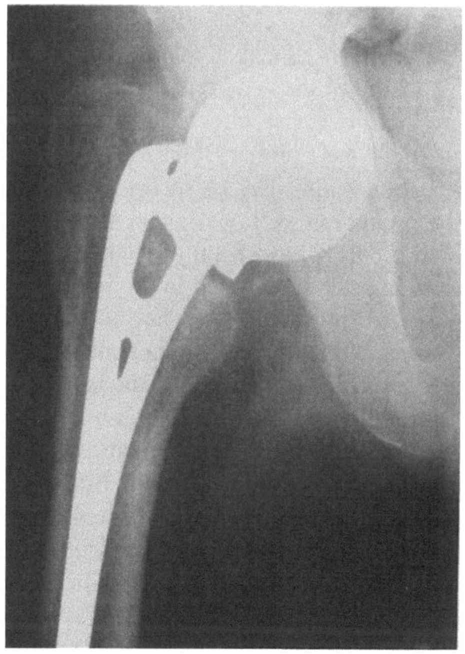

Fig. 8–85 Symmetrical wide border of demineralization with very little sclerosis indicates deep infection around the stem.

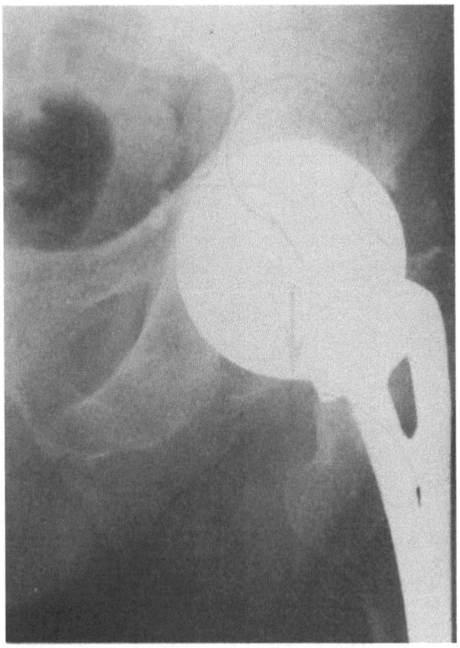

FIG. 8–86 Loss of the joint space within the first year is indicative of a deep infection causing lysis of acetabular cartilage.

proved to be as effective as the old method of open packing of the wound in cases of frank pus. Where there is sparse infected granulation tissue or no frank pus, primary closure of the wound over suction drains may be successful; the drains can be pulled out in 3 or 4 days, after the fluids and loose debris have been evacuated. The acetabulum is seldom involved in the infection.

When the prosthetic stem has been cemented into place, the situation becomes more difficult. If the infection is well contained and is not causing systemic problems, one could wait a few months while the cement becomes more demarcated within the infected bed of bone. Such a delay makes the task of removing the cement en masse much easier. If any of the *distal* particles of cement are well locked into place (indicating that there is no surrounding infection), they need not be disturbed lest the infection be extended to what was once healthy bone.

A promising new method of treating deep infections is emerging with the use of a string of cement beads impregnated with antibiotics such as gentamicin.[224] This method is effective against gram-negative aerobic bacteria as well as gram-positive aerobic bacteria, which represent the most frequent pathogens in prosthetic joint infection. The antibiotic leaches or "elutes" out into the surrounding environment in high localized doses. This phenomenon goes on for 6 weeks, which may be adequate to control the infection.

Operative Femoral Fractures Around the Prosthesis There is a stress riser within the distal one-fourth of a prosthetic stem. With sufficient trauma two types of fracture may occur around the femoral stem: operative and postoperative (traumatic). The first may occur in very osteoporotic bone when the hip is forcefully reduced. It is a long, spiral fracture along the distal half of the prosthesis and on into the shaft (Fig. 8–87). A cracking sound may or may not be heard, and usually the leg becomes hypermobile. This fracture may go undetected at the time of surgery when it is an undisplaced stable fracture. It can be picked up only on the immediate postoperative x-ray film. It is for this reason that a single anteroposterior film should be obtained in the recovery

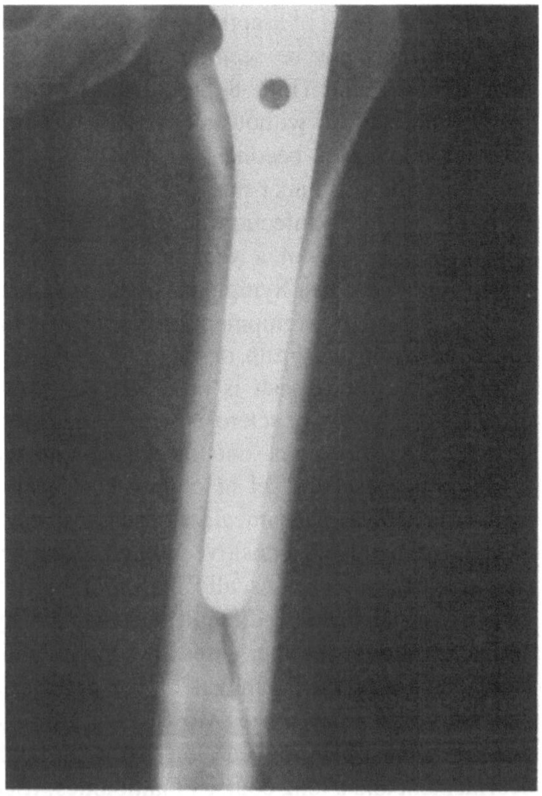

FIG. 8–87 Spiral fracture around prosthetic stem.

room and read promptly by the radiologist or the surgeon. In such a case the strong linea aspera can keep the spiral fracture held together. If the fracture is detected at surgery or in the recovery room, the patient should be promptly taken back to surgery. The incision is extended, and two Parham bands placed around the fracture will hold the fragments together. Two nylon electrician's straps can also be used.

The second type of operative fracture develops during insertion of the prosthesis (Fig. 8–88), with or without the use of cement. This incident may become more frequent as more press-fitted stems are inserted during the present new wave of "canal filling" prostheses. When the prosthesis is too large for the femoral canal, it splits from the inferior neck distally. The posterior upper third with the lesser trochanter is split off, which should be detectable at insertion. The prosthesis must be removed and Parham bands wrapped around the femur or heavy wire around the femur and through the lesser trochanter to prevent the wires from slipping distally. A smaller device is inserted or more reaming is done to accommodate the prosthesis, or both. An x-ray film at this point is prudent.

If the fracture is a long, spiral one, a longer stemmed prosthesis is needed to lend more stability to the fixation of the fracture. If there is only a simple crack in the neck, nothing need be done, but a more cautious rehabilitation period should be followed. Cement could be used once the fragments are precisely brought together, otherwise the cement will flow between the fragments, thereby preventing fracture healing. If cement had been used originally, a long operative procedure must be anticipated. The cement must be chipped away and the fragments reduced and fixed before another prosthesis is reinserted.

Postoperative Fractures Following Trauma Parrish[225] first brought attention to this complicated fracture. It is the result of a fairly violent

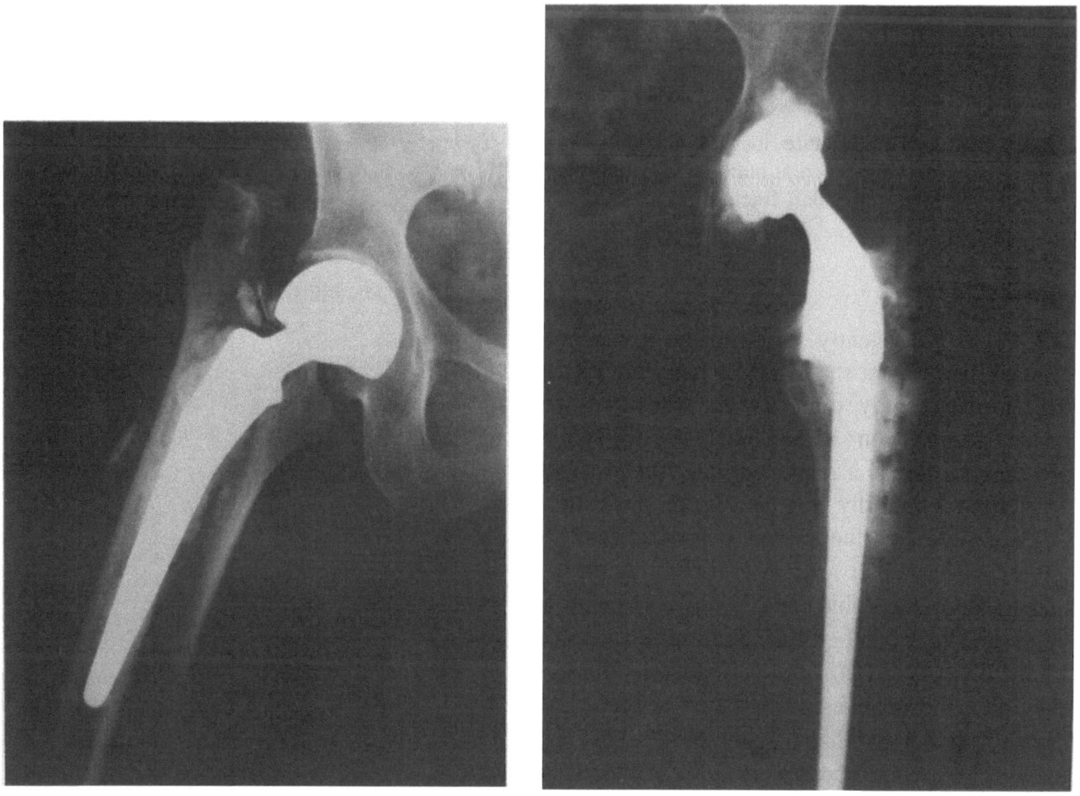

A B

FIG. 8–88 **A** AP and lateral x-rays showing a femur fractured by poor technique while inserting the stem into a bed of cement. The prosthesis was driven down so hard the femur split in half. This case should have been revised at the time of surgery, but it was not. Hence the reconstruction done later was very difficult. **B** A neck replacement prosthesis was used. Note the nylon straps engulfed by bone cement. A total hip replacement was necessary because of an eroded acetabulum from delay in its reconstruction.

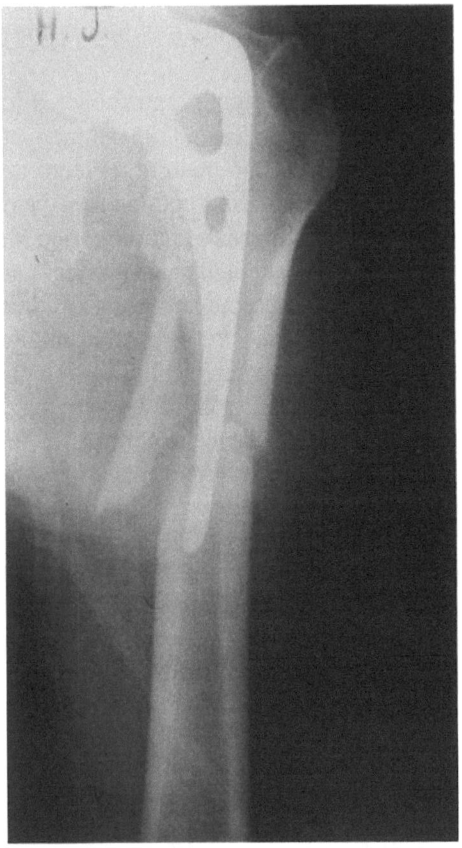

FIG. 8–89 Type I fracture located at distal tip of prosthesis with typical medial butterfly fragment similar to a subtrochanteric/shaft fracture.

fall and is consistently found in the lower one-third of the femoral shaft. Two types were identified from a study done at the University of Pennsylvania[226] on uncemented Austin-Moore prostheses. One is a short, oblique fracture with or without a butterfly fragment in the distal third of the femur with the stem still hooked into the intermedullary shaft (Fig. 8–89). It is relatively undisplaced and stable, and it can be treated in traction. The second type is an unstable situation where there is a long, oblique fracture through the tip of the prosthesis (Fig. 8–90). The distal fragment is not stabilized by the prosthesis. This fracture is treated operatively with a long stem prosthesis passing into the distal fragment and supplemented with cement (Fig. 8–88B). A long plate is another option for the shorter, oblique fractures (Fig. 8–91). The first type could be treated with a plate as well. A third option is to use Ender rods which can be passed up along the prosthesis (Fig. 8–187). An additional question arises as to whether a total hip arthroplasty is an option. If there had been a relatively mediocre arthroplasty up to the time of the trauma with evidence of loosening or acetabular erosion, a total hip prosthesis is done with a long stem porous coated prosthesis if the patient had been robust and ambulatory; cement augmentation is used if the patient had been treated otherwise. In the case of a fracture around cement, use a bone plate as depicted in Fig. 8–92.

Metal Synovitis Surprising enough, particles can rub off the prosthesis and fall into the hip joint causing synovitis. Every experienced surgeon has seen it, although little has been written about it. Its significance has not been thoroughly investigated. To date only failed prostheses have been explored. Successful arthroplasties are left untouched. The process occurs over a long period of time in those cases where the stem had moved about fairly extensively within the femoral canal.

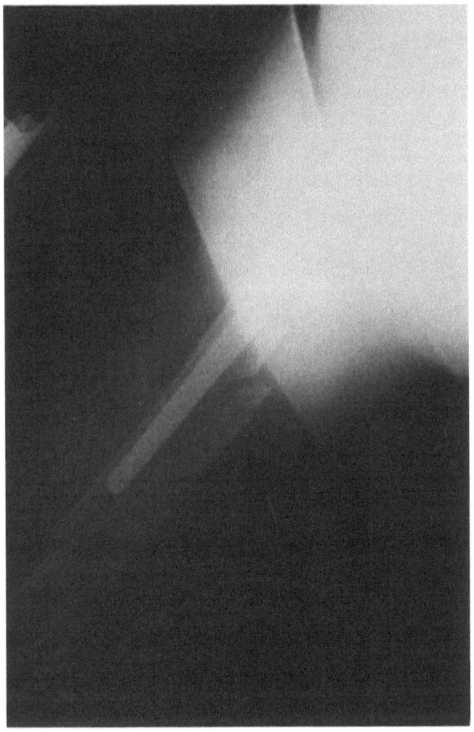

FIG. 8–90 Type II is a long oblique fracture through and past the tip of the prosthesis.

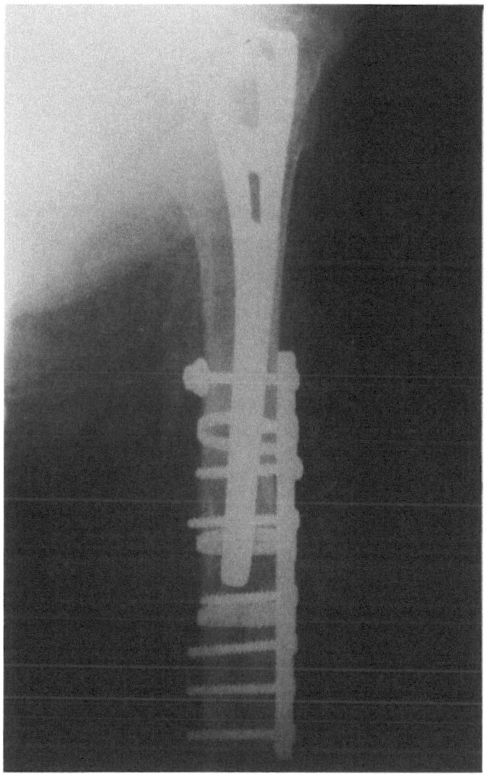

Fig. 8–91 Fracture around an uncemented endoprosthesis treated with a bone plate with bolted screws and Parkam bands as additional fixation in order to firmly hold the typically osteopenic bone.

It may add to the other mechanisms at work that are causing the arthroplasty to fail. The synovial membrane is stained black in this case, and the macrophages contain very fine metal particles. This phenomenon is found unexpectedly when a prosthesis is loose and must be removed. Occasionally the fluid is also black because of the metal particles. There is nothing to do about it except to excise as much of the affected synovium as possible.

Complications of Internal Fixation

Delayed Union Delayed union is highlighted somewhere at the 6-month mark. It is diagnosed when serial x-ray studies show minimal closing of the fracture line, although the line is still apparent at 6 months. With a healing rate between 85 and 95%, the former bleak prognosis of the 1950s must be discarded. The new concept is that femoral neck fractures do heal if given the proper chance to do so.[38–40,64,124,127–133,138–140,142,144,158,161,163,164,227–229] Figure 8–93 is an example of such a fracture which finally showed a solid trabecular pattern after 10 months of waiting. It healed despite a rather poor reduction but in the presence of secure fixation. The patient was 71 years of age, alert, and active, and was asked to ambulate using a cane on the opposite side. The absence of her groin ache matched the onset of consolidation of the fracture.

Figure 8–94 is another example of delayed healing which went on to union after 2 years. The reduction was poor. The Knowles pins were well into the subchondral bone, but one pin was not parallel. The patient was 52 years old and active, with only an ache in her groin that was associated with excessive activity. One pin finally broke 22 months postoperatively, allowing the head to impact onto the femoral neck (Fig. 8–95). Once finally impacted, the fracture healed and the patient's symptoms disappeared.

The hallmark in these cases is a minimal groin ache with the quality of function experienced by the patient considered acceptable. If the ache were to become frank pain to the point of disability,

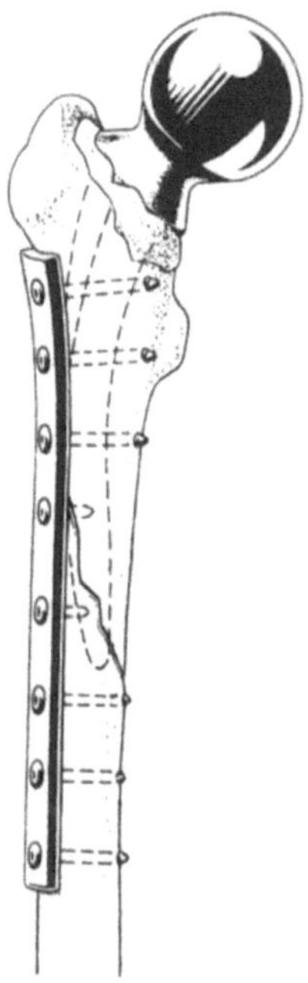

Fig. 8–92 Fracture of the femoral shaft when the prosthesis has been cemented into place can be repaired by extending lateral incision and using a stout ASIF plate for fixation. (Adapted from M. Müller.)

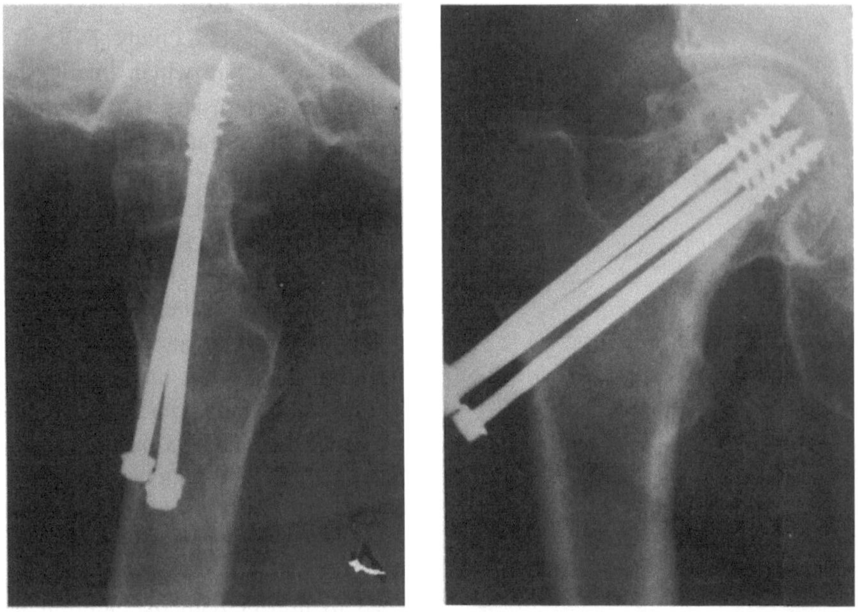

FIG. 8–93 Subcapital fracture with a barely acceptable reduction and fixation. The patient had minimal symptoms with a slight ache in her groin. At 6 months there was still evidence of a fracture line. She was allowed to continue ambulation with a cane. Present pictures illustrate complete union with no necrosis at the end of 10 months.

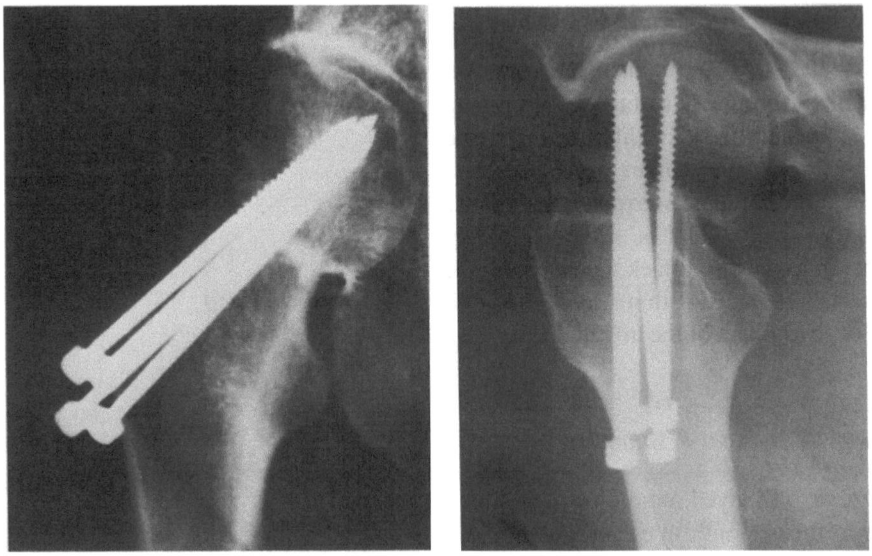

FIG. 8–94 Very poorly reduced subcapital fracture with barely adequate fixation; one pin is not parallel.

a nonunion must be suspected. In that case an aggressive treatment plan would become the order of the day.

Nonunion Fielding[144] thought that femoral neck fractures should be healed by 6 months. Meyers et al.[225] considered any femoral neck fracture not healed by 6 months to be a nonunion. Dooley and Hooper[230] studied 23 nonunions which were treated as such an average of 6 months after the original pinning. Labeling a neck fracture as being nonunited is difficult enough; judging when to intervene is even more difficult.

The reasons for nonunion are usually obvious and preventable. Furthermore, they are treatable. The most glaring cause of nonunion is poor fixation; poorly placed pins should be in a diamond or quadrilateral pattern and up close to the subchondral surface of the femoral head. The pins must be of a heavy-duty variety and deeply threaded so they become well anchored in the head.

Another cause of nonunion is a poor reduction, as pointed out by Garden and colleagues,[24,39] Banks,[103] and Fielding.[38] The most common cause of nonunion is the combination of poor reduction plus poor fixation.

A third major cause of nonunion is avascularity of the femoral head, which also is directly correlated with poor nailing and poor reduction, as shown by Garden.[24] When avascularity is present, as indicated by scan, the chances rise significantly for nonunion along with segmental collapse, as the only blood supply coming up from the metaphysis and neck becomes inadequate for a healing callus to form.[87,88,90,91]

Yet another major cause for nonunion is the inherent instability of the fracture itself. The posterior comminution, which is on the compression side of the fracture, is part of a severe form of osteoporosis. When it is extensive, no meaningful reduction or fixation can be established within such a hollow shell of bone (Fig. 8–96).

Casselbaum and Nugent[33] reported that with an accurate reduction and good internal fixation they could produce union 93% of the time. What causes the remaining 7% to fail? Osteoporosis is the metabolic cause for nonunions in elderly people. Barnes et al.[129] showed that both the rate and the percentage of union decreases with age and with the severity of osteoporosis (Fig. 8–97).

Treatment of Nonunions Dooley and Hooper[230] reviewed the use of a fibular bone graft for treatment of nonunion. The fracture must be reduced exactly if not done so originally. The choice of new internal fixation is chosen so that a path through the center of the neck and into the center of the head must be used. The path for the fibular graft is made with a cannulated drill over a guide pin and with x-ray control. A 3- or 4-inch graft is driven along the channel. Union was obtained in 24 of 26 cases. Their cases were selected on the basis of a vascularized head being present as indicated by a bone scan and no appreciable resorption of either the neck or the head. They concluded that an angulation osteotomy did not contribute to union of the fracture. To them it was deemed an unnecessary procedure. By carefully following the recommended steps outlined by Meyers, Fig. 8–53, good results may be obtained with a posterior muscle pedicle bone graft.[154] The head must be proved viable, and there must be enough residual femoral neck to accommodate the graft. Figure 8–98 is a nonunion that may be successfully treated by a muscle pedicle graft (Fig. 8–99). Figure 8–100 depicts the AO technique for treating a maligned nonunion with an osteotomy and an AO plate. A young patient with a dense femoral neck but a vertical fracture progressing to a nonunion may benefit from a valgus osteotomy alone (Fig. 8–101) using a long angled device through the old nail site which had been well placed.

If conditions are not ideal for bone grafting, arthroplasty becomes a serious consideration. In these cases the acetabulum has not been stressed much because the patient's symptoms enforce no or partial weight-bearing. The subchondral bone becomes friable and the hyaline cartilage on the articular surface atrophic. Such a state of affairs is not ideal for supporting a hemiarthroplasty to a successful endpoint. Total hip replacement is therefore recommended, especially in the older patient. Hip fusion is performed to salvage the hip in a younger patient who may have suffered a complex traumatic injury.

An infected nonunion becomes a complex problem because the situation is grave. In such cases priorities change. Curing the infection becomes so paramount that it may become necessary to convert the hip joint to a pseudoarthrosis. See Chapter 12 by Steinberg on this subject.

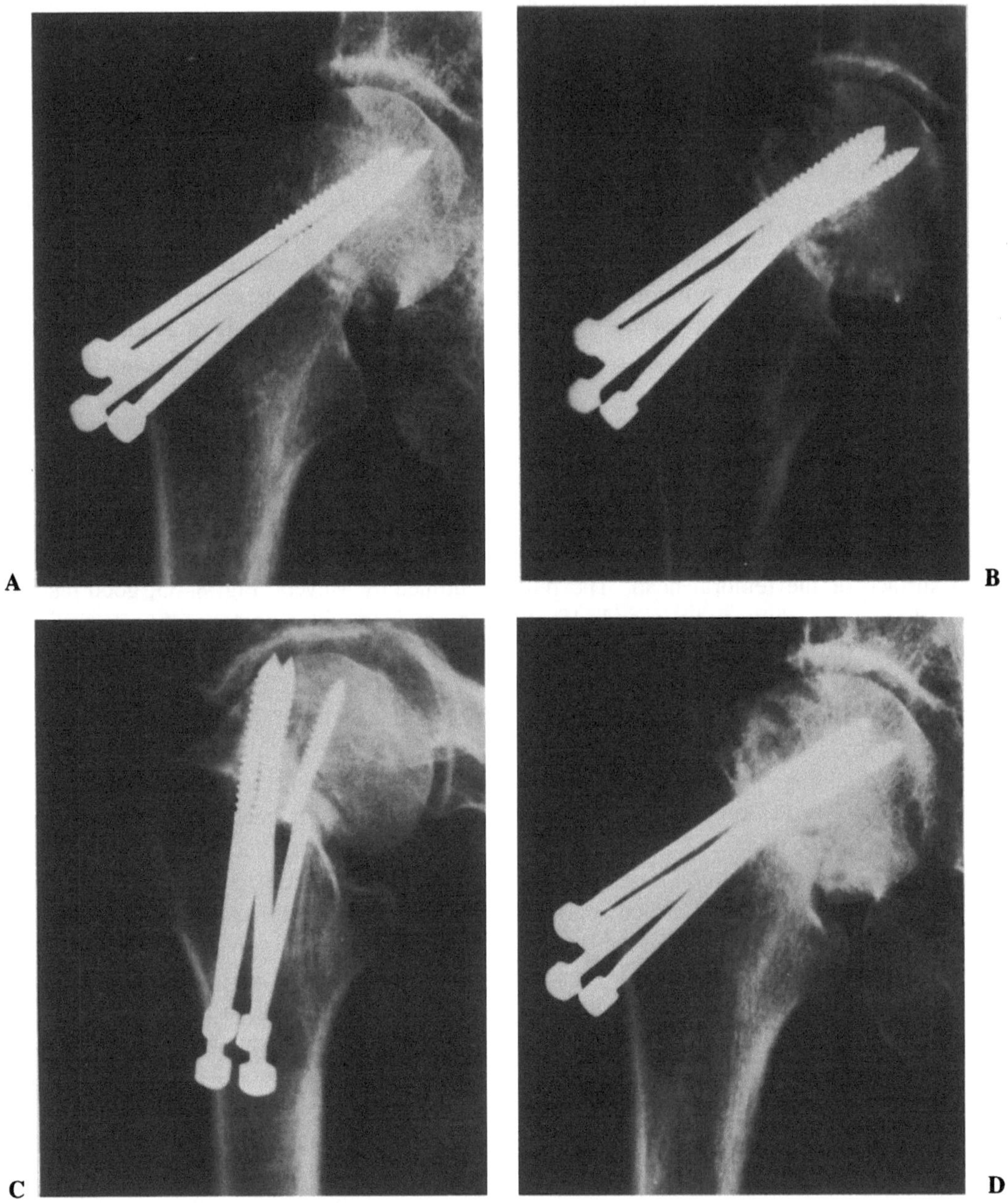

FIG. 8–95 The same fracture as in Fig. 8–94 serial sequence. **A** The head has slipped into varus and **B** posterior angulation. **C** The nonparallel pin finally broke. **D** The head is now beginning to heal.

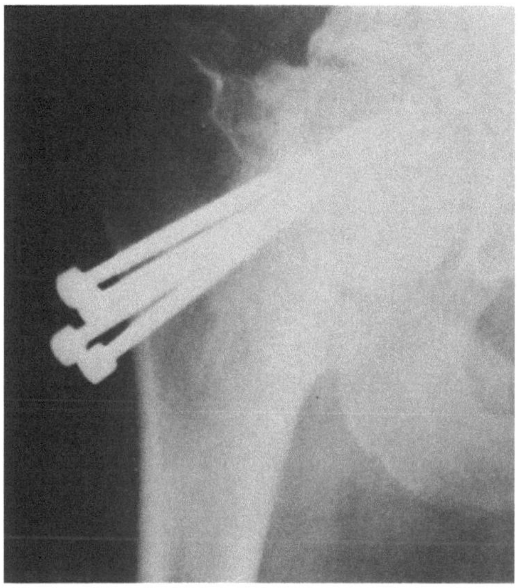

E

FIG. 8–95 **E** Fracture completely healed in marked varus and shortening 5 years after reduction. The patient has no pain, and needs no external support. She has a slight adduction deformity with a relative shortening of 1.25 inches corrected by a heel lift. The patient is happy with her natural hip joint intact.

Femoral Head Necrosis Necrosis of the femoral head is usually an unavoidable and unsolvable complication which singularly stamps femoral neck fractures as bad injuries. A good reduction and a well positioned internal fixation device can reduce its frequency, but such good treatment cannot entirely eliminate it[29,129] (Fig. 8–102). The necrosis is usually segmental at the superoanterior portion of the head. In some cases it becomes total. If it is going to appear, it usually does so within the first 2 years, although it can occur as late as five years; after this time, however, it is a rare event. Not all cases of early necrosis go on to segmental collapse because revascularity may occur spontaneously. Although necrosis is clearly associated with nonunion, it can be completely absent in grossly nonunited fractures (Fig. 8–100). Necrosis is least often seen in undisplaced fractures and most often in displaced valgus fractures. The exact incidence is difficult to calculate. Figures in the literature from the late 1970s and 1980s vary from 7 to 27%.[92]

Garden observed that once a fracture has united

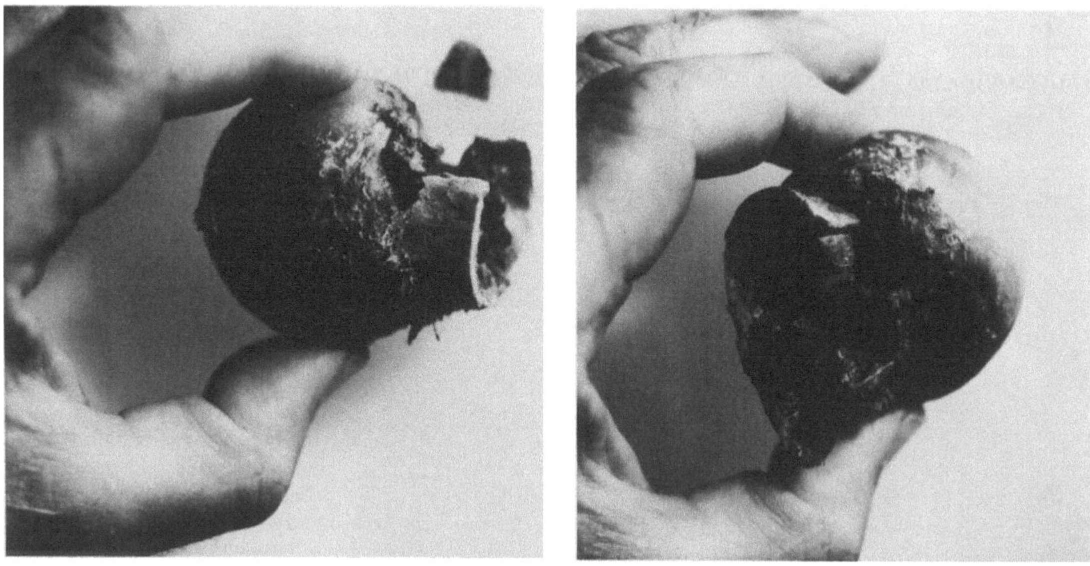

FIG. 8–96 **A** Posterior comminution on the compression side of the fracture may be too severe to expect a stable reduction. **B** The hollow medullary canal of the femoral neck combined with the comminution may render fixation nearly impossible.

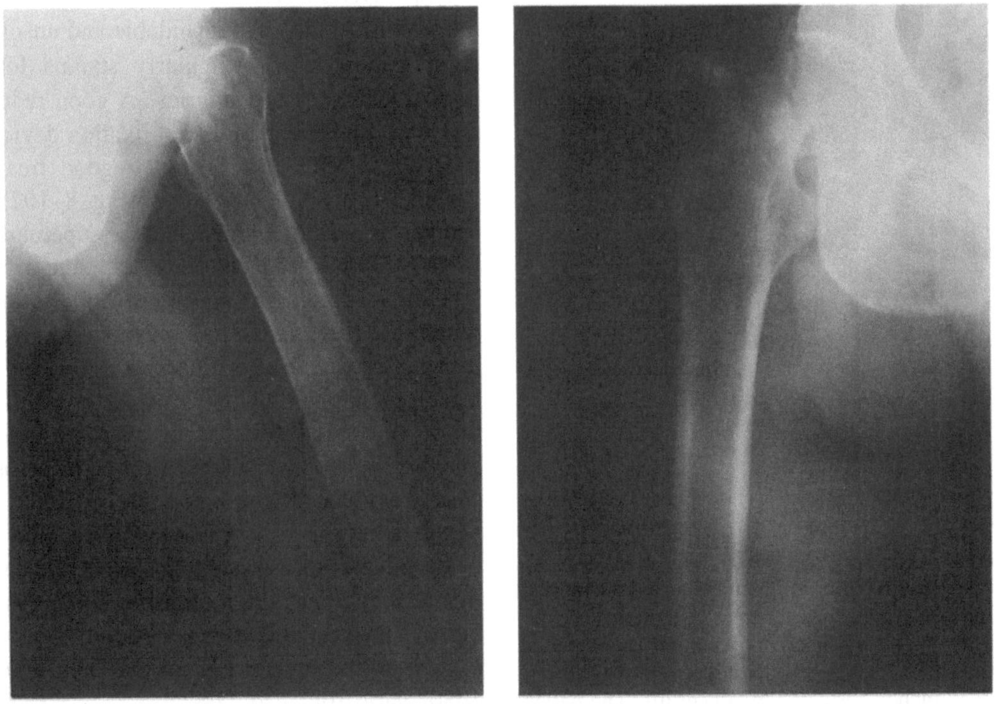

FIG. 8–97 Severe osteoporosis is seen in the femoral shaft of a 77-year-old woman with a femoral neck fracture.

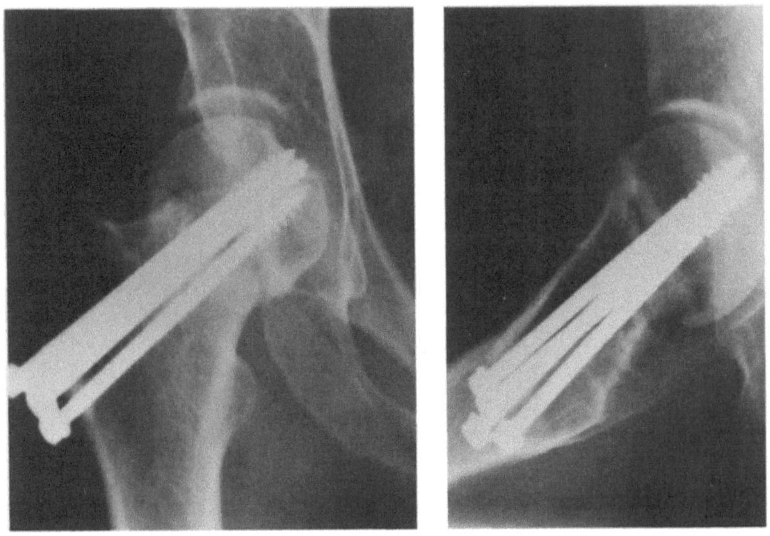

FIG. 8–98 Nonunion of the femoral neck. Note poor reduction appreciated on lateral x-ray. Scleroses at the fracture line establishes it as a nonunion 10 months after reduction.

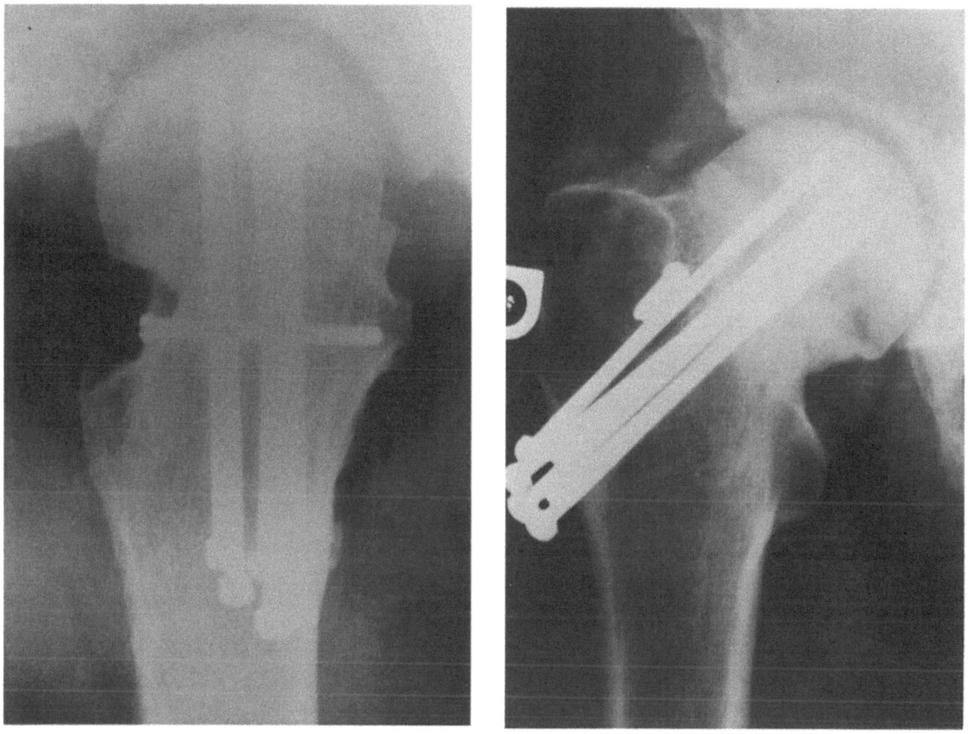

FIG. 8–99 An established nonunion resulting from a poor reduction. Sclerosis on either side of the fracture line clearly establishes it as a nonunion. An example of a nonunion successfully treated by a posterior bone graft.

with any obvious degree of posterior angulation segmental necrosis can be expected to appear. He found a direct relation with a highly distorted alignment index of the fracture reduction. He also noted the highest incidence to occur when the fracture is overreduced in extreme valgus.[29] It is his thesis that malrotation causes such distortion of the biomechanics to the articular surfaces that the segment which is forced to lie outside the new arch of articulation collapses. He challenged the theory that necrosis is due solely to lack of circulation. He, however, does not explain why undisplaced and slightly displaced fractures can foster a necrotic segment (Fig. 8–103). There are other theories too numerous to mention here (see Steinberg, Chapter 1). Phemister most likely had the right idea when he postulated that the fate of the femoral head is established at the moment the fracture occurs.[89]

The hallmark symptom is hip pain, which usually is an ache initially. It may be difficult for the patient to identify as coming from the hip joint itself, especially if it first appears as an ache in the groin. The pain can be acute and severe if the segment collapses suddenly when associated with minor trauma.

Surgical treatment was necessary in only 18% of cases studied by Boyd and Salvatore[32] and in 30% of Barnes et al.'s cases.[129] Brummer made a similar plea that most elderly patients with femoral head necrosis function well enough without further surgical intervention.[197] Younger patients, in their late fifties and sixties, may do well with remodeling of the femoral head and do not need any treatment until secondary arthritic changes become symptomatic years later. Steinberg discusses in detail the treatment options in younger patients in Chapter 1. In this author's opinion, anyone in their sixties would do best with a total hip replacement regardless of the condition of the acetabulum. Too often an acetabulum looks normal and the head appears to be the distorted

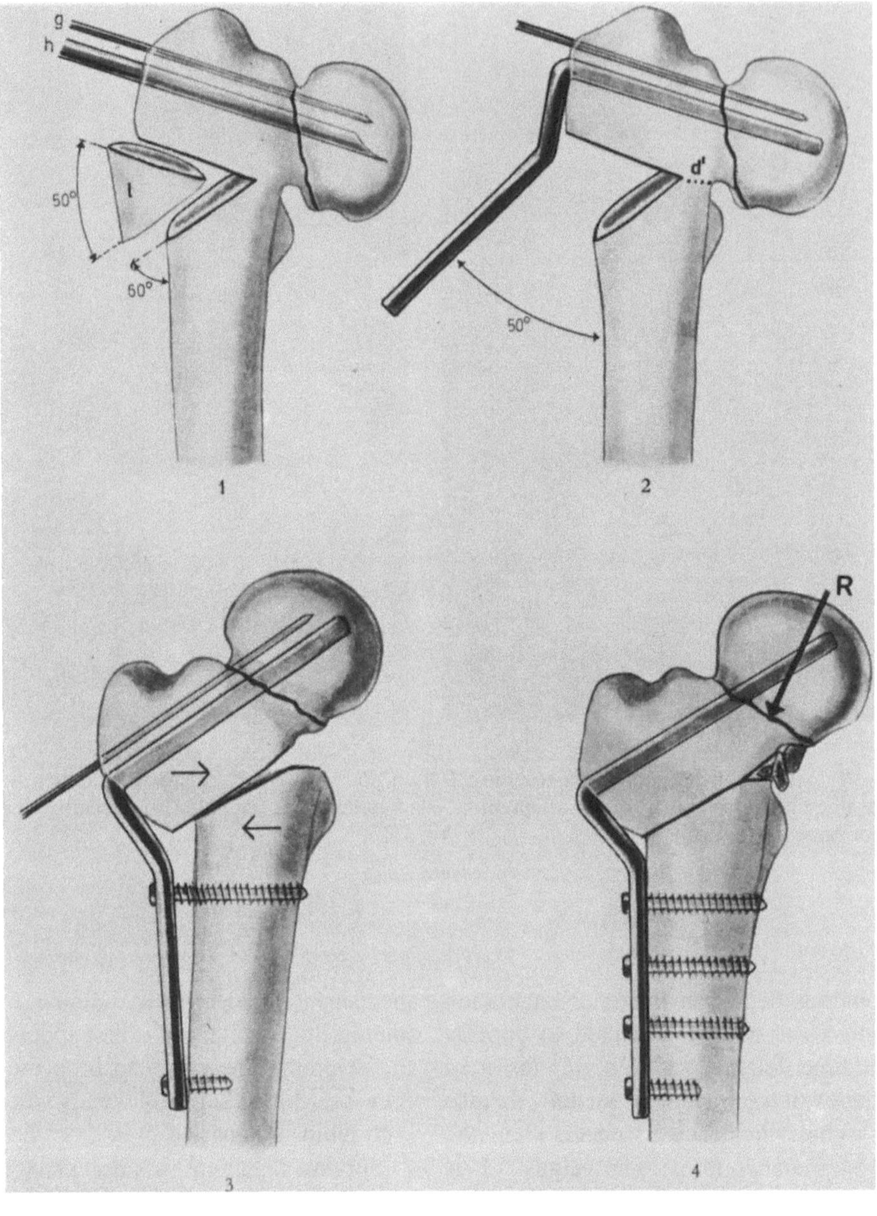

FIG. 8–100 Müller's method of correcting the varus deformity and medially displacing the shaft, both of which increase impaction of the fragments. It was originated by Pauwels. A bone graft from the tibia could be added. (From Müller, Allgower, and Willenegger: Manual of Internal Fixation, New York, Springer-Verlag, 1970.)

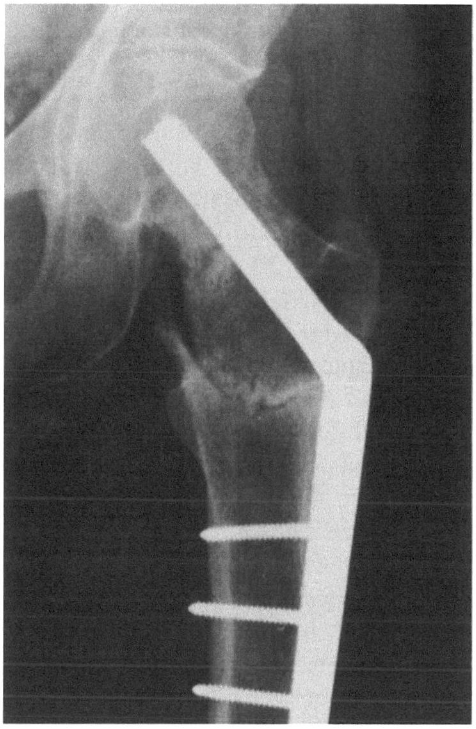

FIG. 8–101 The tension forces can be reversed to compress the forces by a valgus intertrochanteric osteotomy, which may effect complete union without the addition of a bone graft. This procedure is indicated for fractures in young patients where the femoral neck is filled with dense bone and can easily go on to union if a typically vertical fracture line is converted to a more horizontal one by the osteotomy, causing the fragments to be compressed. A compression screw is best here.

culprit when standard x-ray films are reviewed. This is a distortion of the true nature of the articular cartilage because, if inspected carefully, at surgery, it will be found to be abnormal in its dome. When the necrosis is found early by a CT scan or MRI, bone grafting or an osteotomy may offer a successful outcome. These studies should be ordered at the earliest onset of symptoms despite "normal" x-ray studies.

Subtrochanteric Fractures Below the Entrance of the Pins Schmidt and Gregg reported the occurrence of fractures below the entrance of the multiple pins in the subtrochanteric area following pinning of femoral neck fractures.[231] The time of onset in their series was within 6 weeks after surgery.

The fracture occurs at the site of an empty pin hole or at the entrance of pins which originate at the level of the lesser trochanter or just below it. Such a biomechanical situation creates a stress riser effect. The case shown in Figure 8–104 was a 55-year-old patient who had suffered a stress fracture. The pins had been inserted just below the lesser trochanter. The subtrochanteric fracture occurred about 8 weeks after the pinning. It was associated with a minor fall when the patient slipped on a carpet. Minor trauma is another typical aspect of this picture.

Computer studies from the University of Pennsylvania estimated the risk of such a complication in patients following pinning for femoral neck fractures is 1 in 20 patients. To avoid this complication, pins should be inserted just above the lesser trochanter, and no empty holes should be left behind. If an empty hole cannot be filled with another pin or even a shorter pin, the patient should be carefully ambulated, non-weight-bearing, for at least 8 weeks.

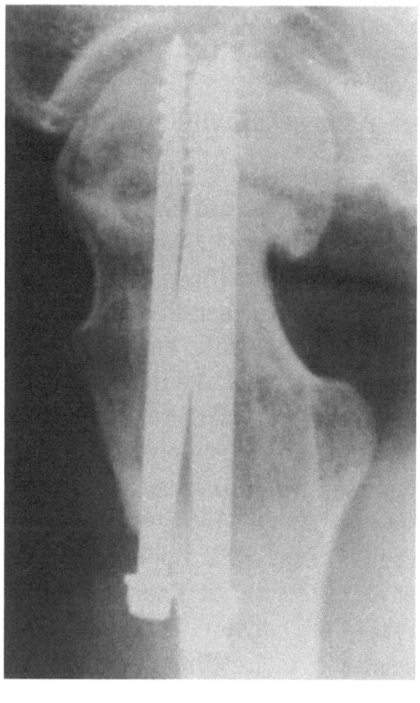

FIG. 8–102 A slightly displaced fracture with a good reduction and a good nailing still went on to necrosis.

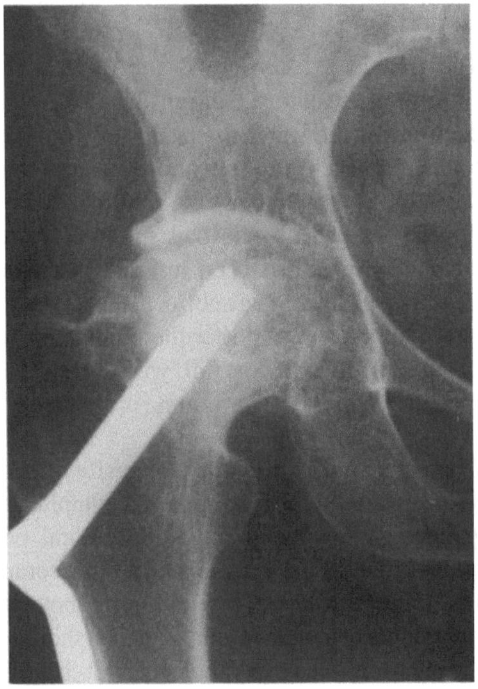

FIG. 8–103 Femoral head necrosis in a fractured femoral neck treated with a solid nail/side plate. Secondary arthritis finally brought the patient to a total hip replacement. Such massive devices may contribute to damaging a delicate network of vessels.

Unique Fracture Situations

Fractures Associated with Arthritis

It is a curious fact that fractures through the femoral neck in an arthritic hip are rare. Figure 8–70 illustrates one of these unusual fractures in an osteoarthritic hip joint. Figure 8–71 shows a patient with bilateral degenerative joint disease who has had a fracture, oddly enough, on the less involved side. Fractures in a rheumatoid hip joint are also uncommon. Hadden et al.[232] found that such complications were more frequent in patients with rheumatoid arthritis than in those with osteoarthritis, and that the former was more difficult to pin because of the softer bone. One could speculate that the osteoarthritic femoral neck is stronger because of the buildup of bone from the arthritic process, and in fact this point proved to be true[233] from a research study recently presented.

In this author's experience such fractures should be treated with a total hip replacement because the acetabulum is abnormal enough to render anything else an unsatisfactory result.

Simultaneous Bilateral Fractures

Simultaneous fractures of the femoral neck are rare. They are sometimes seen in patients with renal failure who were on fluoride therapy.[234] Powell[235] collected 20 cases exclusively caused by electroconvulsive therapy. This author knows of one patient who suffered such an injury following a severe convulsion caused by meningeal irritation from an Amipaque myelogram. In another series Powell found eight cases resulting from severe trauma, such as falling from various heights. Figure 8–105 represents such a case of a nursing home patient. This pair of untreated fractures prompted management with bilateral hemiarthroplasties.

Most of the cases in the literature were markedly displaced unstable fractures which would be difficult to manage with bilateral pinnings. Therefore, hemiarthroplasties are favored. A total hip replacement is a viable option if there is a long life expectancy, because the procedure would outlast the conventional hemiarthroplasty.

Ipsilateral Fracture of the Femoral Neck and Shaft

Since the original description by Delaney and Street,[236] few reports of ipsilateral fracture of the femoral neck and shaft have been published, Fig. 8–106. Such fractures are usually the result of high-speed car or motorcycle accidents. They are more common than reports indicate. Moreover, in the past many were missed.[237,238] When such an oversight happens, it is a disaster. Attention has now been focused on this situation so that fewer are being missed. Any surgeon working with trauma victims routinely obtains x-ray films of all joints above and below the most obvious fracture, especially in the overdrugged or head-injured patient. The reason for the missed diagnosis is that the usual external rotation deformity of the hip fracture is masked by the femoral shaft rotation.

MacKenzie[239] theorized on the mechanism of injury. He noted that there is a longitudinal compression along the axis of the femur with the hip in a position of abduction. Therefore when

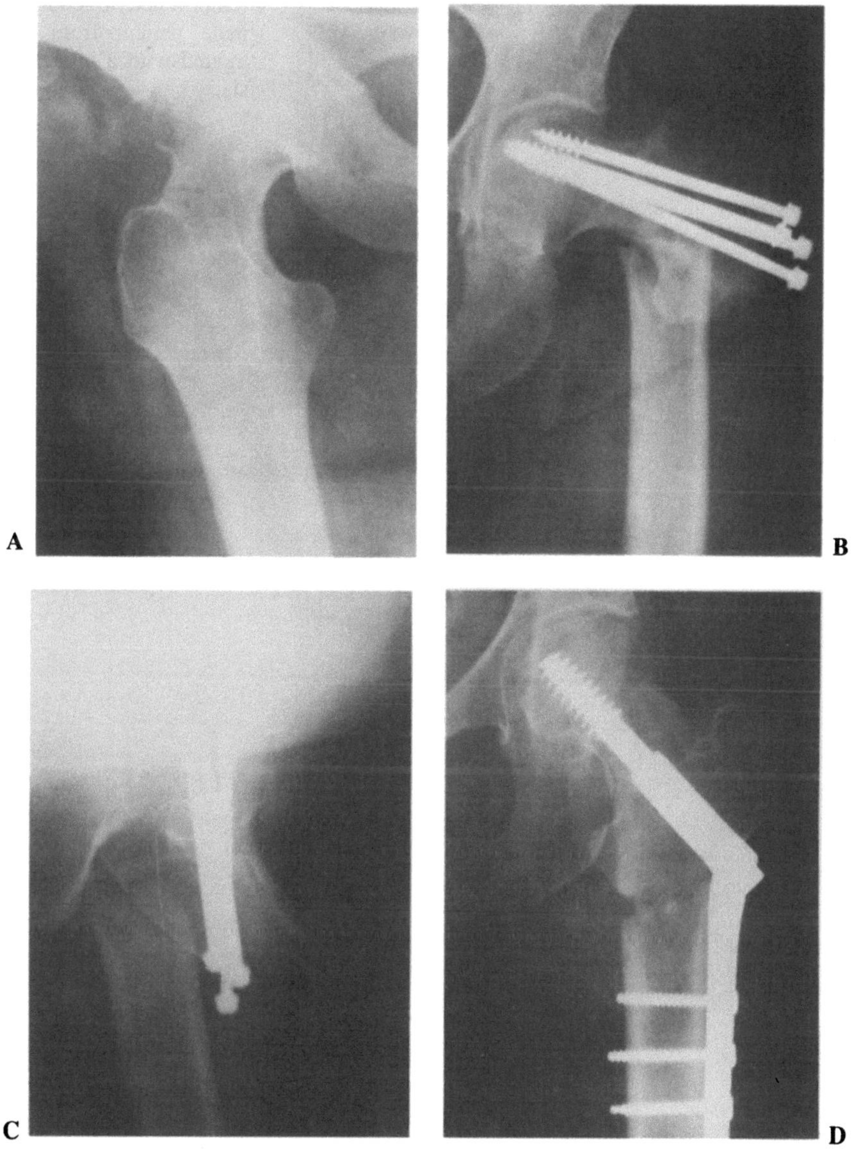

FIG. 8–104 **A** Stress fracture. **B** Treated with multiple pins. An empty pin hole was left at the level of the lesser trochanter, which created a stress riser resulting in a subtrochanteric fracture **(C)**. **D** The complication was treated with a compression screw and a bone graft.

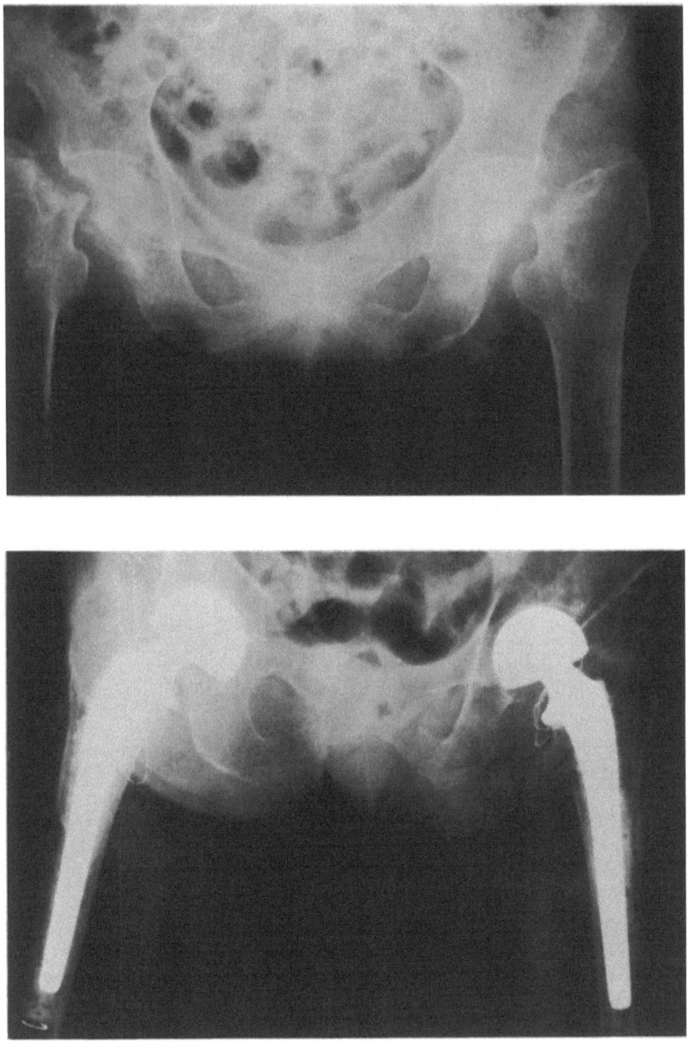

FIG. 8–105 Simultaneous bilateral femoral neck fractures in an elderly female patient from a nursing home treated with a universal head prosthesis.

the hip is forcefully adducted it becomes locked in the acetabulum. If all of the energy is not dissipated at the femoral fracture, a fracture–dislocation of the hip occurs or the femoral neck snaps. Fractures should also be sought in the patella.[236,237] Another mechanism may be simply a double injury, one at impact and the other when the person is catapulted from the car.

Treatment can be complicated especially if the shaft fracture is compounded. If it is a grade III injury, skeletal traction or external fixation may be needed. The neck fracture is usually displaced. Oddly enough, this fracture is one of the more stable types which can and should be reduced as soon as possible and fixed internally. The best overall results ensue when both fractures are internally fixed. There are several options, one of which should be performed as soon as possible.

1. Skeletal traction can be applied until all problems are stabilized.
2. The shaft fracture is fixed first so that the neck fracture can be manipulated into a satisfactory reduction; usually both are treated at the same operation.
   a. A closed curved Küntscher rod followed by Knowles pins are placed on either side of the intramedullary rod.[240] Swinotkowski et al.[240] favor pinning the femoral shaft retrograde first through the medial femoral condyle, followed by pinning the hip fracture. In other cases they fixed the hip first and then rodded the shaft. They presented a protocol

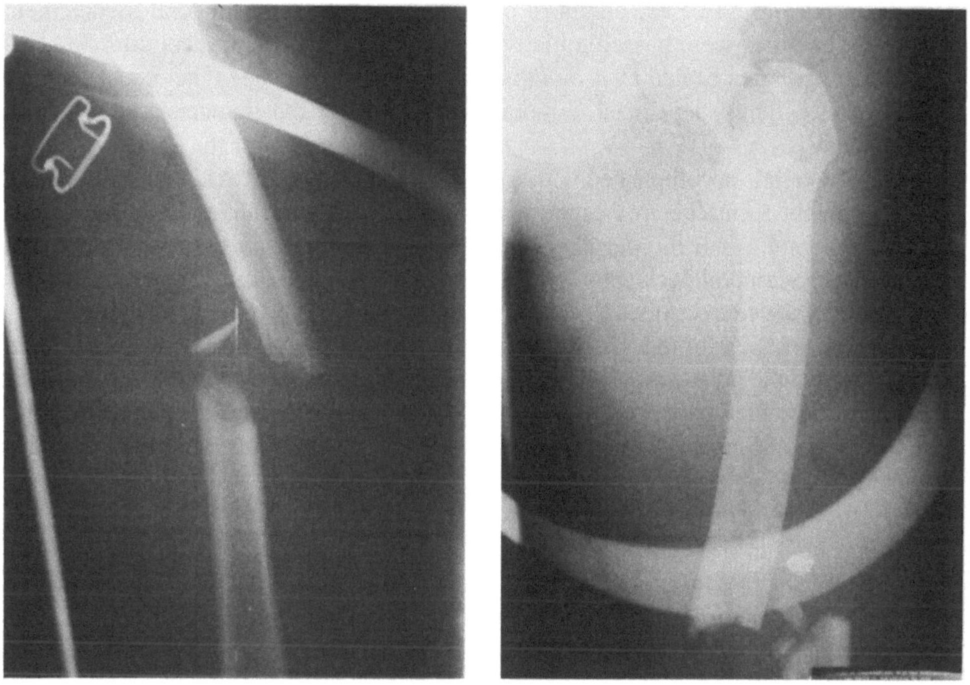

A

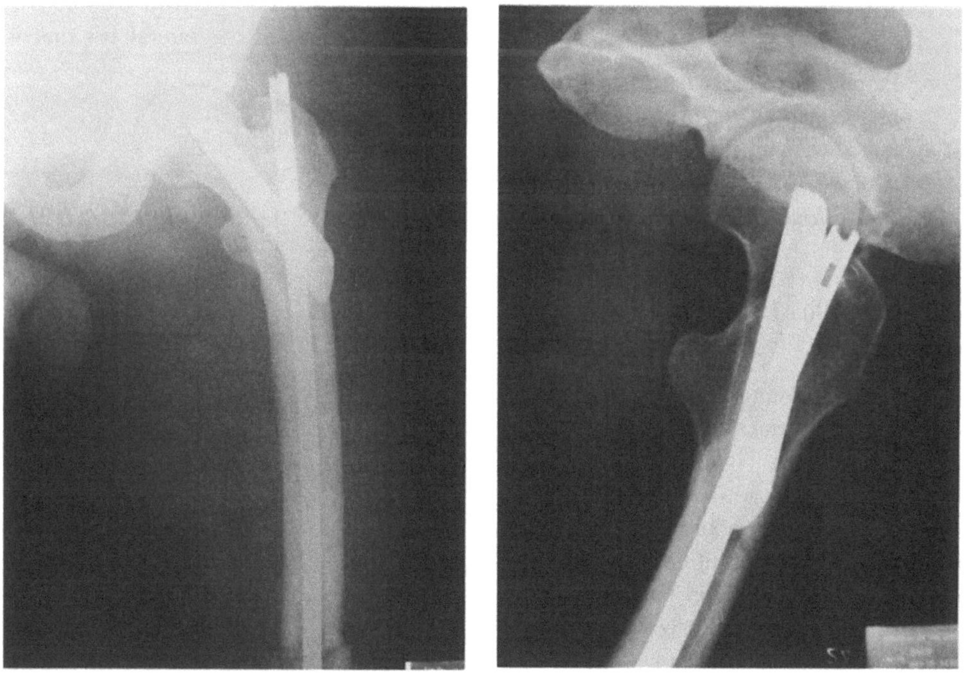

B

FIG. 8–106 **A** Femoral shaft fracture on the same side as a femoral neck fracture, a frequently missed combination. One tip-off is that the upper shaft fracture is adducted. All femoral shaft fractures should have an x-ray study of the upper end in order to avoid missing a femoral neck fracture and/or a hip dislocation. **B** Same case as in Fig. 8–106A fixed by the special Küntscher rod and nail. (Biomet Corp.)

based on their accumulated experience. In their series of 83 cases, one-third of the neck fractures were missed initially. All of the fractures healed by 4 months. Only two patients developed femoral head necrosis.

b. Open reduction is accomplished with either a straight Küntscher rod especially made to accept a nail through the steel shaft into the femoral neck (Fig. 8–106) or a similar device developed by Zickel.
c. Ender rods are used for the shaft without going up into the greater trochanter, followed by Knowles pins, Figure 8–185.
d. A compression hip screw into the neck fracture with a long side plate is used to fix the shaft fracture. This has the least appeal. The shaft fracture must be high for adequate fixation by the plate, and screws for the femoral neck are not as effective as multiple pins, although there are strong devotees for this method.

Caution: Patients with these fractures are often younger people, and both the femoral neck and the shaft are narrower and less resilient than one may be accustomed to, so it may be necessary to ream the femur widely.

Hip Dislocation Plus Femoral Neck Fracture

Hip dislocation plus femoral neck fractures are rare and complex injuries. (Refer to Chapter 5 by Mears and Rubash.) They are called Pipkin grade IV fracture dislocations. Epstein[74] and Pipkin [71] wrote extensively about them. These injuries require open reduction of both the acetabulum and the femoral neck. The latter should be pinned rather than having a hemiarthroplasty, as most of these injuries are in young patients.

Postirradiation Fractures

Fractures of the femoral neck can appear after the patient has been treated for a pelvic malignancy. Fractures may occur in the acetabulum as well but are seen more frequently in the femoral neck.[241–243] They are found most often in women with an average age of 58 who have undergone irradiation for cervical carcinoma. There is a high incidence (40%) of bilateral involvement. Symptoms appear 3 to 20 years after irradiation. The usual interval between the onset of symptoms and treatment for the fracture is about 3 months due to the meagerness of the symptoms. Any middle-aged woman with a history of irradiation who presents with an unheralded onset of aching in her groin, inner knee, or thigh, or even vague sciatica should be carefully checked for a femoral neck fracture by bone scan, laminagram, or a magnetic resonance imaging (MRI) study. Occasionally these symptoms have been ignored, and the patient presents with sudden pain unassociated with trauma, in which case the fracture has become displaced.

An irregular transverse density across the neck is the earliest x-ray sign. It may look like a stress fracture, incomplete in the lateral neck with sclerosis and only slight separation (Fig. 8–107). A complete fracture does not have the distinctly sharp borders of an acute traumatic fracture. Interestingly, the fracture may have some slight varus but little if any of the lateral tilt that is typical

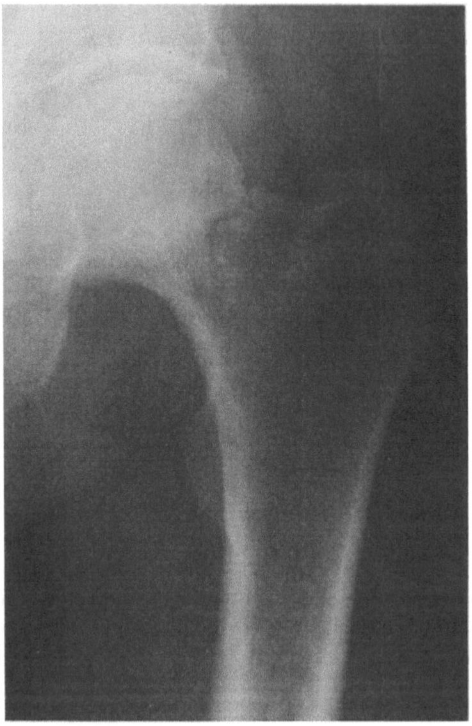

Fig. 8–107 An example of an irradiation fracture with fuzzy borders and no displacement.

of traumatic fractures. This picture is most likely due to the fact that there is no fragmentation of the posterior cortex. The differential diagnosis requires distinguishing it from a fracture through a metastatic lesion. Bone scans, CT scans, and MRI help in the diagnosis.

Pathologically there is an increase in the blood supply, as found by Stephenson and Cohen.[244] They also found a loss of trabecular bulk associated with a loss of cellular elements. Bonfiglio[241] estimated that the amount of radiation these patients receive is less than that which would cause devitalization, thereby accounting for the microscopic evidence of good healing properties. He and his colleagues thought that these fractures are similar to stress fractures; that is, the metabolism of the irradiated bone is sufficiently affected to cause the trabeculae to be so weakened that they cannot withstand the normal shearing stresses of daily activity.

Treatment is geared toward the stage of the condition. If there is significant displacement, total hip replacement is recommended as the acetabulum will have been affected enough to require acetabular reconstruction. If there is minimal displacement, pinning in situ is sufficient because complete healing can be anticipated.

Because there is a high percentage of bilateral disease, one is obligated to keep careful surveillance over the opposite hip.

Femoral Neck Fractures Complicating Metastatic Disease

Metastasis to the upper end of the femur is common, comprising 30 to 50% of all pathological fractures.[245–252] Impending fractures of the femoral neck are common. It is important to treat them early, as the results are better and complications are less, thereby increasing the survival rate.[252] The quality of life can be much improved with aggressive management.

Bone cement, used to fill defects and firmly fix the implant in bone, has been a milestone in orthopedics. Once the bone cracks, the situation changes dramatically because a more extensive operation is then needed and more pain is experienced than may have been necessary. Figure 8–108 illustrates a fracture that was allowed to break through, which is indicative of a far-advanced lesion. Note the uncharacteristic anterior tilt to the femoral neck fracture.

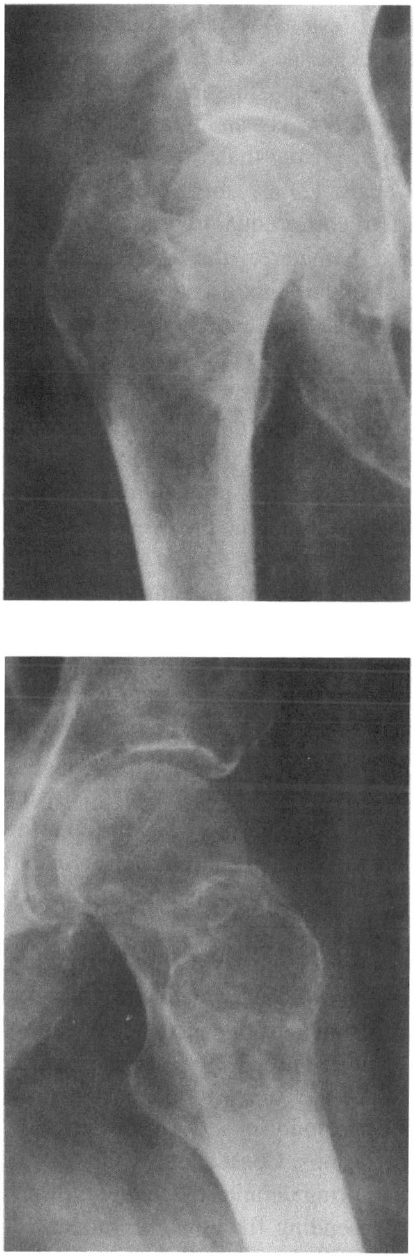

FIG. 8–108 Pathological fracture within the metaphysis of the upper femur going into the neck. *Note* that the head has rolled out in a direction opposite to the typically anterior oriented apex, which is typically seen in the uncomplicated femoral neck fracture.

Cameron et al.[253] recommended prophylactic pinning of lesions which occupy more than 50% of the neck. Lane et al.[252,254] developed a set of criteria for endoprosthetic replacement in the impending lesion: (1) an intramedullary lytic area equal to or greater than 50% of the cross-section of the shaft; (2) a painful lytic lesion involving a length of cortex equal to or more than the cross-sectional diameter of the bone or more than 2.5 cm in the axial length; and (3) a lesion in which pain is unrelieved after a therapeutic dose of radiation.

Murray and Parrish[246] outlined their preoperative plan: (1) The patient's condition must be sufficiently good and life expectancy long enough to justify the surgical procedure. (2) The surgeon must be convinced that the operation is more beneficial than closed treatment. (3) The quality of bone, both proximal and distal to the fracture, should be adequate for stable fixation. (4) The procedure must expedite mobilization of the patient and the reduction of pain or facilitate nursing care significantly. The use of methylmethacrylate has improved the treatment of metastatic lesions considerably.[247–252,254] It has made the use of either a hemiarthroplasty or a total hip arthroplasty more attractive than pinning. If there is any involvement, total hip replacement is best with the lesion filled with cement and reinforced with Steinmann pins as outlined by Harrington.[249]

An overview of the treatment program of these fractures from a major cancer center can be gained from a review article by Lane et al.[252] They reported that the survival rate is increasing with improved techniques and earlier detection of impending lesions. Consequently, the number of patients requiring definitive treatment for pathological or impending fractures has increased. Some 15 to 20% of patients with metastatic disease exhibit identifiable bone metastases during their lifetime. For disseminated breast cancer this figure rises to as high as 60%, or 85% of autopsy cases. Pathological fractures appear in 10 to 15% of patients with x-ray-proved lesions in bone.

About 1.5% of breast cancer patients eventually develop a pathological hip fracture. When they occur, they are particularly debilitating because they cause pain and interfere with walking, which causes further emotional deterioration of their delicate self-image and makes nursing care difficult.

Lane et al.'s patients were all treated at the Memorial Hospital for Cancer & Allied Diseases in New York. The results of 65 consecutive cases were reported. Lane et al. believed that the key to success was use of a long-stem bipolar prosthesis fixed with cement. This approach allowed immediate stability of the fracture site, with subsequent improvement or at least maintenance of ambulatory status in most of the patients. In three cases the lesions were bilateral. The predominant tumor was breast carcinoma (46%, 30 patients), followed by genitourinary and lung cancers; others were sarcomas, multiple myeloma, chronic lymphocyctic leukemia, gastrointestinal tumors, schwannomas, and sweat gland carcinomas. The metastic bone lesion fracture sites were: 34 femoral neck, 17 intertrochanter, and 16 subtrochanter. All but five patients were treated with long-stem bipolar prostheses; the others were treated with long-stem total hip replacement because of acetabular and femoral shaft involvement. All prostheses were cemented. The median survival rate was 7.1%: 86% lived 1 month, 81% lived 2 months, 75% lived 3 months, 56% lived 6 months, 39% lived 12 months, and 16% lived 1 year. Those with breast carcinoma and genitourinary carcinoma survived an average of 12 months, whereas those with lung carcinoma lived only 4 months. Eighty-five percent regained their ability to walk independently or with a walker; 67% of the patients who were not walking prior to surgery were able to walk again.

In 1982 Lane et al. started to follow their patients' PaO_2 more closely and administered 100% oxygen during the cementing stage to compensate for the presumed fat embolus occurrence with methylmethacrylate injection. Serial PaO_2 evaluation during surgery demonstrated a 20 to 30 mm drop in PaO_2 within 10 minutes of cementing in the long-stem implant. Oxygen support, volume replacement, and copious irrigation during surgery brought the mortality rate down to 7% for the first month postoperatively.

The choice of fixation and repair remains unsettled. The use of long-stem implants allows removal of extensive tumor and bridging the gap. It is thought that a bipolar device lessens the wear on the acetabulum (a supposition which must be proved over a longer period of usage). None of the fractures in their series dislocated, nor did any have to be converted to a total hip replacement. Compression hip screws even when supplemented with cement have occasionally failed because of tumor progression beyond the screw and into the remaining head.

Behr et al.[255] studied an older population, averaging 70 years of age. These investigators surgically treated 48 impending or frank fractures. Forty-five percent of these patients had breast cancer, 24% had multiple myeloma, and 11% had lung carcinoma. Flexible rods were used in 64%. Supplemental cement was used in only 24% but is now being used routinely. The use of flexible rods was appealing in such an elderly debilitated population. Technically the method was considered quick and effective, with little blood loss and retaining the ability to institute radiation therapy over the otherwise untouched hip area. Furthermore, the extensively tumor-ridden, demineralized bone could be stress-shielded by the multiple rods. As many rods as possible are stacked in the medullary cavity to prevent upper and/or lower migration of the rod. Pain was relieved in 92% of the patients, and 84% became ambulatory. If the patient survived more than 2 months, the rate of fracture healing was 89%. Their overall survival was 9 months. Behr et al. concluded that the results were encouraging enough to recommend surgery despite their patient's advanced age.

Radiation therapy is not interfered with by the presence of an implant.

Parkinson's Disease

Patients suffering from Parkinson's disease have had high mortality and morbidity rates.[256] Drugs such as levodopa have improved the situation considerably. Because of the patients' tremors, few surgeons are enthusiastic about internal fixation. In anyone with a displaced fracture, a hemiarthroplasty fixed with cement does well if postoperative care is well managed to prevent a dislocation.

Rothermel and Garcia[257] achieved excellent restoration of function when a primary hemiarthroplasty was used for displaced unstable fractures. They found that if the patient's disease was well controlled by such drugs as levodopa, the indications for replacement prosthesis and early ambulation were the same as for the general public. A study from Israel confirmed their recommendations.[258] Early mobilization is the key factor in preventing the many complications that can easily plague these patients.

Spastic Hemiplegia

Fracture of the femoral neck can occur in patients who have had a stroke. It can occur as a complication of the vascular accident. It more commonly happens later when muscular weakness takes its toll along with demineralization and spastic leg deformities. At this stage the spastic limb is more prone to fracture. Because of the spasticity and the contractures, any attempt at reduction is futile. This author[55] and others [259,260] had recommended a primary hemiarthroplasty. The use of acrylic cement has made the procedure even more successful. It is usually not a routine arthroplasty because there must be extensive soft tissue release for better exposure and to keep the hip from dislocating postoperatively.

The most notable correction is for an adductor contracture, which is done with a tenotomy prior to the primary surgical exposure. Any flexion contracture that is present must also be corrected at surgery. The psoas tendon should be released routinely and a wide anterior and posterior capsulectomy done.

These patients must be carefully kept protected in abduction for up to 6 weeks. One of the newer abduction braces should be available immediately postoperatively. Several manufacturers make them as stock items that can be applied to the thigh with plaster to ensure a more dependable grasp of the thigh. They even have adjustable flexion hinges.

Paget's Disease

Femoral neck fracture in a pagetoid femur is less common than fractures in the intertrochanteric or subtrochanteric area.[261] Such fractures develop more commonly in the earlier vascular phase when the bone is softer.[262] It is a formidable type of pathological fracture. Nonunions are common, occurring in up to 75% of cases.[263,264] Such a complication is more typical of the sclerotic phase of the disease. The bone is so hard that impaction of the fragments is difficult, frequently ending up with distraction so that a good reduction is difficult to achieve and firm fixation a struggle to maintain. Because of this complication, hemiarthroplasty is recommended. In one study 78% of the prosthetic patients returned to their preoperative status.[264]

Prosthetic replacement is not as successful in the pagetoid patient as in others. Technical problems are considerable because of the exuberant bleeding and because of the hard bone, which requires laborious reaming. If there is any acetabular involvement, total hip replacement should be performed, as recommended by Stauffer and Sim[264] and DeLee.[36] Only the strictly undisplaced fractures are considered appropriate for pinning. Predrilling with special long drill bits may be necessary. These bits can be "special-ordered" from almost any of the manufacturers. Cementing the prosthesis is highly recommended.

Patients with Renal Failure

Renal osteodystrophy refers to a syndrome of metabolic abnormalities occurring in azotemic patients, especially those on renal dialysis. These patients are at a high risk for fractures in the upper femur. Thornhill and Creasman[265] reported on 48 hip fractures in 43 patients. The patients' mean age of 62 is 10 years younger than that of the general population with similar fractures. Associated trauma was a significant parameter. All of the patients with intertrochanteric fractures[12] had a history of experiencing some form of trauma. All of the fractures healed, but they did so slowly, taking as long as 12 months for union.

Femoral neck fractures were distinctly different. Only about one-third of these patients had some trauma, which was minor, and the rest had no history of trauma, although they did experience some vague ache a few days before the spontaneous onset of the fracture. All neck fractures displaced into varus. Thirty-seven percent of the patients died shortly after the fracture. No one lived long enough to develop clinical necrosis of the head. Eleven neck fractures treated with some form of pinning failed, with a loss of reduction and nonunion. Each in the atraumatic group[14] treated with either nonoperative management[3] or pinning[11] failed. Five of the 15 fractures treated with an endoprosthesis had to have a revision. A primary total hip replacement should be performed on these patients.

These patients can develop secondary hyperparathyroidism and osteomalacia, and so their vitamin D and calcium stores must be maintained. They can also develop refractory osteomalacia due to deposition of iron from multiple transfusions and to aluminum deposits from the dialysis solutions.

Trochanteric Fractures

Lesser Trochanteric Fractures

Fractures of the lesser trochanter are usually avulsion injuries that are generally seen in teenagers who are engaged in competitive sports (Fig. 8–4). They are caused by a forceful contracture of the iliopsoas muscle, which is attached to the lesser trochanteric apophysis. It is an acute injury that produces pain on flexion. It can also occur in an elderly patient as a complication of severe osteoporosis. In either age group it is a rare lesion.

There is tenderness in the femoral triangle. Pain is reproduced with resistance against hip flexion. When there is complete separation of the apophysis, the Ludloff sign is positive. This sign is elicited by having the patient in a seated position so as to demonstrate his inability to lift his leg off the ground, indicating iliopsoas insufficiency. In the most common form the separation is incomplete. Treatment in these cases is bed rest, sometimes for 3 to 4 weeks, with the hip flexed and "iced down" for comfort.

If there is a wide separation with a positive Ludloff sign, open reduction and reattachment with a malleolar AO screw are necessary to restore better flexion without a prolonged period of disability. In the elderly patient with limited demands of the iliopsoas, simple rest in a chair is usually sufficient treatment for fibrous union.

Isolated Lesser Trochanteric Fractures Without Trauma

A unique situation exists when there is no trauma associated with a fracture of the lesser trochanter. *It can be the first manifestation of an otherwise unrecognized metastatic malignancy.* Bertin et al. highlighted this unique syndrome. Their comprehensive report can be reviewed for more details.[266] This fracture is uncommon at any age but especially in adults, so great suspicion should be aroused when it is seen. It may well herald the presence of a metastatic malignancy. For treatment to be effective its importance must be recognized early. The diagnostic evaluation should include a bone scan, tomography, and a computed tomography (CT) scan. A biopsy may have to be done to prove its malignant contents. If so, it should be performed through the medial approach of Ludloff (see Vol. I, p. 111). The biggest threat is to have the fracture convert to a subtrochanteric fracture. Should the lesion be allowed to enlarge beyond the medial femoral cortex, a subtrochanteric fracture will evolve. A subtrochanteric fracture through a pathologic lesion is a serious complication because it is difficult to reduce. Strong internal fixation is needed and supplemented with methylmethacrylate. For these reasons early internal fixation is strongly recommended.

Greater Trochanteric Fractures

Isolated fractures of the greater trochanter are uncommon but are more frequently seen than those of the lesser bone. When an isolated incident it is benign, but it may disguise an intertrochanteric fracture, which may appear suddenly as a displaced fracture when its obtuse existence is left unsuspected.

This fracture assumes two variations: It may be an avulsion fracture from a sudden abductor pull that is triggered when a patient braces to prevent a fall (Fig. 8–3). This form usually responds to bed rest and crutch walking gauged on an individualized basis. The other, more common, variety occurs from a direct fall or from a direct blow to the lateral side of the hip. Bed rest may be needed for 2 to 3 weeks with the patient keeping the leg abducted as much as possible for comfort. The symptoms may take longer to abate than the situation seems to warrant. The second type should be monitored carefully for any associated intertrochanter fracture component. A laminogram is done to clarify its true nature.

Intertrochanteric Fractures

An intertrochanteric fracture is one of two major fractures of the hip joint. In our series of 200 consecutive hip fractures, this type comprised 56% of all diagnoses. In some series these patients are about 3 years older as a group than those in the femoral neck group. In our group there was no age difference.

The outlook for intertrochanteric fractures has improved steadily as they became grouped into a more sophisticated system based on their behavior patterns. Improvements in fixation have been made, greatly brightening their potential outcome.

Kyle et al.[267] analyzed 622 fractures both retrospectively and prospectively. They modified Massie's classification, which is now known as the Kyle classification. They compared their results using a solid nail (Jewett) with those using a sliding device in the form of a Massie nail. In the latter group early weight-bearing, anticoagulation, and prophylactic antibiotics were used. The mortality rate dropped from 12% to 4%. These authors had an overall "good" result in 96% of their cases compared with an 80% rate in the early series. They had a nonunion rate of 2%, an infection rate of 2%, and an avascular necrosis rate of 0.8%. Any report today would have to refer to their work as a benchmark study. As one would expect, nail penetration in the joint occurred in 11% with a Jewett nail and in 2% with the Massie nail (the barrel was too long, preventing the nail from fully collapsing, thus piercing the neck fragment.)

A working classification is essential to the true understanding of these fractures. An important parameter toward this end is the type of fracture based on behavioral patterns in relation to the type of fixation and reduction needed. The early classifications were based on how the fracture behaved when fixed with a solid nail and/or sideplate.[268,269] Evans coined the idea of "stable" and "unstable" fractures (Fig. 8–109). Boyd and Griffin around the same time grouped fractures by their difficulty in reduction, with the most difficult type being a combination of intertrochanteric and subtrochanteric fractures[270,271] (Fig. 8–110). Massie appreciated the fact that the outcome of unstable fractures could be improved with the use of his collapsible nail.[272] The Kyle or Hennepin County Hospital classification is a further refinement of the Massie concepts[267] (Fig. 8–111). Cram at the University of Pennsylvania was the first to describe a method of managing unstable fractures by pushing the distal fragment under the neck as a means of stabilizing the fracture complex.[273] His method was to be described later as "medial displacement." An oversimplified description of an unstable fracture came from Dimon and Hughston[274] (Fig. 8–112). They subcategor-

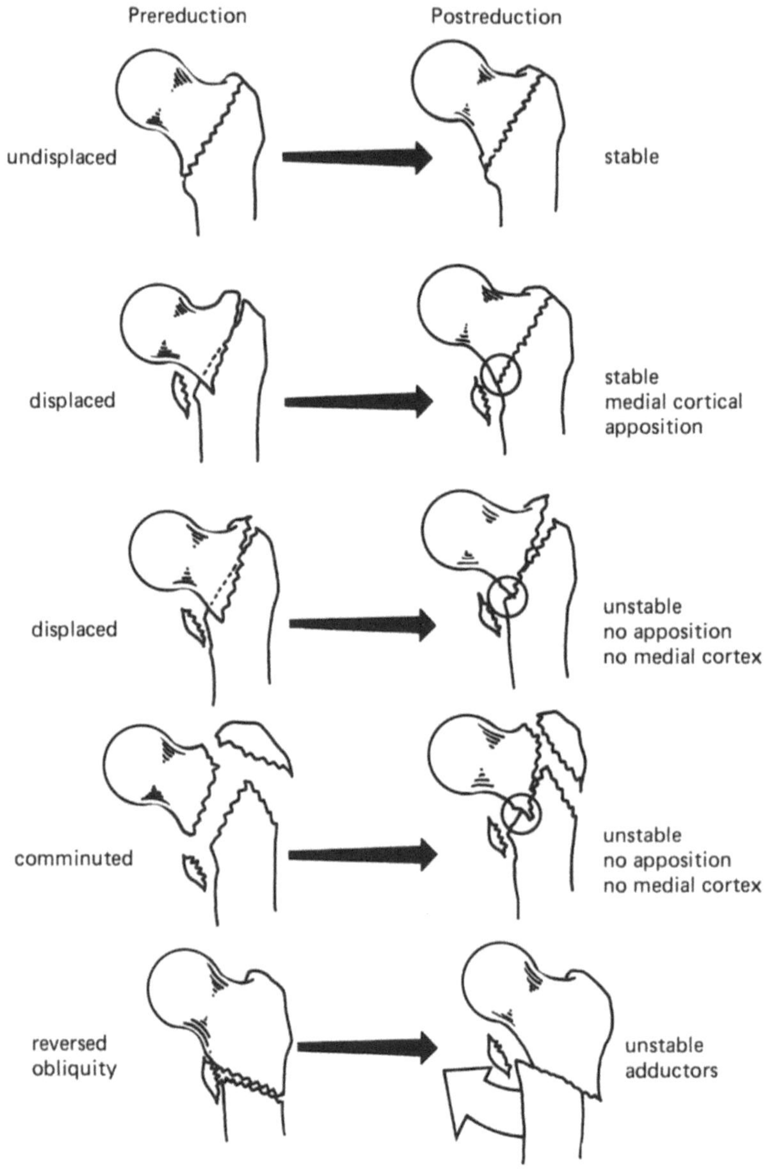

FIG. 8–109 Evan's classification into stable and unstable groups. When the medial cortex is comminuted, instability can be expected to cause failure of fixation and loss of reduction. The classification does not fully appreciate the important role of posterior comminution in producing instability. (Adapted from Dohee.[36])

FIG. 8–111 The Kyle or Hennepin County Hospital classification clarified Massie's expansion of Evan's classification. Types I and II are stable fractures, undisplaced and displaced with a little comminution; types III and IV are unstable with increasing comminution at the medial cortex. (Adapted from Kyle, J. A., Gustillo, R. B., Premer, R. F.: An analysis of 622 intertrochanteric hip fractures. J. Bone Joint Surg., 61A:216, 1979).

FIG. 8–110 Boyd and Griffin's classification is based on the ease or difficulty of obtaining a reduction. The most difficult fracture to reduce is type IV in which there is a subtrochanteric component. ▶

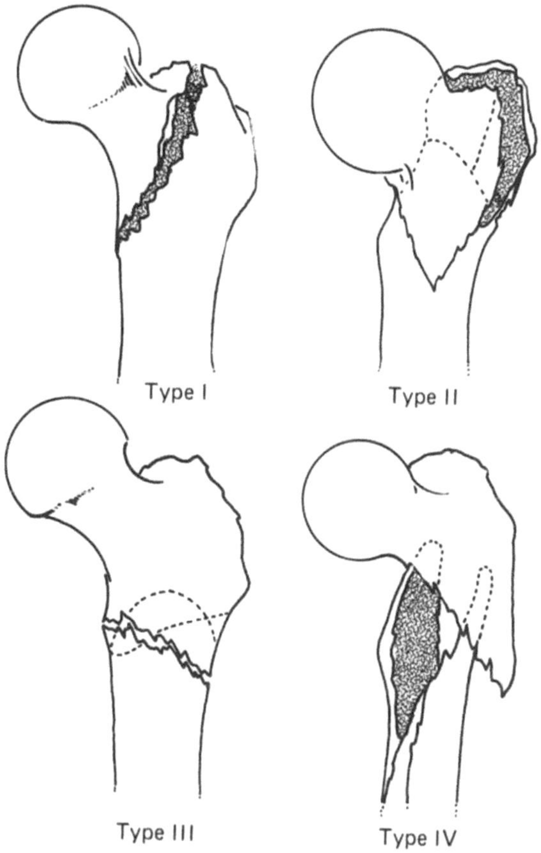

ized the fracture using simple numbered parts and coined the term "four-part fracture." Their medial displacement osteotomy (Fig. 8–113) was made necessary only while the use of solid nails (Jewett types) were in vogue for fixation of these fractures. A short, solid Jewett nail became a necessary part of the displacement osteotomy. This idea is fine if one still uses a solid nail and side-plate, but it has no relevance when such a fracture is fixed with a sliding nail where the fracture is allowed to medially displace itself spontaneously, or to telescope upon itself, as described by Tronzo[55] (Fig. 8–114). The latter is accomplished without the added morbidity and technical gymnastics of an artificial osteotomy. As the advantages and improvements of the compression hip screw expanded, and as more understanding of the anatomy of the trochanteric fracture was appreciated, a functional classification emerged from Tronzo.[55,275] The author's newest refined version is presented in this section. Its

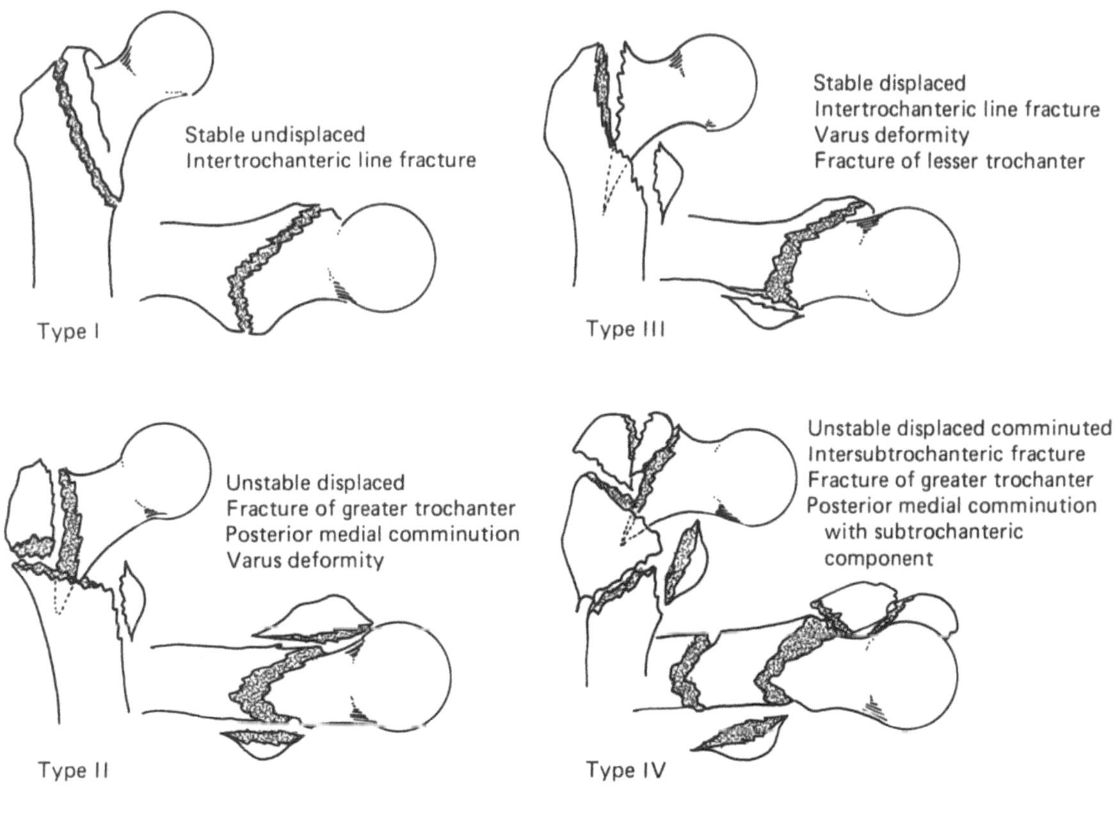

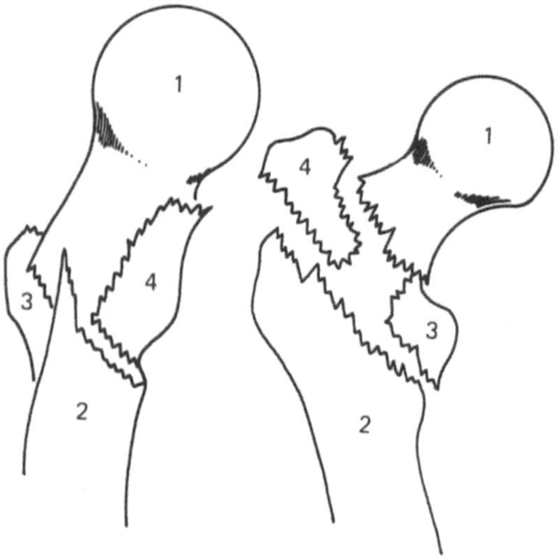

FIG. 8–112 Dimon and Hughston's "four-part" fracture concept for identifying the composition of an unstable fracture. (Adapted from Dimon, J. H., Hughston, J. C.: Unstable intertrochanteric fractures of the hip. J. Bone Joint Surg., 49:440, 1967.)

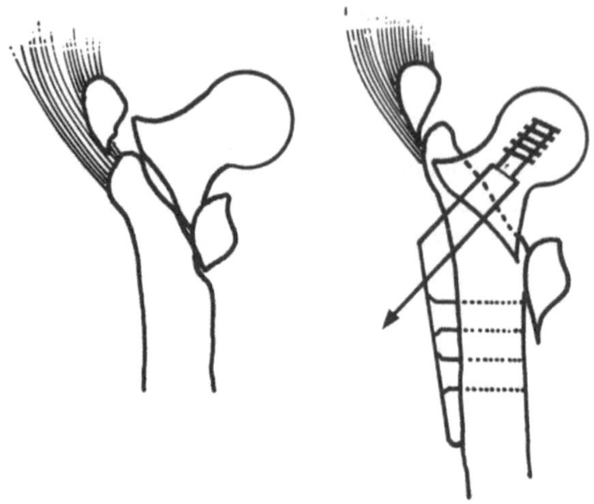

FIG. 8–114 Tronzo's telescoped reduction for spontaneous stabilization *without an osteotomy* as a feature of the compression hip screw system.

intended use is to help the surgeon (1) predict the behavior of any given intertrochanteric fracture when an open reduction is planned and (2) understand what mechanics will render the fracture stable once fixed.

Upper Femoral Anatomy

The following observations have been made at the operating table during open reductions and arthroplasties for fresh femoral neck fractures. The *capsule* and *iliofemoral ligament* play important roles in the fragmentation patterns in intertrochanteric fractures. These two structures blend together to form a strong buttress anteriorly as they are attached superiorly at the acetabulum and distally to a distinct ridge of bone along the intertrochanteric line (Fig. 8–115A). In a husky normal man this combined mass can be as thick as 10 mm. Posteriorly the anatomy at the base of the neck is quite different. The iliofemoral ligament does not attach to any such ridge of bone. It becomes rolled up into a thick, tough ring called the *zona orbicularis,* which acts like a sling or noose around the femoral neck (Fig. 8–31B). The capsule anteriorly blends into the iliofemoral ligament but becomes distinct posteriorly as it passes under the ligament and slightly

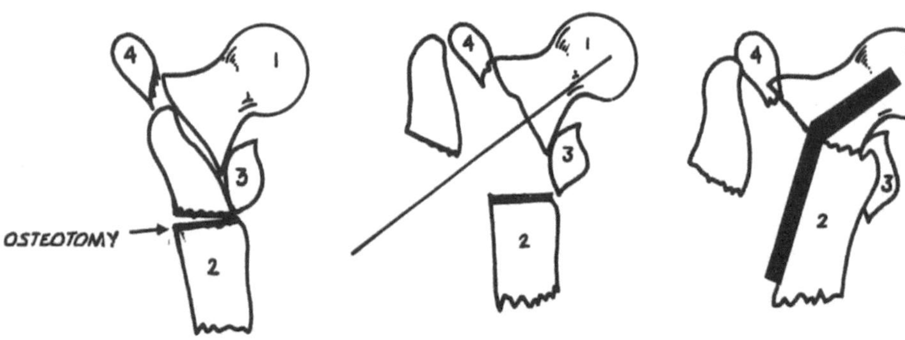

FIG. 8–113 Dimon and Hughston's medial displacement osteotomy necessitated by use of the Jewett nail. Modern-day collapsible screws have changed this concept by obviating further morbidity created by such additional surgery.

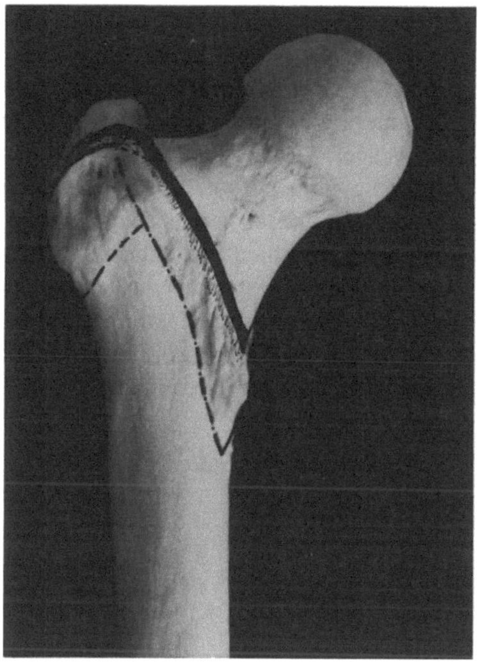

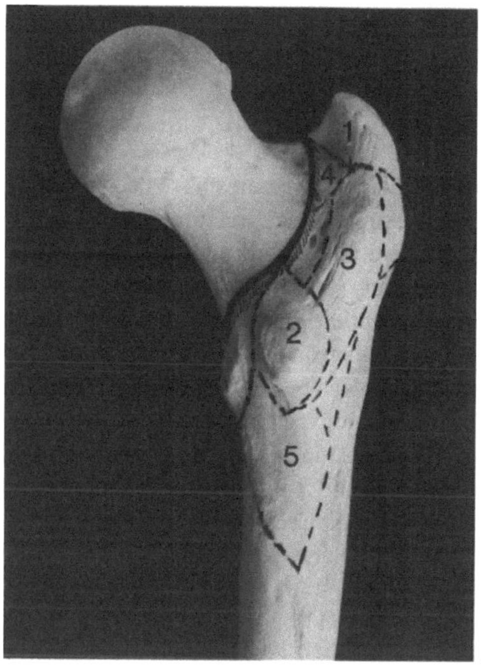

FIG. 8–115 **A** Anterior anatomy of the upper femur shows a thick, roughened ridge of bone where the tough iliofemoral ligament attaches. It constitutes the intertrochanteric line. The solid line follows the intracapsular portion of stable fractures. The broken line indicates the extracapsular portion of the fracture. **B** Posterior osteology of the upper femur. 1, Greater trochanter. 2, Lesser trochanter. 3, Trochanteric crest connecting the posterior overhang of the greater trochanter and the posteriorly placed lesser trochanter. 4, Periformis fossa. 5, Medial extension of the iliofemoral ligament, an all important postero-medial cortical wall.

beyond to attach to the periosteum at the midportion of the neck. For this reason the front of the femoral neck is completely covered and protected by the capsule and ligament, whereas posteriorly its distal part is uncovered and unprotected. The important ligamentous anatomy allows a wide range of circumferential motion in flexion but locks it almost completely when the leg is extended. The stand-up stance therefore is stable, whereas the bent or flexed stance is much less so. If a person's leg is forced beyond the 180° of extension the upper femur fractures, but when forced into flexion it is nearly impossible to fracture.

Half of the greater trochanter is posterior, while the entire lesser trochanter sets posteriorly. The posterior bone that connects the two trochanters is a smooth, rounded hump called the *trochanteric crest* (Fig. 8–115B). It is important to realize that its cortical wall is thin and much weaker than its anterior counterpart because it is unstressed by any ligamentous strains. On the other side, though, the mass of bone that extends from the base of the lesser trochanter around anteriorly to the greater trochanter is a thick, strong cortical ridge called the linea intertrochanterica, the *intertrochanteric line* (Fig. 8–115A). In a stripped-down cadaver specimen it is a jagged ridge where the capsule and iliofemoral ligament tenaciously attach (Fig. 8–115A). The lesser trochanter sits posteriorly on the shaft as an eccentric cantilever for pull of the iliopsoas tendon (see Fig. 8–32). The tendon acts like a bowstring across this part of the upper femur pulling it into a flexed position which fractured.

All of these anatomical characteristics of the femoral neck and upper trochanteric area come together, causing it to buckle posteriorly with varying degrees of comminution. Torsional stresses added to a direct blow against the greater trochanter produce an intertrochanteric fracture. The trochanteric crest explodes with various configurations of comminution. The severity of the explosion and the amount of extension into and around the lesser trochanter and trochanteric crest determine the degree of inherent stability of any given fracture (Fig. 8–115B). Comminution around the greater trochanter is relatively insignificant because it is not a weight-bearing area.

Defining Fracture Types

All intertrochanteric fractures have been traditionally called extracapsular fractures, but it will be developed here that not all intertrochanteric fractures are purely outside the capsule. It is the author's conception that *stable* fractures are intracapsular, whereas *unstable* fractures are extracapsular. It can be shown at surgical exploration that the stable type fractures occur just proximal to the intertrochanteric line and lay well within the capsule anteriorly with only minor extracapsular comminution posteriorly (Fig. 8–116). These fractures are held captured within the strong ligamentous boundaries, similar to a Chinese finger trap, which makes them easy to reduce and fix. When the bone fractures just beyond the iliofemoral ligament (beyond the intertrochanteric line), the entire fracture becomes extracapsular. The fragments all lay outside the stabilizing influence of the iliofemoral ligament and capsule and so are unstable, rendering the fracture more difficult to reduce and fix. Simple traction does not spontaneously align the fragments; therefore instrumentation must be used to reduce them into a telescoping posture in order to render them a stable complex.

Characteristics of a Stable Fracture

Figure 8–116 depicts the following features of stable intertrochanteric fractures:

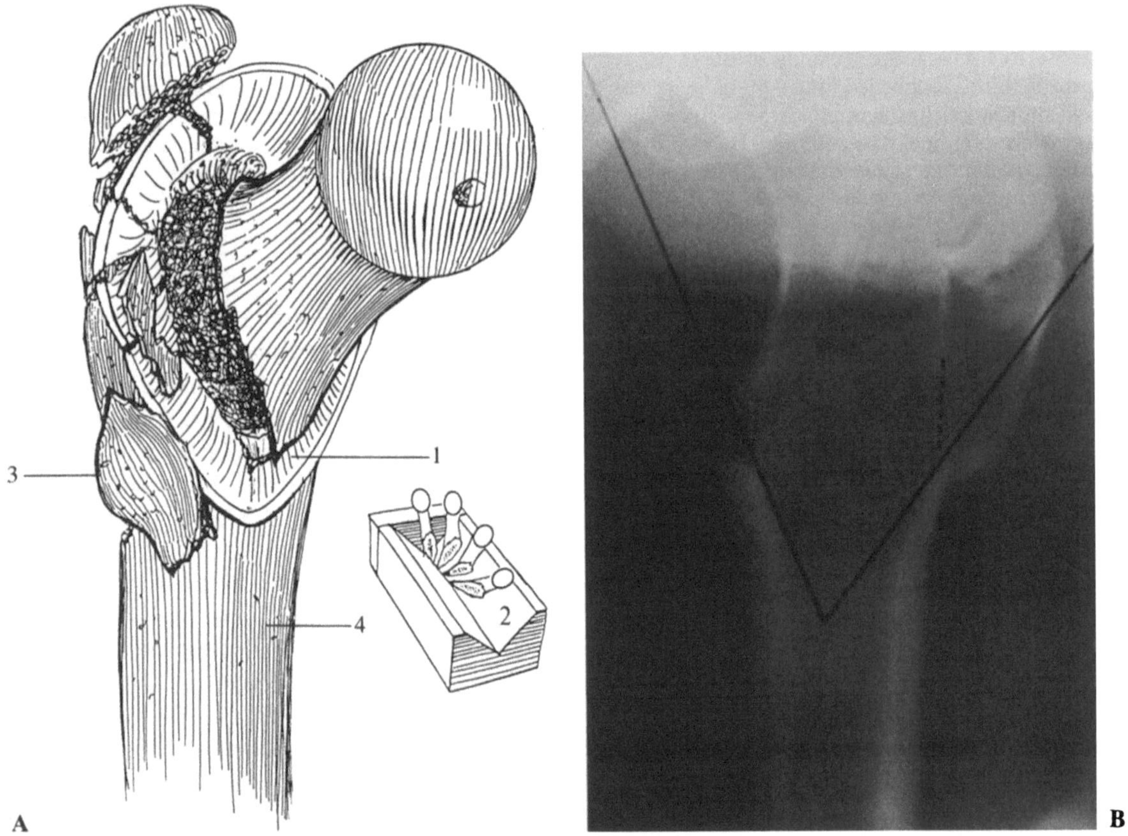

FIG. 8–116 **A** Characteristics of a stable intertrochanteric fracture: 1. The fracture occurs inside of the capsule. Even though the capsule is opened or unattached posteriorly, the main fracture complex lies within the boundaries of the capsular structures. 2. Lateral displacement is minimal but angulation into varying degrees of varus takes place within the confines of an unshattered medullary trough (inset). 3. The lesser trochanter is usually small because it simply pulls away from an intact medial cortex (4). **B** Lines are drawn to accentuate trough boundaries into which the neck remains confined. *Note* minimal posterior comminution.

1. The stable fracture is created proximal to the intertrochanteric line, keeping the main upper fragment inside the capsule (intracapsular). The capsule is open posteriorly but the fracture line passes within the confines of the capsular borders.
2. There is some displacement, but angulation in the anteroposterior (AP) view varies from minimal to marked varus. There is only slight angulation in the lateral view or coronal plane. NOTE: *The neck fragment does not shift laterally but only angulates with its apex anteriorly.*
3. The lesser trochanteric fragment is usually small and minimally displaced. It can be a long, oblique fragment without displacement. It merely comes off the surface of the cortical wall.
4. The posteromedial cortex remains a solid buttress because of the minimal posterior comminution. The proximal fragment remains in its femoral shaft trough where it remains confined by the intact anterior and posterior walls (Fig. 8–116B).
5. On the A/P x rays the neck appears as a short, oblique fragment with a blunted inferior beak due to its intracapsular rotation. Once reduced, it assumes its real orientation and appears sharper. Its fracture surface is fairly perpendicular, which makes reduction and impaction easy.
6. Only simple leg traction with internal rotation to neutral position is necessary to achieve a proper reduction. Direct manipulation of the fracture is seldom necessary. A limited exposure of the lateral cortex is all that is needed for the introduction of a fixation device. This fracture is inherently stable.

Stable Fracture Varieties Figure 8–117 is a diagrammatic composite of the five varieties of stable fractures which can be used as a reference atlas.

1. High intertrochanteric fractures (formerly called ''basicervical'' fractures) are seen in Fig. 8–117A, and 8–118. The neck fragment is short with a squared base breaking off just distal to the intertrochanteric line at the lesser trochanter. The greater trochanter may or may not be fractured. The lesser trochanter is intact. Mild to moderate varus with a degree of external rotation is characteristic. There is angulation with its apex *anterior* (Fig. 8–118C).

The reduction of these fractures can be tricky. First, the nail or screw must go all the way to the subchondral bone, otherwise the short neck fragment can easily lose its reduction by having the device cut out of the head. These fractures should never be treated with an Ender nail system. Second, the base of the fragment may have a sharp spike that can be trapped under the tendon of the iliopsoas (Fig. 8–119). Occasionally the tendon must be cut to allow the fragment to be adequately reduced before it can be pinned. To accomplish this the leg must be severely rotated externally to bring the lesser trochanter into view. This maneuver also serves to disengage the fragments. Internal rotation is then applied, without abduction, with straight traction. Occasionally direct force must be applied with an instrument on the neck to correct the angulation while it is being pinned.

2. Undisplaced fractures are straightforward enough (Fig. 8–117B). They are easily pinned in situ. Unlike their counterpart in neck fractures, they displace if not pinned or fixed (Fig. 8–120).

3. Minimal to moderately displaced fractures are shown in Fig. 8–117C. The neck fragment is seen in varus with varying degrees of angulation. The lesser trochanter is simply avulsed away from an intact cortex and may not be seen if the leg is severely rotated (Fig. 8–121). The greater trochanter is only slightly fragmented and displaced. Simple traction quickly pulls all the fragments together with the knee rotated into a neutral position. The fracture is quickly fixed through a short, lateral incision just below the trochanter.

4. The most common of the intertrochanteric fractures is shown in Fig. 8–117D and 8–122. The neck fragment is in marked varus and angulated, and both trochanters are obviously fractured. Its distinction is that the main posterior medial wall is intact. The lateral x-ray film shows the neck to be angulated but not displaced. The lesser trochanter is not a major fragment, and there is no significant comminution around it (Fig. 8–122B). This fracture is the most misunderstood of the intertrochanteric fractures and is frequently considered a treacherous unstable complex. It therefore undergoes mutilation by being inflicted with a ''displacement osteotomy.'' If traction is applied first in external rotation and then in internal rotation, the fracture reduces well. Heavy traction is unnecessary. With a compression hip screw in place, the fragments telescope or collapse

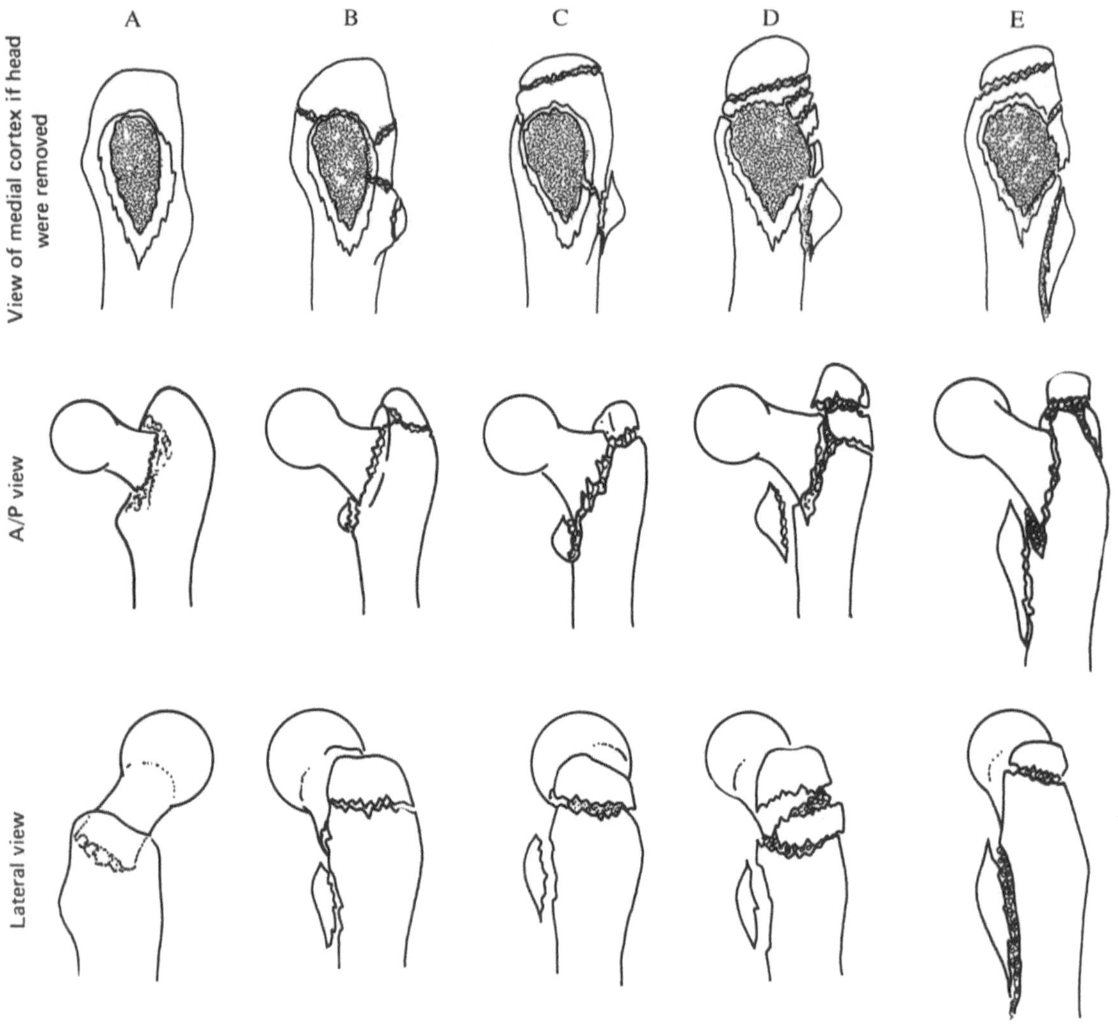

FIG. 8–117 Composite of five varieties of stable fractures. This illustration can serve as an atlas for a reference in analyzing x-rays.

on themselves with an automatic medial displacement. They become well impacted and stabilized.

5. Fractures in the group shown in Fig. 8–117E are uncommon. They look like a complicated unstable type because of the large size of the lesser trochanteric fragment, Figure 8–123. Note, however, that they are relatively undisplaced. The fractured bone splits away from the surface of the shaft only as an avulsion fragment, leaving the posterior medial wall unopened. When examined closely, all of the component fragments are relatively undisplaced in the lateral x-ray (Fig. 8–123C). With straight traction the angulation is fully corrected. The fracture is simply fixed through a straight lateral incision that exposes only the lateral cortex at the base of the greater trochanter.

Characteristics of an Unstable Fracture

Figure 8–124 is a sketch of unstable fracture characteristics.

1. The unstable fracture's line is distal to the intertrochanteric line, which places the main upper fragment outside the capsule (extracapsular.
2. Displacement is marked in both the coronal and sagittal planes (in both AP and lateral views). NOTE: The neck fragment typically shifts laterally to a significant degree as seen on the lateral x-ray film (Fig. 8–125). It also angulates and rotates with its long inferior beak pointing anteriorly as it makes a major shift (displacement).

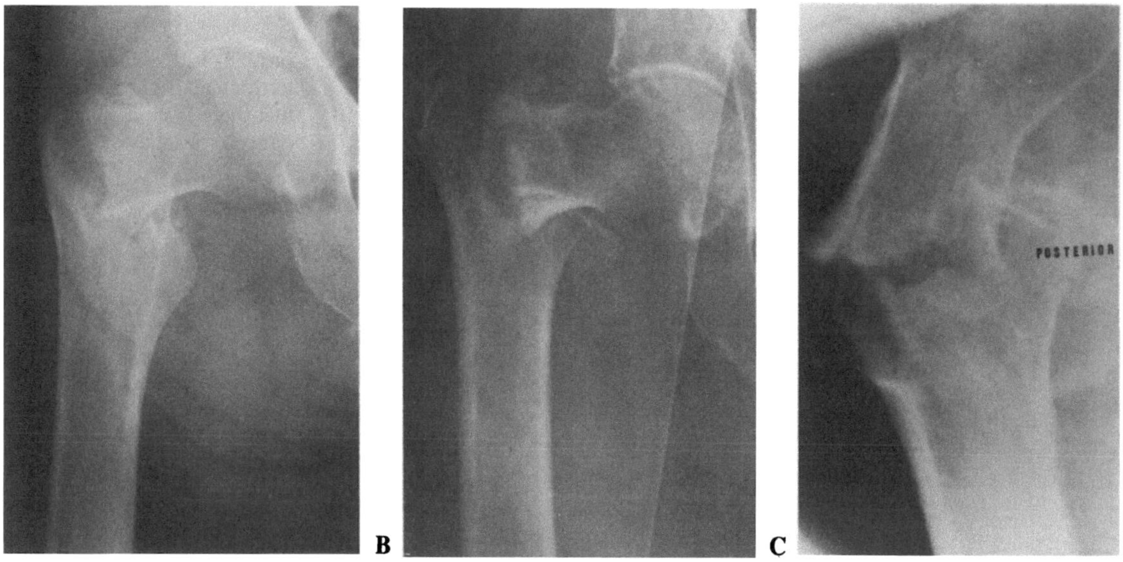

FIG. 8–118 High intertrochanteric fracture (old basicervical). **A** AP view of the short neck. The base is scooped out distal to the intertrochanteric line; both trochanters are basically intact. **B** AP view showing slight comminution of the lesser trochanter as another variation of the same theme. **C** Lateral x-ray, typical with the angulation in reverse of the usually posterior direction; the apex is typically anterior. An instrument such as a bone tamp may be needed to push the neck back down into its properly reduced position.

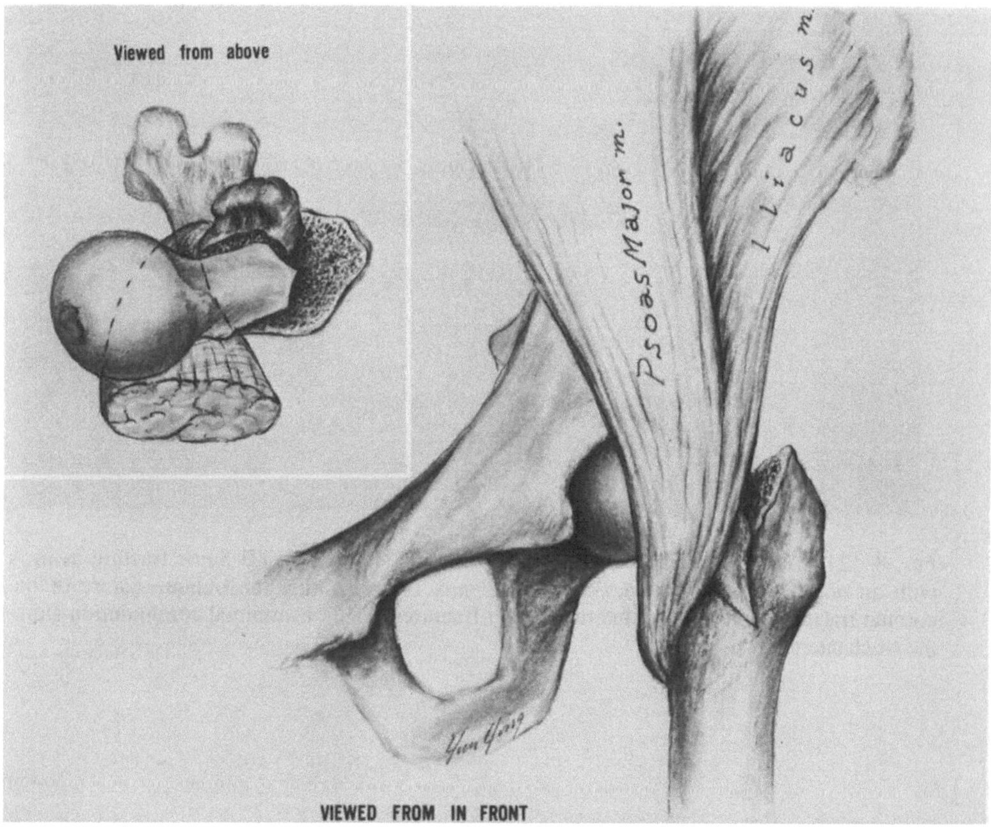

FIG. 8–119 Special type-I fracture must be treated by detachment of the iliopsoas tendon when the inferior spike on the neck fragment is long and sharp, causing it to be caught under the tendon much like a Chinese finger-trap. The best way to release the tendon is to osteotomize it with a curved osteotomy.

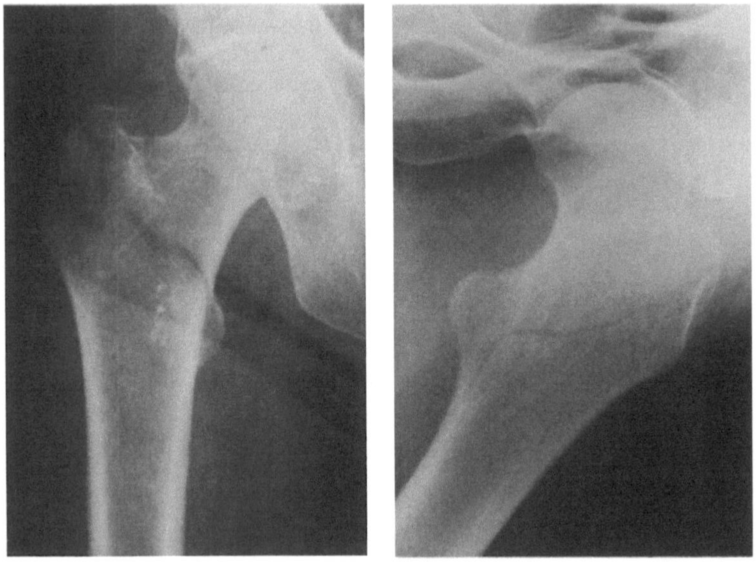

Fig. 8–120 Undisplaced intertrochanteric fractures. Note that there is no displacement in either x-ray view.

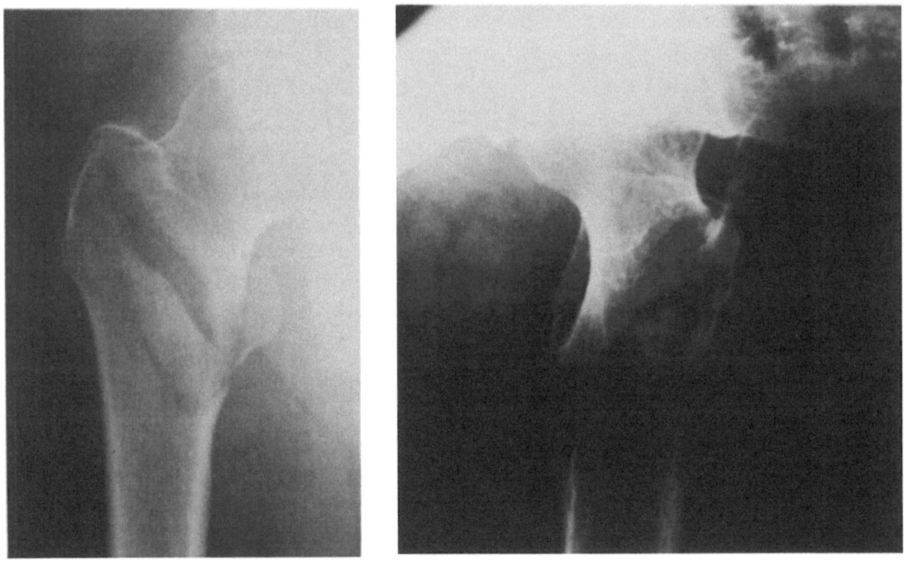

A B

Fig. 8–121 **A** Intertrochanteric fracture displaced in slight varus. **B** Same fracture as in A with an unusually good lateral x-ray film clearly demonstrating the oblique nature of the coronal fracture line typical of intertrochanter fractures. There is minimal comminution along the trochanteric crest.

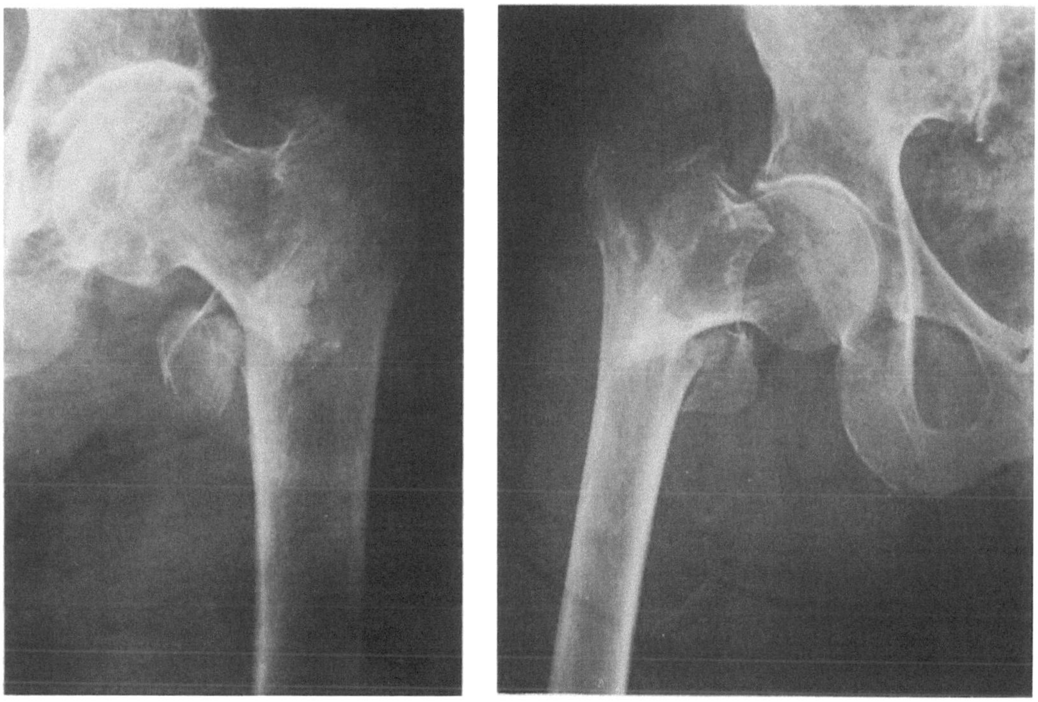

A B

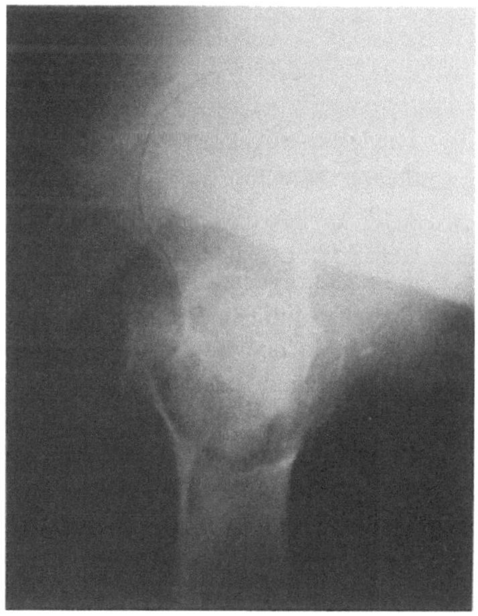

C

FIG. 8–122 The most common type of intertrochanteric fracture is shown in two variations **(A)** and **(B)**. They have an identical lateral x-ray picture **(C)** illustrating an intact posterior femoral shaft despite higher or more proximal comminution. The fracture remains confined inside its trough of cortical bone. (See inset Fig. 116) without any displacement. This is the hallmark of stable fractures.

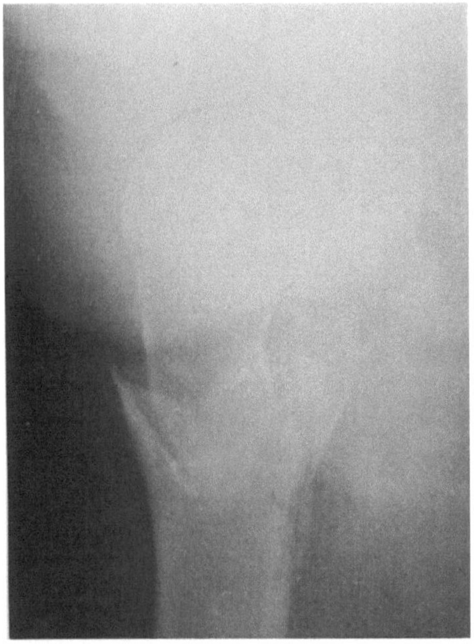

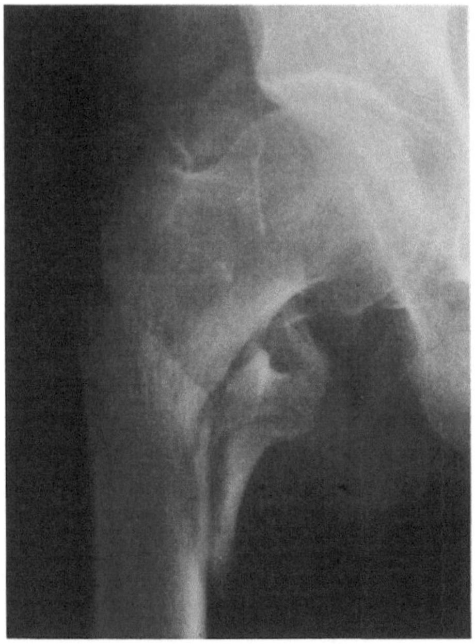

FIG. 8–123 **A** Uncommon fracture of the long lesser trochanter, which has been avulsed from the medial shaft, leaving the main portion of the cortex intact. **B** Lateral view confirms that the solid cortical trough is keeping the neck fragment confined.

3. The lesser trochanter is usually a long, sharp, major fragment with separation from the posterior cortex; alternatively, it may be quite fragmented into smaller parts as it splits off the posteromedial cortex.
4. There is significant posteromedial loss of cortical bone due to the severe comminution. The proximal fragment shifts, rotates, angulates, or displaces out of the femoral shaft trough for there are no walls left to confine it.
5. The neck fragment is elongated and sharp, or it can be a short comminuted piece when seen on an A/P x ray. Its fracture surface is oblique, which makes anatomical reduction nearly impossible.
6. Reduction can be treacherous if a master plan is not mapped out. An extensive incision is needed to afford a wide exposure of the fracture so that instruments can be used to manipulate the fragments into alignment. Most of the time the main fragments must be released from their soft tissue tethers before they can be reduced properly. Introduction of the fixation device can be difficult. These fractures are inherently unstable.

The key difference between stable and unstable fractures is best appreciated on the lateral x-ray film:

1. Stable fractures show no lateral displacement, only angulation (Fig. 8–116).
2. Unstable fractures show marked lateral displacement and rotational angulation (Fig. 8–126). CT scans are not usually needed, although they vividly demonstrate the unstable qualities of these comminuted osteoporotic fractures (Fig. 8–127).

Fracture Atlas

A diagramatic scheme illustrates five varieties of unstable fracture complexes, Fig. 8–129. The general characteristics of unstable fractures are illustrated by the author's old type III fracture (Fig. 8–128). The degree of comminution is severe with an explosion of the posterior medial wall. Both trochanters are comminuted, displaced, and rotated. The neck fragment not only goes into varus but is displaced outside its cortical trough by slipping anteriorly or posteriorly as it angulates. Its inferior beak is usually long and

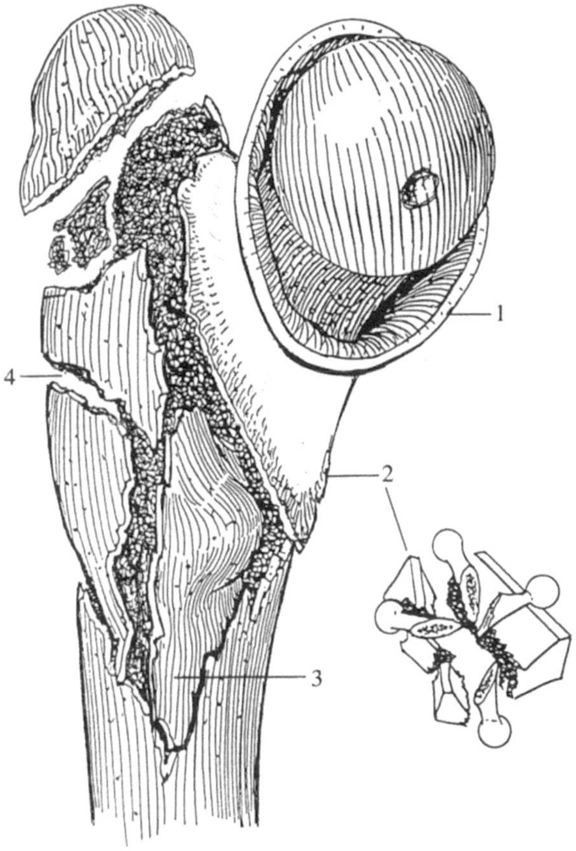

FIG. 8–124 Characteristics of an unstable intertrochanteric fracture: 1. The fracture occurs outside of the capsule and just distal to its attachment to the intertrochanteric line. 2. There is marked lateral displacement as well as rotation and angulation into varus as it moves freely in a shattered medullary trough (inset). 3. The lesser trochanter is a major fragment because it is part of the medial cortex. 4. Posterior comminution is severe.

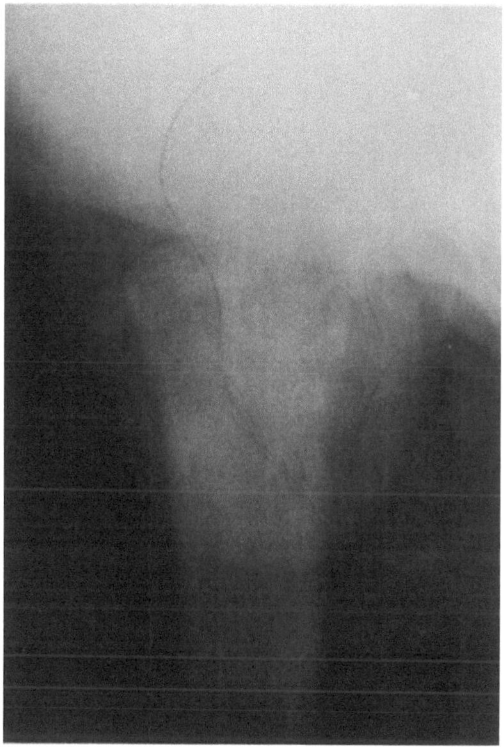

FIG. 8–125 Example of an essential lateral x-ray film to illustrate the unstable fracture type with an exploded femoral shaft trough. The neck has shifted and rotated out of the widely opened femoral shaft.

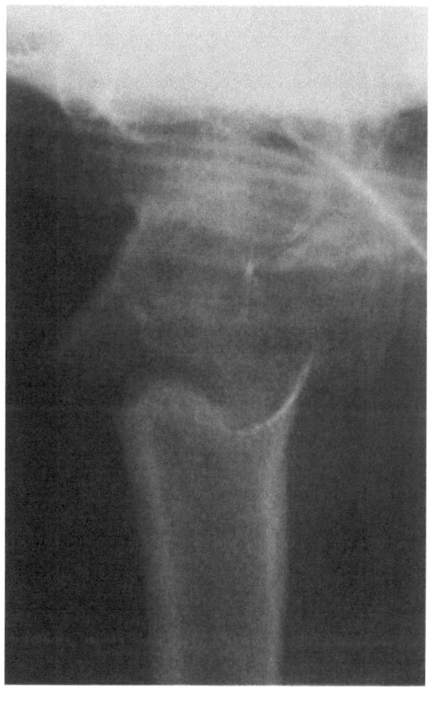

FIG. 8–126 The fracture surface of the head fragment is oblique and has rotated and shifted outside of the comminuted cortical trough. ▶

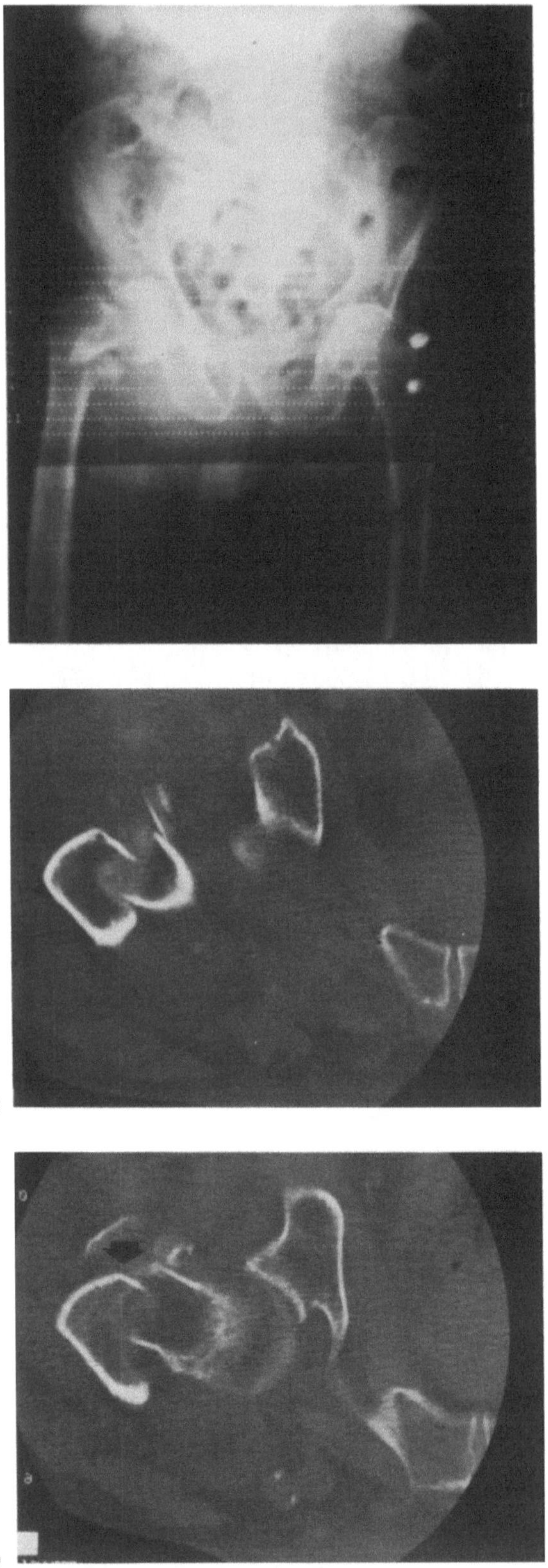

A

B

C

◄

Fig. 8–127 **A** The complexities that make up an unstable intertrochanteric fracture can be appreciated on a CT scan. **B** At the level of the lesser trochanter a large medial wall of cortical bone is split longitudinally; the posterior cortex is comminuted; the fragments are displaced one from the other. **C** As the x-ray moves toward the greater trochanter, one can see more posterior comminution; the hollow osteoporotic intermedullary canal is very evident; the head fragment is displaced outside of the intermedullary trough. Note the thin cortices which would make any attempt at an anatomical reduction futile.

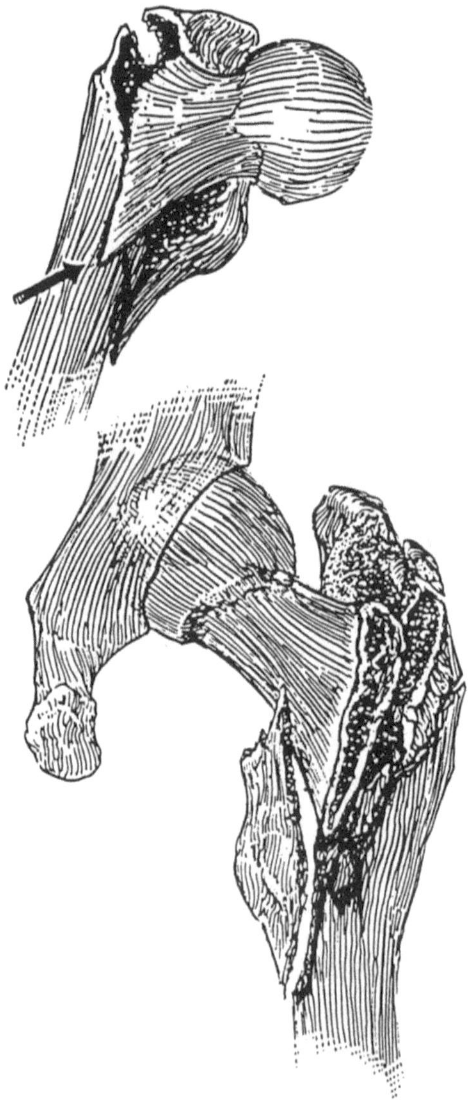

▲

Fig. 8–128 Common characteristics of a type III fracture are explosion of the posterior medial cortex, marked varus displacement, and angulation outside of the intermedullary cavity. No restraining cortex is present. (This is Tronzo's old type III.)

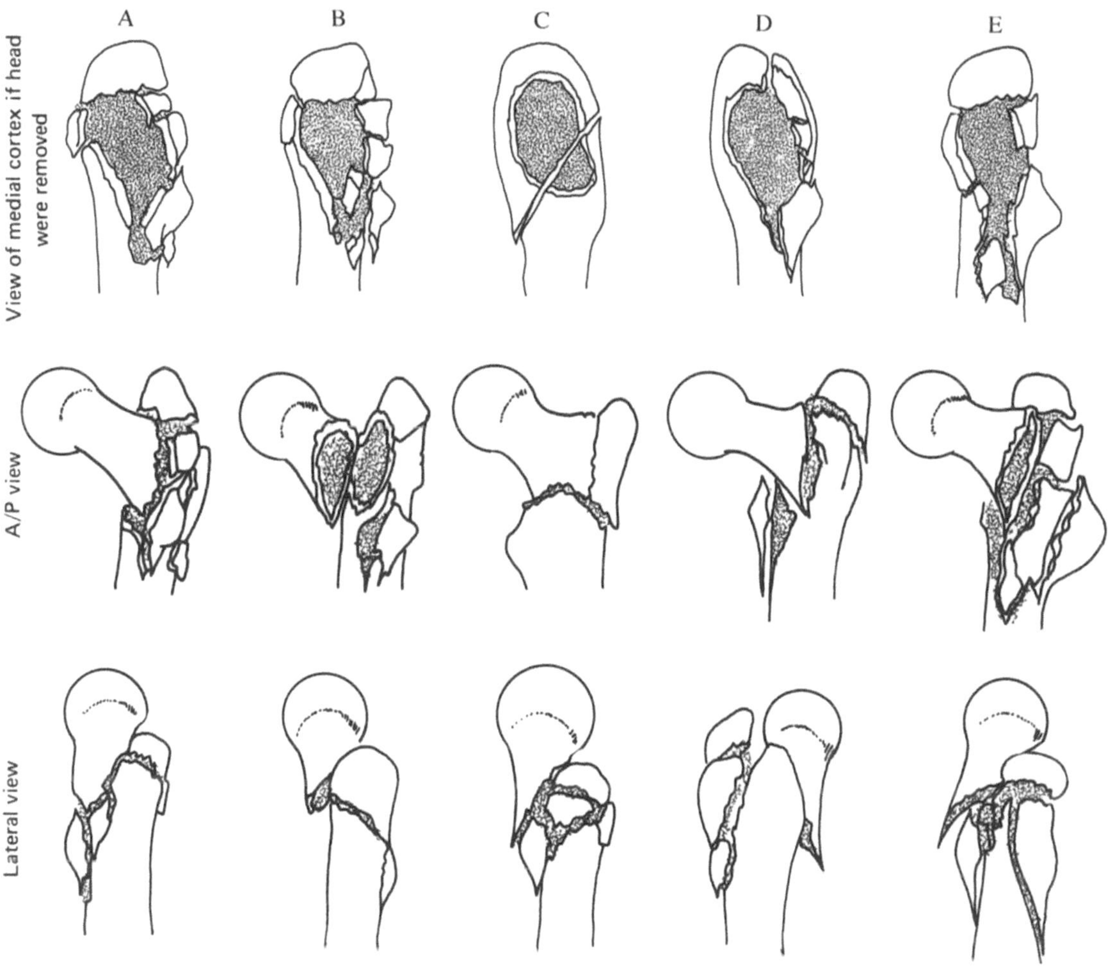

FIG. 8–129 Unstable fracture varieties.

sharp. In some varieties it can be broken up into smaller fragments along with its medial wall. Simple traction and internal rotation do not reduce these fractures. They must be opened widely and manipulated into a telescoping posture by forcefully tucking the inferior portion of the neck into what is remaining of the shaft before any meaningful reduction can be accomplished.

1. The most common fracture of this group is illustrated in Fig. 8–129A. The neck fragment goes into marked varus. It droops posteriorly to the shaft with its inferior beak pointing anteriorly as it is rotated by the pull of the iliofemoral ligament. The medial wall is only partially violated, but the posterior cortex is severely fragmented. The lesser trochanter is usually a large fragment. It is displaced medially by the pull of the iliopsoas tendon. The greater trochanter is comminuted with some upward displacement (Fig. 8–130).

2. An uncommon type of unstable fractures is the second one depicted in Fig. 8–129B. Most of the medial wall is intact, but little is left of the posterior cortex. The lesser trochanter is pulled upward and laterally so that it is superimposed on the femur and is not easily seen on x-ray film (Fig. 8–131). The abductors on the upper shaft and the strong adductors on the medial side of the shaft pull it upward and laterally, leaving the neck displaced away from it medially. The neck–head segment (Fig. 8–131C) appears to be floating by itself. It is a very difficult fracture to reduce by telescoping or tucking the neck into the shaft. If there is any fracture suited to the

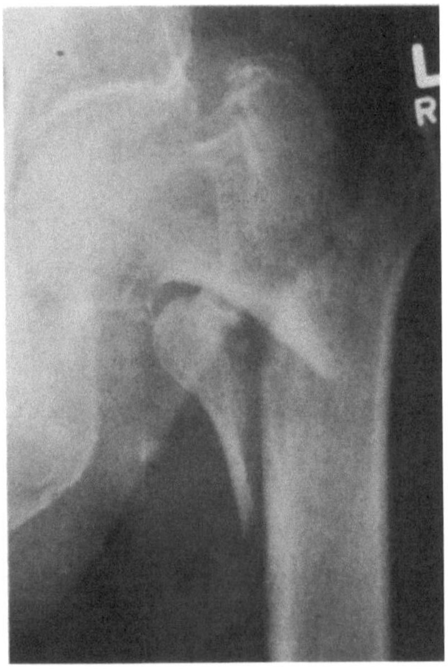

A

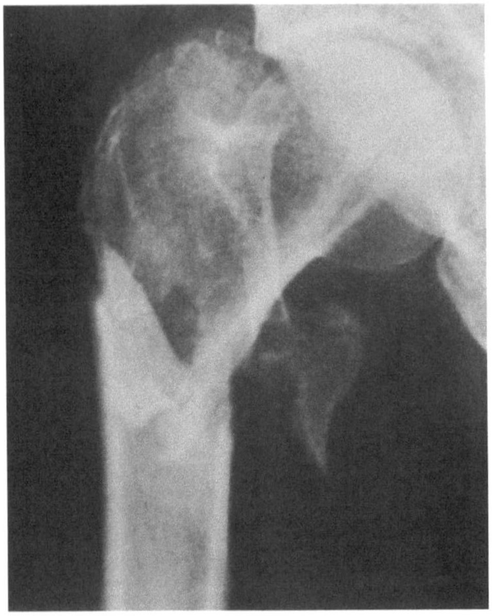

B

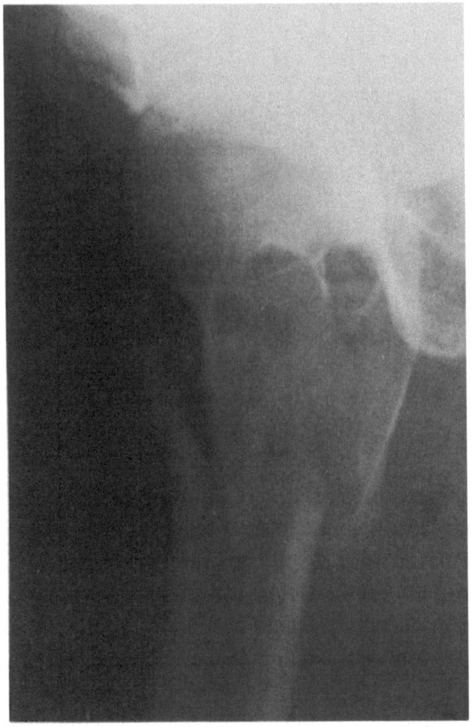

C

FIG. 8–130 **A, B** X-ray film of the most common unstable type, which has a long inferior spike to the neck. There is posterior comminution, some loss of the medial wall, and a large lesser trochanter. A and B are two variations. **C** In the lateral x-ray film the posterior shift of the neck can be appreciated outside the confines of the femoral canal.

use of the Ender system, it is this one. The Ender rods pass directly into the neck, which is displaced outside the shaft with an unobstructed path to the femoral head.

3. Another problematical fracture in this category is seen in Fig. 8–129C. The fracture lines are in reverse of the usual direction (Fig. 8–132). The lesser trochanter is untouched, but the posterior cortex above it is quite fragmented, rendering it a very unstable complex. The neck is sheared off from the shaft, leaving a large fragment of greater trochanter above it. In some cases the greater trochanter appears to be attached to the neck; it is an illusion, however, because a fracture between the two always exists. The neck fragment looks deceivingly blunted only because it has rotated into an anteroposterior orientation. The lateral x-ray film is difficult to obtain because the leg is markedly rotated externally. Reduction and fixation are not easy. The author has worked out a master plan for it as depicted in Fig. 8–133. Many times the shaft must be notched to permit telescoping of the neck. The lateral side of the greater trochanter cannot be drilled out in the usual manner, otherwise it can become displaced. A rongeur is used to clear a path for the compression hip screw.

4. A fourth variety occurs when the neck fragment is large (Fig. 8–129D). It contains a major

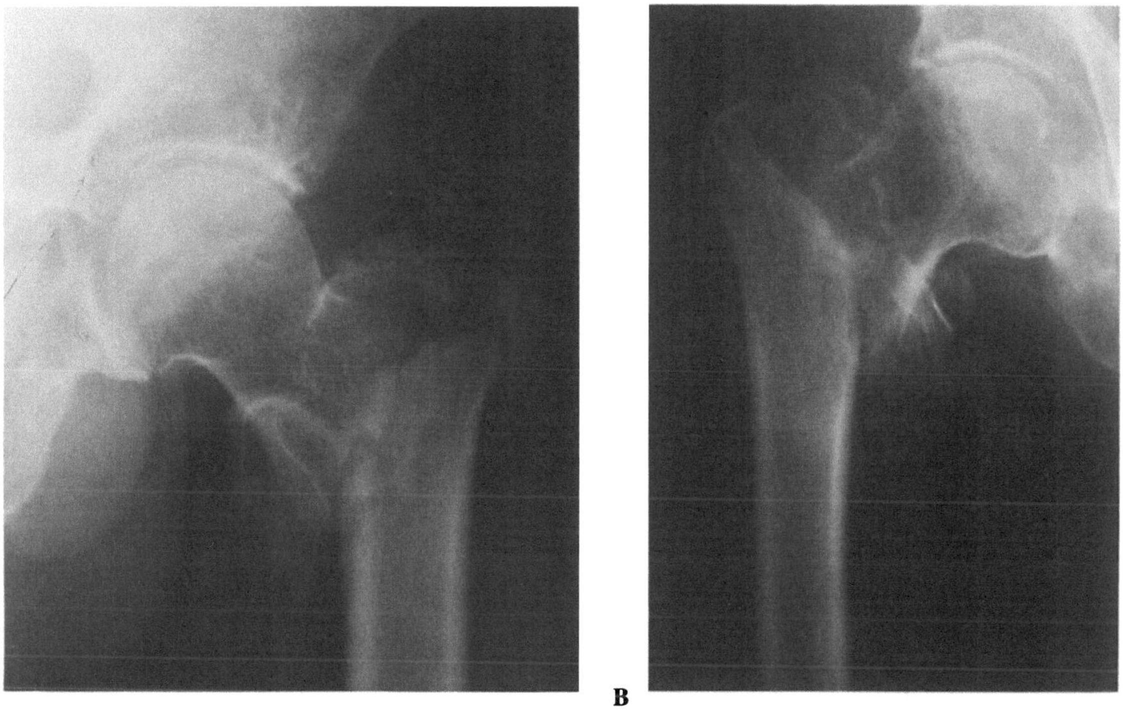

A B

portion of the posterior cortex as one large piece of bone. The spike is displaced anteriorly, with its inferior sharp beak pointing upward. The spike portion is so sharp that the operator can cut his glove on its edges while trying to maneuver it back into a reduced position. Only the upper part of the greater trochanter is comminuted. The lesser trochanter is a long, oblique fragment that is displaced medially (Fig. 8–134). To get the inferior beak tucked back into the shaft may require ronguering it so as to blunt it enough to be manageable.

5. The most treacherous fracture complex is transitional between intertrochanteric and subtrochanteric (Fig. 8–129E). When the fracture begins to extend down into the subtrochanteric region, an obliquity occurs causing the shaft to split in the coronal plane. A good lateral x-ray film can show it (Fig. 8–135). The area fractured involves both regions; consequently these fractures are the most unstable and the most difficult to reduce and stabilize.

Internal Fixation

The benchmark of internal fixation for intertrochanteric fractures is the sliding compression

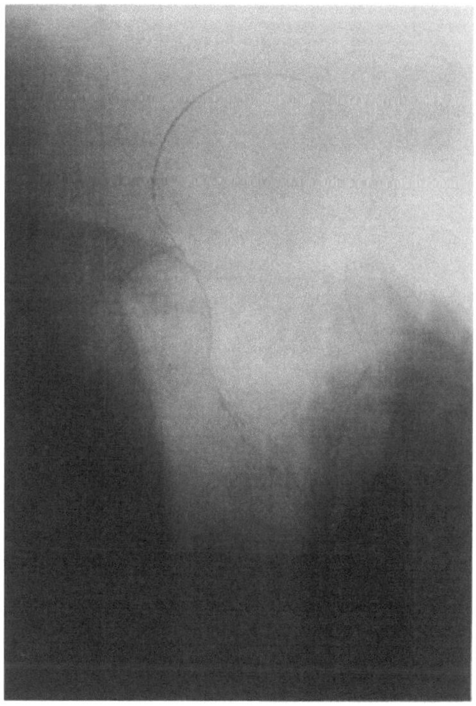

C

FIG. 8–131 A very sinister fracture lurks in variety B. The neck fragment appears to be floating by itself medial to the shaft. The shaft appears to be pulled upward while the neck is pulled downward past the medial cortex. The neck lies outside of the intermedullary cavity (**A** and **B**). There is a marked shift laterally as seen in the x-ray view, **C**.

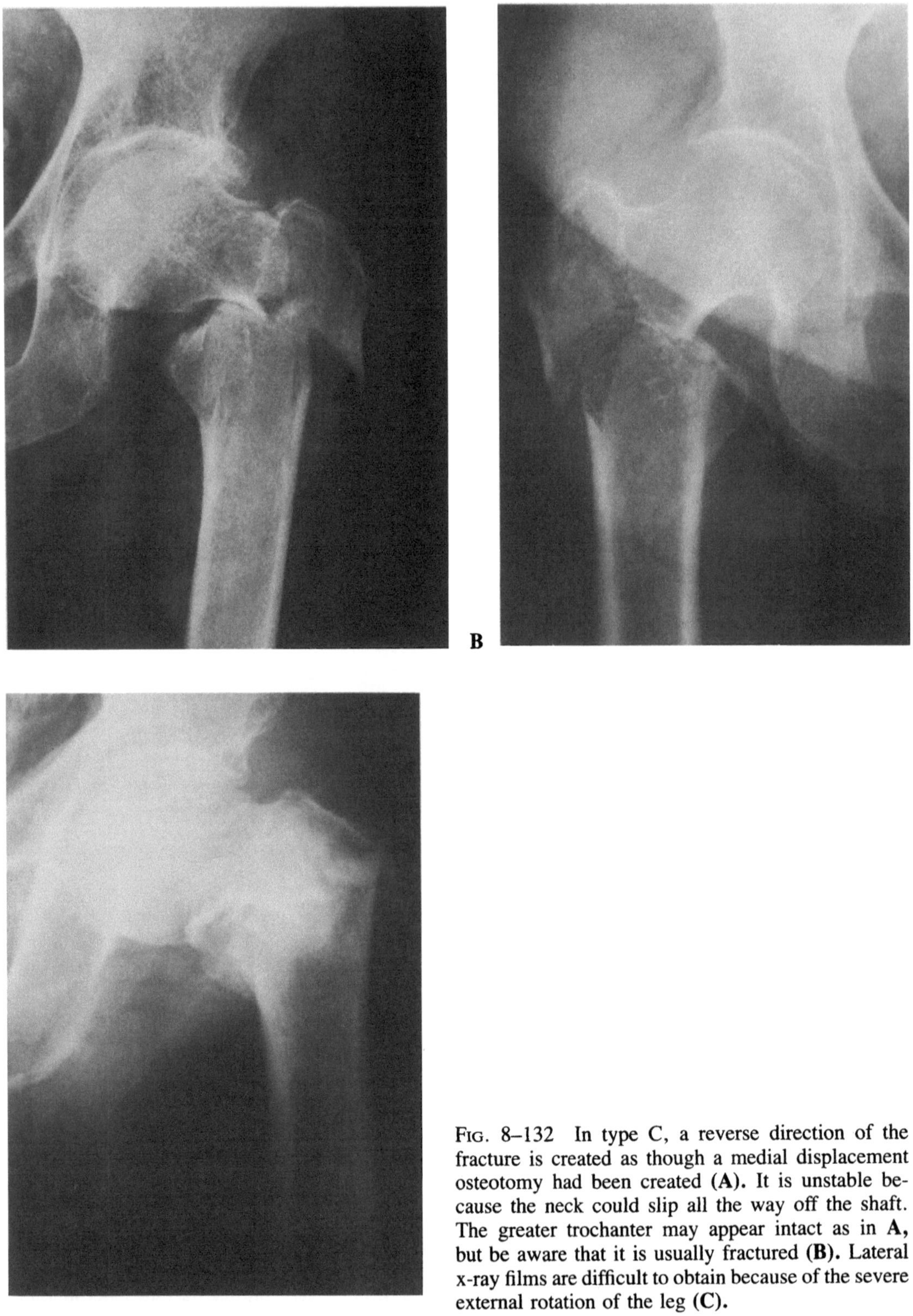

A B C

Fig. 8–132 In type C, a reverse direction of the fracture is created as though a medial displacement osteotomy had been created **(A)**. It is unstable because the neck could slip all the way off the shaft. The greater trochanter may appear intact as in **A**, but be aware that it is usually fractured **(B)**. Lateral x-ray films are difficult to obtain because of the severe external rotation of the leg **(C)**.

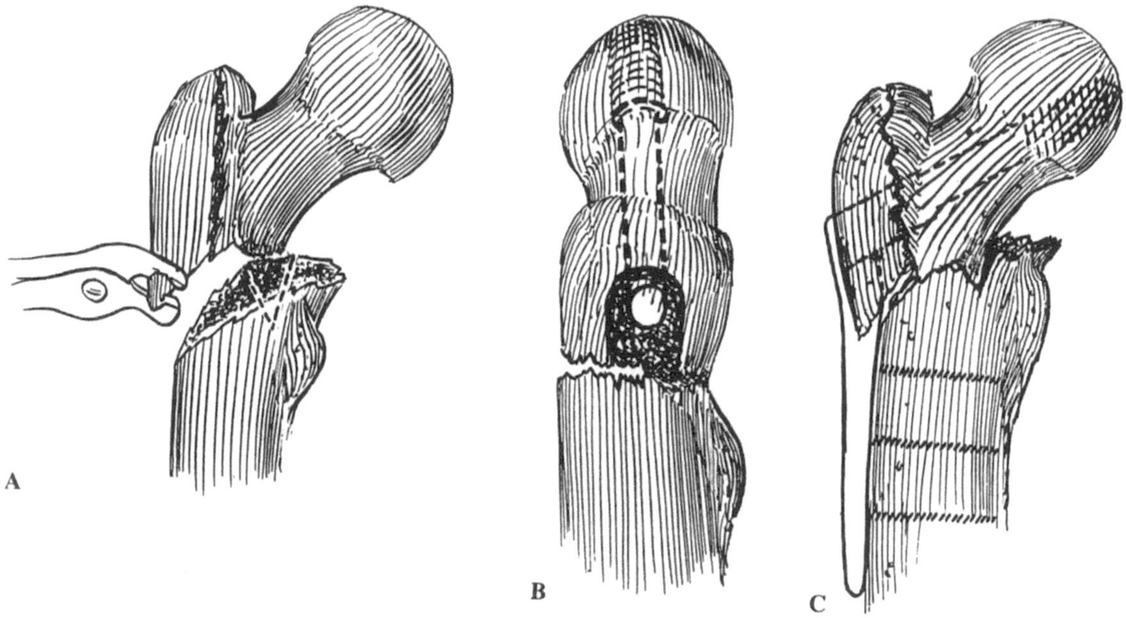

D
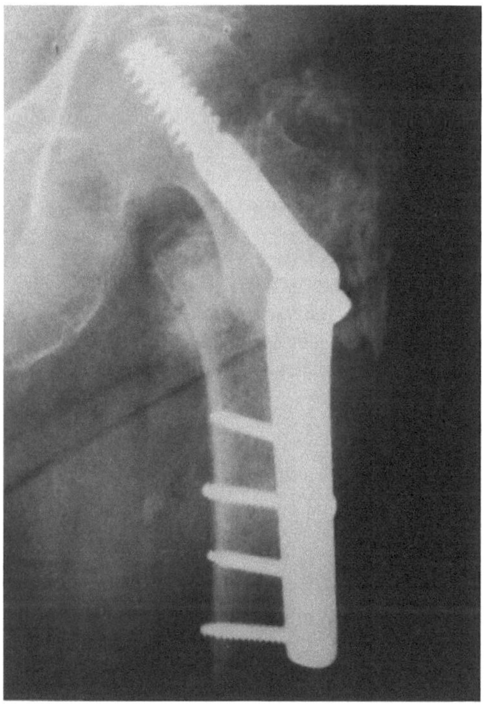

FIG. 8–133 **A** Tronzo's technique of stabilizing fractures with reverse obliquity. Because the greater trochanter is a thin shell, drilling may cause it to shatter. It is best to use a rongeur to open a path for the side plate (**B**). Notch the shaft fragment (**A**) so that the neck can be tucked into it (**C**). Once so stabilized the fracture will heal promptly (**D**).

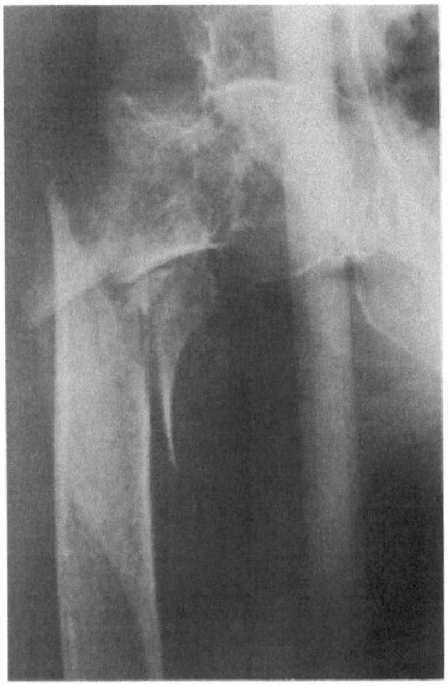

A

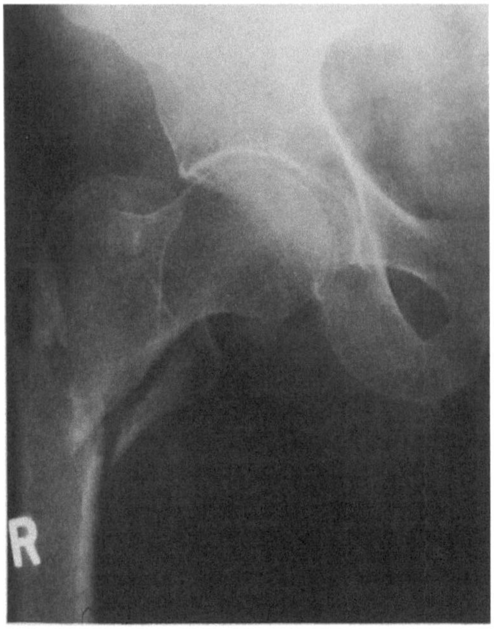

B

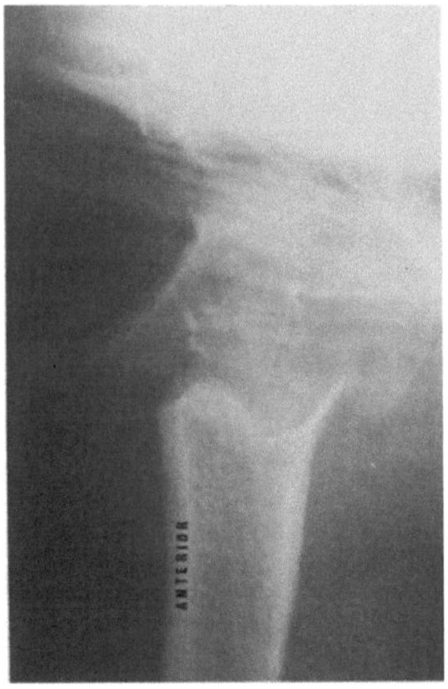

C

FIG. 8–134 Type D fracture characteristically has a long, oblique neck component (**A**). It is rotated and displaced anteriorly (**B**). The lesser trochanter is also a long, oblique fragment which is markedly displaced. The lateral x-ray film (**C**) shows the rotation of the upper fragment as it shifts outside of the cortex. Its spike is typically projected anteriorly. Note how it is superimposed on the A-P x-ray.

screw.[276–281] It has undergone evolutionary improvements, especially spearheaded by the Richards Manufacturing Company, Figure 8–133D. This screw has gone from a relatively lightweight device to a strong, massive one that can withstand even the stresses of a subtrochanteric fracture.[282] The other major improvement is the keyless, or key-free, system that was contributed by Southwick and first produced by Zimmer.[283] All other makes had a slot in the barrel of the screw that was intended to prevent rotation of the fragments. Southwick and his colleagues noted that the fragments interdigitated so well after being compressed that rotation was inherently prevented. To many the keyed device now seems superfluous. The side plate is massive, and its screw holes are larger to accept the AO screw system for better anchorage to the femoral shaft. In the past, side plates were known to pull away from the shaft when stressed by weight-bearing, which

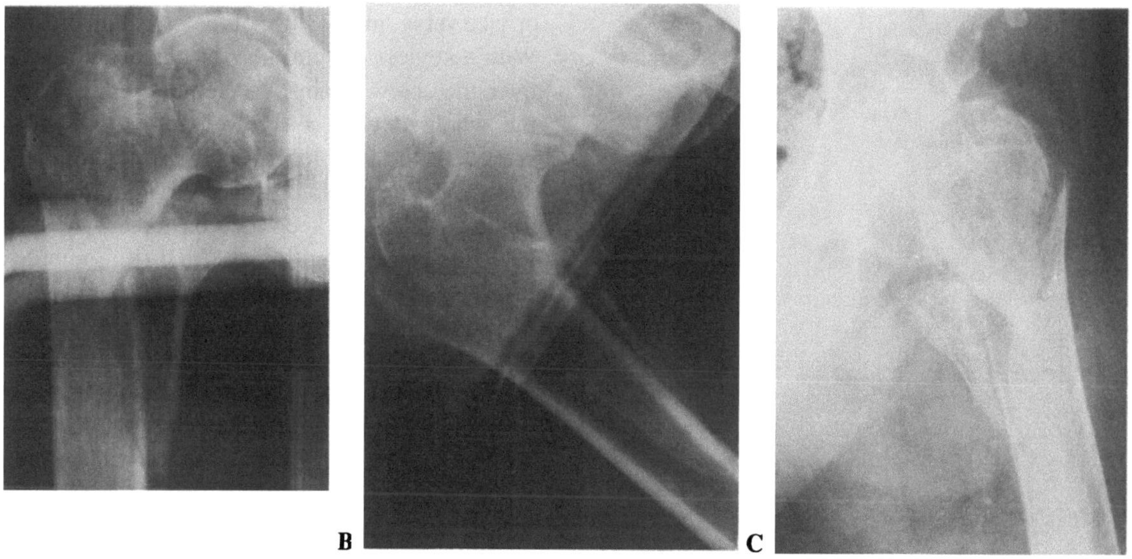

FIG. 8–135 Type E fracture. **A** The most unstable and complex of the groupings is seen when there is a transitional fracture extending from the greater trochanter into the subtrochanteric region. **B** There is seldom much varus displacement, but the lesser trochanter is a major component taking with it the whole posterior and medial wall. **C** The lateral x-ray film is important in order to appreciate the oblique split in the coronal plane where the posterior shaft and lesser trochanters are divided.

caused the smaller screws to break. Another improvement is the use of a larger guide pin. The old guide pins were small, and they bent easily when being inserted, causing them to break or get stuck inside the screw.

The overall major advantage of a sliding compression screw is that it allows the fragments to impact on one another in a controlled manner during the reduction as well as during the healing process, Fig. 8–146. A very stable complex is accomplished which encourages prompt healing.[55] When the reduction is well done (the head angles at least 135°, the head fragment is tucked into the shaft or telescoped); immediate weight-bearing by the patient is encouraged.[55,277] Rehabilitation and recovery are shortened considerably. With the newest devices few mechanical failures have occurred. Jensen and associates compared four methods of internal fixation.[284] They concluded: "Sliding screw fixation was found to be the only suitable fixation method for unstable trochanteric fractures because of a low failure rate, a low reoperation rate, and with the added advantage of secondary impaction for early weight-bearing and early union."

In the early, weaker models implant failures occurred. The commonest failure happened when the plate fractured at the neck/shaft angle. This author has had a rare failure when a Zimmer screw fractured within the lag threads which were weakened because they cut deeper into the barrel than is necessary (Fig. 8–136). The threads should begin at the diameter of the screw shaft and then flair out as a lag screw, which is the case of all other manufacturers. In the keyed versions the screw can jam at the key mechanism inside the barrel, causing it to be converted to a solid nail system.

Another failure of the older models was breakage of the screw at the level of the side plate barrel. In an ongoing study, Dr. L. Latta, at the University of Miami, and the author found that at high loads the shaft of the screw proximal to the side plate barrel bent, which could be another cause for some sliding screws to become bound inside their barrels, like a solid nail. The author has had such a case in a keyless system. Placing the head into slight valgus prevents such an occurrence. It has been shown in the laboratory that these devices slide better in valgus. There can be an iatrogenic failure, when the screw slides out of the side plate barrel, causing a loss of

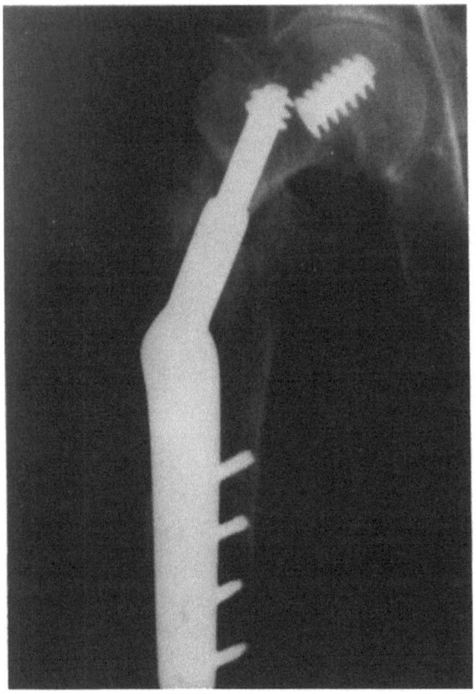

FIG. 8–136 Zimmer screw fractured within the threads (a rare occurrence).

that would fit into the female slot on the shaft or vice versa, making use of the nail cumbersome. With a keyless system the side plate can be fitted over the screw against the femoral cortex while the whole device is screwed into place. Once impacted, the fragments become so interdigitated that they cannot rotate. Some surgeons still cling to the old idea. To keep their customers satisfied, Richards came up with the AMBI (i.e. ambidextrous) system, which provided the quick option of placing a key into the screw after it has been fully inserted. The author has yet to see the advantage of a keyed device after treating hundreds of fractured hips with the keyless system.

Solid Nails Solid nails or two-piece (nonsliding) devices have no place in modern orthopedics. With their use the fragments cannot physiologically impact for self-stabilization. The failure rate is high with their use. The nail penetrates the joint when the fracture collapses, with a "shish kabob effect." The nail broke all too frequently at the nail plate junction. Immediate weight-bear-

reduction (Fig. 8–137). The length of the screw should be so measured as to leave about 0.5 inch inside the barrel for proper sliding without fear of the parts separating.

Sliding Triflanged Nails These devices (e.g., the Ken/Pugh, Massie, or Haig nails) are slowly becoming passé. They have the unique disadvantage of slipping out of the head, as seen in Fig. 8–138. With the use of a screw, the implant is so well anchored in the head that it can be gently pulled into the shaft by the compressing device. With sliding nails impaction can be achieved only by pounding against the femoral shaft, which could lead to avascular necrosis of the head if it were to damage the delicate articular cartilage. In younger patients the pounding can cause distraction of the fragments.

Keyed Versus Keyless System It was originally thought that it was necessary to have a mechanism in the sliding implant that would prevent the fragments from rotating. Either the barrel had a key

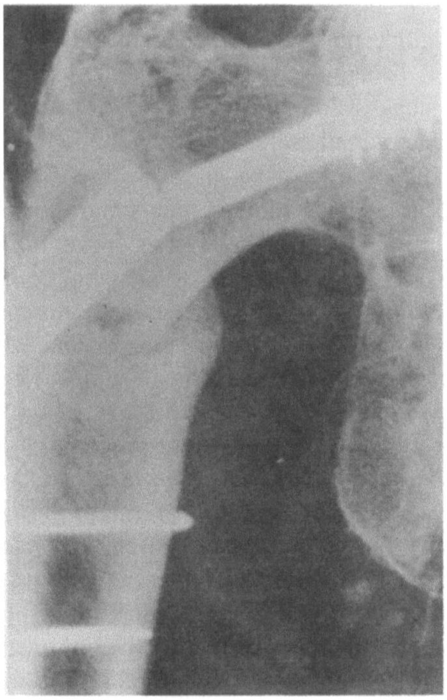

FIG. 8–137 If the length of the screw is not properly sized within the barrel, it can become distracted. There should be about 0.5 inch inside the barrel.

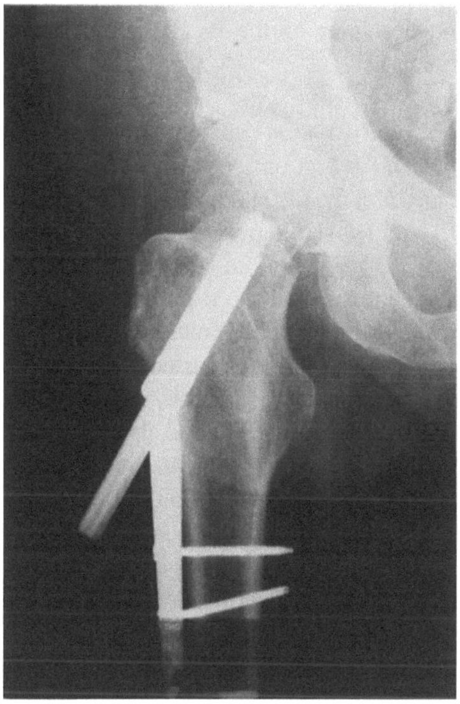

FIG. 8–138 Triflanged sliding nails have the disadvantage of sliding out of the head.

ing by the patient could not be permitted until the fracture was well healed, and rehabilitation could take up to 4 to 6 months.

Length of the Side Plate The length of the side plate for uncomplicated intertrochanteric fractures has been a moot point for years. Osteotomy plates used by the Swiss system have only three screw holes. Experimentally it has been shown that four holes are sufficient.[285] The standard side plate for the Richards system is four holes; none of their standard plates are any shorter. To use a six-hole side plate on a stable fracture creates unnecessary operative morbidity. Most unstable fractures are adequately fixed with a four-hole side plate. Only in unstable type V fracture, where there is a subtrochanteric component, is a longer side plate needed.

Ideal Placement of the Screw into the Head Proper placement of the screw in the femoral head is the most crucial part of the operation. Gesler and Goldberg[286] found that poor placement of the screw was the most significant failure in their series review. The densest bone is in the center of the head. Even in heads severely affected by osteoporosis this area of concentrated bone remains the best anchoring point (Latta and Tronzo, unpublished data). The worst area for placement is the superior one-third of the head. Loads normally concentrate at this spot to such magnitudes that they themselves are responsible for failure of the implant or loss of reduction of the fracture (Fig. 8–139). Despite studies indicating that this area has superior "holding potential,"[137] allowing the implant to remain in the superior zone under such loads is courting failure. Placement into the inferior one-third of the head is quite acceptable because loads are minimal and there is usually sufficient bone to keep the screw anchored.[287] To reach the central location one must imagine the femoral neck as being a funnel-shaped structure. Two points are chosen: the center of the neck at its base and the center of the head. If one parallels the inferior cortex of the

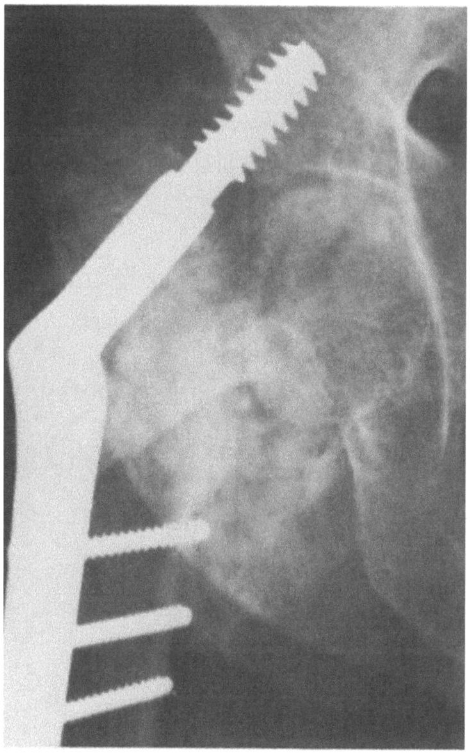

FIG. 8–139 Superiorly placed implant in the head will surely cut itself out especially in elderly osteoporotic bone with subsequent loss of reduction because there is so much stress concentration on the superior portion of the head.

neck, the screw ends up in the superior part of the head. There is little leeway in the coronal plane (lateral x-ray film) for placement of the screw. In the past it was thought that the implant should be placed in the posterior section of the head, which would help prevent posterior migration of the fracture. The screw is best seated in the bull's-eye spot in the lateral x-ray film, otherwise the reduction is at risk for failure; this is especially true if the screw is left sitting in the anterior part of the head where load stresses are maximal. The screw's final destination must be at the subchondral level to ensure its anchorage in the best part of the head where the bone is most dense.

Modes of Reduction There are basically four modes of reduction: anatomical, appositional (Wayne County), medial displacement osteotomy, and physiological telescoping reduction (Fig. 8–140). An anatomical reduction is practical only in undisplaced or slightly displaced types of fracture. In displaced fractures of any classification, only the anterior surfaces can be brought together anatomically, but they quickly subluxate one on top of the other due to their comminution posteriorly. In the Wayne County reduction[288] the neck fragment is pushed or pulled up against the medial wall of the shaft (Fig. 8–141). This reduction has limited application—in only a small percentage of cases, where there is relatively little medial wall comminution. The medial displacement osteotomy proposed by Dimon and Hughston[274] is still frequently done today (Fig. 8–142), even though it was originally designed to prevent solid nails from penetrating the femoral head when anatomical reductions were still being attempted for the highly collapsible, unstable frac-

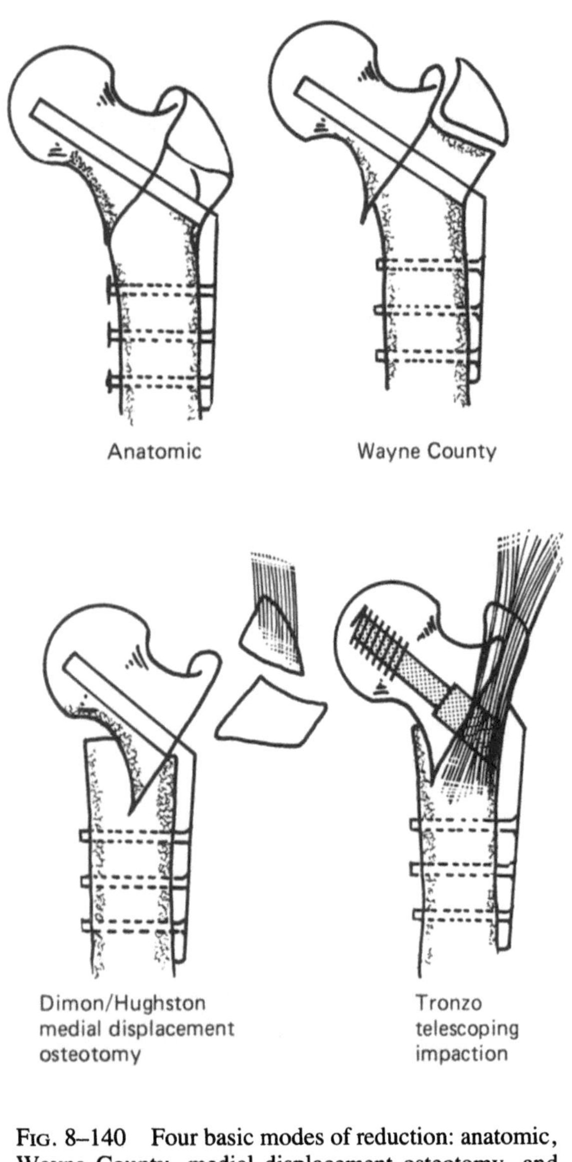

FIG. 8–140 Four basic modes of reduction: anatomic, Wayne County, medial displacement osteotomy, and physiological impaction (telescoping) with sliding screw.

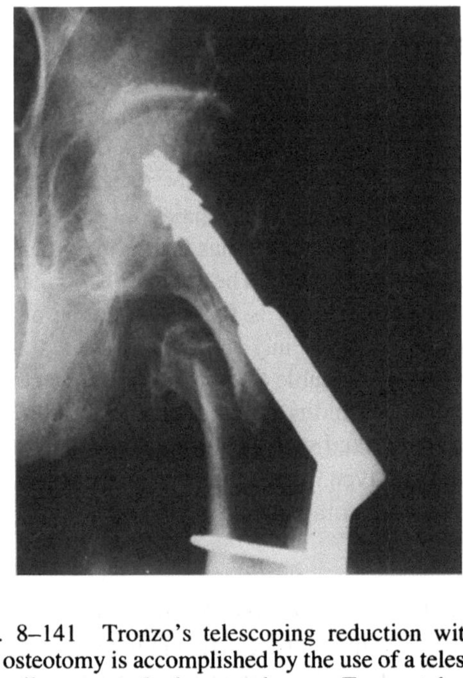

FIG. 8–141 Tronzo's telescoping reduction without any osteotomy is accomplished by the use of a telescoping nail or screw. In the case shown a Tronzo telescoping nail was used. In this method the fracture impacts itself into a stable complex.

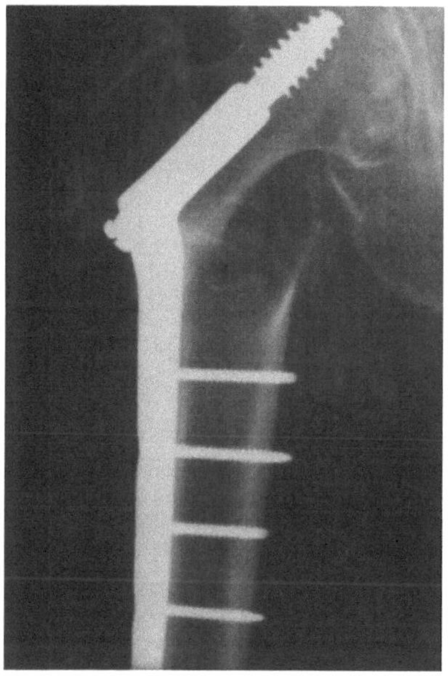

FIG. 8–142 An example of a medial displacement osteotomy. Note the jeopardized bony contact and the shortened length. It is an unnecessary step when a sliding screw is used.

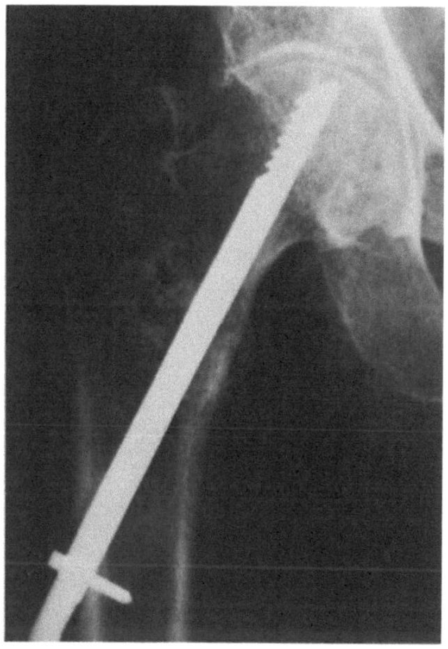

FIG. 8–143 Küntscher "low angle" nail. This x-ray film, given to the author by Professor Kuntscher, demonstrates the first valgus nail for valgus reductions.

tures. Since the advent of sliding hip screws, the collapse at the fracture site can be easily controlled without adding to the morbidity of the operation. Such displacement adds unnecessary time to the procedure, increases blood loss, makes insertion of the implant more difficult because very short screws with especially short barrels must be available, and slows healing because of compromised bone contact. It was a wonderful concept to help correct the deficiencies of a solid nail.

Küntscher pioneered the idea of valgus reduction with valgus nails (Fig. 8–143). It was later promoted by Boyd and Anderson[289] and Massie.[271] He called this device his "low angled nail." Its cross section was similar to his famous cloverleaf rod. Undoubtedly, placing the fracture into valgus reduces the bending loads on the fracture and the implant, thereby reducing the number of failures, Fig. 8–144. However, 155° is extreme. The fracture must be overreduced, or the end of the implant will end up in the superior part of the head (Fig. 8–145). The exposure is too extensive, and drilling into the hard lateral cortex at that low level (Fig. 8–145) is likewise difficult and adds to the morbidity of the operation. Getting the head to shift into such a valgus angle is not easy either, and once done the patient's knee will have been thrown into valgus giving the patient an unnecessary knock-knee deformity. Experimentally, it has been shown that a sliding nail slides better in valgus[276] (as one would expect to happen); 135° has proved to be a very practical angle to work with clinically.

The author has developed an easy technique for reducing the head fragment in slight valgus with the use of a 135° device. It takes advantage of a posture that is not so extreme in order to help minimize the loads on both the device and the fracture complex. It allows the fragments to become apposed, as in Fig. 8–146, or to become telescoped naturally in whatever way the particular fracture cares to follow, as in Fig. 8–133. The steps of this technique are as follows:

1. A limited lateral incision is used for *stable* fractures where only the lateral cortex of the shaft needs to be exposed. An extended Watson-Jones approach is needed for a more extensile exposure when treating *unstable* fractures that require manipulation of the fragments (Fig. 8–147). Do not hesitate to lift off the entire vastus intermedius

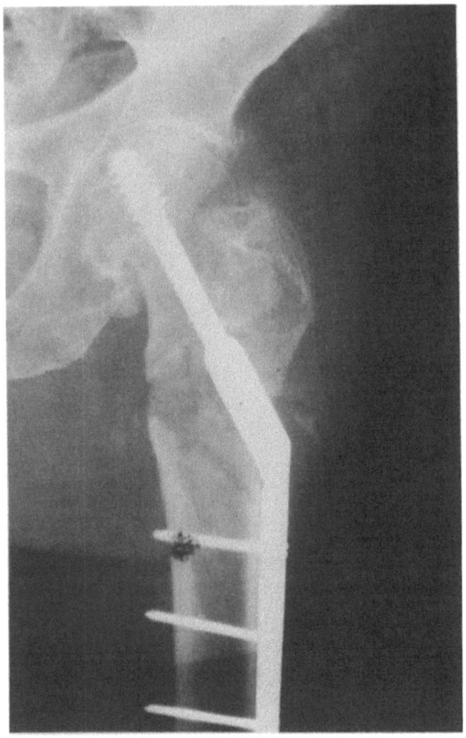

FIG. 8–144 Valgus reduction using a valgus implant (155°). The head must be forced into valgus to meet the nail in its central zone.

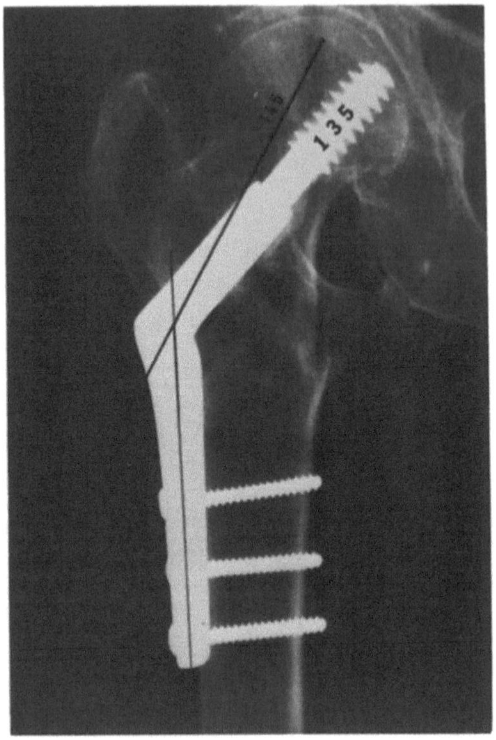

FIG. 8–146 Tronzo's method of achieving a slight valgus reduction of the fracture with the use of a 135° implant.

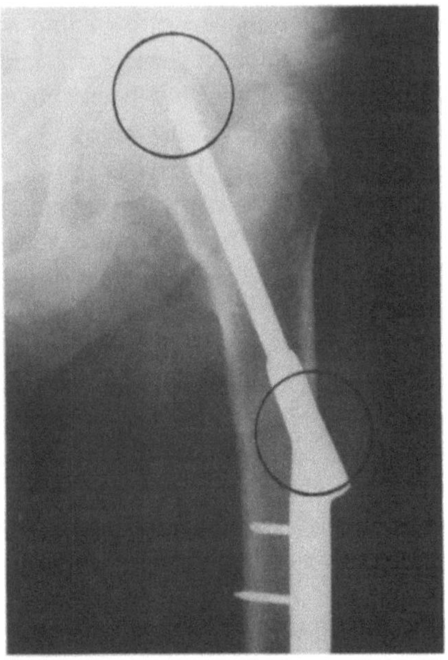

FIG. 8–145 Valgus nailing, but the head was not reduced into valgus, leaving the tip of the implant in a poor position in the superior neck. Note that the low ankle side plate must be drilled into the thick hard cortex. This is not a valgus reduction.

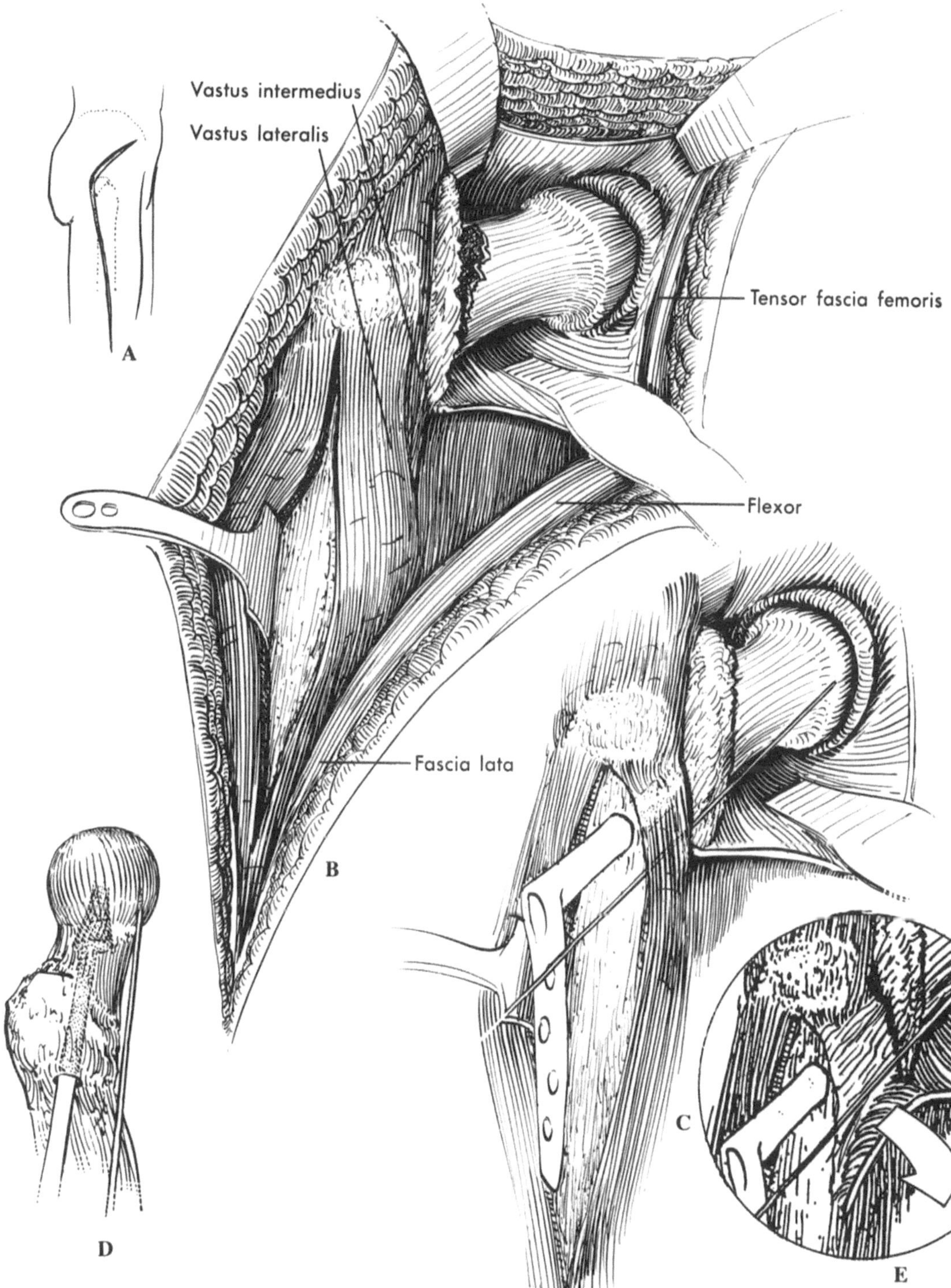

FIG. 8–147 Incision and technique for open reduction of trochanteric fractures: A modified Watson-Jones incision is used. It is brought posterior to the greater trochanter for better access to the posterior shaft and for the release of the tight tensor fascia attached to the gluteus maximus **(A)**. The capsule is opened by a vertical incision so that the reduction and the entire upper fragment are visualized **(B)**. A guide pin is aligned over the neck. The shaft is drilled parallel to the guide pin, followed by the nail; this will produce a perfect lateral position for nail placement without the multiple x-rays necessary with the old method of intermedullary guide pins **(C)**. The author's extramedullary guide-pin technique can ensure an ideal placement of the screw through the central part of the head in the lateral view **(D)**. In difficult comminuted cases of unstable fracture complexes, more exposure will be necessary by folding back the vastus intermedius **(E)**.

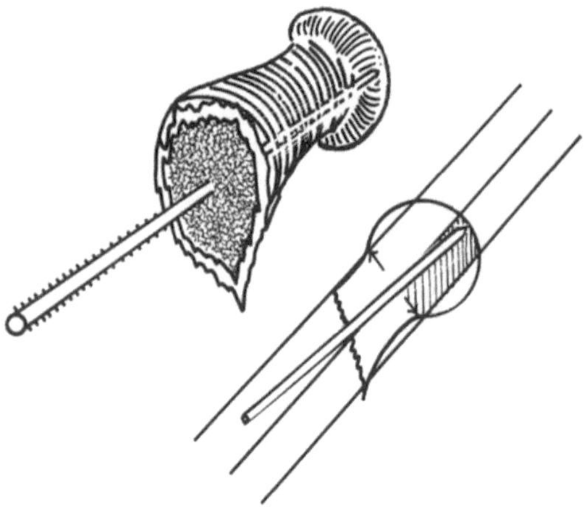

FIG. 8–148 The first priority is to firmly fix the head with a well placed screw. Once this is accomplished the final reduction becomes much easier: *the head is fixed first, the fracture is reduced second.* Imagine the head fragment as a single unit; isolate it in your mind. Run the guide pin from the *center of the neck to lower third of the head.*

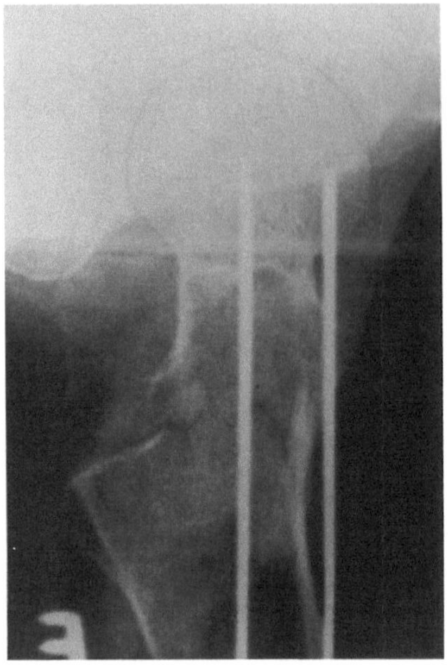

FIG. 8–150 Lateral x-ray film of guide pins in place.

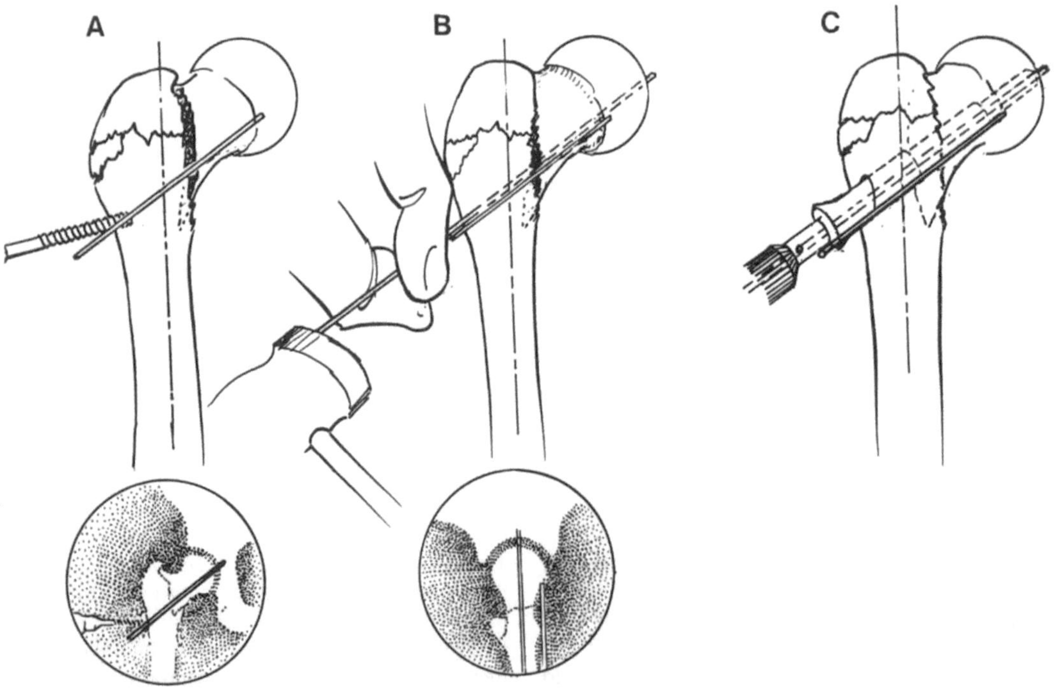

FIG. 8–149 Tronzo's method of drill guide placement for achieving precision placement of screw into the femoral neck and head in the all important lateral plane.

for better exposure of the fracture site (Fig. 8–147E) for unstable fractures.

2. Reduce the displaced fracture so that the inferior beak on the neck fragment is tucked into the intermedullary cavity of the shaft. At this point it is not necessary to align the fragments into anything further than what casually appears to be about 135°. This is an important departure from the traditional method of getting all of the fragments into a finalized mode of reduction first and then pinning it. *In this method the first priority is to accurately place the screw into an ideal position in the head and then finalize the reduction by bringing the fragments to the plate.*

3. Placement of a heavy guide pin is crucial to the technique because it will not bend as it is inserted. The extramedullary pin placement developed by the author[55] works well here. The use of an image intensifier is essential for accurate reduction. Precision pin placement is crucial to this technique. The surgeon must isolate the femoral head and neck as a single imaginary unit. His goal for final pin placement implant is (1) in the center at the base of the neck and (2) in the inferior one-third of the head (Fig. 8–148). Slide the guide pin *under* the capsule along the femoral neck until it stops at the edge of the head, which it will pierce (Fig. 8–149A). If the guide pin slides past and goes on top of the head into the acetabulum, an erroneous placement laterally will ensue. Start the pin at what should be the *center of the neck* (Fig. 8–148), and aim downward toward the inferior one-third of the femoral head (Fig. 8–149B). With a quick check using the image intensifier, the pin is reset as needed. The pin is tapped into the edge of the *head.* Drill an oversize hole in the lateral cortex immediately below the outside guide pin (Fig. 8–149A). A second pin is tapped into the intramedullary canal of the neck paralleling the outside pin (Fig. 8–149B). Once this step is completed a perfect position in the head and neck laterally should have been accomplished (Fig. 8–149B). A special drill is used next to channel out a path for the screw (Fig. 8–149C). The lateral x-ray should look like Figure 8–150. Note that no angled guide is used because the fracture was not precisely aligned as yet; only a visual estimate had been made at 135° because up to this point all efforts have been focused on getting the pin ideally positioned in the head. The reduction follows as a separate step. Traditionally, reduction and nailing have been attempted as a single step, which is less sophisticated and ends up with a 135° implant piercing the superior part of the head fixed in varus.

4. After choosing an appropriately sized screw, drill it well into the head, to the subchondral level. Place a four-hole, 135° side plate over the screw. There will be a gap between the side plate and the shaft (Fig. 8–151A), representing the amount of valgus shift of the head. Note that the final amount of valgus is equivalent to the angle of the pin from the midline of the neck (Fig. 8–151C). Use a single-pronged Lowman clamp to bring the shaft to the plate, (Fig. 8–151C), which places the head into slight valgus (140°–145°) (Fig. 8–146). This maneuver may cause the remaining part of the greater trochanter to crack. However, it is of no consequence as it plays no important part in the stability of the reduction. The fragments are pulled together and interdigitated with only an internal compression screw. Once this is done the loads on the implant and its side plate are reduced while compression on the fracture is increased so as to improve its stability by continued physiological impaction. Compression devices are not recommended because they apply so much force on the screw that it can be easily ripped out of the head. The head–neck telescope into the shaft and impact in a controlled manner, ensuring a stable reduction in slight valgus (Fig. 8–146).

Special Techniques Required for Unstable Fractures Unstable fracture complexes require a wide surgical exposure because they must first be dismantled piece by piece before they can be put back together. The various muscle attachments that pull the fragments in several directions can be appreciated in Fig. 8–152. The iliofemoral ligament and capsule distort the neck by pulling it upward, and in some cases the short external rotators are still attached so well that the neck is pulled under the shaft. When the base of the neck slips posteriorly, a wider exposure is necessary to visualize all of the pieces as they are related to each other. The vastus intermedius may have to be peeled from the shaft (Fig. 8–147E). The linea aspera and even the broad tendon of the gluteus maximus must be released in order to free the shaft enough so that it can be manipulated properly (Fig. 8–153). There are times when the beak of the inferior neck fragment blocks any

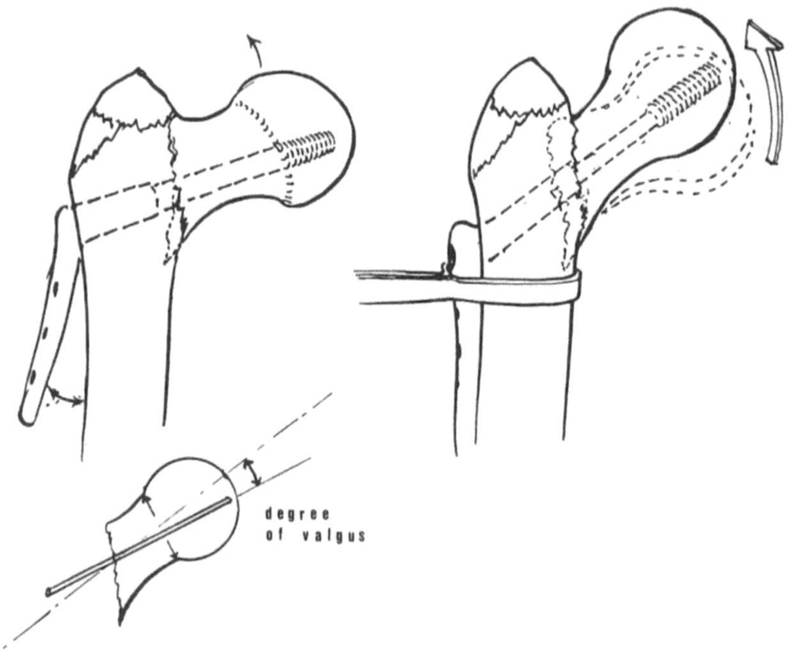

FIG. 8–151 Once the guide pin is properly placed into the head and the screw is well inserted to the subchondral level, reduction into slight valgus becomes automatic. The fragments are compressed together thus unloading the implant. Therefore, the priorities are: *First fix the head with a well placed screw and secondly reduce the fracture.*

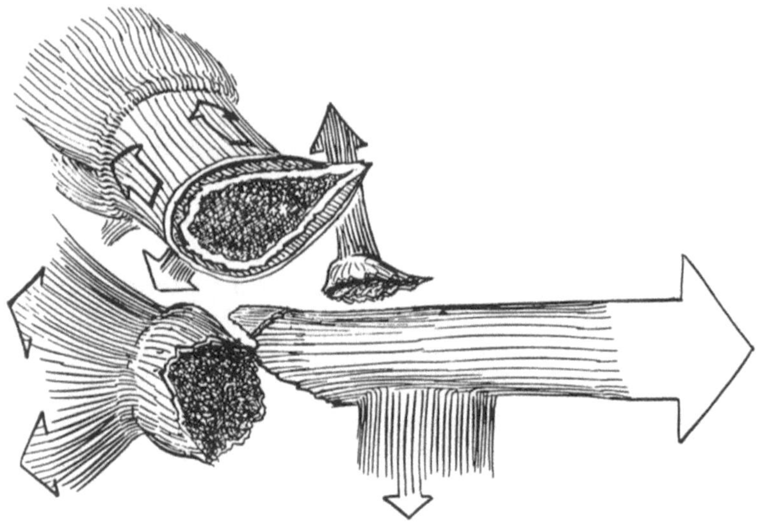

FIG. 8–152 In comminuted fractures the fragments are pulled in various directions. The neck gets pulled upward by the iliofemoral ligament and externally rotated by remnants of the short rotators; the lesser trochanter is pulled medially and upward by the iliopsoas muscle. The greater trochanter does not move much, but if it does it is moved upward and inward by the gluteus medius and minimus; the shaft can be held down by the tendon of the gluteus maximus.

reduction (Fig. 8–154) so that the sharp point must be clipped away before it can be tucked into the intermedullary canal. The tethering effect of the iliofemoral ligament may need to be cut away in order to free up the femoral neck (Fig. 8–155). Externally rotate the leg to disengage the fragments for better exposure so that it can be maneuvered back into the medial femoral canal for a telescoping reduction (Fig. 8–146B). Hohmann retractors are excellent instruments to help manipulate the fragments into their reduced position. When the neck shifts anteriorly as in *type IV* unstable fractures (Fig. 8–156), the spike of the Hohmann retractor is inserted into the shaft. Lift it up to the neck and hold it there while a guide pin is inserted to maintain the position. When the neck droops down behind the shaft as in type I and II unstable fractures (Fig. 8–157),

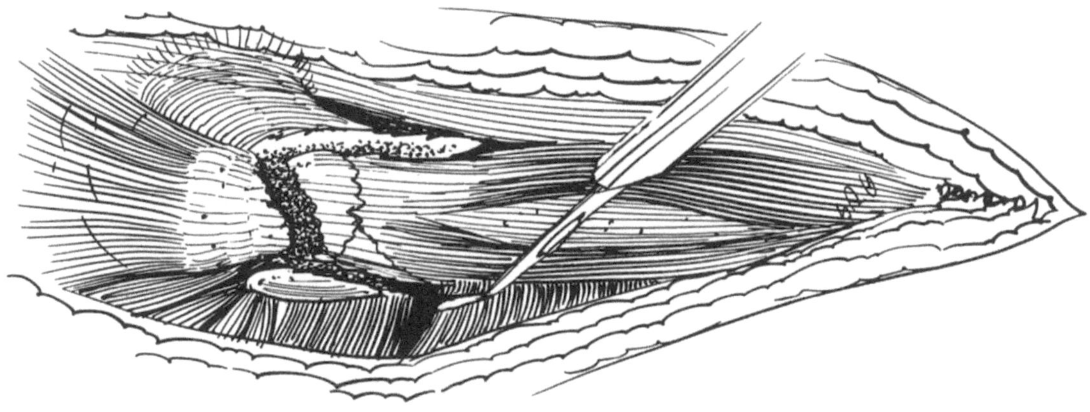

Fig. 8–153 With unstable fracture complexes, the fragments must be released from their incarcerating soft tissues. Here the tethering effect of the gluteus maximus tendon and some of the linea aspera is being severed.

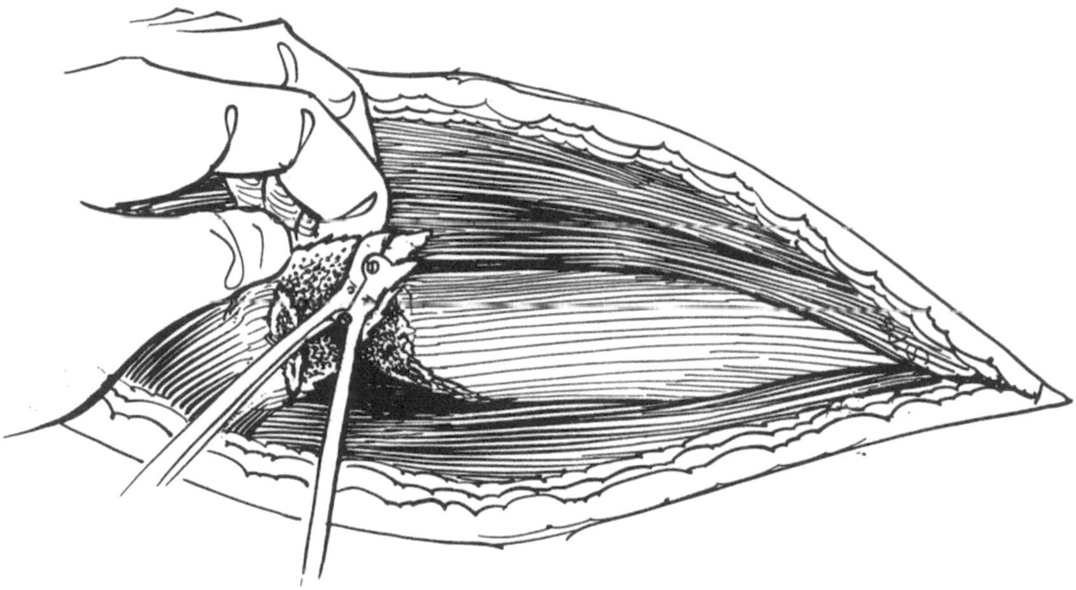

Fig. 8–154 The sharp beak on the inferior neck may refuse to be inserted into the femoral canal, so it must be shaved off with a rongeur.

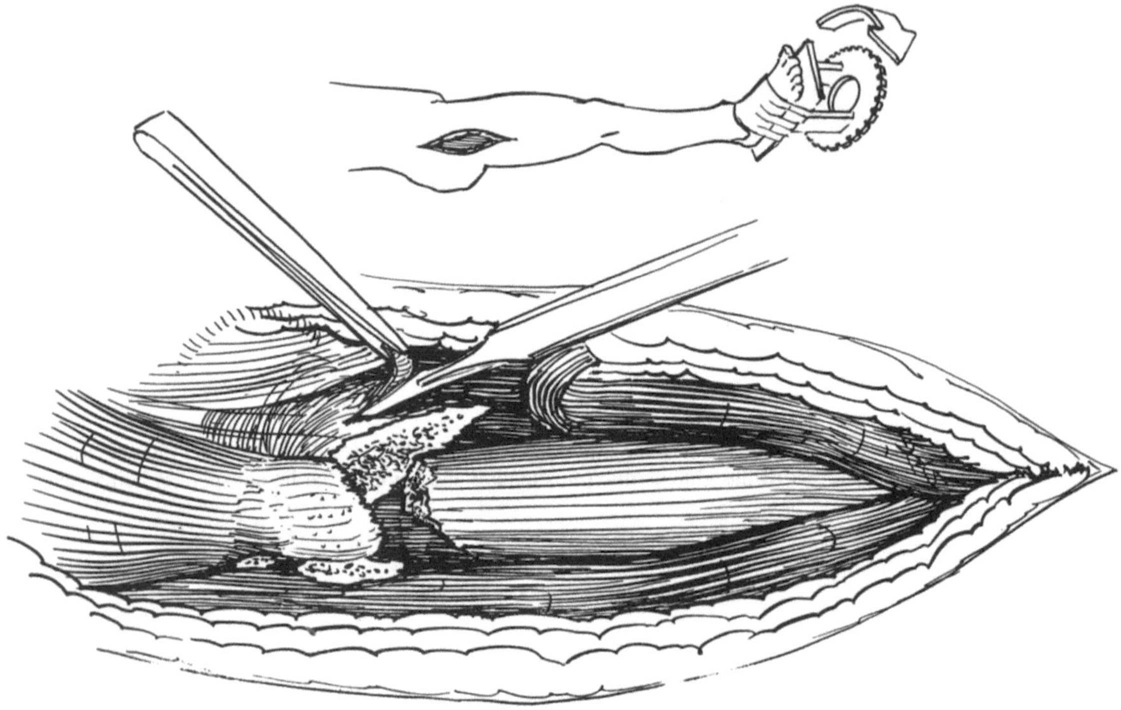

FIG. 8–155 The iliofemoral attachment on the inferior beak may also need to be shaved away before it can be tucked inside the medullary canal. The fracture will have to be opened up by externally rotating the leg.

the retractor can be used to pierce the neck and lever it up out of its depths and then pushed inside the shaft.

Too much traction can be detrimental because it causes the fragments to separate into several free agents (Fig. 8–152), which is especially true of types IV and V. Only *light traction in slight abduction* is needed with the leg freely movable.

Surgical Requirements by Unstable Fracture Type
Most of the principles laid down for unstable fractures applies in general to all of *type I* fractures.

Type II fractures have a long inferior neck segment that may be difficult to get tucked into a telescoping mode. There are two options. If the sharp beak is too long, rongeur it away until it fits into the medullary canal (Fig. 8–154). The other option is to abut it up against the medial femoral cortex (Fig. 8–158). In the maneuvers, the placement of the pin screw must be very precise.

Type III fractures are not as common as the others but can be intimidating. See Fig. 8–133 for the author's technique of creating a slot for the neck to engage itself into the femoral canal.

Type IV fractures are very challenging because the inferior portion of the long beak has rotated outwardly and anteriorly. It must be derotated and brought into alignment and held there by fixation, otherwise the reduction is lost postoperatively by a poorly executed operation (Fig. 8–159). An oblique screw directed up into the medial fragment might work, but frequently it merely splits the fragment. Cerclage wires or Parham bands are better, but they can be cumbersome to apply. The author prefers nylon electrician's straps (Fig. 8–160). They can be autoclaved and purchased at hardware stores or electrician depots. They are easier and quicker to use because they are self-locking (Fig. 8–161).

Unstable type V fracture is the most challenging of all the intertrochanteric fractures because it extends into the subtrochanteric region. The subtrochanteric component is a spiral fracture

FIG. 8–156 **A** The neck may be anterior to the shaft and must be lifted up. **B** A Hohmann retractor serves as a levering device.

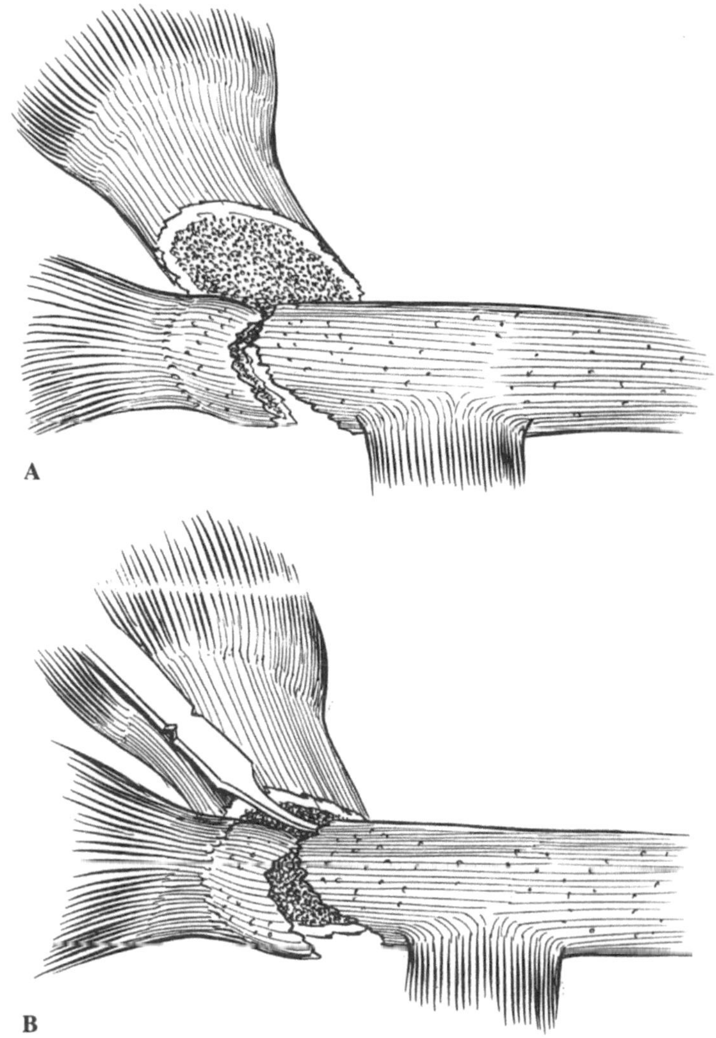

through the coronal plane of the femoral shaft. If the complex is reduced in steps, it can be stabilized back together like a jigsaw puzzle. The key step is the use of nylon bands with or without additional screws placed perpendicular to the femoral fracture plane. The subtrochanteric portion of the complex must be reduced and stabilized first. The neck fragment is externally rotated to a marked degree. With bone clamps, preferably a three-pronged Lowman clamp, first reduce the spiral shaft fracture by rotating it externally and then clamp the fragments together. When it is reduced, the fracture line is even more appreciated as a vertical spiral dividing the lateral cortex. Hold this fracture together with two or three nylon straps (Fig. 8–160). Use the bone clamps as handles to control the shaft and rotate the femur back to a neutral position by turning it internally.

The neck fracture can then be reduced by correcting any residual valgus angulation. Following the author's extramedullary guide pin technique fix the upper fragment with an appropriately sized screw. Take off the Lowman clamp while the fracture is being held together by the nylon strap. Fit a six- or eight-hole side plate over the nylon strap or straps, (Fig. 8–161B). Try to angle the

Fig. 8–157 When the head droops under the shaft **(A)**, use the sharp point of a Hohmann retractor to pull is up out of its hold **(B)**.

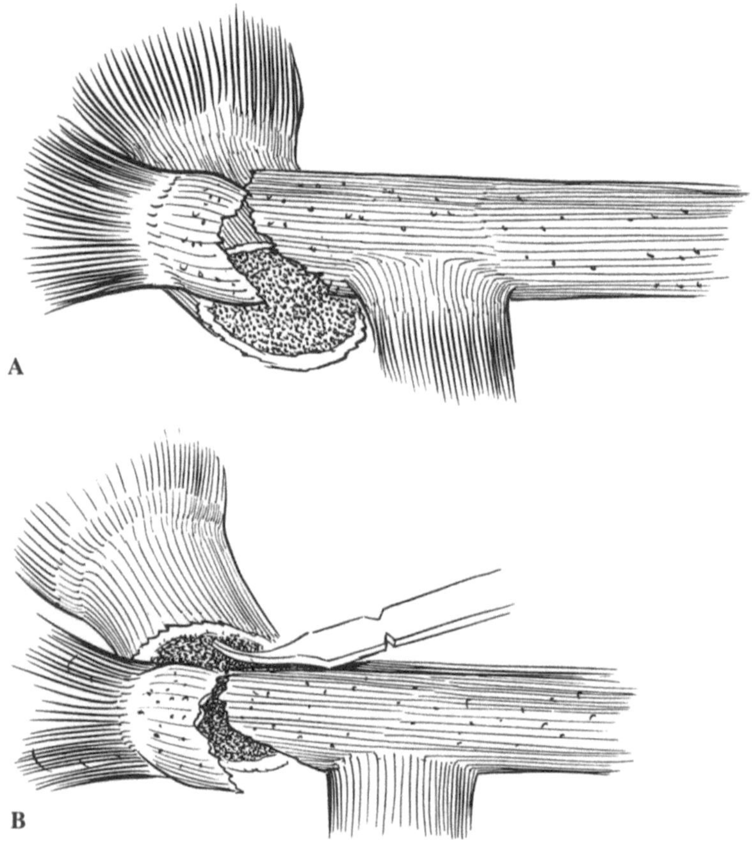

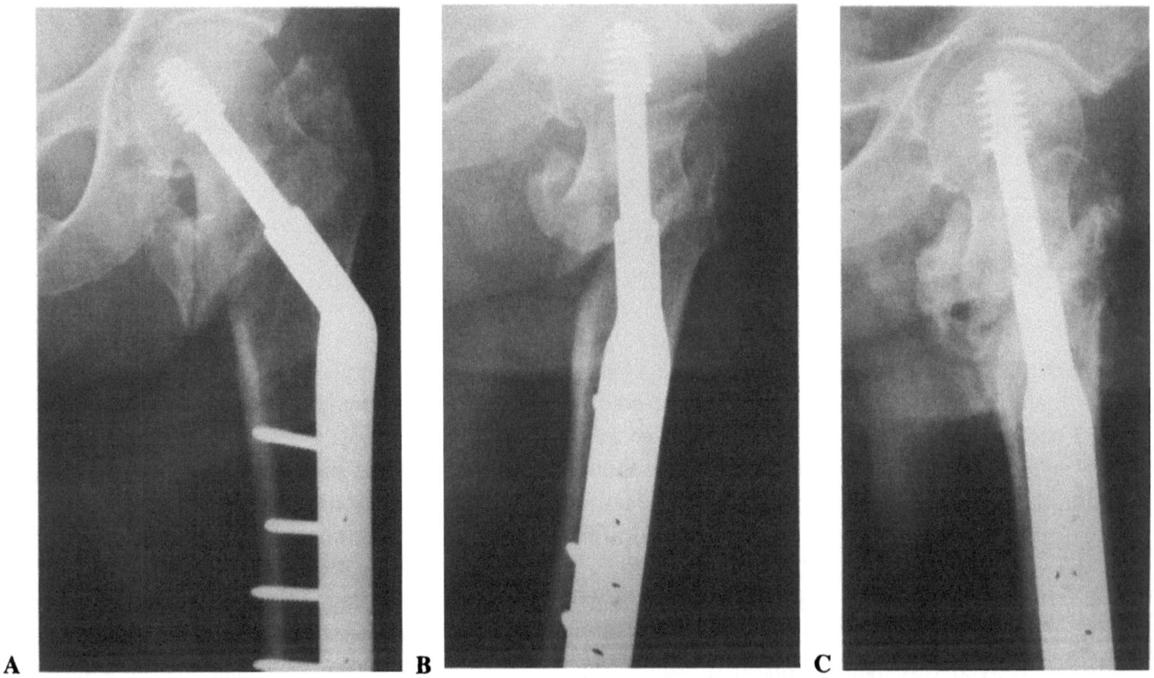

Fig. 8–158 When there is sufficient medial cortex left, it may be possible to oppose the neck against it and compress them firmly together with the hip compression system **(A)**. Note the extreme obliquity to this fracture **(B)**. They will heal quickly when so well stabilized **(C)**.

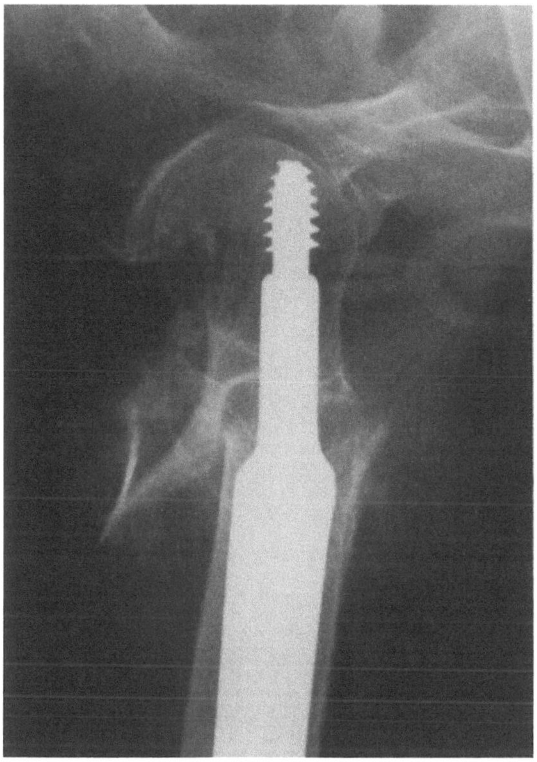

Fig. 8–159 When the long inferior beak is not controlled by forcing it into the femoral canal, reduction is compromised by its spinning on the shaft as seen in this lateral x-ray film. This is a poor reduction and poor placement of the screw.

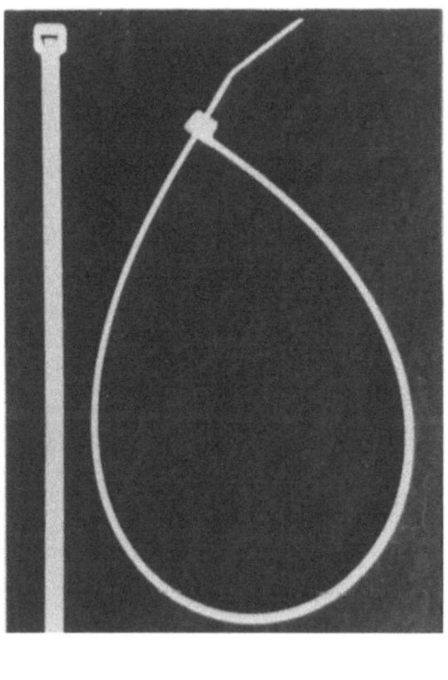

Fig. 8–160 A nylon strap used by electricians to wrap cables comes in various sizes. It is self-locking and easily autoclaved.

screws going into the side plate so that they avoid passing through the split in the cortex. An additional nylon strap is wrapped around the shaft and over the side plate (Fig. 8–161C). (The straps, being nylon, do not create a potential hazard of different metal reaction as is the case with Parham bands.) These patients must *not* bear weight until the fracture is healed, otherwise the implant will break under the stresses directed into the subtrochanteric area. A heavy-duty plate such as the Richards plate or its equivalent is obligatory (Fig. 8–162).

Fractures Complicated by Arthritis An intertrochanteric fracture complicated by arthritis of the hip and treated by a Tronzo total hip system is shown in Fig. 8–163. This was once a rare combination but it is seen more frequently as patients live longer. It is a difficult fracture to treat. One option is to fix it and perform a total hip arthroplasty later when it is healed. The other is to do a primary replacement as was done here. When it is more severely comminuted, a neck replacement implant must be employed. In the case shown, the segment between the fracture and the osteotomized neck becomes a bony ring down through which the prosthesis is passed, a tricky bit of surgery.

Severe Comminution At times the comminution is so extensive the fracture is one mass of bone fragments, more than can be appreciated from preoperative x-ray films, or the manipulation initially causes the comminution of otherwise delicate fragments. There should be a master plan for such occasions. Try to think of the complex as being composed of only two fragments: the head–neck and the shaft (Fig. 8–164A). Secondly, think of the task ahead as creating a stable reduction by inserting the neck into the femoral canal at an angle of 135°. Clear away a path so the neck can be clearly seen on end. Get control of it by inserting a guide pin down its own short intramedullary canal (Fig. 8–164A). With the aid of the heavy-duty guide pin, jam the inferior part of the neck into the shaft (Fig. 8–164A). At this point do not be concerned about the head–shaft angle. Insert an appropriately sized screw about 0.5 inch longer than what protrudes beyond the base of the neck (usually about a 3-inch screw). Insert a four-hole, 135° side plate over the shaft of the screw (Fig. 8–164B). The complex will

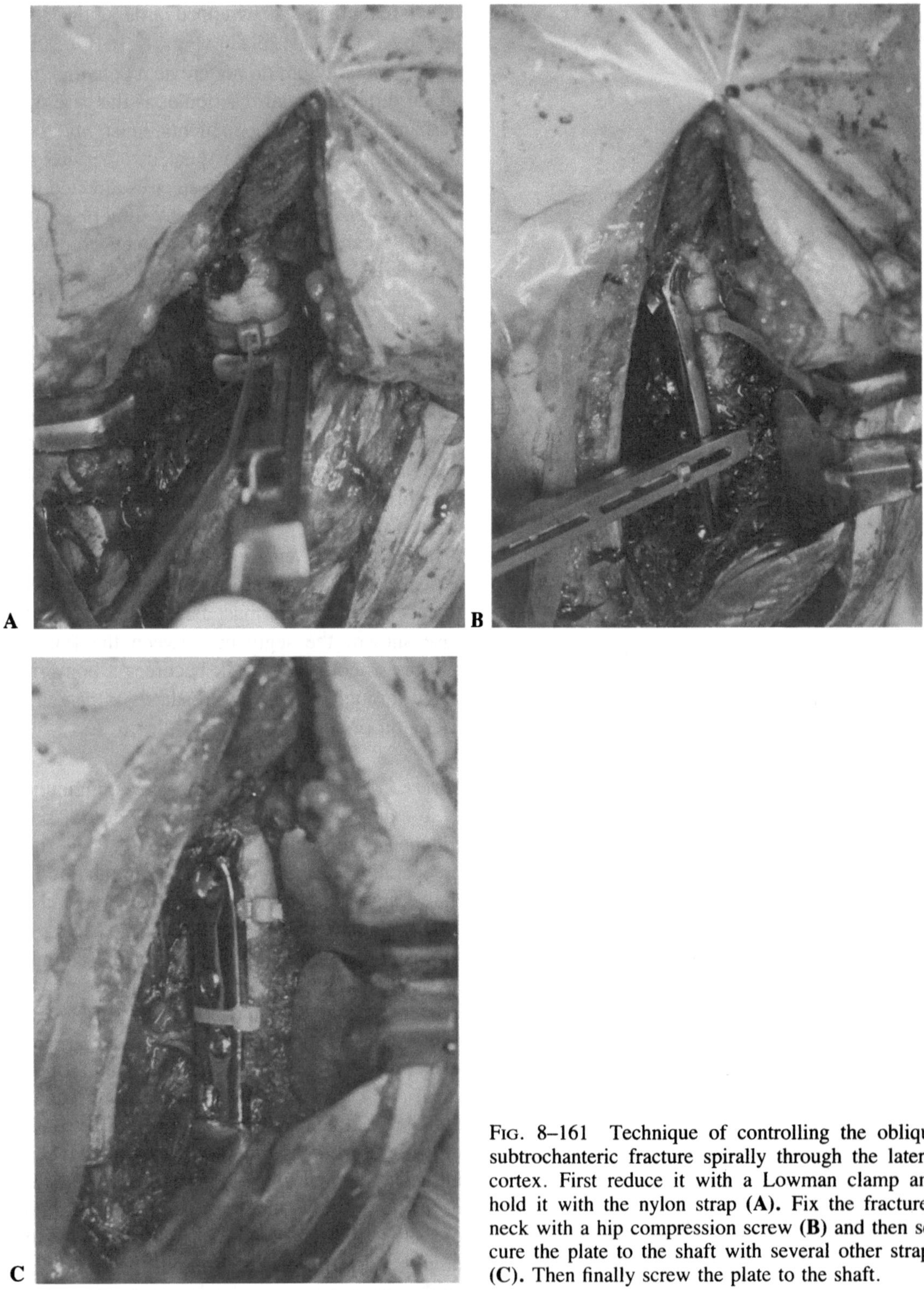

FIG. 8–161 Technique of controlling the oblique subtrochanteric fracture spirally through the lateral cortex. First reduce it with a Lowman clamp and hold it with the nylon strap **(A)**. Fix the fractured neck with a hip compression screw **(B)** and then secure the plate to the shaft with several other straps **(C)**. Then finally screw the plate to the shaft.

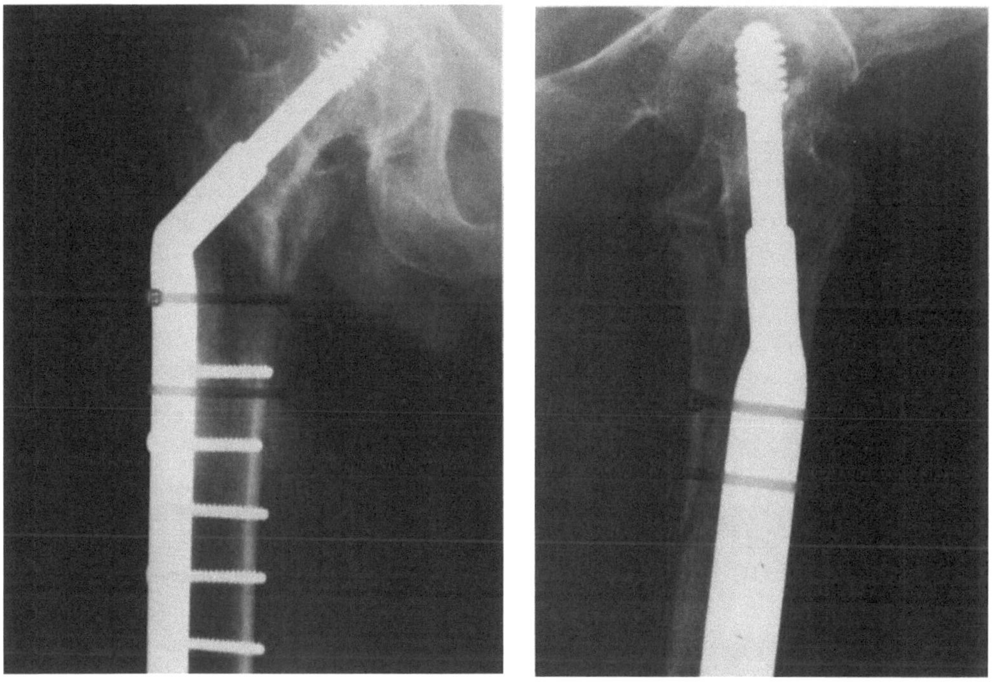

A B

FIG. 8–162 X-ray film of a Type V fracture firmly secured by a heavy side plate supplemented with nylon straps **(A)** and a well placed screw in the lateral x-ray. **(B)**, centrally positioned.

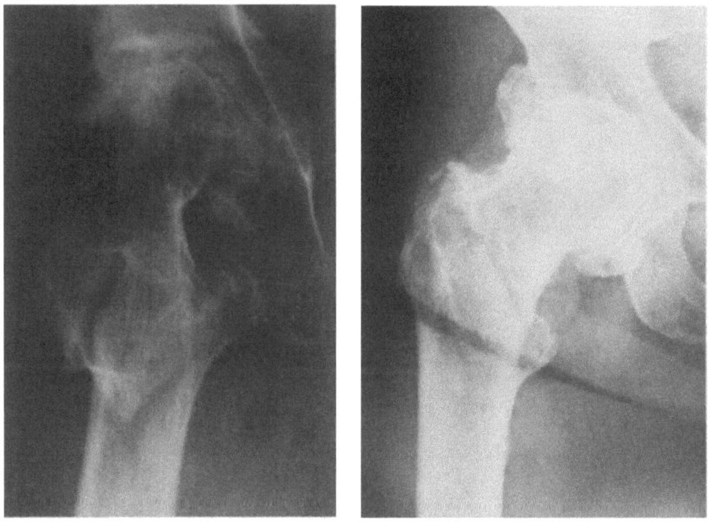

A B

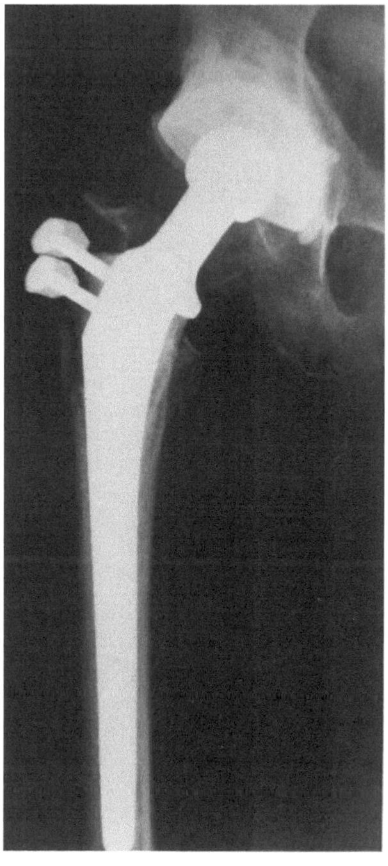

C

FIG. 8–163 **A, B** An intertrochanteric fracture complicated by arthritis of the hip. It has been replaced with a Tronzo total hip system **(C)**.

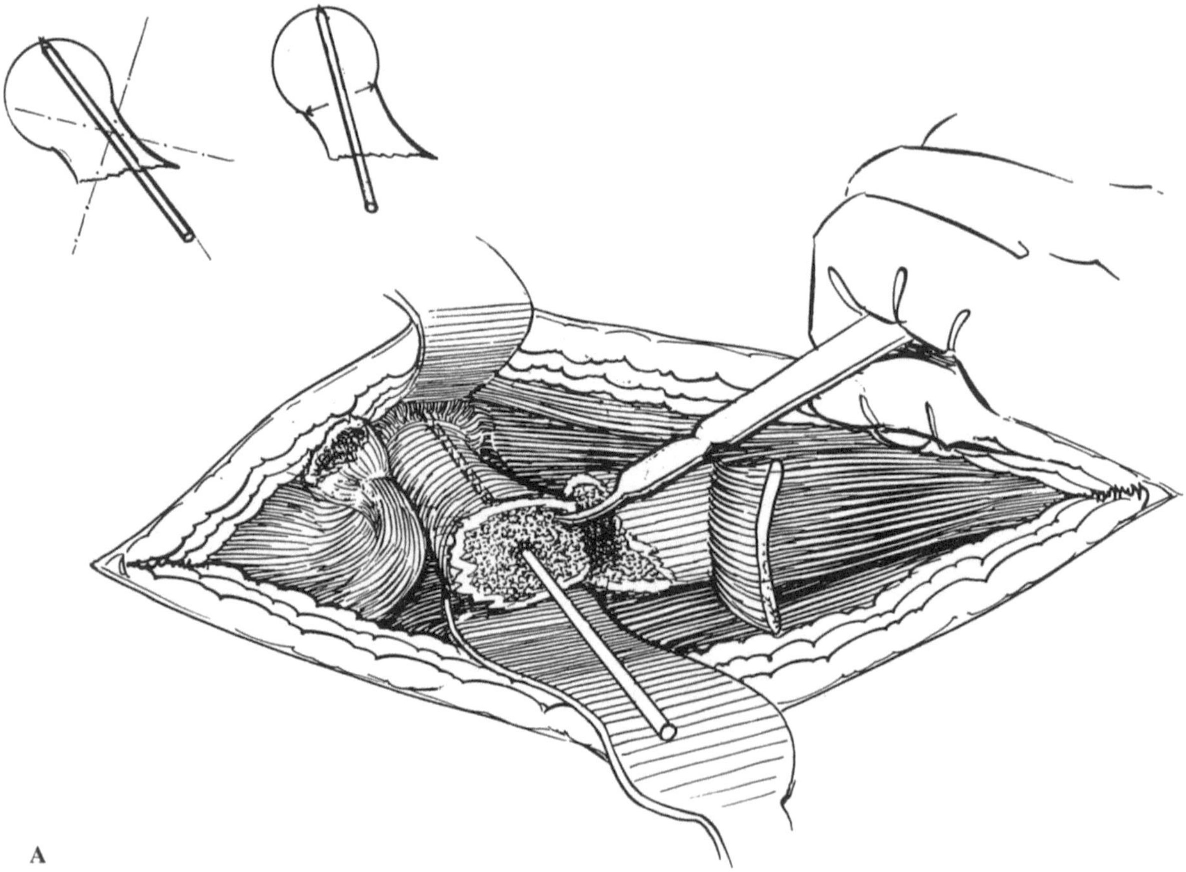

A

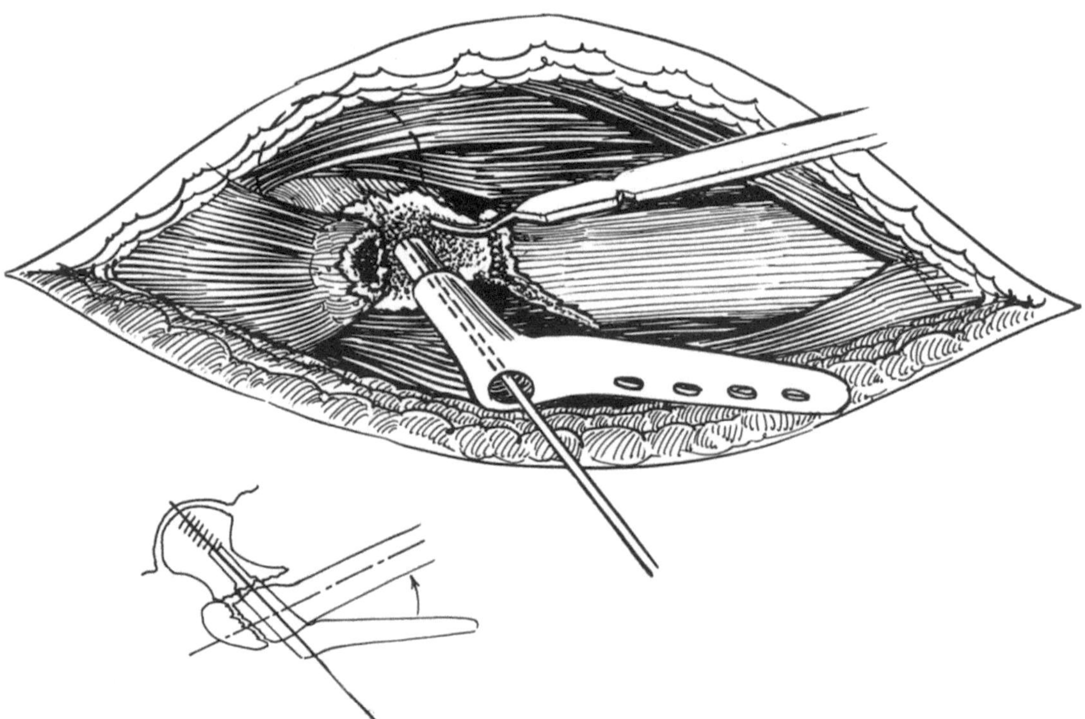

B

FIG. 8–164

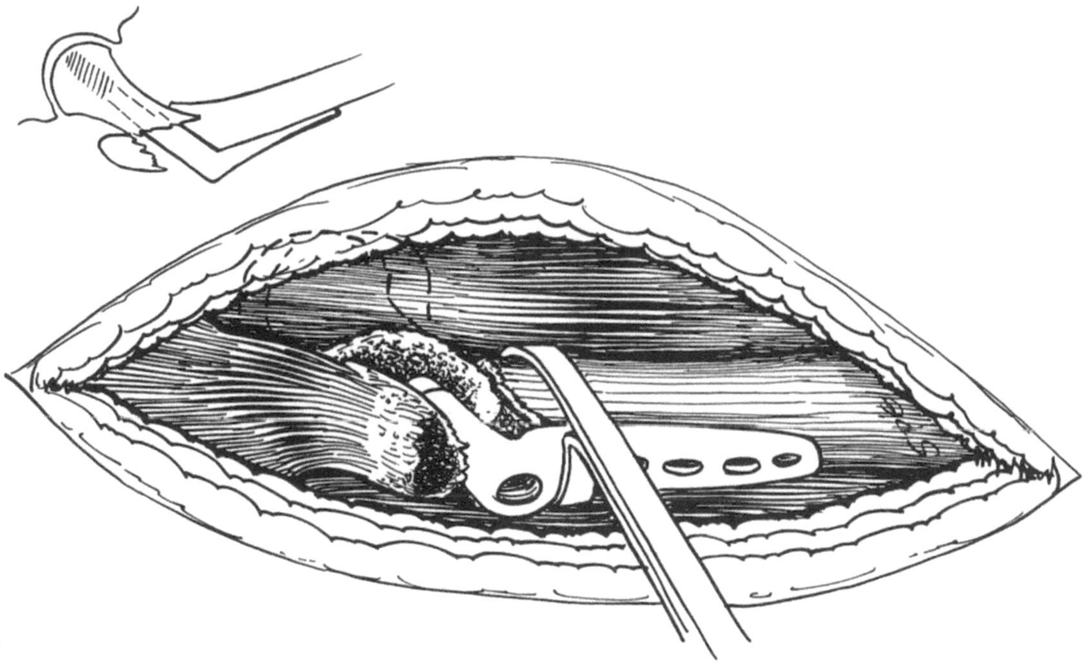

C

FIG. 8–164 **A** In severely comminuted fractures concentrate first on controlling the head and neck by an ideally placed screw. To do this, dismantle the fracture so that the base of the neck is exposed. Place the guide pin down the center of the neck into the center of the head or slightly inferior (see inset). **B** Screw over the guide pin and slide a four to five hole, 135° sideplate over it. Keep the neck controlled by a Hohmann speared into its base. Ignore the greater trochanter. **C** The fracture complex is finally reduced by controlling the head with the screw, which can then be forced inside of the intermedullary canal while the shaft comes into alignment as it is squeezed against the plate by a Lowman clamp (see insert).

appear on an x-ray film as it is depicted in the inset of Fig. 8–164B). When the side plate is pushed onto the femoral shaft, an excellent reduction will have been achieved in slight valgus (Fig. 8–164C). Once compressed together the loads on the implant will have been minimized and the fracture well stabilized (see insert, Fig. 8–164C).

Alternatives to Open Reduction

A patient medically too ill to undergo surgical treatment presents a serious problem. Skeletal traction with a pin through the upper tibia is one option. Balanced suspension is impractical because nursing care and groin ulceration from the Thomas frame compound the problem. Skeletal traction with the leg on two pillows suffices. The author described his modified Russell's traction which has been proved successful (Fig. 8–165).[55] Another possibility is the use of an external fixation frame for these patients or use a cast brace.[293] Skeletal traction is a good alternate for treating type V fractures where surgical stabilization may be a task beyond the experience of the treating surgeon.

Management of Associated Fractured Trochanters Neither trochanteric fragments are specifically treated. An osteotomized greater trochanter as part of a total hip arthroplasty can be a major complication when it becomes avulsed. The situation is quite different with intertrochanteric fractures. The trochanter never presents a problem because the short external rotators are still attached to it in whole or in part. Consequently, they control the fragment, holding it in position and supplying it with a generous blood supply for eventual healing. Likewise, the lesser trochan-

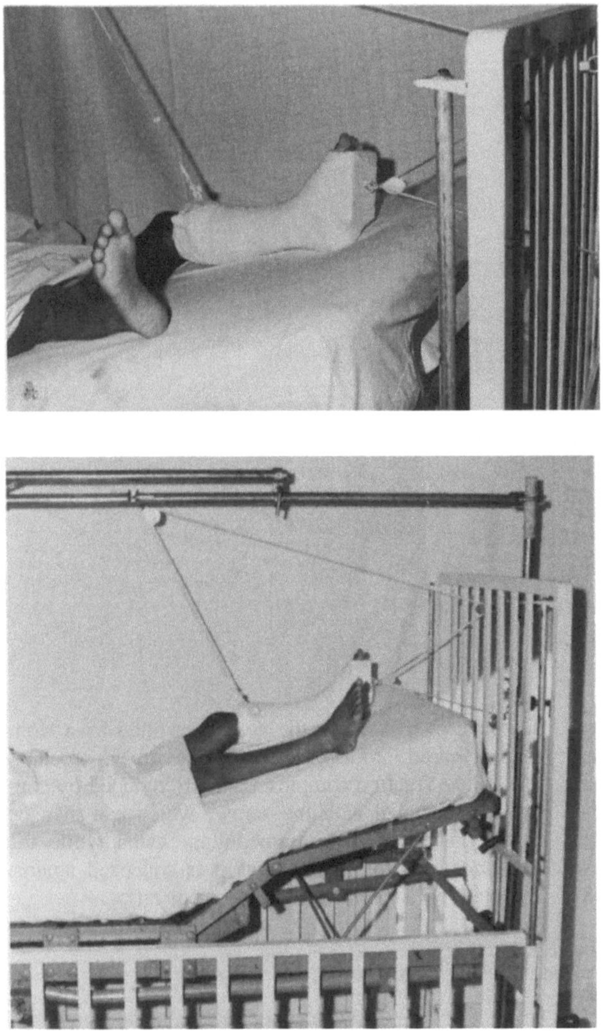

Fig. 8–165 Author's modified Russell's traction using skeletal traction and a short leg cast. Rotary deformities are well corrected and controlled. Be sure the heel is well padded with a pillow under the heel cord!

ter is ignored. The tendon of the iliopsoas muscle may pull it proximally where it will heal solidly into the medial shaft without any loss of flexor power.

Endoprosthetic Replacement The author was the first to report the use of a long, straight-stem Moore prosthesis in the treatment of unstable intertrochanteric fractures[290] (Fig. 8–166). It has since been used and recommended as primary treatment.[291] The procedure has not become popular because as a surgical exercise it is complicated. With the more refined use of compression screws, as advocated, such an arthroplasty is no longer attractive. However, in cases of failure with primary screw fixation (loss of reduction with nonunion *and* a nonviable head) an endoprosthesis, cemented into place, can be an excellent salvage procedure in an elderly patient.

Postoperative Care

Except for the more complicated unstable fractures such as type V, all of the fractures should be stabilized well enough with one of the new sliding nails to allow immediate weight-bearing.[277–279,292] Even the unstable fractures heal rapidly *when well reduced and well fixed* (Fig. 8–167). Stable fractures heal in 8 to 12 weeks, and unstable fractures heal in 3 to 6 months. Just

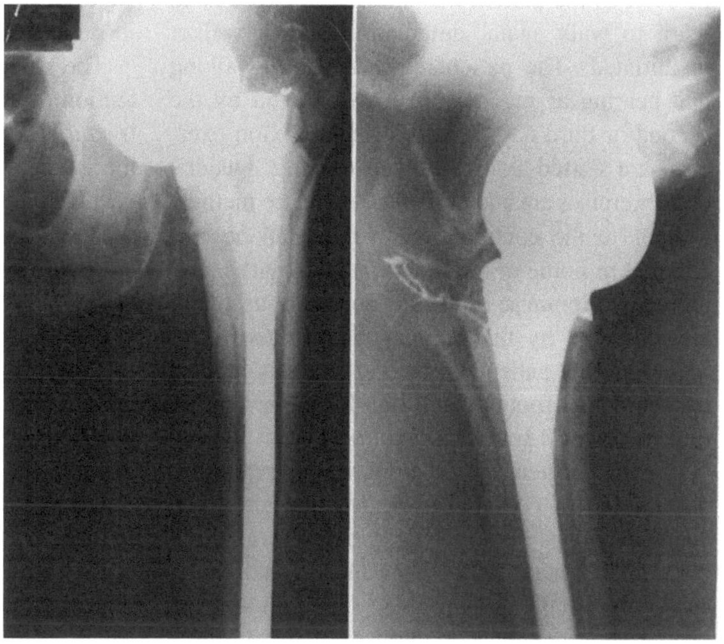

FIG. 8–166 Straight stem Austin-Moore prosthesis cemented in as a replacement for an unstable fracture first reported in 1974 by Tronzo. Today this method is not as good as a well executed open reduction. Saving the natural femoral head should be the surgeon's primary goal of treatment.

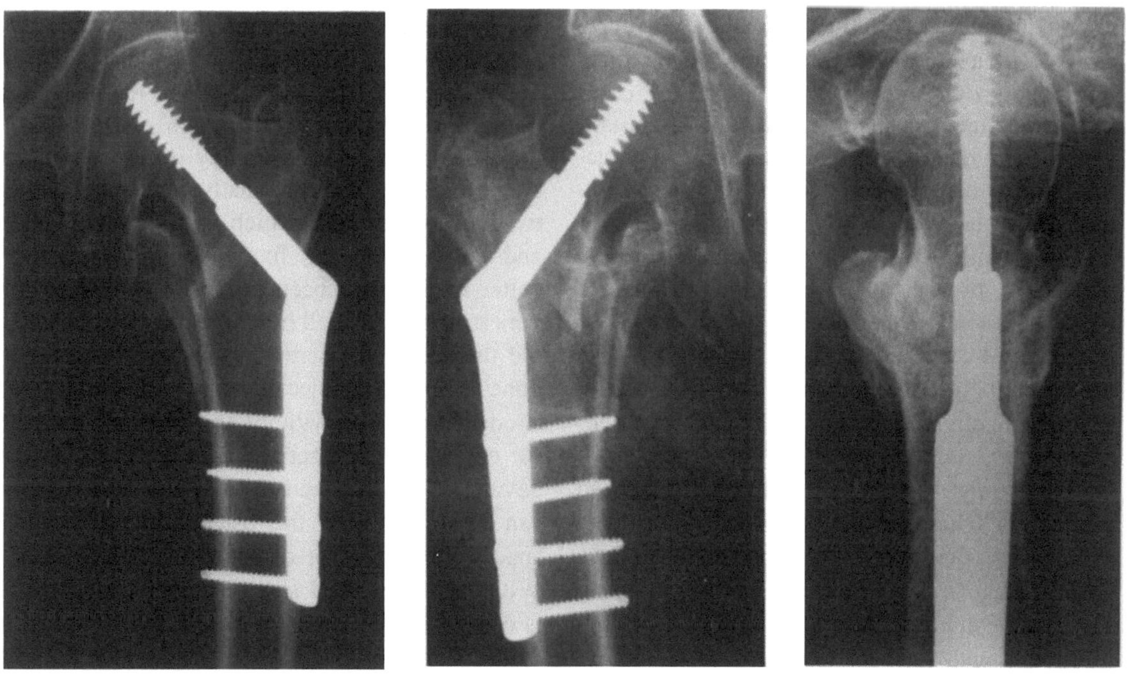

FIG. 8 167 Even unstable fractures heal promptly when well reduced and well fixed. Healing is seen here to be well established at 6 weeks. Nylon strapping was used to secure the lesser trochanter. It was put under the plate to keep it from slipping down the oblique edge of the fracture.

as soon as the patient has the mental capacity to learn to walk again, ambulation with a walker is initiated. The patient should be up walking and bearing as much weight as tolerated by the second or third day. Abduction and flexion exercises are started along with gait training. Quadriceps exercises are added. Unless there are medical reasons to the contrary, the patient can be discharged to home or a nursing facility by the seventh day. Hemovac drains are routinely used and are extracted by the second postoperative day. Switching the patient to jogging shoes is helpful to secure their footing. In Romash's cases healing time averaged 12 weeks.[293] In most cases the patient's leg shortens to some degree depending on the amount of collapse at the fracture site. The average collapse in our stable cases is about 1 cm, which when translated into functional shortening becomes unnoticeable. The amount of shortening from the collapsed segment is minimized by the fracture being reduced in valgus. Unstable fractures can collapse more, requiring corrective heel and sole lifts. Cast braces may be tailored to aid rehabilitation in the younger patient with a type IV or V fracture.[293]

Complications

A model study for assessing the results of modern-day management of intertrochanteric fractures treated with a hip compression screw can be found in the work by Rao et al.[280] A total of 162 cases of unstable intertrochanteric (unspecified classification) were treated with a near-anatomical reduction with a compression screw. They were followed for an average of 19 months. Loss of reduction with varus angulation occurred in five patients, a 4% incidence of failure; 110 patients were bearing all of their weight by 3 weeks. The fractures were healed on an average of 18 weeks postoperatively. The fractures were reduced in anatomical alignment, the screw was inserted, and compression was applied. Ninety percent of their fractures displaced medially and stabilized themselves. These authors concluded: "Displacement osteotomies after Dimon and Hughston have no advantage over the present method of using a compression hip screw and spontaneous settling of the fragment." There were no nonunions, except in five cases that were improperly treated. There were no cases of avascular necrosis. The hospital mortality rate was 3.2%. Five failures were iatrogenic, with poor screw placement and inadequate depth of insertion.

The role of osteoporosis is receiving more attention as the main culprit in failure of unstable fracture complexes.[282,283] Singh et al.[14] pioneered the concept of measuring the quality of the trabecular pattern in the upper end of the femur as an attempt to quantify osteoporosis. The greater the degree of osteopenia, the greater is the risk of fracture. The more osteoporotic hips have unstable fractures. It is not a practical tool for clinical use, however, because it is difficult to obtain ideal x-ray films for comparison. The most severely osteoporotic bone is grade I and the least is grade V.

Despite a well placed screw, the head can be so osteoporotic that the screw withdraws itself or cuts out of the head *causing loss of reduction,* Figure 8–168. There are also iatrogenic problems which compound the problem of osteoporosis. Such a situation can develop when the surgeon penetrates the head with a nail or screw more than once, so that the anchorage is severely jeopardized. Also, when too much compression is applied to the screw by an external compression device, it can be pulled out of the head, which further jeopardizes the quality of any fixation at that site. An implant placed too superiorly in the head of an osteoporotic patient will surely migrate out of it with load-bearing. In these cases the screw can be withdrawn, the channel filled with methylmethacrylate, and the device realigned and reinserted. When using this method, the cement must be carefully packed away from the fracture site, otherwise, it can be inadvertently forced between the fragments, which will prevent healing and compromise the fixation (Fig. 8–169). A better method has been proposed by Tronzo.[202] Fenestrations or small holes can be made between the threads of the screw which allow the liquid bone cement to be injected at any time the surgeon chooses to do so without the mess of packing the cavity with cement and having to reinsert the device. With the fenestrated screw the cement can be forced into the osteoporotic trabecular spaces ensuring firm cementation (Fig. 8–170). With the fenestrated screw, only the upper end is cemented into place.

Breakage of the new sliding screw devices are rare today. Keyed systems can still jam and become solid nails with subsequent failures typical of solid nail systems. The side plate was the

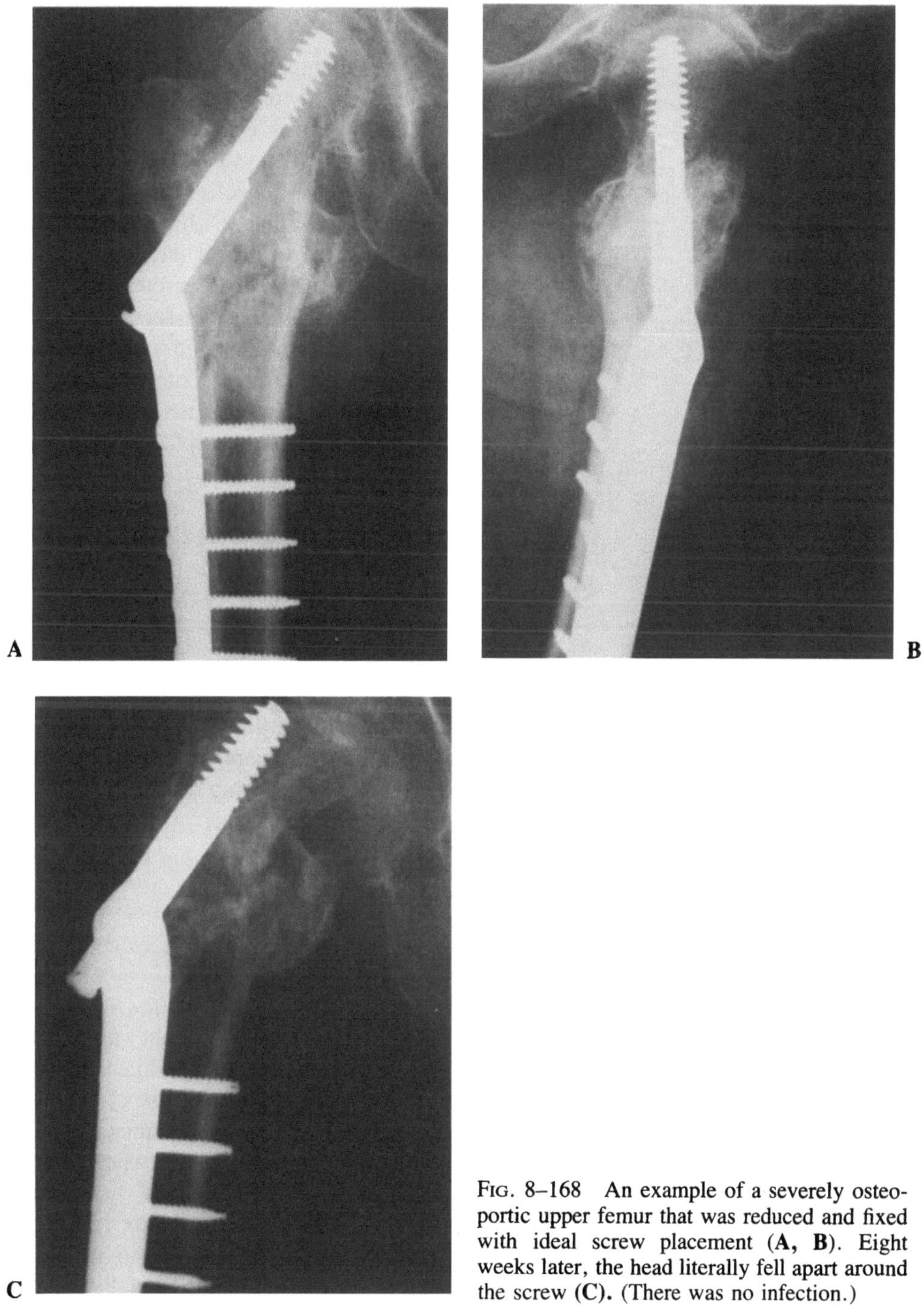

FIG. 8–168 An example of a severely osteoportic upper femur that was reduced and fixed with ideal screw placement (**A, B**). Eight weeks later, the head literally fell apart around the screw (**C**). (There was no infection.)

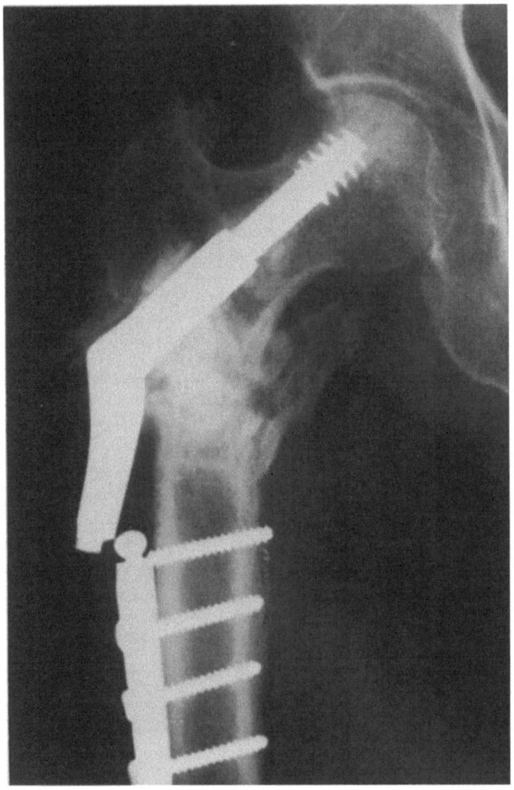

FIG. 8–169 When cement is allowed to creep between the fragments, healing is prevented. In this case, the patient literally walked on cement and fractured the plate onto which all of the load had been transferred.

site of most failures, breaking typically at the nail plate junction or at one screw hole below it. The new heavy-duty side plates seem to have solved this problem. When the smaller screws were used the plate could pull away as the screws fractured, which rarely is seen with the heavy AO screws. At least 2 to 3 cm of the screw shaft should remain inside the barrel of the side plate, otherwise there is a chance of the screw becoming disengaged from the barrel, especially if the internal compression screw is not used. A loss of reduction follows.

Persistent *external rotation* of the foot is due to improper reduction of the fragments at surgery, especially with the unstable fracture. An internal rotational deformity exists where excessive internal rotation past the midplane was used to reduce a stable type of fracture. If an open reduction is done a few days after injury, the fracture fragments should visually match up well, thereby avoiding such a deformity. Internal rotatory deformities are due to excessive internal rotation at the time of reduction.

Extrusion of the shaft of the screw beyond the side plate may cause a *painful* bursa. Most of the time this is only to a slight degree and seldom causes any trouble. If the internal compression screw is left in place, it can protrude as the device collapses. It becomes a sharp prominence, which in a frail, elderly woman requires its removal. For this reason most surgeons use the screw to impact the fragments and then remove it. In severely comminuted cases, however, collapse at the fracture site can be considerable, and the whole implant may have to be removed after healing has taken place.

Nonunions are rare in intertrochanteric fractures when good technique has been followed. Bernasek et al. analyzed seven nonunions at the University of New Mexico.[294] Two were with Jewett nails. In three of the four cases with sliding screws the placement was poor. The seventh case utilized Ender rodding. Each of the patients had an average of three operations in the treatment of their initial fracture that led to the nonunion. Six of the seven were alcoholics. Their cases were salvaged by a total hip replacement using a calcar replacement prosthesis.

Treatment of Failures

Loss of reduction due to osteoporosis or poor placement of the screw can be corrected by reinsertion in the proper position in the lower one-third of the head with slight valgus reduction of the fracture plus augmentation with bone cement either with or without the use of the newer fenestrated hip screw for cement injection. Bone grafts are seldom needed except where gaps must be filled in by locally harvested iliac crest bone.

Nonunions without a loss of reductions are uncommon and are usually due to the sliding device becoming blocked, converting the unit into a solid nail thus preventing the fragments from impacting into each other. The solution is either to screw the tip further into the head or use a side plate with a shorter barrel, or both. Using a fenestrated screw system or packing the channel with bone cement first and then screwing in the device allows the neck to be impacted by force of the internal compression screw. Once this is done, union is prompt. Another consideration is to os-

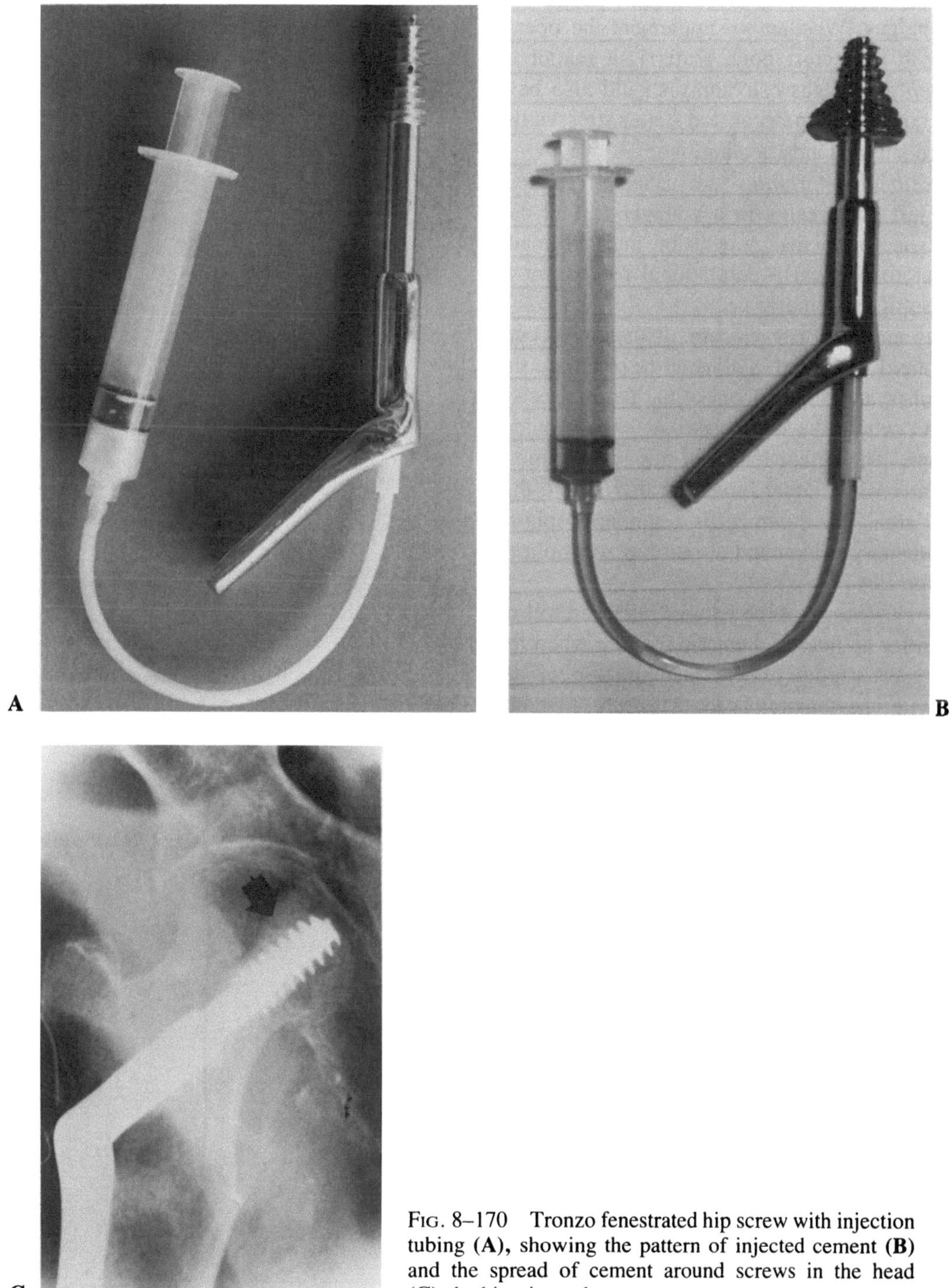

FIG. 8–170 Tronzo fenestrated hip screw with injection tubing (**A**), showing the pattern of injected cement (**B**) and the spread of cement around screws in the head (**C**), locking into place.

teotomize the intertrochanteric area and correct any varus deformity by turning the fracture into slight valgus. Whether to supplement the operation with iliac crest bone grafts is a matter of judgment. A valgus osteotomy should also be a prime consideration because it better stresses the fracture site and aids healing.

Rotational deformities are usually tolerated, but if left uncorrected in a younger patient can cause knee problems. A decision must be made whether to perform a derotational osteotomy at the base of the femoral neck.

Avascular necrosis is rare. It usually occurs when the device used is allowed to penetrate the superior or anterior segment of the femoral head, or both, where the main vascular supply enters the bone. The author has seen this happen more frequently when Ender pins were driven into this critical area. The treatment is a hemiarthroplasty in a sedentary person and a total hip arthroplasty in a vigorous person.

Stress fractures of the femoral neck can follow fixation for an intertrochanteric fracture when the nail or screw goes only to the junction of the neck with the femoral head. This was first de-

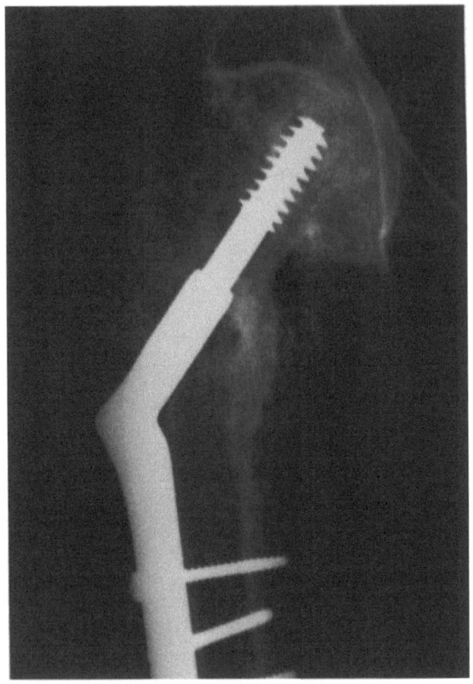
A

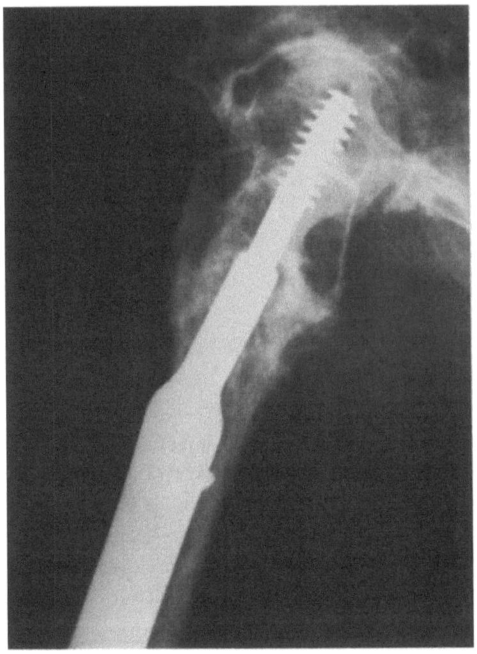
B

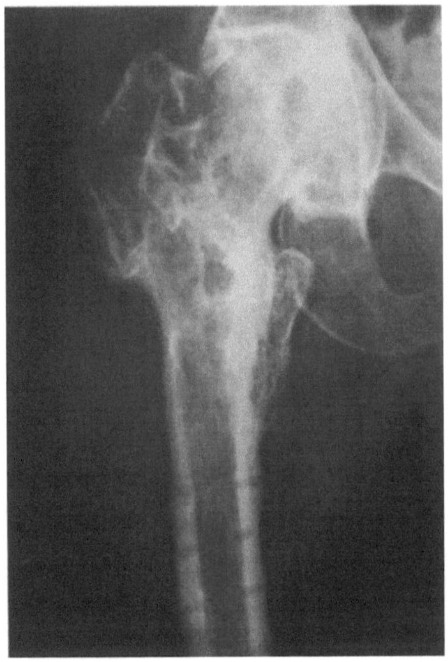
C

FIG. 8–171 **A** Example of chronic infection with cysts formed surrounded by sclerotic bone. **B** Once the implant is removed, the infection has a good chance to heal with appropriate antibiotics **(C)**.

scribed by Tronzo. It has been subsequently called the "Tronzo fracture"[55,295] (see page 181, Fig. 8–25, for details).

Postoperative Infection The diagnosis and management of early and late infections are similar to those defined for femoral neck fractures (see earlier in this chapter). The most common organism is *Staphylococcus*.

Intravenous and intraoperative lavage with antibiotics is routine today and a very effective means of preventing infections. Usually the implant can stay in place for open drainage of an infected hematoma. In a more chronic case the implant must be removed (Fig. 8–171). Before removing an implant an appraisal of bone union must be made. In chronic cases the bone in the intertrochanteric area heals despite a deep infection, which distinguishes it from infected femoral neck fractures, which do not heal. If not united there is usually enough fibrous union to permit extraction of the device with protective non-weight-bearing postoperatively. Skeletal traction may be an option for an unstable union.

Subtrochanteric Fractures

Subtrochanteric fractures are defined by this author as those fractures whose central impact occurs in the region bounded by the lesser trochanter above and the isthmus of the femoral shaft below. From this point of reference they usually extend in either direction. Only short, oblique varieties remain strictly confined to this region (Fig. 8–172). The region in question is unique for several reasons: (1) The forces that zero in on this region are great,[98] causing the femoral cortex to develop to its greatest width. In 1917 Koch, using theoretical static figures, accurately calculated the stress on the medial cortex of the proximal femur under static loading of 100 pounds and found it to be 1200 pounds per square inch.[296] These figures have yet to be found in error with dynamic loading studies using strain gauges.[297] (2) Vascularity is less abundant in hard cortical bone; therefore healing is slow with nonunions high. (3) The magnitude of the impact required to produce these fractures is considerably greater than for any of the other upper femoral fractures.[298] (4) These same stresses cause frequent failure of the implant with subsequent loss of fixation and delayed or frank nonunions.[299]

Because of its shape, the femur is subjected to eccentric loading. In vivo this bending force loads the medial cortex in compression and the cortex in tension. The forces are not in equilibrium. Strain gauge studies show that compressive loads are considerably greater than the tensile loads. This dissimilar loading pattern is of great importance in selecting internal fixation devices and in understanding the causes and prevention of failure on internal fixation devices. Such a loading pattern further emphasizes the importance of prestressing of the implant in tension, which in turn increases axial compression and increases the stability of the implant into a functional unit.[298]

Younger patients who suffer this fracture have been injured in a high-energy collision. For this reason there is a wide age range, bringing the average age down significantly compared to those with intertrochanteric fractures. In Munson's large series the age ranged from 20 to 90 with an average of 55.5.[300] It is difficult to understand the mechanism in the elderly patient, as the fracture can occur in a patient who simply tripped going down a simple step.

In Fielding's study of fractured hips, subtrochanteric fractures comprised 7% of all upper femoral fractures. These patients stayed in the hospital three times longer than other fractured hips. The patients' average age was 67 years, which confirms the lower than average age for hip fractures.[301] Such patients require three times the amount of time for healing, and most importantly the patients cannot be allowed to bear weight until there is absolute proof of bone union by a laminogram.

Classification of these fractures have been attempted by several interested people.[55,270,298,302–306] Seinsheimer's classification appears to be the most popular (Fig. 8–173). The transverse and short, oblique types are straightforward (Fig. 8–172). They are often best classified only after they have been opened and reduced. There are two basic fracture components: (1) a butterfly fragment medially and varying degrees of comminution posteromedially, especially in the upper end; figures 8–172 *or* (2) a long, oblique fracture line in the coronal plane (a long vertical split in the lateral cortex) (Fig. 8–174). The fracture line spiralling through the coronal plane can be a de-

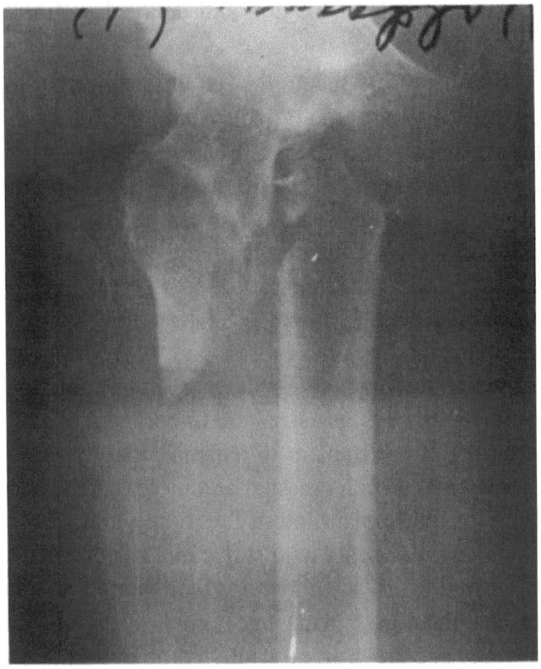

FIG. 8–172 Short oblique subtrochanteric fracture.

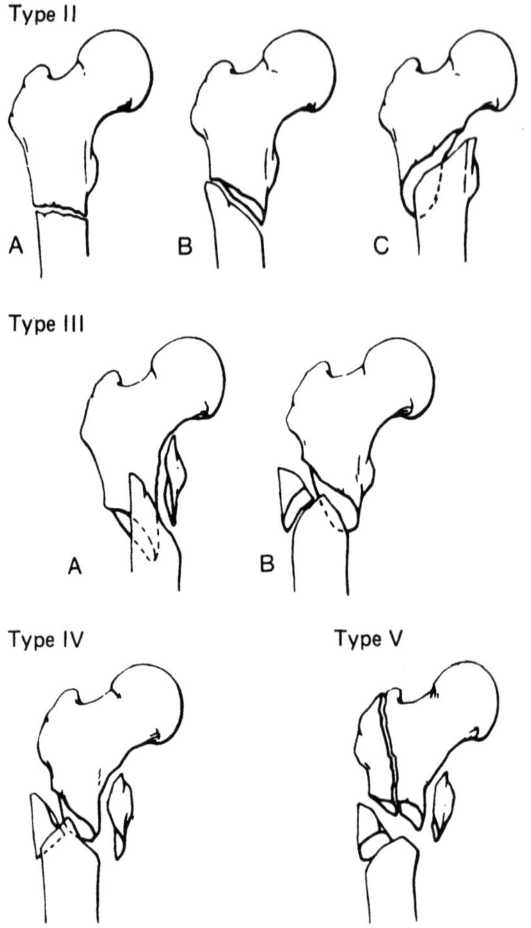

FIG. 8–173 Seinsheimer's classification of subtrochanteric fractures. (Adapted from Seinsheimer, F.: Subtrochanteric fractures of the femur. J. Bone Joint Surg., 60A: 300–306, 1978.)

ceivingly complex feature of all subtrochanteric fracture types. They frequently need supplemental bone grafts placed along the medial cortex in order to reestablish the compression bands of the femoral shaft.

Subtrochanteric stress fractures have been reported, but they are rare. Seven cases were studied by Butler and associates.[307] Their description of a stress fracture is quite good: "A stress fracture is an example of a bone remodeling process in response to repeated stress." Bone scans are essential in making the diagnosis in a patient with thigh pain unrelated to any trauma. All of their cases were treated with varying degrees of rest with gradual partial weight-bearing. All healed without surgery within a period of 4 to 6 weeks. See Figure 8–104 for an example of a subtrochanteric fracture complicating multiple pin fixation when used for repairing a femoral neck fracture.

In order to decide on the type of fixation to be used, it is crucial to determine the site of the major instability, which is where comminution is most extensive. If the major fragmentation is trochanteric, a strong device such as the Richards AMBI does well.[318] If the explosion occurred mainly within the isthmus area and below, an intramedullary device such as the Zickel system is more appropriate.[306] When in doubt, use an intramedullary device.

Surgical Technique

An open reduction must be done with a generous set of instruments and implants being available (Figs. 8–160, 8–161, 8–162). The author uses nylon strappings routinely. If they are not available, Parham bands should be on the operating room setup. AO screws should also be available. The author's technique for unstable type V fractures where there is a intertrochanteric–subtrochanteric combination is also followed in these fractures. Figure 8–175 is an example of a spiral fracture within the coronal plane whose shaft

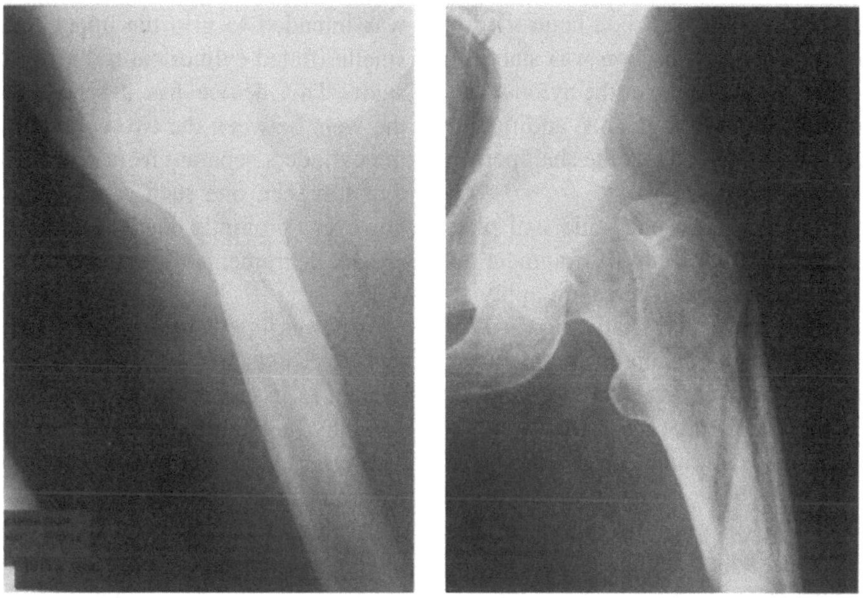
A B

FIG. 8–174 **A** Long spiral subtrochanteric fracture without a medial butterfly component. **B** Fracture line passes through the coronal plane of the femoral shaft which makes subtrochanteric fractures so difficult to fix.

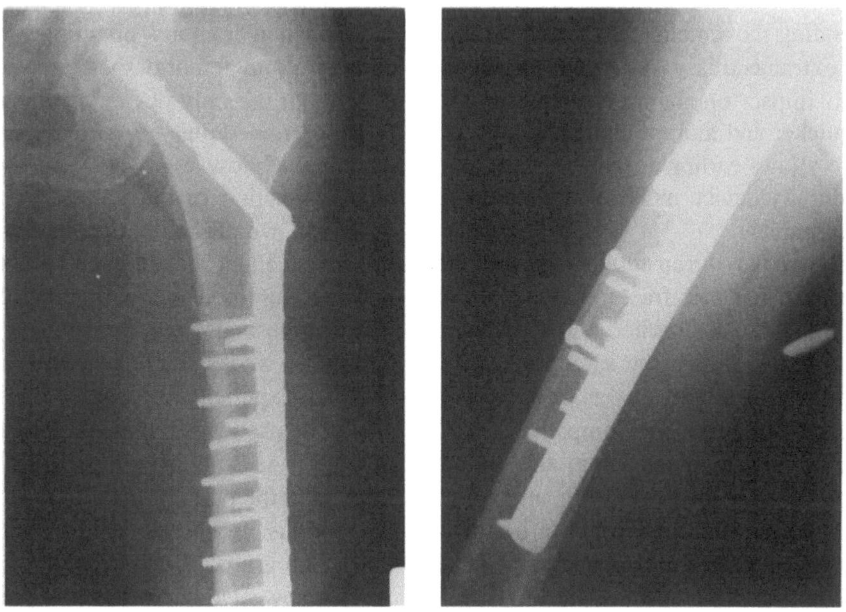

FIG. 8–175 An example of a subtrochanteric fracture in an AP and Lateral x-ray fixed with an AMBI plate and screw. Nylon straps and supplemental screws were used to add fixation to the oblique fragments first. *Note* that if this type of device is to be used, the side plate should be one of special design and material to carry the extraordinary loads of such an unstable fracture site.

component was first fixed with a series of nylon straps. The neck portion was then controlled by a sliding screw. The shaft portion was stabilized with a long heavy side plate over the nylon straps, and finally the oblique fragments additionally fixed with AO screws drilled into the shaft perpendicular to its long axis.

The Swiss use a very strong solid nail plate. They first reduce a major butterfly fragment and fix it with cortical screws. Then they apply the plate to the upper femur and shaft (Fig. 8–176). In the comminuted cases the major fragments are brought together with cortical screws, and the nail plate is then applied. They strongly advise supplementing the comminuted posteromedial wall with cancellous bone from the patient's iliac crest (Fig. 8–177). It is essential to replace bone loss with iliac bone, which augments bone healing at a point where stresses are greatest at the posteromedial segment and where cortical hypertorphy will develop (Fig. 8–178). The work of Cecg and Sosna[309] should be reviewed for principles that apply for using bone grafts in fresh subtrochanteric fractures and in nonunions of these fractures.

Special Intramedullary Devices

An intramedullary rod has the advantage of spreading the stresses over a wide area by neutralizing the bending movements that would ordinarily load an extramedullary system. It allows the fragments to impact on themselves like a shish kabob for quicker and more reliable healing. The latter feature allows earlier weight-bearing. With an extramedullary device much of the loading is borne by the implant.

The most popular intramedullary system designed for subtrochanteric fractures is the Zickel nail[310] (Fig. 8–179). Küntscher much earlier in 1942 had designed almost the same device and called it the "Y" nail.[311,312] It was manufactured by the Orthopedic Equipment Company. A modern version is now available from the Biomet Corp. It was a Küntscher rod with an oblique hole at its upper end through which a hollowed hip pin passed into the femoral neck and head. The intramedullary rod controlled the shaft fragment, and the hip pin controlled the upper femoral segment, a concept copied into the Zickel system.[313]

Another special device, the Samson rod, was reported by Allen and Burstein.[314] The upper metaphyseal portion is a large fluted cylinder that was intended to grip the upper femur while the smaller fluted cylindrical rod gripped the femoral shaft. This device has a serious defect in that the weld between the two cylinders is weak, and the cylinders separate from one another. This author has seen one such case. The manufacturer, however, promptly lends technical support and special instruments for extraction of the separated pieces.

A newer fluted design comes from Hungary.[315] It is a Küntscher rod with three tapered fins welded to its upper one-fourth. The fins grip the metaphysis while the rod fixes the femoral shaft. The report is a worthwhile thesis to review for its biomechanical analyses.

At this writing a Zickel II has been introduced by the Howmedica Company. The rod portion has four deeper flutes. Anteversion has been built into the hip nail portion. The new system is stronger and easier to insert. The surgical details are illustrated in the technical bulletin prepared by Zickel for the Howmedica Company.

Thomas and Villar[316] studied 135 consecutive patients with subtrochanteric fractures. They concluded that the Zickel nail was superior to other devices, but they warned: "The Zickel nail's use should be reserved for surgeons of reasonable experience." The device is especially valuable in segmental fractures affecting both the subtrochanteric and femoral shaft areas (Fig. 8–179). It is about the only device available to salvage a failed extramedullary system. Figure 8–180 is an example of how overwhelming the stresses are at this junction in the femur. It is a case of a 93-pound woman with rheumatoid arthritis who had an excellent reduction and pinning for a comminuted subtrochanteric fracture. She was very cooperative and went from wheel chair to bed. Within 10 weeks she returned for a visit because she was experiencing progressive leg pain. The side plate used was the heaviest made by Zimmer in 1985. As shown in Fig. 8–180, it began to fracture at the point of maximum stress just above the isthmus. It was salvaged by a Zickel rod and iliac bone grafts.

The newest device that has great promise is the interlocking medullary nail such as the Brooker-Wills and the Grosse-Kempf systems.[284,317] They, too, are modified Küntscher rods. In the Brooker-Wills device a special set of blades is passed through the rod and are spread

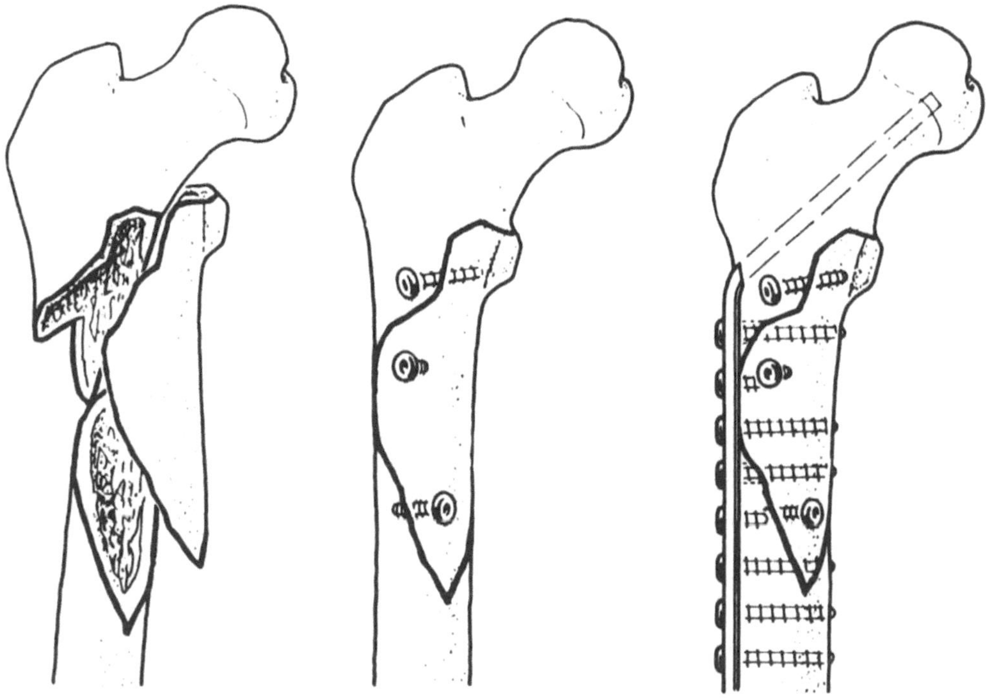

FIG. 8–176 Technique of first screwing together the large medial butterfly fragment and then inserting the main implant. (From Müller, Allgöwer and Willenegger: *Manual of Internal Fixation*. New York, Springer-Verlag, 1970.)

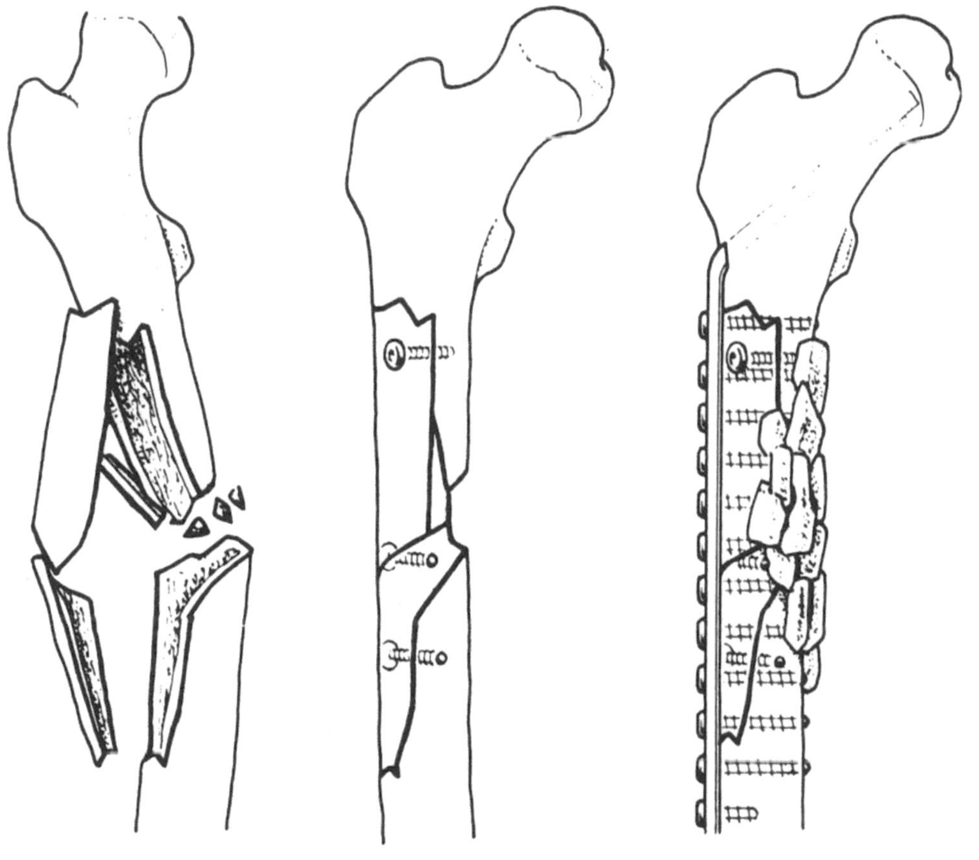

FIG. 8–177 An example of fragments first screwed together and then fixed with a long side-plated nail. Iliac-crest bone grafts must be used to fill any medial gaps. (From Müller, Allgöwer and Willenegger: *Manual of Internal Fixation*. New York, Springer-Verlag, 1970.)

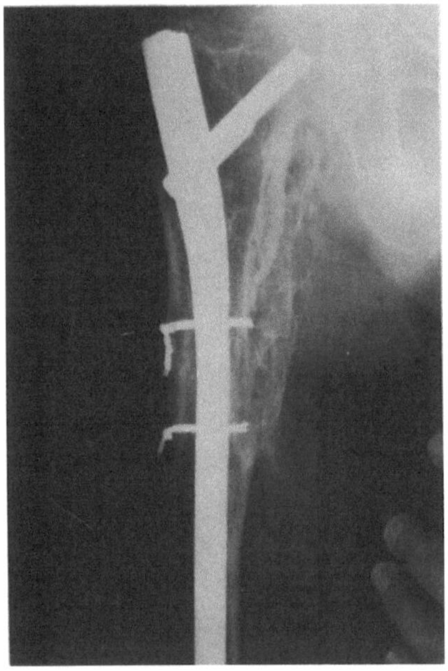

FIG. 8–178 The medial cortex hypertrophies as healing takes place. Stress is transferred to it via an intramedullary rod. The device used here is the Zickel system.

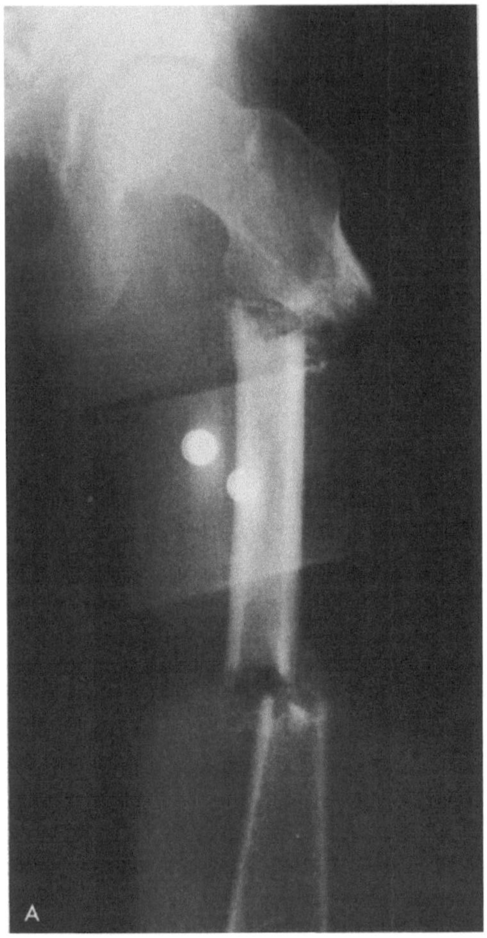

FIG. 8–179 **A** Segmental fractures of the shaft combined with a subtrochanteric fracture is best treated with an intermedullary device such as the Zickel system, **B.** Note the slower rate of healing of the subtrochanteric segment, **C.**

out into the supracondylar area, anchoring the distal femur. A heavy screw is passed obliquely down into the lesser trochanter. The device can be used for subtrochanteric fractures by reversing the screw and turning the nail around 180° so that the screw can be placed into the femoral neck and head, thereby rigidly controlling both fragments from rotation.

Preventing rotation of the distal fragment in a large femur is a defect with the Zickel system. An advantage of the interlocking nail systems is that they prevent the severe comminution from collapsing. Leg length is restored and maintained, which is a feature of no other intramedullary system.

Another interlocking nail is the Grosse-Kempf system, which requires two heavy screws placed perpendicular to the shaft through holes in the nail. Use of this implant is not as easy to master as the Brooker-Wills nail. Both of these systems are presently undergoing clinical trials for the treatment of subtrochanteric fractures with gradual improvement in the learning curve and modification to the system to accommodate these difficult fractures.

Shotgun injuries in the trochanteric and subtrochanteric areas are ideally treated with the new interlocking nails (Fig. 8–181), because the comminution can be so severe that putting the fragments together plus treating the open wound is too tedious to justify traditional surgery other than the necessary débridement.

Subtrochanteric fractures through a pathological lesion of the lesser trochanter is discussed on page 72.

Postoperative Management Postoperative management must be individualized. In general, this fracture must be protected for at least 12 weeks, less so with transverse or short oblique fractures. A fracture brace may be a prudent supplement to the internal implant.[293] Union usually takes 6 to 8 months to be complete. Partial weight-bearing can usually be commenced at about 4 months. Consideration should be given to the use of a

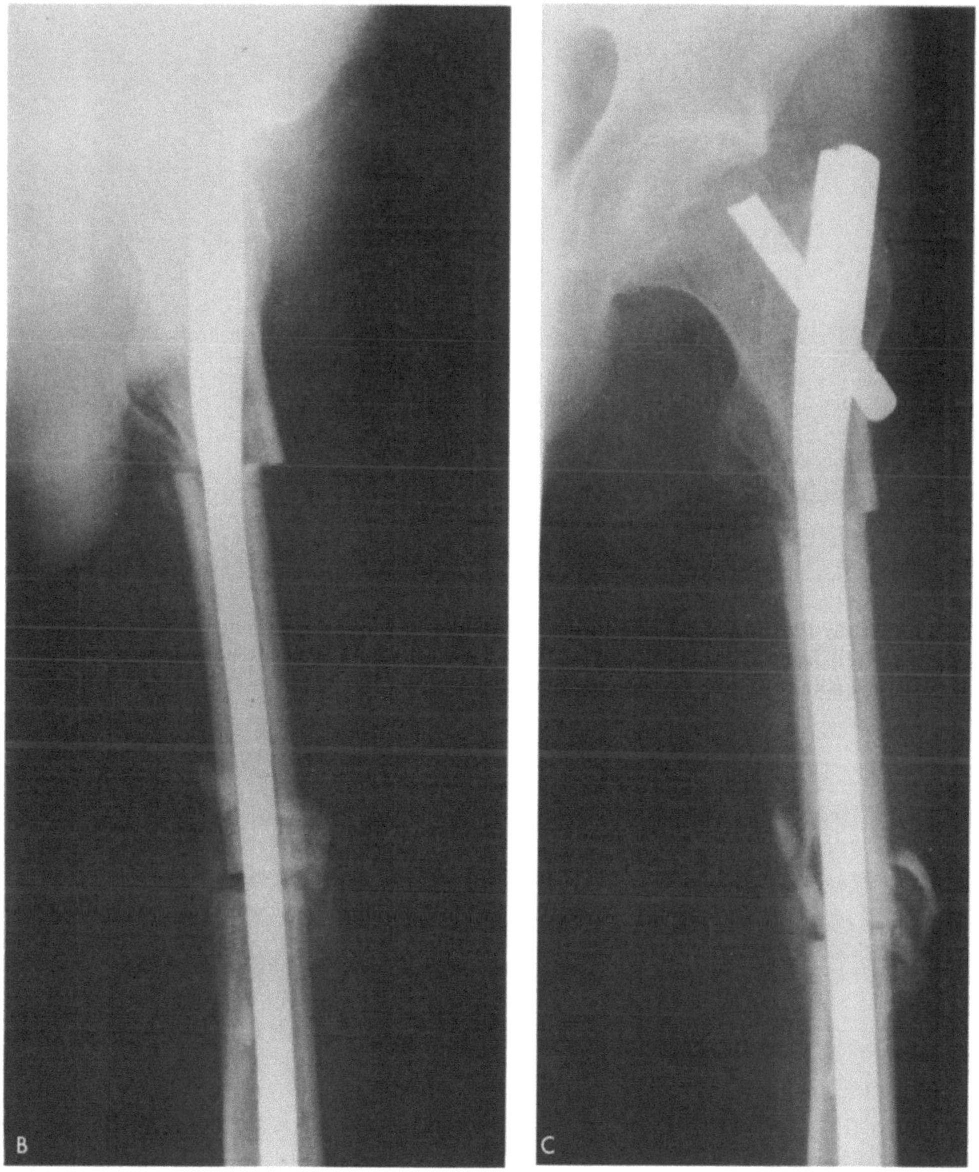

FIG. 8–179 *Continued*

cast brace for the more unstable comminuted variety especially when treated with Ender rods.[318]

Complications

Aside from wound infections, the most frequent complications are loss of reduction from implant failure, delayed union, and nonunion, which is usually accompanied by fracturing of the side plate. The best treatment for these problems is to convert the fixation to an intramedullary system plus application of a bone graft. At this time the Zickel II system is best. Munson had a 100% union with the Zickel nail as a primary method of treatment.[296]

Ender Rods

Ender pins are flexible rods that are threaded up into the intramedullary cavity and into the upper

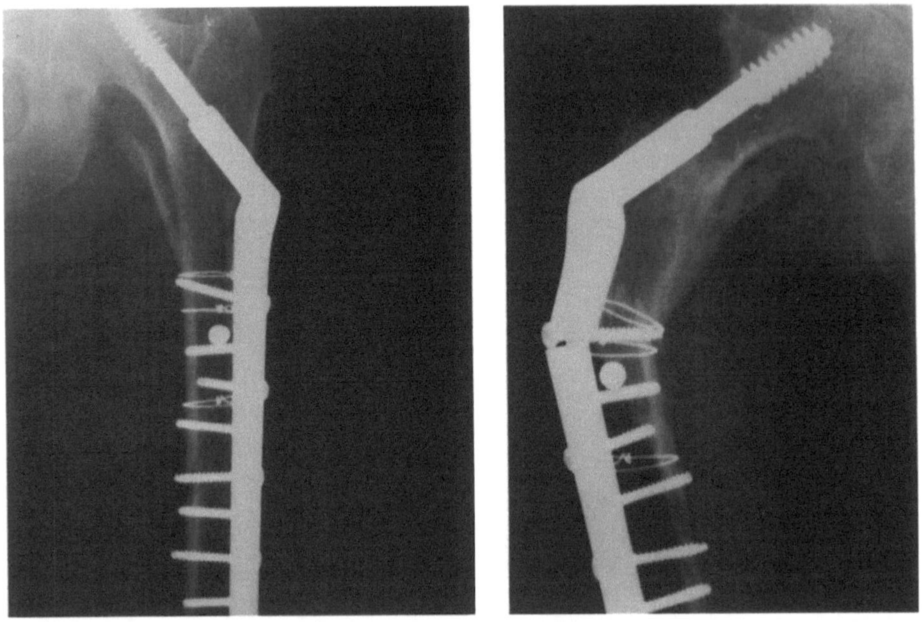

A B

FIG. 8–180 X-ray film of a slightly built rheumatoid patient with a comminuted subtrochanteric fracture well fixed and reduced **(A)** that fell apart 10 weeks later after the side plate failed **(B)** at the point of highest stress concentration.

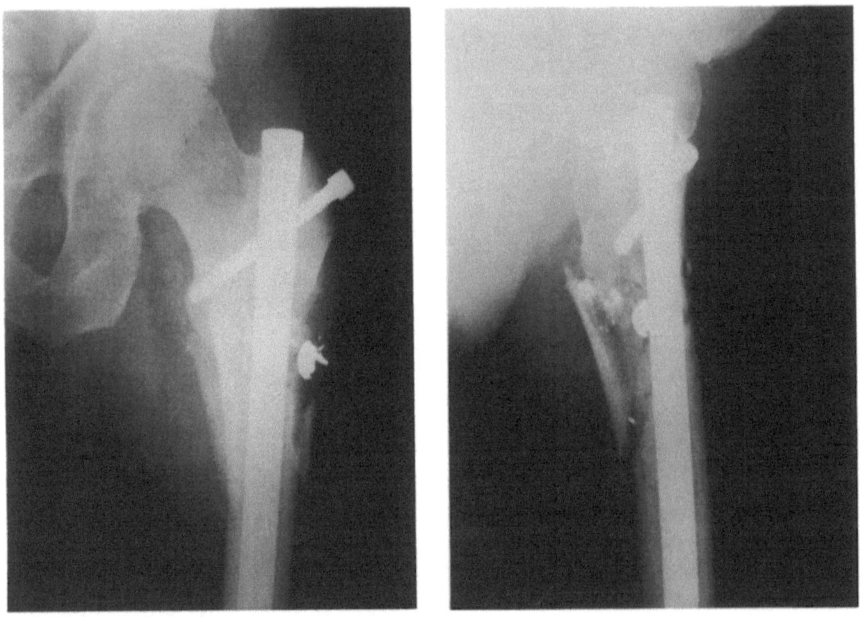

FIG. 8–181 Shotgun injury with loss of lateral skin. The fracture was well fixed with the Brooker-Wells intramedullary rod.

end of the femur via an entrance hole in the femoral condyle. They became popular from 1981 to 1984 for the treatment of trochanteric fractures. The system was designed by the senior Ender in 1969 and promoted by his son 10 years later.[319] The rods have been likened to Rush rods, which are more rigid and thicker. Ender claimed that the unique steel requirements for flexibility are strict.

Like the Zickel nail being a variation of the Küntscher "Y" nail, the Ender concept is a variation of the Küntscher curved condylocephalic nail.[320] The former consists of three to five flexible curved rods, whereas the latter was one heavy curved rod. The modern day copy of Küntscher's implant is the Harris nail, which has a slight second curve in an attempt to restore some anteversion to the reduction.[321] It comes in only one size so it cannot be used for slightly built, small women. The short, stubby femurs with narrow canals such as are seen in Oriental people do not accept the heavy, thick Harris rod with its double curves. Trafton and associates compared it with the hip compression screw on a prospective randomized study.[321a] They found that the Harris rod incurred more fixation reoperations, pressure sores, longer acute hospitalizations, and more systemic complications than did the compression hip screw. To this author such findings would make it an unacceptable system with nothing special to justify its use. Sherk and Foster found the same problems with the Harris idea and could not recommend its use.[322] There is also a Hansen-Street version with similar drawbacks.

The younger Ender used his father's system extensively at the Böhler Trauma Center[323,324] (Fig. 8–182). They used it as an alternative to a nonsliding nail, which had more than enough of its own problems, notably implant failures.[325] With this point of reference the Ender system had an attractive mechanical advantage.[326] Such an intramedullary implant lies exactly in the line of forces applied to the femur where stresses would become entirely axial so that there would be no bending loads on the nail whether a medial buttress is present or not. It was touted as having other advantages: easy to use with less operative time needed, less blood loss, immediate weight-bearing, lower morbidity, and no infections at the fracture site.[324,327,328]

Böhler warned of disadvantages clinically: (1) There can be difficulties in introducing the nail; (2) the tip of the nail only rarely reaches the head of the femur; and (3) the insertion at the medial epicondyle can injure the medial collateral ligament and thus cause limitation of knee motion.[323] As time passed and the American experience grew, other serious problems emerged: (1) The pins had a frequent habit of backing out, causing knee pain, which occurred 76% of the time in Levy et al.'s series[329] (Fig. 8–183); (2) frequent painful bursitis at the knee (insertion site pain) without the pins extruded; (3) perforation of the pins through the femoral head; and (4) fracturing of the femur at the site of entrance, which is common and, although not usually a problem, unfortunately can be the site of a supracondylar fracture of the femur both intraoperatively and later. (Fig. 8–184). The Ender system, moreover, cannot be used in comminuted unstable fractures unless the patient is treated in skeletal traction postoperatively (H. Ender, personal communication); it definitely is not an easy technique to master and has an unacceptably long learning period; infections and hematomas at the knee can occur; migration of the foot into external rotation commonly develops because the pins fail to control rotation of the fragments; an imaging machine is essential; closed manipulation of the fragments into valgus and displacing the neck fragment medially (reverse of the usual routine) can require more anesthesia time than is worth any mechanical advantage; and an open reduction can be required unexpectedly.[324]

Seventy percent of the patients reviewed by Raugstad et al.[328] and 50% of those reviewed by Kuderna et al.[324] suffered residual external rotatory deformities at the knees. Jensen concluded that the Ender rods were inadequate fixation for any comminuted trochanteric fracture because in his series 64% of the cases had secondary displacement of the rods and 46% required reoperation.[330] There may be a place for the routine use of Ender nails for the stable uncomplicated fracture. A long period is required to master its use, and the question is whether a community surgeon and his or her patients can afford such a long learning period. Migration of the pins can occur even in very stable fractures, as shown by Nelson et al.[331]

The complication rate in trained hands for the Ender system is still too high and cannot compare

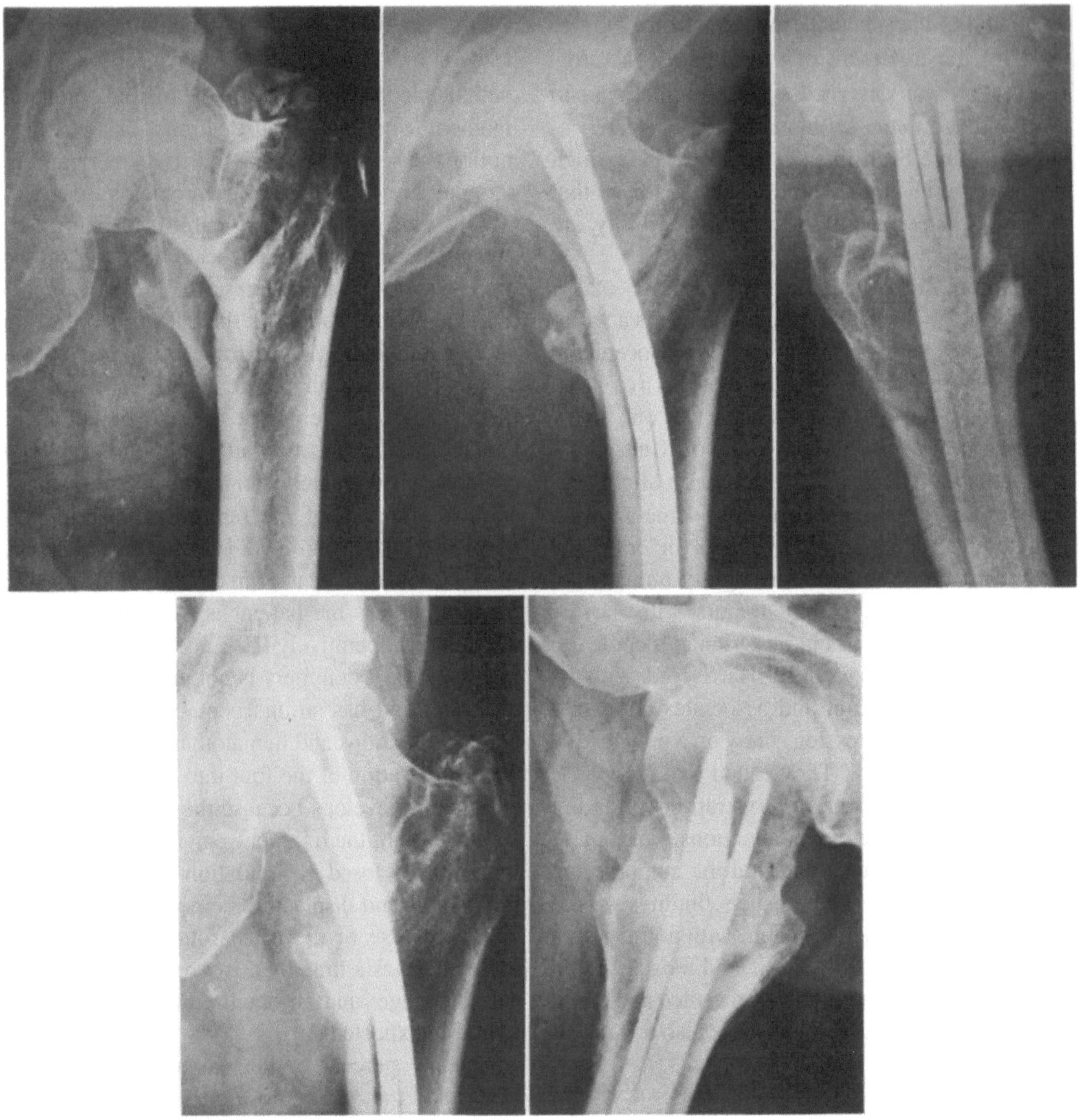

FIG. 8–182 Ender rod fixation. A minimum of three rods are used and fanned out in the lateral view and centered in the femoral head. Four rods are better as seen here.

with the versatility and efficiency of the newest hip compression srews.[332,333] There are some who disagree with this conclusion,[334] but they are few in number. Schaumberg believed that the complication rate is directly related to one's skill and experience.[334]

There are special indications for the use of Ender nails, i.e., specific problems that are untreatable by an open reduction with a hip screw.

1. Skin problems about the hip can prohibit any surgical procedure such as an open reduction. Pressure sores over the greater trochanter can occur in the debilitated patient. Dermatitis, infected abrasions, and infected traumatized tissue can prevent traditional surgery. The

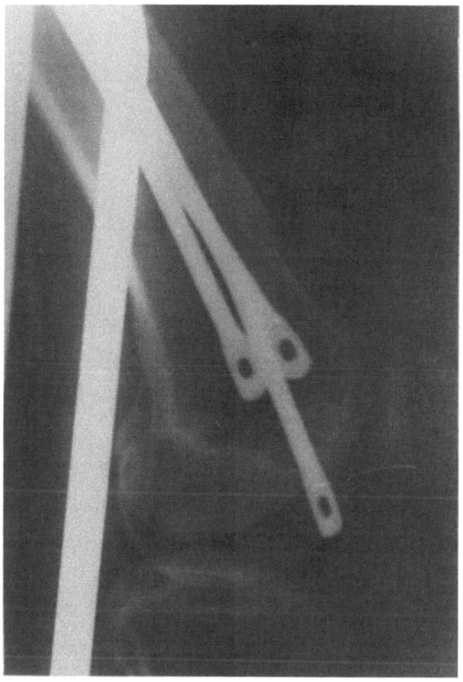

FIG. 8–183 A frequent complication is the rod backing out at the knee. Subsequent knee pain and bursitis are frequent disturbing problems.

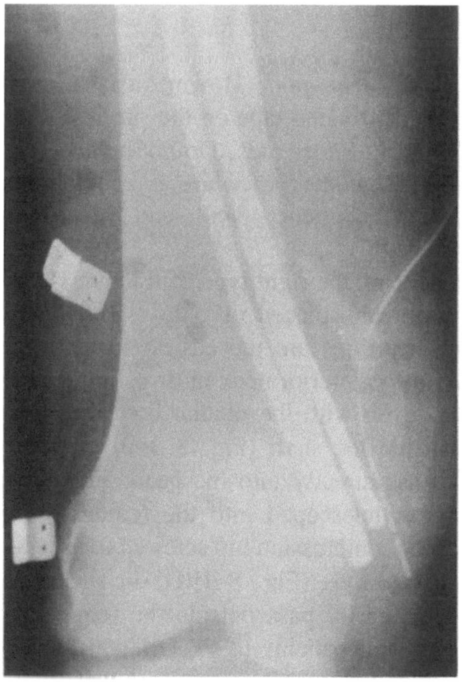

FIG. 8–184 Fracture at the point of entrance in the medial femoral cortex is disturbing. It can act as a stress riser causing a supracondylar fracture.

Ender system proved valuable in treating a drug addict who had multiple infected injection sites about her hip, which she had fractured during a drug episode.

2. Ipsilateral femoral shaft and femoral neck or trochanteric fractures are complex injuries (Fig. 8–185). They usually occur in the multiple trauma patient. With Ender rods both fractures can be treated simultaneously.
3. In open injuries with massive soft tissue damage, Ender pins can be superior to external fixation devices.[333,335] They circumvent the damaged tissue at the hip by being introduced at the knee (Fig. 8–186).
4. Femoral shaft fractures below an *uncemented* prosthesis or nail plate can be treated rather well with Ender pins when driven up the shaft from both the medial and lateral condyles[333,336] (Fig. 8–187).
5. Certain uncomplicated, relatively undisplaced subtrochanteric fractures may be fixed relatively well with Ender rodding (Fig. 8–188). The more typically comminuted displaced subtrochanteric fractures are not recommended because two sites of entry are needed for cross pins medially and laterally (Fig. 8–189). When so fixed, the reduction remains inadequate.

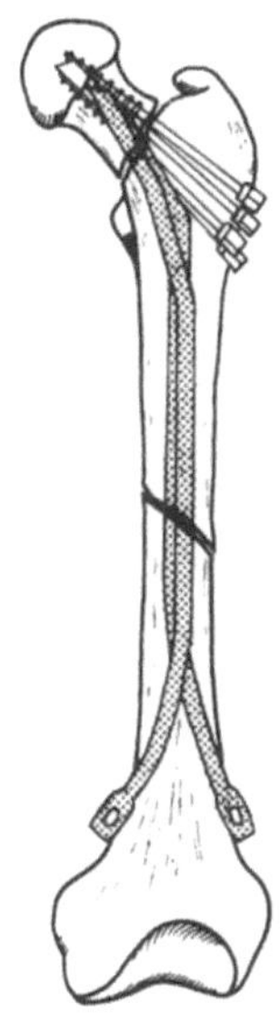

FIG. 8–185 Ender rods are excellent for fixing a femoral shaft fracture complicated by a femoral neck fracture. (Courtesy of Orthopedic Equipment Company from their product bulletin.)

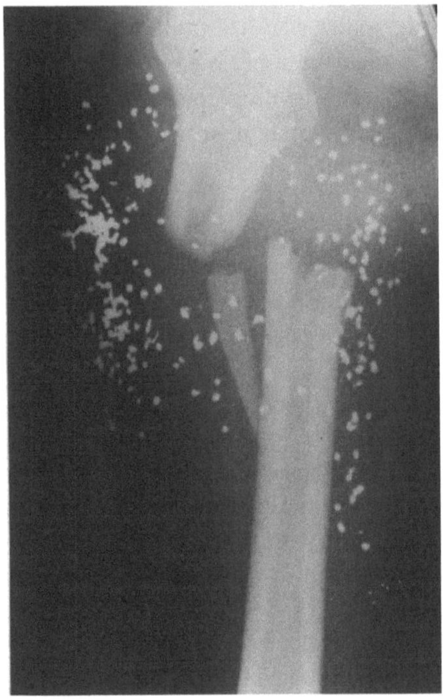

FIG. 8–186 Massive tissue damage from trauma (gunshot wounds). The wounds can be treated by Ender rods, which circumvent the area by going to the tissue.

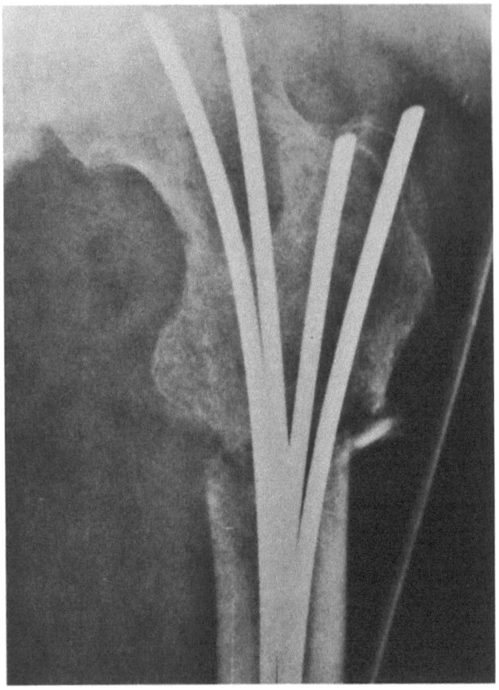

FIG. 8–188 Undisplaced or slightly displaced, short, oblique, subtrochanteric fractures can be treated with Ender rods.

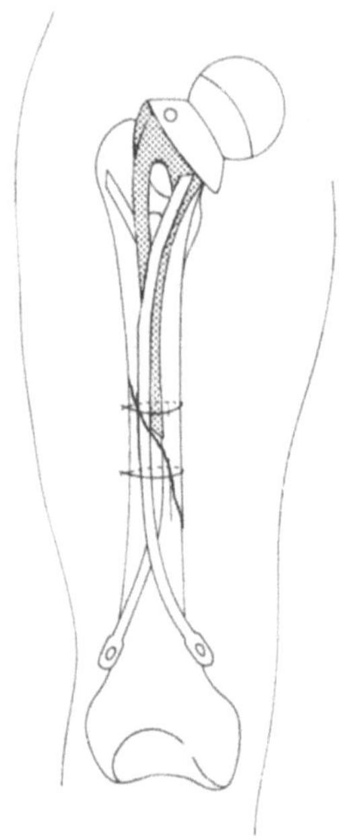

FIG. 8–187 Fractures below an *uncemented* endoprosthesis can be fixed with Ender rods.

Surgical Technique Howmedica has produced an excellent video tape on the surgical technique of inserting Ender rods. Do not be deceived into thinking that the procedure is easy; it requires patience, experience, skill, and a long learning curve.

Choosing the right type of fracture is very important. Undisplaced or only slightly displaced stable fractures are the easiest to manage. The beak of the inferior neck must be reduced so that it lies even with the medial cortex of the shaft or outside the shaft (Fig. 8–190), and the pins then pass directly into the head. Fractures with the neck telescoped into the femoral canal are ideal for compression hip screws but are not good for Ender rods (Fig. 8–191). In such fractures the pins easily pass outside the femur (Fig. 8–192). Small patients (e.g., Orientals) may have canals that do not accept more than two pins. Young patients have a very tough constricted canal that is technically difficult to manage with this system.

The pin length is determined by placing a pin

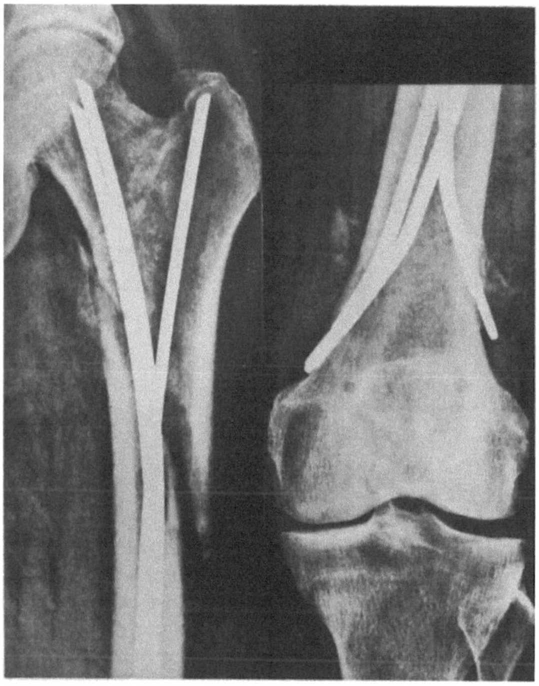

FIG. 8–189 Displaced subtrochanteric fractures are not recommended because two sites of entry must be used to insert medial and lateral rods. When finished, the fixation is still inadequate and traction must be used for at least six weeks.

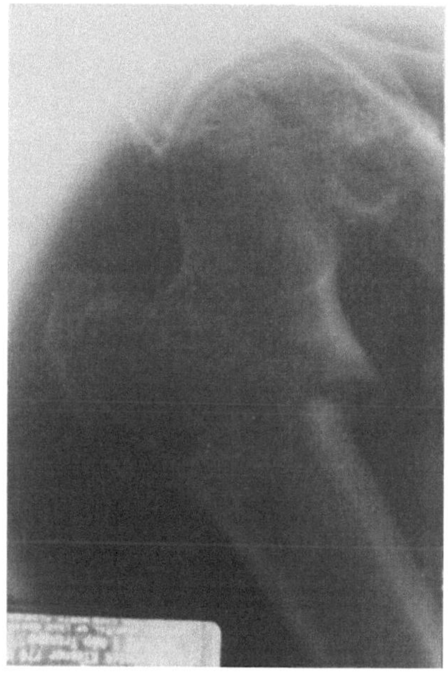

FIG. 8–190 Fracture type ideally suited for Ender rodding because the inferior neck is outside the femoral canal, making it easy for the rods to pass directly into the head.

of an estimated length over the thigh and checking it with an imaging x-ray study. It should go from well within the head and just to the side of the medial cortex at the site of the entrance hole. It should be slightly short because there will be some collapse of the fracture after the traction has been finally removed.

The incision is a slow curve over the medial epicondyle, about 6 to 10 cm long (Fig. 8–193). Start at the adductor tubercle if it can be felt. The inferior edge of the vastus medialis muscle is identified. Slip a Hohmann elevator under its edge and retract it anteriorly. Avoid violating the intermuscular septum because it protects the femoral vessels. The bone is a flat surface and is called "Adam's arch." A 0.25-inch drill is used to make a hole into the femur just proximal to the lateral genicular artery. The cortex should be thin and easily entered. A special curved awl is used next to create a path for the pins. The upper part of the hole should be enlarged to a generous oval with a duckbill rongeur to prevent the pins from splitting the cortex. The first pin

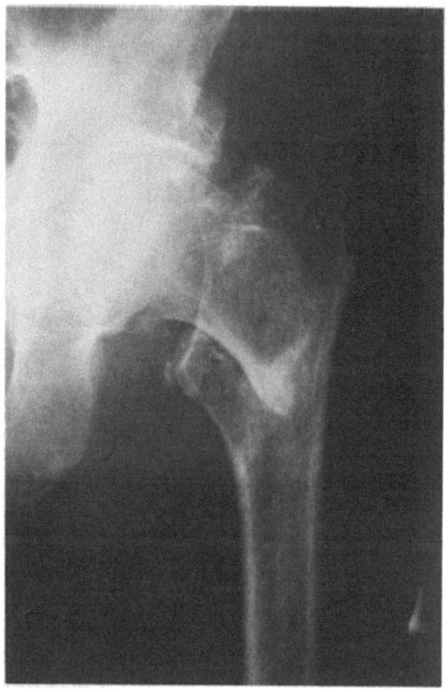

FIG. 8–191 Fractures impacted deeply into the femoral canal are poorly suited for Ender rods, which are likely to pass outside along the medial cortex, unless the fracture is opened as proposed by Böhler (323).

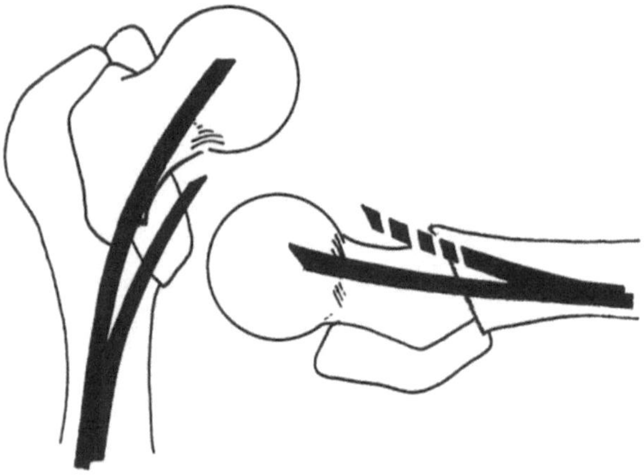

Fig. 8–192 Greatest shortcoming in the Ender technique: the rod slips outside the head. Considerable manipulation maneuvers may be needed. The learning curve for this device is long and may not be justified when compared to a hip compression screw.

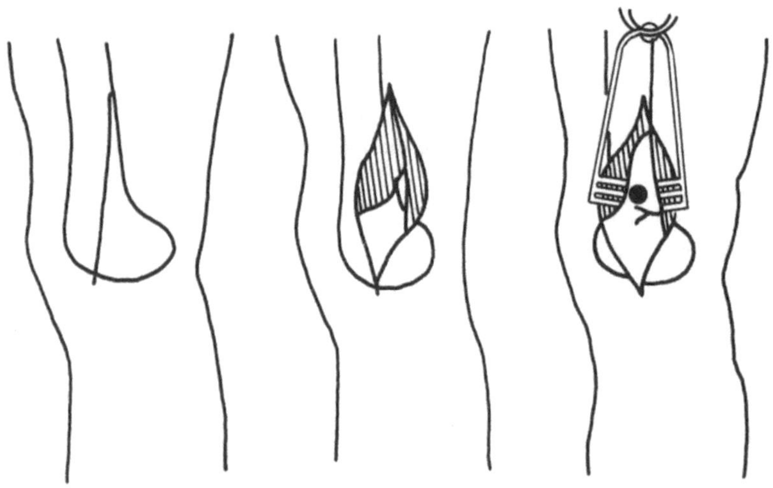

Fig. 8–193 Incision is along the medial femoral condyle. Lift the vastus medialis up, and penetrate the cortex at Adam's arch, just proximal to the branch of the medial genicular artery. Widen the hole into the oblong entrance with a rongeur, and then enter the canal with a curved awl.

is the most difficult to insert into the head. *The head must be in valgus so the pins pass into the center of the head* (not the superior region where fixation is poorest and the blood supply is in jeopardy). To get the rod into the middle of the head several maneuvers may be tried (Fig. 8–194). Pass the rod just to fracture site and then have an assistant force the head into valgus by pushing on the trochanter with a crutch (Fig. 8–194) or with stockingette.

The entire canal must be filled with tightly fitting rods. With a severely osteoporotic bone, five pins may be necessary to secure firm fixation. They must be turned as they are driven up the shaft so as to fan out as they enter the head (Fig. 8–195). Use a Hemovac drain because occasionally the medullary cavity hemorrhages more than one would expect.

Avoiding the Pitfalls Unfortunately, backing out of the pins cannot always be prevented. There are two ways to help prevent it. First try to drive the pins in as tightly as possible. The author has created what has become known as a "blocking pin." If the last curved pin does not go all the way up because it becomes too tightly bound in the canal, take a shorter pin and straighten it out; it should be long enough to pass just beyond the isthmus (Fig. 8–196). Driving this last pin up into the shaft serves to tighten the stack of pins

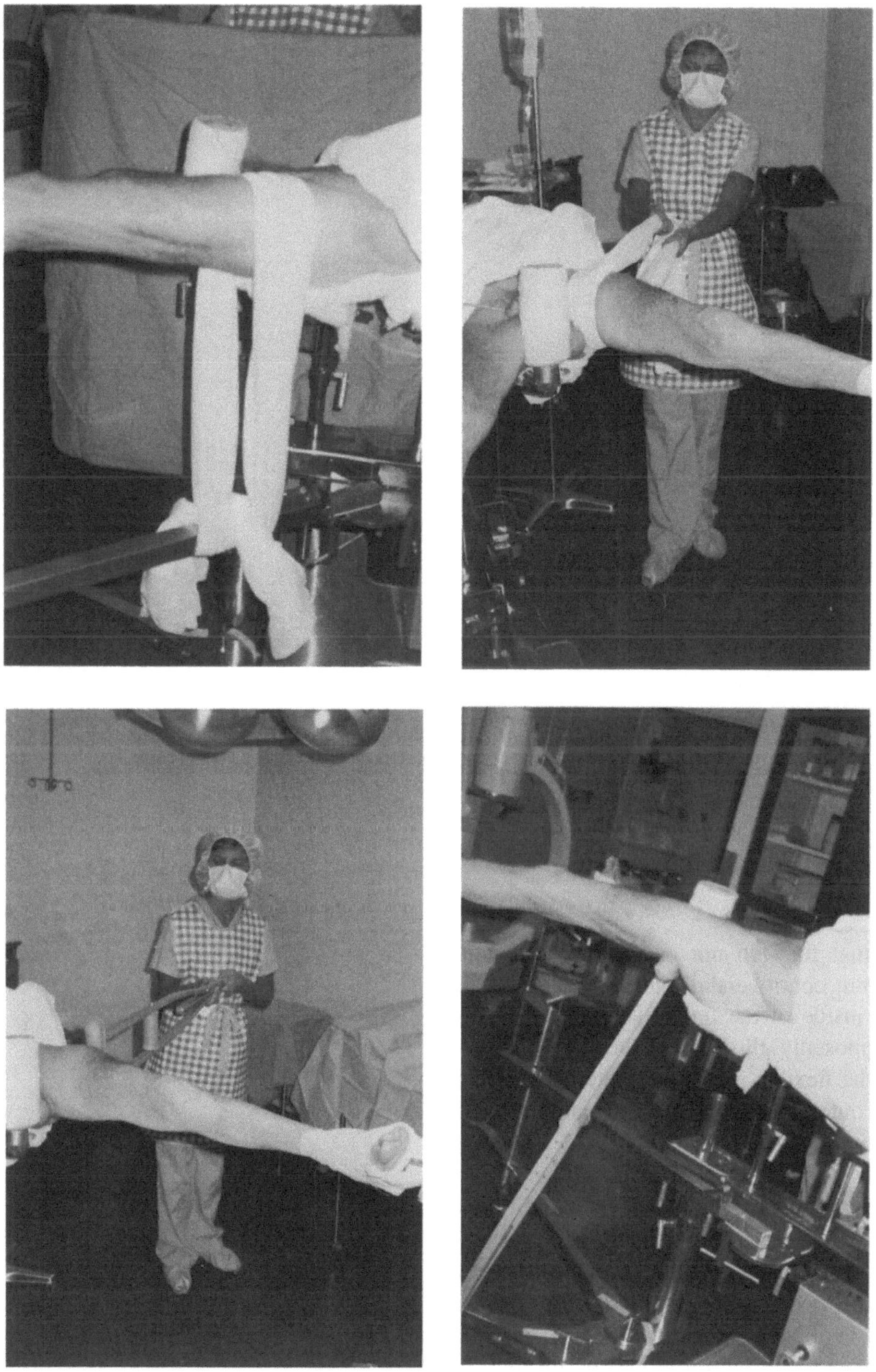

Fig. 8–194 Various maneuvers with a crutch or straps are needed to manipulate a fracture into valgus while attempting to pin an intertrochanteric fracture with Ender rods.

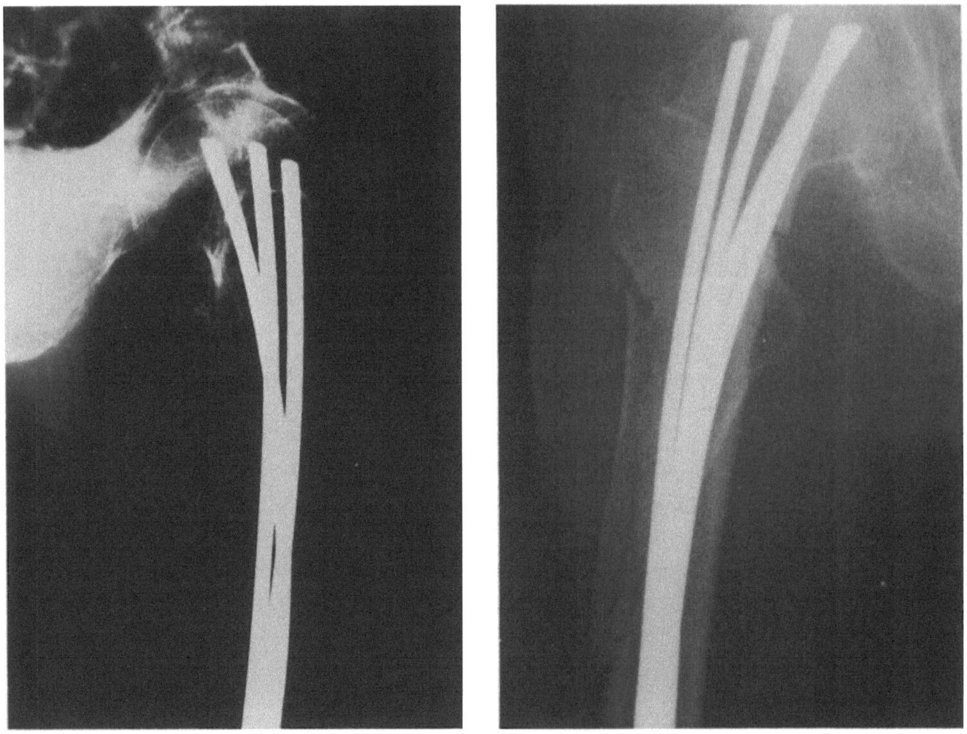

FIG. 8–195 To prevent migration and to accomplish firmer fixation, the rods should fan out in both lateral and AP planes. Each rod should be hand-bent before their insertion.

so well that they do not easily slip backward. Another but controversial maneuver is to let the pins flip inside of the femoral condyle (Fig. 8–197). Supposedly, this loosens the three-point fixation of the flexible pins: head, lateral inner cortex, and outer medial cortex. In reality there is only two-point fixation if they are driven in tightly: the isthmus and the head.

Do not use any screws or cement at their distal point as an attempt to prevent extrusion. Such a fixed point will surely cause the pins to pass through the head as the fracture naturally and expectedly collapses on itself.

Loss of reduction is prevented by driving the pins well up into the inferior subchondral bone of the head. Fan out the pins, be sure the head is reduced in valgus, and be sure that the fracture is not a high trochanteric one (the previously labeled "basicervical" fracture) because there will be insufficient bone to anchor the pins. Levy et al. reported a 100% failure rate for basicervical fractures treated with Ender rods.[329]

External rotation of the foot occurred in 50%

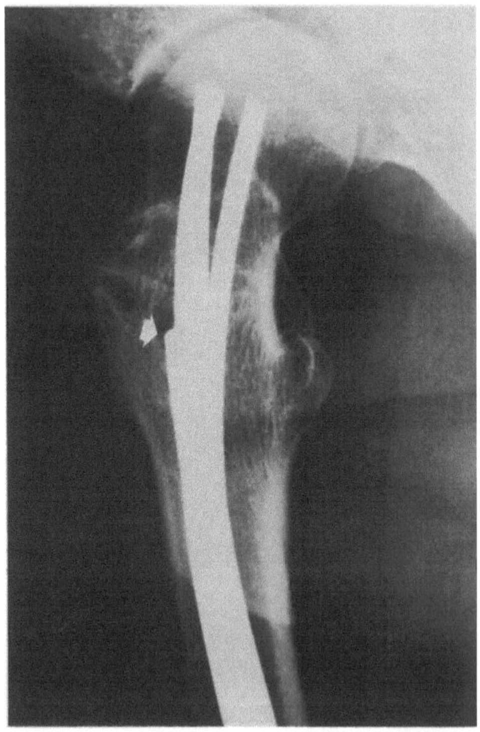

FIG. 8–196 Tronzo's "blocking pin" (indicated by arrow) is a short rod, straightened at its proximal end so as to stack the rods in as tightly as possible in the isthums.

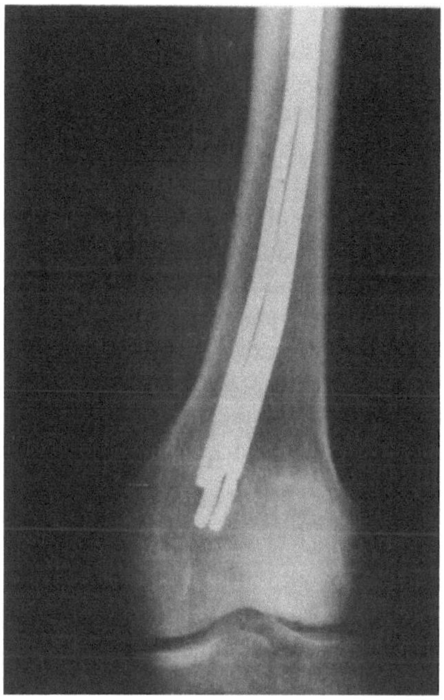

FIG. 8–197 If the pins are tight at the isthmus, it is permissible to allow the ends to flip inside of the femoral canal in order to avoid knee pain from pins backing out under the skin.

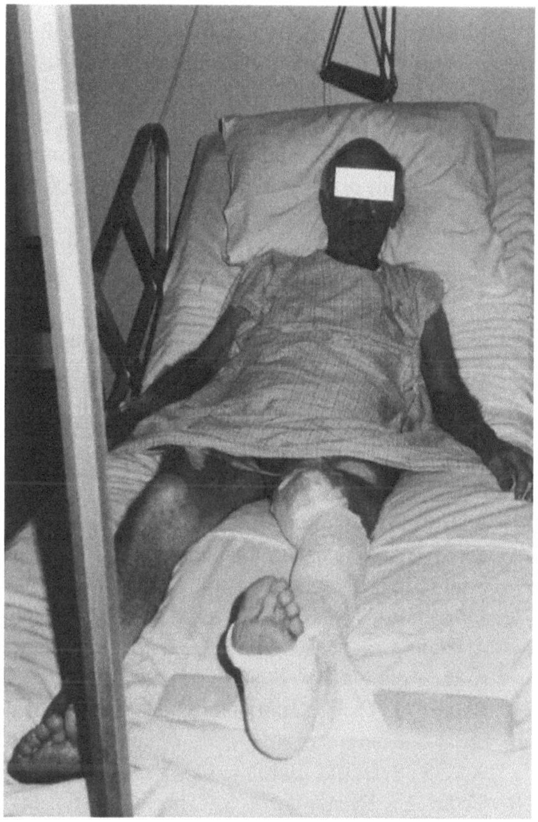

FIG. 8–198 Derotation boot used to control rotary deformities.

of the cases reported by Kuderna et al.[324] Raugstad et al.[337] reported that external rotation exceeded 10° in 36% of their cases. With experience they nailed the fractures in an overcorrected (internally rotated) position, which reduced the deformity to 17%.

Postoperative rotational deformities are difficult to prevent, as pointed out by Levy et al.[329] The following procedures may be tried: tight pins; fanning out the pins; reducing the fracture with the knee internally rotated. Adding a third bow to the pin at its proximal end in an attempt to recreate anteversion has been recommended.[338] Tencer and associates reported some excellent radiographic studies to prove this point and urged that all Ender rods be made with an anteverted upper bow.[339] If the foot flops out externally a great amount by the end of the first or second week, anesthetize the patient and try to derotate the leg. Apply a derotation cast to the leg holding the foot corrected for about 6 to 8 weeks (Fig. 8–198).

If Ender rods are to be used with subtrochanteric fractures, a combined closed–open procedure must be anticipated.[324] Cerclage wiring works, but Parham bands are better in bringing large butterfly fragments tightly reduced before the rods are passed down the shaft.[317] Furthermore, be prepared to add skeletal traction through the tibial tubercle for 3 to 4 weeks while the fragments heal well enough to remain stable.

Postoperative management is geared toward early weight-bearing in the uncomplicated stable fractures similar to the program followed by a well reduced well fixed fracture when a compression screw is used. Caution must be exercised in the complex unstable types. Most of the time these fractures must be treated with skeletal traction for a minimum of 3 weeks until some union has developed to help keep the fragments together enough to prevent their collapse. It has been suggested that a cast brace be fitted in these cases, but beware of pin migration at the knee, which is aggravated by the brace.

References

1. Miller, C. W.: Survival and ambulation following hip fracture. J. Bone Joint Surg., 60A:930, 1978.
2. Lewinnek, G. J., Kelsey, J., White, A. A., Krieger, N. J.: The significance and a comparative analysis of the epidemiology of hip fractures. Clin. Orthop., 152:35, 1080.
3. Knowelden, J., Buhr, A. J., Dunbar, O.: Incidence of fractures in persons over 35. Br. J. Prevent. Soc. Med., 18:130, 1964.
4. Kofoed, H., Alberts, A.: Femoral neck fractures. Acta Orthop. Scand., 51:127, 1980.
5. Kenzora, J. E., McCarthy, R. E., Lowell, J. D., Sledge, C. B.: Hip fracture mortality. Clin. Orthop., 186:45, 1984.
6. Crane, J. G., Kernek, C. B.: Mortality associated with hip fractures in a single geriatric hospital and residential health facility. J. Am. Geriatr. Soc., 31:472, 1983.
7. Johnell, O., Nilsson, B., Obrant, K., Sernbo, I.: Four time periods as related to hip fracture risks. Acta Orthop. Scand., 55:290, 1984.
8. Bauer, G. C. H., Hansson, L. I., Lidgren, L., et al.: Comprehensive care of hip fractures. AAOS, Scientific Exhibit, Las Vegas, 1985.
9. Ceder, L., Svensson, B. S., Thorngren, K.: Statistical prediction of rehabilitation in elderly patients with hip fractures. Clin. Orthop., 152:185, 1980.
10. Mullen, J. O.: Mortality in hip fractures—its relationship to mental status and hospital confusion in a prospective study. Presented to the American Academy of Orthopedic Surgeons, Las Vegas, 1985.
11. Milton, L. S., Ilstrup, D. M., Beckenbaugh, R. D.: Hip fracture recurrence. Clin. Orthop., 167:131, 1982.
12. Older, M. W., Edwards, D., Dickerson, J. W.: A nutrient survey in elderly women with femoral neck fractures. Br. J. Surg., 67:884, 1980.
13. Elabdien, B. S. Z., Olerud, S., Karlstrom, G.: The influence of age on the morphology of trochanteric fractures. Arch. Orthop. Trauma Surg., 103:156, 1984.
14. Singh, M., Nagrath, A. R., Maini, P. S.: Changes in the trabecular pattern of the upper end of the femur as an index of osteoporosis. J. Bone Joint Surg., 52A:457, 1970.
15. Khairi, M. R. A., Cronin, J. H., Robb, J. A., et al.: Femoral trabecular pattern index and bone mineral content measurement by photon absorption in senile osteoporosis. J. Bone Joint Surg., 58A:221, 1976.
16. Kranendonk, D. H., Jurist, J. M., Lee, H. G.: Femoral trabecular patterns and bone mineral content. J. Bone Joint Surg., 54A:1472, 1972.
17. Freeman, M. A. R., Todd, R. C., Pirie, C. J.: The role of fatigue in the pathogenesis of senile femoral neck fractures. J. Bone Joint Surg., 56B:698, 1974.
18. Garrett, M. W., Vernon-Roberts, B.: Absence of metabolic bone disease in the proximal femur in patients with fractures of the femoral neck. J. Bone Joint Surg., 64B:319, 1982.
19. Lips, P., Tacones, W. K., van Ginkel, F. C.: Radiologic morphometry in patients with femoral neck fractures and elderly control subjects. Clin. Orthop., 183:64, 1984.
20. Genant, H. K.: Assessing osteoporosis: CT's quantitative advantage. Diagn. Imaging, 7:54, 1985.
21. Kaplan, S. S., Stegman, C. J.: Transient osteoporosis of the hip. J. Bone Joint Surg., 67A:490, 1985.
22. Levine, S., Makin, M., Menczel, J., et al.: Incidence of fractures of the proximal femur in Jerusalem. J. Bone Joint Surg., 52:1193, 1970.
23. Brooklehurst, J. C., Exton-Smith, S. M., Barber, L., et al.: Fracture of the femur in old age: Two-center study of associated clinical factors and cause of the fall. Age Ageing, 7:2, 1978.
24. Garden, R. S.: Reduction and fixation of subcapital fractures of the femur. Orthop. Clin. North Am., 5:683, 1974.
25. Key, J. A., Conwell, H. E.: *The Management of Fractures, Dislocations and Sprains,* 7th ed. St. Louis, Mosby, 1961.
26. Watson-Jones, R.: *Fractures and Joint Injuries,* 4th ed. Baltimore, Williams & Wilkins, 1955.
27. Klenerman, L., Marcuson, R. W.: Intracapsular fractures of the neck of the femur. J. Bone Joint Surg., 52B:514, 1970.
28. Askin, S. R., Bryan, R. S.: Femoral neck fractures in young adults. Clin. Orthop., 114:259, 1976.
29. Garden, R. S.: Reduction and fixation of subcapital fractures of the femur. Orthop. Clin. North Am., 5:683, 1974.
30. Linton, P.: On different types of intracapsular fractures of the femoral neck. Acta Chir. Scand. [Suppl. 86], 90:1, 1944.
31. Pauwels, F.: Der Schenkenholsbruck, em mechanisches Problem. Grundlagen des Heilungsvorganges: Prognose und kausale Therapie. Stuttgart, Beilageheft zur Zeitschrift fur Orthopaedische Chirurgie, Ferdinand Enke, 1935.
32. Boyd, H. B., Salvatore, J. E.: Acute fracture of the femoral neck: Internal fixation or prosthesis? J. Bone Joint Surg., 46A:1066, 1964.
33. Casselbaum, W. H., Nugent, G.: The predictability of bony union in displaced intracapsular fractures of the hip. J Trauma, 3:421, 1963.

34. Halpin, P. J., Nelson, C. L.: A system of classification of femoral neck fractures with special reference to choice of treatment. Clin. Orthop., 152:44, 1980.
35. London, P. S.: Classification of fractures of the neck of the femur and the technique of reduction. In: *The Hip. Proceedings of Fifth Meeting of the Hip Society,* 1977, p. 13
36. DeLee, J. C.: Fractures and dislocations of the hip. In: *Fractures in Adults,* 2nd ed. (C. A. Rockwood and D. P. Green, eds.) Philadelphia, Lippincott, 1984, Ch. 24.
37. Fielding, J. W.: Displaced femoral neck fractures. Orthop Rev., 2:11, 1973.
38. Fielding, J. W.: The telescoping Pugh nail in the surgical management of the displaced intracapsular fracture of the femoral neck. Clin. Orthop., 152:123, 1980.
39. Barnes, R., Brown, J. T., Garden, R. S., Nicoll, E. A.: Subcapital fractures of the femur. J. Bone Joint Surg., 58B:2, 1976.
40. Smyth, E. H. J., Shah, V. M.: The significance of good reduction and fixation in displaced subcapital fractures of the femur. Injury, 5:197, 1973–1974.
41. Swinotkowski, M. F., Umquist, R. A., Hansen, S. T.: Fractures of the femoral neck in patients between the age of twelve and forty-nine years. J. Bone Joint Surg., 66A:837, 1984.
42. Jeffrey, C. C.: Spontaneous fractures of the femoral neck. J. Bone Joint Surg., 44B:543, 1962.
43. Devas, M.: *Stress Fractures.* New York, Churchill Livingstone, 1975.
44. Kaltas, D. S.: Stress fractures of the femoral neck in young adults: A report of seven cases. J. Bone Joint Surg., 63B:33, 1981.
45. Howland, J.: Stress fractures of the femoral neck. Am. J. Orthop. Surg., 11:46, 1969.
46. Wolfgang, G. L.: Stress fracture of the femoral neck in a patient with open capital femoral epiphyses. J. Bone Joint Surg., 59A:680, 1977.
47. Miller, L. F.: Bilateral stress fracture of the neck of the femur. J. Bone Joint Surg., 32A:695, 1950
48. Nand, S., Shukla, R. K.: Fatigue fracture of the femoral neck. Int. Surg., 61:31, 1976.
49. Hajek, M. R., Noble, H. B.: Stress fractures of femoral neck in joggers. Am J. Sports Med., 10:112, 1982.
50. Blecher, A.: Uber den Einfluss des Parade-Marsches auf die Entstehung der Fuss Geschwulst. Med. Klin., 1:305, 1905.
51. Morris, J. M., Blickenstaff, L. P.: *Fatigue Fractures.* Springfield, Ill., Charles C Thomas, 1967.
52. Ernst, J.: Stress fracture of the neck of the femur. J Trauma, 4:71, 1965.
53. Prather, J. L., Nusynowitz, M. L., Snowdy, H. A., et al.: Scintigraphic findings in stress fractures. J. Bone Joint Surg., 59A:869, 1977.
54. Walsh, R. J.: Displaced stress fractures of the neck of the femur treated with bone grafting. Surg. Gynecol. Obstet., 132:503, 1971.
55. Tronzo, R. G.: *Surgery of the Hip Joint.* 1st ed. Lea & Febiger, Philadelphia, 1973.
56. Baker, D. M.: Fractures of the femoral neck after healed intertrochanteric fractures: A complication of too short a nail plate fixation. J. Trauma, 15:73, 1975.
57. Cameron, H. U., Pilliar, R. M., Hastings, D. E., Fornasier, V. L.: Iatrogenic subcapital fracture of the hip. Clin. Orthop., 112:218, 1975.
58. Baksi, D. P.: Internal fixation of ununited femoral neck fractures combined with muscle-pedicle bone grafting. J. Bone Joint Surg., 68B:239, 1986.
59. Pankovich, A. M.: Primary internal fixation of femoral neck fractures. Arch. Surg., 110:20, 1975.
60. Eklund, J., Eriksson, F.: Fractures of the femoral neck: With special regard to the treatment and prognosis of stable abduction fractures. Acta Chir. Scand., 127:315, 1964.
61. Ohman, U., Bjorkegren, N., Fahlstrom, G.: Fracture of the femoral neck. Acta Chir. Scand., 135:27, 1969.
62. Crawford, H. B.: Experience with the nonoperative treatment of impacted fractures of the neck of the femur. J. Bone Joint Surg., 47A:830, 1965.
63. Bunata, R. E., Fahey, J. J., Drennan, D. B.: Factors influencing stability and necrosis of impacted femoral neck fractures. JAMA, 223:41, 1973.
64. Hansen, B. A., Solgaard, S.: Impacted fractures of the femoral neck treated by early mobilization and weight-bearing. Acta Orthop. Scand., 49: 180, 1978.
65. Lowell, J. D.: Results and complications of femoral neck fractures. Clin. Orthop., 152:162, 1980.
66. MacAusland, W. R., MacAusland, A. R., Lee, H. G.: Fractures of the neck of the femur. Surg. Gynecol. Obstet., 58:679, 1934.
67. Fielding, J. W.: The telescoping Pugh nail in the surgical management of the displaced intracapsular fracture of the femoral neck. Clin. Orthop., 152:123, 1980.
68. Bentley, G.: Treatment of nondisplaced fractures of the femoral neck. Clin. Orthop., 152:93, 1980.
69. Aufranc, O. E.: Fractures and dislocations of the hip. In: *Fractures and Dislocations of the Hip.* (Cave, E. F., ed.) Chicago, Year Book, 1958, Ch. 25.
70. Thompson, V., Epstein, H.: Traumatic disloca-

tion of the hip joint. J. Bone Joint Surg., 33A:746, 1951.
71. Pipkin, G.: Treatment of grade IV fracture-dislocation of the hip. J. Bone Joint Surg., 39A:1027, 1957.
72. Stewart, M.: Management of fractures of the head of the femur complicated by dislocation of the hip. Orthop. Clin. North Am., 5:793, 1974.
73. Roeder, L. F., DeLee, J. C.,: Femoral head fractures associated with posterior hip dislocations. Clin. Orthop., 147:121, 1980.
74. Epstein, H. C.: *Traumatic Dislocation of the Hip*. Baltimore, Williams & Wilkins, 1980.
75. Butler, J. E.: Pipkin type II fractures of the femoral head. J. Bone Joint Surg., 63A:1292, 1981.
76. DeLee, J. C., Evans, J. A., Thomas, J.: Anterior dislocation of the hip and associated femoral head fractures. J. Bone Joint Surg., 62A:960, 1980.
77. Dowd, G. S., Johnson, R.: Successful conservative treatment of a fracture-dislocation of the femoral head. J. Bone Joint Surg., 61A:1244, 1979.
78. Speed, K.: The unsolved fracture. Surg. Gynecol. Obstet., 60:341, 1935.
79. Dickson, J. A.: The "unsolved" fracture. J. Bone Joint Surg., 35A:805, 1953.
80. Barnes, R.: The diagnosis of ischemia of the capital fragment in femoral neck fractures. J. Bone Joint Surg., 44B:760, 1962.
81. Harty, M.: Blood supply of the femoral head. Br. Med. J., 2:1236, 1953.
82. Walmsley, T.: The articular mechanism of the diarthroses. J. Bone Joint Surg., 19:40, 1928.
83. Chung, S.: The arterial supply of the developing proximal end of the human femur. J. Bone Joint Surg., 58A:961, 1976.
84. Claffey, T. J.: Avascular necrosis of the femoral head. J. Bone Joint Surg., 42B:802, 1960.
85. Trueta, J., Harrison, M. H.: The normal vascular anatomy of the femoral head in adult man. J. Bone Joint Surg., 35B:442, 1953.
86. Wertheimer, L., Fernandes Lopes, S.: Arterial supply of the femoral head. J. Bone Joint Surg., 53A:545, 1971.
87. Phemister, D. B.: Fractures of the neck of the femur, dislocation of the hip and obscure vascular disturbances producing aseptic necrosis of the head of the femur. Surg. Gynecol. Obstet., 59:415, 1934.
88. Sherman, M., Phemister, D. B.: The pathology of ununited fractures of the neck of the femur. J. Bone Joint Surg., 29:19, 1947.
89. Phemister, D. B.: Repair of bone in the presence of aseptic necrosis resulting from fractures, transplantations, and vascular obstruction. J. Bone Joint Surg., 12:769, 1930.
90. Phemister, D. B.: The pathology of ununited fractures of the neck of the femur with special references to the head. J. Bone Joint Surg., 21A:681, 1939.
91. Phemister, D. B.: Treatment of the necrotic head of the femur in adults. J. Bone Joint Surg., 31A:55, 1949.
92. Sevitt, S.: Avascular necrosis and revascularization of the femoral head after intracapsular fractures. J. Bone Joint Surg., 46B:270, 1964.
93. Backman, S.: The proximal end of the femur. Acta Radiol. [Suppl.], (Stockh.), 146:1, 1957.
94. Frankel, V. H.: *The Femoral Neck Function: Fracture Mechanism and Internal Fixation*. Springfield, Charles C Thomas, 1960.
95. Frankel, V. H., Buratein, A. H.: Force and energetics of femoral neck fractures. In: Proceedings Dixieme Congress International de Chirugie, Orthopaedique et de Traumatologie, Paris, 1966.
96. Fredensborg, N., Nisson, B. E.: The bone mineral content and cortical thickness in young women with femoral neck fracture. Clin. Orthop., 124:161, 1977.
97. Rydell, N.: Forces acting on the femoral head prosthesis. Acta Orthop. Scand. [Suppl.], 88:7, 1966.
98. Rydell, N.: Biomechanics of the hip joint. Clin. Orthop., 92:6, 973.
99. Radin, E. L.: Biomechanics of the human hip. Clin. Orthop., 152:28, 1980.
100. Scheck, M.: Intercapsular fractures of the femoral neck. J. Bone Joint Surg., 41A:1187, 1959.
101. Scheck, M.: Management of fractures of the femoral neck. J. Bone Joint Surg., 47A:819, 1965.
102. Scheck, M.: The significance of posterior comminution in femoral neck fractures. Clin. Orthop., 152:138, 1980.
103. Banks, H. H.: Factors influencing the results in fractures of the femoral neck. J. Bone Joint Surg., 44A:931, 1962.
104. Klenerman, L., Marcuson, R. W.: Intracapsular fractures of the neck of the femur. J. Bone Joint Surg., 52B:514, 1970.
105. Urovitz, E. P. M., Fornasier, V. L., Risen, M. I., MacNab, I.: Etiological factors in the pathogenesis of femoral trabecular fatigue fractures. Clin. Orthop., 127:275, 1977.
106. Todd, R. C., Freeman, M. A. R., Pirie, C. J.: Isolated trabecular fatigue fractures of the femoral head. J. Bone Joint Surg., 54A:723, 1972.
107. Griffiths, W. E. G., Swanson, S. A., Freeman, M. A. R.: Experimental fatigue fracture of the human cadaveric femoral neck. J. Bone Joint Surg., 53B:136, 1971.
108. Linton, P.: On different types of intracapsular fractures of the femoral neck. Acta Chir. Scand. [Suppl. 96], 90:1, 1944.
109. Linton, P.: Types of displacement in fractures of the neck of the femur. J. Bone Joint Surg., 31B:184, 1949.
110. Stromqvist, B., Hansson, L. I., Ljung, P., et

al.: Preoperative and postoperative scintimetry after femoral neck fracture. J. Bone Joint Surg., 66B:49, 1984.
111. Stromqvist, B., Brismar, J., Hansson, L. I., Palmer, J.: Technetium-99m–methylenediphosphonate scintimetry after femoral neck fracture. Clin. Orthop., 182:177, 1984.
112. Fitzgerald, R. H.: Editorial comment. J. Bone Joint Surg., 66B:49, 1984.
113. Holmberg, S., Thorngren, K. G.: Preoperative ^{99m}Tc-MDP scintimetry of femoral neck fractures. Acta Orthop. Scand., 55:430, 1984.
114. Sherk, H. H., Snape, W. J., Loprete, F. L.: Internal fixation versus nontreatment of hip fractures in senile patients. Clin. Orthop., 141:196, 1979.
115. Lyons, L. L., Nevins, M. A.: Nontreatment of hip fractures in senile patients. JAMA, 239:1175, 1977.
116. Hyams, D. E.: Letter to the editor: Nontreatment of hip fractures. JAMA, 239:1492, 1978.
117. Dorr, L. D.: Treatment of hip fractures in elderly and senile patients. Orthop. Clin. North Am., 12:153, 1981.
118. Mikhael, S. F., Sonn, M., Lawton, H. H.: Optimism in the management of hip fracture in elderly patients. J. Am. Geriatr. Soc., 26:39, 1978.
119. Leadbetter, G. W.: A treatment for fracture of the neck of the femur. J. Bone Joint Surg., 15:931, 1933.
120. Whitman, R.: A new method of treatment for fractures of the neck of the femur, together with remarks on coxa vara. Ann. Surg., 36:746, 1902.
121. Massie, W. K.: Treatment of femoral neck fractures emphasizing long term follow-up observations on aseptic necrosis. Clin. Orthop., 92:16, 1973.
122. Flynn, M.: A new method of reduction of fractures of the neck of the femur based on anatomical studies of the hip joint. Injury, 5:309, 1973–1974.
123. Compton, E. H.: Accuracy of reduction of femoral subcapital fractures. Injury, 9:71, 1977–1978.
124. Deyerle, W. M.: Manipulation for reduction of femoral neck fractures. In: *Surgery of the Hip Joint,* 1st ed. (Tronzo, R. G., ed.) Philadelphia, Lea & Febiger, 1973, pp. 542–543.
125. Zickel, R. E., Asnis, S. E., Haberman, E. T., et al.: Symposium: Transcervical fractures of the femoral neck. Contemp. Orthop., 10:101, 1985.
126. Swinotkowski, M. D., Winquist, R. A., Hansen, S. T.: Fractures of the femoral neck in patients between the ages of twelve and forty-nine years. J. Bone Joint Surg., 66A:837, 1984.
127. Meyers, M. H., Harvey, J. P., Moore, T.: The muscle pedicle bone graft in the treatment of displaced fractures of the femoral neck: Indications, operative technique, and results. Orthop. Clin. North Am., 5:779, 1974.
128. Meyers, M.: Treatment of displaced femoral neck fractures with internal fixation and a muscle pedicle graft. In: *The Hip, Proceedings of Fifth Open Scientific Meeting of the Hip Society,* 1977, Ch. 4.
129. Barnes, R., Brown, J. T., Garden, R. S., Nicoll, E. A.: Subcapital fractures of the femur—a prospective review of 1503 cases. J. Bone Joint Surg., 58B:2, 1976.
130. Gruder, J. L., Horowitz, M.: Clinical evaluation of the sliding compression screw in hip fractures. South. Med. J., 73:1343, 1980.
131. Bauer, G., Weber, D. A., Ceder, L., Lennart, D., Egund, N., Hansson, L. I., Stromqvist, B.,: Dynamics of technetium—99m methylenediphosphonate imaging of the femoral head after hip fractures. Clin. Orthop., 152:85, 1980.
132. LaMont, O.: Treatment of femoral neck fractures with sliding screw and two Knowles pins. Clin. Orthop., 190:158, 1984.
133. Rubin, R., Trent, P., Arnold, W., Burstein, A.: Knowles pinning of experimental femoral neck fractures: A biomechanical study. J. Trauma, 21:1036, 1981.
134. Tronzo, R. G.: Hip nails for all occasions. Orthop. Clin. North Am., 5:479, 1974.
135. Austin-Moore, T.: Fracture of the hip joint (intracapsular); a new method of skeletal fixation. J. S. C. Med. Assoc., 30:199, 1934.
136. Hogh, J., Jensen, J., Lauritzen, J.: Displaced femoral neck fractures. Follow-up study of 98 cases treated with multiple AO (ASIF) cancellous bone screws. Acta Orthop. Scand., 53:245, 1982.
137. Crowell, R. R., Edwards, W. T., Hayes, J. J.: Holding power of fixation devices in trabecular bone of the femoral head. Orthopedic Research Society, 1985, Las Vegas.
138. Asnis, S. E.: The guided screw system in intracapsular fractures of the hip. Contemp. Orthop., 10:33, 1985.
139. Van Audekercke, R., Martens, M. D., Muher, J. C., Stuyck, J.: Experimental study on internal fixation of femoral neck fractures. Clin. Orthop., 141:203, 1979.
140. Brodetti, A.: The blood supply of the femoral neck and head in relation to the damaging effects of nails and screws. J. Bone Joint Surg., 42B:794, 1960.
141. Tronzo, R. G.: Use of an extramedullary guide pin for fractures of the upper end of the femur. Orthop. Clin. North Am., 5:525, 1974.
142. Pankovich, A. M.: Intracapsular fractures of the femur. In: *Surgery of the Musculoskeletal System,* Vol. 2. (Evarts, M. C., ed.) New York, Churchill Livingstone, 1983, Ch. 4.
144. Arnold, W. D.: Percutaneous Knowles pinnings:

primary treatment for femoral neck fractures. In: *The Hip. Proceedings of the Fifth Open Scientific Meeting of the Hip Society,* 1977, pp. 21–34.
145. Buch, R. G., et al.: Intrapelvic migration of Knowles pin through the external iliac vein. Orthopedics, 8:1023, 1985.
146. Kleinman, S. Z., Russen, L. A.: Migration of left hip pin with involvement of left ureter. Urology, 16:396, 1980.
147. Alpers, D. D.: Migration of broken hip pin into urinary bladder. JAMA, 212:2123, 1970.
148. Altner, P. D.: How not to pin a hip. Int. Surg., 63:22, 1978.
149. Shaw, J. A.: Preventing unrecognized pin penetration into the hip joint. Orthop. Rev., 13:45, 1984.
150. Tronzo, R. G.: Augmented internal fixation with a fenestrated hip screw and cement. Orthop. Rev., 12:59, 1983.
151. Judet, R.: Traitement des fractures du col de femur por graffe pediculae. Acta Orthop. Scand., 32:421, 1962.
152. Meyers, M. H.: The unsolved fracture. Contemp. Orthop., 9:13, 1984.
153. Meyers, M. H.: The role of posterior bone grafts in femoral neck fractures. Clin. Orthop., 152: 143, 1980.
154. Meyers, M. H., Harvey, J. P., Moore, T. M.: Delayed treatment of subcapital and transcervical fractures of the neck of the femur with internal fixation and a muscle pedicle bone graft. Orthop. Clin. North Am., 5:743, 1974.
155. Chacha, P. B.: Vascularized Pedicular bone grafts. Int. Orthop., 8:127, 1984.
156. Morwessel, R., Evarts, M. C.: The use of a quadratus femoris muscle pedicle bone graft for the treatment of displaced femoral neck fractures. Orthopedics, 8:972, 1985.
157. Lloyd, E. I.: Quoted from Watson-Jones, R.: *Fractures and Joint Injuries,* ed. 3, Vol. II. Edinburgh, Livingstone, 1946.
158. Johnston, C. E., Ripley, L. P., Bray, C. B., Shaffer, L. W., Strong, T., Henning, G. D., Pruner, R. A.: Primary endoprosthetic replacement for acute femoral neck fractures. Clin. Orthop., 167:123, 1982.
159. Bray, T. J., Chapman, M. W.: Percutaneous pinning of intracapsular hip fractures. Instruct. Course Lect., 33:168, 1984.
160. Calandruccio, R. A.: Biomechanics, classification, and treatment of fractures of the neck of the femur. Presented at AOA Third International Symposium, San Francisco, 1982.
161. Welch, R. B.: The rationale for primary hemiarthroplasty in the treatment of fractures of the femoral neck in elderly patients. In: *The Hip. Proceedings of the Eleventh Open Scientific Meeting of the Hip Society,* 1983, p. 42.
162. Soreide, O., Moster, A., Raugstad, O. J.: Internal fixation versus primary prosthetic replacement in acute femoral neck fractures: A prospective, randomized clinical study. Br. J. Surg., 66:56, 1979.
163. Sikorski, J. M., Barrington, A.: Internal fixation versus hemiarthroplasty for the displaced subcapital fracture of the femur. J. Bone Joint Surg., 63B:357, 1981.
164. Dorr, L.: Treatment of hip fractures in elderly and senile patients. Orthop. Clin. North Am., 12:153, 1981.
165. Christiansen, T.: A new hip prosthesis with a trunion bearing. Acta Chir. Scand., 135:43, 1969.
166. Bowman, A. J. et al.: Experience with the bipolar prosthesis in hip arthroplasty. Orthopedics, 8:460, 1985.
167. Drinker, H., Murray, W. R.: The universal proximal femoral endoprosthesis. J. Bone Joint Surg., 61A:1167, 1979.
168. Steinberg, M. E., Unger, A. S.: Femoral endoprosthetic replacement in younger patients. Paper 132. Presented at the Scientific Meeting of the American Academy of Orthopedic Surgeons, Las Vegas, January 26, 1985.
169. Charnley, J.: Personal communication. Proposed to the author during a panel discussion in 1974.
170. Kwoh, D. C., Cruess, R. L.: Effect of the cemented femoral component on the articular cartilage of the acetabulum in dogs. Presented to the Canadian Orthopaedic Research Society, Kingston, Ontario, June 1982.
171. Cabanela, M. E., Van Demark, R. E.: Bipolar endoprosthesis. In: *The Hip. Proceedings of Twelfth Open Scientific Meeting of the Hip Society,* 1984, Ch. 6.
172. Murray, W. R.: Bipolar endoprosthesis. In: *The Hip. Proceedings of Twelfth Open Scientific Meeting of the Hip Society,* 1984, Ch. 7.
173. Sim, F. H.: Displaced femoral neck fractures: The rationale for primary total hip replacement. In: *The Hip, Proceedings of the Eleventh Open Scientific Meeting of the Hip Society,* 1983, Ch. 4.
174. Gingras, M. B., Clarke, J., Evarts, C. McC.: Prosthetic replacements in femoral neck fractures: Cemented versus noncemented. Clin. Orthop., 152:147, 1980.
175. Ordway, C. B., Kleiman, R., Garroway, R.: A retrospective study of fixation of hip prosthesis, cement versus noncemented stems. Presented as a scientific exhibit at the 1981 AAOS meeting.
176. Korthauer, K. M.: Endoprosthetic replacement for acute femoral neck fractures. Presented at the Western Orthopedic Association, 1983.

177. Glousman, R., Dorr, L., Sew Hoy, A., Vanis, P.: Treatment of femoral neck fractures with total hip replacement versus cemented and noncemented hemiarthroplasty. Presented at the Western Orthopedic Association, 1984.
178. Welch, R. B., Taylor, L. W., Wynne, F., White, A.: Results with the cemented hemiarthroplasty for displaced fractures of the femoral neck. Read at the Fifth Open Scientific Meeting of The Hip Society, 1977, Ch. 8.
179. Jaffe, W. L.: Editorial comment for the paper by Lane et al.[169]
180. Charnley, J.: The elimination of slip between the prosthesis and the femur. J. Bone Joint Surg., 47B:56, 1956.
181. Follocci, F. M., Charnley, J.: A comparison of the results of femoral head prosthesis with and without cement. Clin. Orthop., 62:156, 1969.
182. Hardinge, K.: The direct lateral approach to the hip. J. Bone Joint Surg., 64B:17, 1982.
183. Bauer, R., Kerschbaumer, F., Porsel, S., Oberthaler, W.: The transgluteal appraoch to the hip joint. Arch. Orthop. Trauma Surg., 95:47, 1979.
184. Gustke, K.: Hemiarthroplasty and total arthroplasty in the treatment of intracapsular fractures. III. Fractures of the hip. Inst. Course Lect., 33:195, 1984.
185. Johnson, R., Bendjelloul, H., Ekelund, L., et al.: Comparison between hemiarthroplasty and total hip replacement following failure of nailed femoral neck fractures focused on dislocations. Arch. Orthrop. Trauma Surg., 102:187, 1984.
186. Roberts, J. M., Fu, F., McClain, E., Ferguson, A. B., Jr.: A comparison of the posterolateral and anterolateral approaches to total hip arthroplasty. Clin. Orthop., 187:205, 1984.
187. Iyer, K. M.: A new posterior approach to the hip joint. Injury, 13:76, 1981.
188. Sim, F. H.: Displaced femoral neck fractures: The rationale for primary total hip replacement. In: *Proceedings of the Eleventh Open Scientific Meeting of the Hip Society,* 1983, Ch. 4.
189. Kofoed, H., Kofoed, J.: Moore prosthesis in the treatment of fresh femoral neck fractures: A critical review with special attention to secondary acetabular degeneration. Injury, 14:531, 1983.
190. Coates, R., Armour, P.: Treatment of subcapital fractures by primary total hip replacement. Injury, 11:132, 1979.
191. Bryan, R. S.: Editorial comment on Coates and Armour's article (ref. 268). In: *Yearbook of Orthopedics,* Chicago, Year Book, 1980, p. 223.
192. Klein, L.: Quoted in the *Wall Street Journal,* front page, October 9, 1984, "New question in race [Presidential campaign]: Is oldest U.S. President now showing his age?"
193. Merkow, R. L., Pellicci, P. M., Hely, D., Sabati, E. A.: Total hip replacement for Paget's disease of the hip. J. Bone Joint Surg., 66A:752, 1984.
194. Yurt, R. W., Ehrenkranz, N. J., Rogers. W., Finegold, S. M.: What's new in cephalosporin prophylaxis and therapy. Infect. Surg., 3:631, 1984.
195. Karam, G. H.: Antibiotic review for the orthopedic surgeon. Orthopedics, 7:1546, 1984.
196. Arnold, W. D.: The effect of early weight-bearing on the stability of femoral neck fractures treated with Knowles pins. J. Bone Joint Surg., 66A:847, 1984.
197. Brummer, R.: Natural course in nailed fractures of the femoral neck. Arch. Orthop. Trauma Surg., 103:52, 1984.
198. DeLee, J. C., Rockwood, C. A.: Current concepts review: The use of aspirin in thromboembolic disease. J. Bone Joint Surg., 62A:149, 1980.
199. Harris, W. H., Athanasoulis, C. A., Waltman, A. C., Salzman, E. W.: High and low-dose aspirin prophylaxis against venous thromboembolic disease in total hip replacement. J. Bone Joint Surg., 64A:63, 1982.
200. Snook, G. A., Chrisman, O. D., Wilson, T. C.: Thromboembolism after surgical treatment of hip fractures. Clin. Orthop., 155:21, 1981.
201. Zeckert, F., Khon, P., Vormittag, E.: Prophylaxis of thromboembolic diseases in traumatological patients: A randomized double-blind study with acetylsalicylic acid. Presented to the Fourth International Congress on Thrombosis and Hemostasis, Vienna, 1973, p. 281.
202. Day, L.: Pulmonary embolism and deep vein thrombosis in patients with hip fractures. In: *Fractures of the Hip,* 1st ed. (Meyers, M. H., ed.) Chicago, Year Book, 1985, Ch. 25.
203. Johnson, R., Green, J. R., Charnley, J.: Pulmonary embolism and its prophylaxis following total hip replacement. Clin. Orthop., 127:123, 1977.
204. Dalen, J. E., Alpert, J. S.: Natural history of pulmonary embolism. Prog. Cardiovasc. Dis., 17:259, 1975.
205. Browse, N.: Diagnosis of deep vein thrombosis. Br. Med. Bull., 342:163, 1978.
206. Moser, K. M., LeMoine, J. R.: Is embolic risk conditional by location of deep venous thrombosis? Am. Intern. Med., 94:439, 1981.
207. LeQuesne, L. P.: Relation between deep vein thrombosis and pulmonary embolism in surgical patients. N. Engl. J. Med., 291:1292, 1974.
208. Kakkar, V. V., Spindler, J., Flute, P. T.: Efficacy of low doses of heparin in prevention of deep vein thrombosis after major surgery. Lancet, 2:101, 1972.
209. Lunt, H. R.: The role of prosthetic replacement

of the head of the femur as primary treatment for subcapital fractures. *Injury,* 3:107, 1971.
210. Sikorski, J. M., Barrington, R.: Internal fixation versus hemiarthroplasty for the displaced subcapital fracture of the femur. J. Bone Joint Surg., 63B:357, 1981.
211. Sharma, S., Sankaran, B.: Primary replacement arthroplasty of the hip in femoral neck fractures. Int. Surg., 65:259, 1980.
212. Soreide, O., Molster, A., Raugstad, T. S.: Internal fixation versus primary prosthetic replacement in acute femoral neck fractures: a prospective study. Br. J. Surg., 66:56, 1979.
213. Soreide, O., Antti, A., Rietti, D.: Internal fixation versus endoprosthesis in the treatment of femoral neck fractures in the elderly. Acta. Orthop. Scand., 51:827, 1980.
214. Salvati, E. A., Wilson, P. D.: Long term results of femoral head replacements. J. Bone Joint Surg., 54A:1355, 1972.
215. Ratliff, A. H. C.: Vascular and neurologic complications following total hip replacements. In: *The Hip, Proceedings of the Hip Society,* St. Louis, Mosby, 1981, p. 276.
216. Hoaglund, F. T., Law, W. D. L.: Anatomy of the femoral head and neck. Clin. Orthop., 152:10, 1980.
217. Radin, E. L.: Biomechanics of the human hip. Clin. Orthop., 152:48, 1980.
218. Cathcart, R. F.: The shape of the femoral head and results from clinical use of a more normally shaped nonspherical hip replacement prosthesis. J. Bone Joint Surg., 43A:1559, 1972.
219. Clarke, I. C., Amstutz, H. C.: Human hip joint geometry and hemiarthroplasty selection. In: *The Hip, Proceedings of the Hip Society,* St. Louis, Mosby, 1975, Chap. 4.
220. Harris, W. H., Rushfeldt, P. D., Carlson, C. E., et al.: Pressure distribution in the hip and selection of a hemiarthroplasty. In: *The Hip, Proceedings of the Hip Society,* St. Louis, Mosby, 1975, Chap. 5.
221. Salvati, E. A., Artz, T., Aglietti, P., Asnis, S. E.: Endoprosthesis in the treatment of femoral neck fractures. Orthop. Clin. North Am., 5:757, 1974.
222. Ornahold, J., Espersen, J. O.: Para-articular ossifications after primary prosthetic replacement ad modum Austin-Moore. Acta Orthop. Scand., 46:643, 1975.
223. Whittaker, R. P., Abeshaus, M. M., Scholl, H. W., Chung, S.: Fifteen years experience with metallic endoprosthetic replacement of the femoral head for femoral neck fractures. J. Trauma, 12:799, 1972.
224. Nelson, C. L., Fitzgerald, R., Nelson, J. P., et al.: Symposium on antibiotic impregnated acrylic cement. Contemp. Orthop., 12:85, 1986.
225. Parrish, T. F., Jones, J. F.: Fractures of the femur following prosthetic arthroplasty of the hip. J. Bone Joint Surg., 50B:743, 1964.
226. Whittaker, R. P., Sotos, L. N., Ralston, E.: Fractures of the femur about femoral endoprostheses. J. Trauma, 14:675, 1974.
227. Zickel, R. E.: An intramedullary fixation device for the proximal part of the femur. J. Bone Joint Surg., 58A:866, 1976.
228. Chapman, M. W., Stehr, J. H., Eberle, C. F., et al.: Treatment of intracapsular hip fractures by the Deyerle method. J. Bone Joint Surg., 57A:735, 1975.
229. Arnold, W. D., Lyden, J. P., Minkoff, J.: Treatment of intracapsular fractures of the femoral neck. J. Bone Joint Surg., 56A:254, 1974.
230. Dooley, B. J., Hooper, J.: Fibular bone grafting for nonunion of femoral neck fractures. Aust. N. Z. J. Surg., 52:134, 1982.
231. Schmidt, R. G., Gregg, J. R.: Subtrochanteric fractures complicating multiple pin fixation of the hip. Read at the 1985 Scientific Meeting of the American Academy of Orthopedic Surgery.
232. Hadden, W. A., Abernathy, P. J., Haw, C.: Hip fractures of rheumatoid arthritis. Clin. Orthop., 170:252, 1982.
233. Distefano, M., Suda, M., Habermann, E. T.: A histomorphometric comparison of the femoral head in femoral neck fracture and osteoarthritis. Orthopedic Research Society, Las Vegas, January 1985.
234. Gerster, J. C., Charhon, S. A., Jaeger, P., Boivin, D.: Bilateral fractures of femoral neck in patients with moderate renal failure receiving fluoride for spinal osteoporosis. Br. Med. J., 287:723, 1983.
235. Powell, H. D. W.: Simultaneous bilateral fractures of the neck of the femur. J. Bone Joint Surg., 42B:235, 1960.
236. Delaney, W. M., Street, D. M.: Fracture of the femoral shaft with fracture of neck of same femur. J. Int. Coll. Surg., 19:303, 1953.
237. Bernstein, S. M.: Fractures of the femoral shaft and associated ipsilateral fractures of the hip. Orthop. Clin. North Am., 5:799, 1974.
238. Kimbrough, E.: Concomitant unilateral hip and femoral shaft fracture—a too frequently unrecognized syndrome. J. Bone Joint Surg., 43A:443, 1961.
239. MacKenzie, D. B.: Simultaneous ipsilateral fracture of the femoral neck and shaft: Report of 8 cases. S. Afr. Med J., 45:459, 1971.
240. Swiontkowski, M. F., Sigvard, T. H., Kellam, J.: Ipsilateral fractures of the femoral neck and shaft—a treatment protocol. J. Bone Joint Surg., 66A:260, 1984.

241. Bonfiglio, M.: The pathology of fracture of the femoral neck following irradiation. AJR, 70:449, 1953.
242. Goodman, A. H., Sherman, M. S.: Postirradiation fractures of the femoral neck. J. Bone Joint Surg., 45A:723, 1963.
243. Kotani, P. T., Oonishi, H., Shikita, T., Hamaguchi, T.: Study on the surface shape and contours of the femoral head and acetabulum of the human joint. Bull. Hosp. Bone Joint Dis., 36:81, 1975.
244. Stephenson, E. H., Cohen, B.: Post-irradiation fractures of the neck of the femur. J. Bone Joint Surg., 38B:830, 1956.
245. Jensen, T. M., Dillon, W. L., Reckling, F. W.: Changing concepts in the management of pathological and impending pathological fractures. J. Trauma, 16:496, 1976.
246. Murray, J. A., Parrish, F. F.: Surgical management of secondary neoplastic fractures about the hip. Orthop. Clin. North Am., 5:887, 1974.
247. Harrington, K. D., Sam, F. H., Enis, J. E., Johnston, J. O., Dick, H. M., Gristina, A. G.: Methyl methacrylate as an adjunct in the internal fixation of pathologic fracture. J. Bone Joint Surg., 58A:1047, 1976.
248. Harrington, K. D.: Specific problems of pathologic fractures. In: *Complications of Fracture Management.* (Gossling, M. R., Pillsburg, S. L., eds.) Philadelphia, Lippincott, 1984, pp. 187–212.
249. Harrington, K. D.: The management of acetabular insufficiency secondary to metastatic malignant disease. J. Bone Joint Surg., 63A:643, 1981.
250. Haberman, E. T., et al.: The pathology and treatment of metastatic disease of the femur. Clin. Orthop., 169:70, 1982.
251. Sabato, S., Stein, H.: The surgical management of pathological fractures. Int. Orthop., 7:65, 1983.
252. Lane, J. M., Glasser, D. B., McCormick, R. R.: Endoprosthetic replacement for pathologic fractures of the hip. In: *Mediguide to Orthopedics,* Vol. 5. Cranbury, N.J., Wallace Laboratories, 1984, pp. 1–5
253. Cameron, H. U., Fornasier, V. L., McNab, I.: Pathological fractures of the femoral neck. Can. Med. Assoc. J., 111:791, 1974.
254. Lane, J. M., Sculco, T. P., Zolan, S.: Treatment of pathologic fractures of the hip by endoprosthetic replacement. J. Bone Joint Surg., 62A:954, 1980.
255. Behr, J. T., Dobozi, W. R., Bodrina, K.: The treatment of pathological and impending pathological fractures of the proximal femur in the elderly. Clin. Orthop., 198:173, 1985.
256. Coughlin, L., Templeton, J.: Hip fractures in patients with Parkinson's disease. Clin. Orthop., 148:192, 1980.
257. Rothermel, J. E., Garcia, A.: Treatment of hip fractures in patients with Parkinson's syndrome on levodopa therapy. J. Bone Joint Surg., 54A:1251, 1972.
258. Eventov, I., Moreno, M., Geller, E., et al.: Hip fractures in patients with Parkinson's syndrome. J. Trauma, 23:98, 1983.
259. Gingras, M. B., Clarke, J., Evarts, C. M.: Prosthetic replacement in femoral neck fractures. Clin. Orthop., 152:147, 1980.
260. Sisk, T. D.: Fractures. In: *Campbell's Operative Orthopedics* (Edmondson, A. S., Crenshaw, A. H., eds.) St. Louis, Mosby, 1980.
261. Barry, H. C.: Fractures of the femur in Paget's disease of bone in Australia. J. Bone Joint Surg., 49A:1359, 1967.
262. Lake, M.: Studies of Paget's disease (osteitis deformans). J. Bone Joint Surg., 33B:323, 1951.
263. Milgram, J. W.: Orthopaedic management of Paget's disease of bone. Clin. Orthop., 127:63, 1977.
264. Stauffer, R. N., Sim, F. H.: Total hip arthroplasty in Paget's disease of the hip. J. Bone Joint Surg., 58A:476, 1976.
265. Thornhill, T. S., Creasman, C.: Hip fractures in patients with renal failure. Presented to the AAOS, Las Vegas, January 24, 1985.
266. Bertin, K. C., Horstman, J., Coleman, S. S.: Isolated fracture of the lesser trochanter in adults: An initial manifestation of metastatic malignant disease. J. Bone Joint Surg., 66A:770, 1984.
267. Kyle, J. A., Gustillo, R. B., Premer, R. F.: An analysis of 622 intertrochanteric hip fractures. J. Bone Joint Surg., 61A:216, 1979.
268. Evans, E. M.: The treatment of trochanteric fractures of the femur. J. Bone Joint Surg., 31B:190, 1949.
269. Evans, E. M.: Trochanteric fractures. J. Bone Joint Surg., 33B:182, 1951.
270. Boyd, H. B., Griffin, L. L. Classification and treatment of trochanteric fractures. Arch. Surg., 58:853, 1949.
271. Massie, W. K.: Fractures of the hip. J. Bone Joint Surg., 46A:658, 1964.
277. Massie, W. K.: Functional fixation of femoral neck fractures with a telescoping nail technique. Clin. Orthop., 12:230, 1959.
273. Cram, R. H.: The unstable intertrochanteric fracture. Surg. Gynecol. Obstet., 101:15, 1955.
274. Dimon, J. H., and Hughston, J. C.: Unstable intertrochanteric fractures of the hip. J. Bone Joint Surg., 49A:440, 1967.
275. Sisk, D.: Fractures. In: *Cambell's Operative Orthopedics,* 6th ed. St. Louis. Mosby, 1980, p. 617–620.

276. Kyle, R. F., Wright, T. M., Burstein, A. H.: Biomechanical analysis of the sliding characteristics of compression hip screws. J. Bone Joint Surg., 62A:1308, 1980.
277. Ecker, M. L., Joyce, J. J., Kohl, E. J.: The treatment of trochanteric hip fractures using a compression screw. J. Bone Joint Surg., 57A:23, 1975.
278. Wolfgang, G. L., Bryant, M. H., O'Neill, J. P.: Treatment of intertrochanteric fractures of the femur using sliding screw plate fixation. Clin. Orthop., 163:148, 1982.
279. Jensen, J. S.: Trochanteric fractures. Acta Orthop. Scand. [Suppl.], 188:1, 1981.
280. Rao, J. R., Rao, J. P., Banzon, T., Weiss, A. B., Rayhack, J.: Treatment of unstable intertrochanteric fractures with anatomic reduction and compression hip screw fixation. Clin. Orthop., 175:65, 1983.
281. Treharne, R. W.: The compression hip screw—the 25th anniversary of its development. Orthop. Rev., 11:45, 1982.
282. Tronzo, R. G.: Augment internal fixation with fenestrated hip screw. Orthop. Rev., 12:59, 1983.
283. Bartucci, E. J., Bartucci, E., Gonzalez, M. H., Cooperman, D. R., Freedberg, H. I., Barmada, R., Laros, G. S.: The effect of methyl methacrylate on the healing and function in osteoporotic intertrochanteric fractures. Presented at the 1985 AAOS meeting, Las Vegas. To be published.
284. Jensen, J. S., Sonne-Holm, S., Tondevold, E.: Unstable trochanteric fractures. Acta Orthop. Scand., 51:949, 1980.
285. Seinsheimer, F.: Concerning the proper length of femoral side plates. J. Trauma, 21:42, 1981.
286. Gesler, J. W., Goldberg, V. M.: An analysis of failures of the sliding compression screw in intertrochanteric fractures. Presented at the 1981 AAOS meeting, Las Vegas.
287. Doherty, J., Lyden J. P.: Intertrochanteric fractures of the hip treated with the hip compression screw—an analysis of problem. Clin. Orthop., 141:184, 1979.
288. Sonstegard, D. A., Kaufer, H., Matthews, L. S.: A biomechanical evaluation of implant, reduction, and prosthesis in the treatment of intertrochanteric hip fractures. Orthop. Clin. North Am., 5:551, 1974.
289. Boyd, H. B., Anderson, L. D.: Management of unstable trochanteric fractures. Surg. Gynecol. Obstet., 112:633, 1961.
290. Tronzo, R. G.: The use of an endoprosthesis for severely comminuted trochanteric fractures. Orthop. Clin. North Am., 5:629, 1974.
291. Pinder, C. R., Durnin, S. W., Cook, D. A.: The Leinbach prosthesis in the treatment of complex intertrochanteric fractures. Presented at the 1981 AAOS meeting, Las Vegas.
292. Harrington, K. D.: The use of methyl methacrylate as an adjunct in the internal fixation of unstable comminuted intertrachonteric fractures in osteoporotic patients. J. Bone Joint Surg., 57A: 744, 1975.
293. Romash, M., La Follette, B. F.: Cast brace management of intertrochanteric and subtrochanteric fractures with immediate ambulation. Presented at the 1981 AAOS meeting, Las Vegas.
294. Bernasek, T., Marcus, N. A., Pratt, W.: Intertrochanteric nonunions. Presented at the American Orthopedic Association Resident's Conference, New Orleans, 1985. To be published.
295. Wilson-MacDonald, J.: Subcapital fracture complicating an intertrochanter fracture. Clin. Orthop., 201:147, 1985.
296. Koch, J. C.: The laws of bone architecture. Am. J. Anat. 21:177, 1917.
297. Frankel, V. H., Burstein, S. H.: *Orthopedic Biomechanics,* Philadelphia, Lea & Febiger, 1970.
298. Schatzker, J., Waddell, J. P.: Subtrochanteric fractures of the femur. Orthop. Clin. North Am., 11:539, 1980.
299. Velasco, R. U., Comfort, T. H.: Analysis of treatment problems in subtrochanteric fractures of the femur. J. Trauma, 18:513, 1978.
300. Munson, M.: The operative treatment of subtrochanteric fractures. Orthopedics, 6:874, 1983.
301. Waddell, J. P.: Subtrochanteric fractures of the femur. J. Trauma, 19:582, 1979.
302. Watson, H. K., Campbell, R. D., Wade, P. A.: Classification, treatment and complications of the adult subtrochanteric fractures. J. Trauma, 4: 457, 1964.
303. Fielding, J. W., Magliato, H. J.: Subtrochanteric fractures. Surg. Gynecol. Obstet., 122:555, 1966.
304. Fielding, J. W., Cochran, G. V. B., Zickel, R. E.: Biomechanical characteristics and surgical management of subtrochanteric fractures. Orthop. Clin. North Am., 5:629, 1974.
305. Zickel, R. E.: An intramedullary fixation device for the proximal part of the femur. J. Bone Joint Surg., 58A:866, 1976.
306. Zickel, R. E.: Subtrochanteric femoral fractures. Orthop. Clin. North Am., 11:555, 1980.
307. Butler, J. E., Brown, S. L., McConnell, B. G.: Subtrochanteric stress fractures in runners. Am. J. Sports Med., 10:228, 1982.
308. Wright, P. H., Wainer, R., Gilbert, J., et al.: Biomechanical characteristics of Ender rods, Zickel nails and the AMBI compression screw. Presented at the 52nd Annual Meeting of the

American Academy of Orthopedic Surgeons, Las Vegas, Jan. 28, 1985.
309. Cecg, O., Sosna, A.: Principles of the surgical treatment of subtrochanteric fractures. Orthop. Clin. North Am., 5:651, 1974.
310. Zickel, R. E.: A new fixation device for subtrochanteric fractures of the femur. Clin. Orthop., 54:115, 1967.
311. Küntscher, G.: Die stabile osteosynthese bei der Osteotome. Chirurg, 14:161, 1942.
312. Cuthbert, H., Howat, T. W.: The use of Kuntscher "Y" nail in the treatment of intertrochanteric and subtrochanteric fractures of the femur. Injury, 8:135, 1976.
313. Ruszkowski, I., Muftic, O.: Modifizierter Kuntwscher nagel suz fixierung des proximalen teiles des femurs nach korrektiven osteotomien bei kindern. Arch. Orthop. Unfallchir., 89:239, 1977.
314. Allen, W. C., Burstein, A. H.: A fluted femoral intramedullary rod. J. Bone Joint Surg., 32A: 506, 1978.
315. Scherfel, T.: A new type of intramedullary nail for the internal fixation of subtrochanteric fractures of the femur. Int. Orthop., 8:255, 1985.
316. Thomas, W. G., Villar, R. N.: Subtrochanteric fractures—Zickel nail or nail/plate. J. Bone Joint Surg., 68B:255, 1986.
317. Hagglund, G., Lidgren, L., Nordstrom, B.: Intramedullary Ender nailing combined with Parham's modified bands in the treatment of subtrochanteric femoral fractures. Arch. Orthop. Trauma. Surg., 100:131, 1982.
318. Archer, J. H., Murphy, C., D'Ambrosia, R.: Treatment of fractures of the femur with Grosse-Kempt rods. Orthopedics, 8:1393, 1985.
319. Ender, J.: Probleme bei frischen per- und subtrochanteren Oberschenkelbruchen. Hefte Unfallheilkd., 106:2, 1970.
320. Küntscher, G.: Zur operation Behandlung der pertrochanteren Fraktur. Z. Chir., 91:281, 1966.
321. Pugh, W. L.: A self-adjusting nail-plate for fractures about the hip joint. J. Bone Joint Surg., 37A:1085, 1955.
321a. Trafton, G., Day, L. J., Cohen, H. A., Kaye, R. A., Bovill, E. G.: Harris nail versus compression hip screw for intertrochanteric fracture—a prospective randomized comparison. Presented at the 1984 AAOS meeting.
322. Sherk, H. H., Foster, M. D.: Hip fractures treated with Harris rods vs. compression hip screws. Clin. Orthop., 192:255, 1985.
323. Bohler, J.: Percutaneous intramedullary nailing of intertrochanteric fractures. In: *Proceedings of the Hip Society,* St. Louis, Mosby, 1975, Chap. 11.
324. Kuderna, H., Bohler, N., Collon, D. J.: Treatment of intertrochanteric and subtrochanteric fractures of the hip by the Ender method. J. Bone Joint Surg., 58:604, 1976.
325. Hall, G. H., Ainscow, D.: Comparison of nail-plate fixation and Ender's nailing for intertrochanteric fractures. J. Bone Joint Surg., 63B:24, 1981.
326. Hayward, S. J., Lowe, L. W., Tzevelekos, S.: Intertrochanteric fractures—a comparison between fixation with a two piece nail plate and Ender's nails. Int. Orthop., 7:153, 1983.
327. Russin, L. A., Sonni, A.: Treatment of intertrochanteric and subtrochanteric fractures with Ender's intramedullary rods. Clin. Orthop., 148:203, 1980.
328. Raugstad, T. S., Molster, A., Haukeland, W., Hestenes, O., Olerud, S.: Treatment of pertrochanteric and subtrochanteric fractures of the femur by the Ender method. Clin. Orthop., 138: 231, 1979.
329. Levy, R. N., Siegel, M., Sedlan, E. D.: Complications of Ender pin fixation in basicervical, intertrochanteric, and subtrochanteric fractures of the hip. J. Bone Joint Surg., 65A:66, 1983.
330. Jensen J. S., Sonne-Holm, S.: Critical analysis of Ender nailing in the treatment of trochanteric fractures. Acta Orthop. Scand., 51:817, 1980.
331. Nelson, B., Tondevold, E.: Limitations of Ender's nails in the stabilization of femoral shaft fractures. Presented at the 1985 AAOS meeting, Las Vegas.
332. Wilson, J. K., Chapman, M. W.: Ender pins in the treatment of fractures of the hip and femoral shaft—a second look. Presented at the 1985 AAOS meeting, Las Vegas
333. Bray, T. J., Chapman, M. W.: The use of Ender nail fixation for extracapsular fractures about the hip. In: *Fractures of the Hip* (Meyers, M. H., ed.) Chicago, Year Book, 1985, Chap. 18.
334. Schaumberg, E. W.: Ender nailing of the proximal femur. Presented at the 1985 AAOS meeting, Las Vegas.
335. Hallman, B. W., Iftikhar, T. B.: Ender nail fixation for concomitant unilateral hip and shaft fracture. Orthopedics 8:1003, 1985.
336. Pankovich, A. M., Tarabisky I., Barmada, R.: Fractures below non-cemented femoral implants—treatment with Ender pins. J. Bone Joint Surg., 63A:1024, 1981.
337. Raugstad, T. S., Molster, A., Haukeland, W., Hostenes Olerud, S.: Treatment of pertrochanteric and subtrochanteric fractures of the femur by the Ender method. Clin. Orthop., 138:231, 1979.
338. Olerud, S., Stark, A., Gillstrom, P.: Malrotation following Ender nailing. Clin. Orthop., 147:139, 1980.

339. Tencer, A. G., Johnson, K. D., Johnston, W. E.: A biomechanical comparison of various methods of stabilization of subtrochanteric fractures of the femur. J. Orthop. Res., 2:297, 1984.
340. Hirsh, J.: Prophylaxis of venous thromboembolism, J. Am. Heart Assoc. 53:25, 1984.

CHAPTER 9

Pathological Fractures of the Upper End of the Femur Secondary to Metastatic Disease

STEVEN GITELIS, MITCHELL B. SHEINKOP, KIM HAMMERBERG, AND MICHAEL GITELIS

The management of metastatic lesions in the region of the hip has become a more frequent orthopedic problem in recent years. This increase is due to prolonged survival of patients with malignant disease and reflects advances made in the oncological treatment of these patients. Classically, the orthopedic objectives when treating secondary neoplastic deposits to the hip are the alleviation of pain and the preservation of function.

Metastatic skeletal lesions can be expected in 15 to 30% of patients with malignancies. The incidence of metastasis to bone can be as high as 60% in patients with disseminated breast carcinoma.[2,18,24,26,28,39,47] Breast carcinoma is responsible for the majority of skeletal metastases encountered. Over the past two decades, however, there has been an increase in the incidence of skeletal metastases from carcinoma of the lung. At the present time, breast, lung, prostate, and kidney probably account for more than 80% of all the metastases to bone.[13,18,37,39] The incidence of femoral involvement by metastatic carcinoma is between 10 and 25%.[6,13] Although metastases to the spine and pelvis are more frequent than those to the femur, catastrophic pathological fractures with acute changes in ambulatory function are most common in the proximal one-third of the femur.[6,7,21,23]

Pathological fractures involving the proximal femur present major difficulties in stabilization. In this area there is a problem of high-stress requirements frequently associated with extensive bone loss with concomitant loss of strength and substance. Until recently, the evolution of the treatment of pathological hip fractures has been slow and often discouraging. The dismal prognosis for a patient with a pathological hip fracture at the turn of the century was expressed by Grunert. In 1905 he reported that in carcinomatosis union of the fragments can never occur, and there has never been a reported case of such a recovery.[17] During the first half of the century, the treatment of pathological hip fractures remained predominantly palliative and, except for amputation, was strictly nonsurgical. A variety of techniques were used to provide external immobilization including traction, splintage, plaster, and sand bags. Adjunctive therapy was primarily directed toward the alleviation of pain. During this time, however, advancements in the oncological treatment of metastatic disease improved with hormonal manipulation, radiation therapy, and chemotherapy.[29,42–44] Despite these advances, patients who presented with a pathological fracture of the hip were severely disabled with pain and the inability to ambulate, and death remained imminent.

The technical advancements made in internal fixation of fractures during the 1940s may have prompted the more aggressive surgical treatment of pathological fractures.[1,10,16] Since that time, internal fixation of a pathological hip fracture with any one of a variety of devices has become the standard treatment.[3,4,8,13,22,29] The advantages of aggressive intervention are the relief of pain, facilitation of nursing, reduced hospitalization, and return of functional ambulation. These benefits have been documented by many reports in recent years.[9,30,32,33,38]

In order to overcome the failures of conventional fixation devices resulting from extensive cortical bone loss in the area of the metastatic lesion, the diseased bone can be replaced by methyl methacrylate.[5,11,45] Harrington has reported a large series of pathological hip fractures treated with internal fixation and augmented with methyl methacrylate, with a high percentage regaining the ability to ambulate.[20,21]

Despite augmentation with bone cement, standard internal fixation devices are not always of sufficient strength to withstand failure. The development of reinforced devices such as the Zickel nail have improved stabilization for the difficult subtrochanteric fracture.[31,46] The problems of fracture stabilization and fixation failure can be circumvented by resection of the diseased bone and reconstruction with hip arthroplasty. With this technique the diseased bone is removed until mechanically sound bone is encountered that allows seating of a prosthetic device. The efficacy of hemiarthroplasty for pathological fractures of the femoral head and neck has been demonstrated by Poigenfurst et al.[34] The concept of prosthetic replacement has expanded to include total hip arthroplasty and replacements of the proximal one-third of the femur.[21,30,33,40,41] Total joint replacement also allows reinforcement of the acetabulum, which is frequently involved by metastases.[19]

Despite the trend toward more aggressive surgical intervention in the treatment of pathological hip fractures, the acceptance of prophylactic fixation has been slower to occur. As early as 1947, Greissman and Schutemyer reported the prophylactic fixation of impending femur fractures.[16] Since then, others have recognized that prophylactic fixation of an impending fracture can be technically easier, improve stabilization, facilitate rehabilitation, alleviate pain, and reduce morbidity.[2,3,12,14,25,35,38] The substantial benefits produced certainly outweigh the relatively low morbidity and mortality encountered with prophylactic surgery. The problem of dealing with an impending fracture of the hip is deciding which patients need prophylactic stabilization. In the past, the guidelines were mostly radiographic, including (1) involvement of one-half of the cortex, (2) lesions greater than 2.5 cm in diameter, (3) purely lytic lesion without demonstrable bony repair, and (4) a demonstrable metastatic lesion that is rapidly progressing radiologically or which was not previously seen. Although these radiological criteria add some objectivity to the decision about which lesions represent an impending fracture, it still is a difficult decision about operative indications. Tronzo in the past has stated that "when you first see it, nail it!" This emphasizes the need for aggressive surgical treatment of impending fractures of the proximal femur.

Role of Prophylactic Surgery in the Management of Metastatic Hip Disease

We reviewed our experience with the management of metastatic lesions of the proximal one-third of the femur[15] seeking to determine if prophylactic surgery plays any role in the management of metastatic hip disease. We retrospectively reviewed 53 patients treated prophylactically for a metastatic lesion involving the proximal one-third of the femur from 1971 to 1979. This represented a consecutive series of patients. The majority of these patients were ambulatory prior to surgical intervention but were incapacitated by severe and progressive hip pain. Their functional ambulatory status was characteristically decreasing, and increasing amounts of pain medications were required. The average patient was 61 years of age (Fig. 9–1). Eighty-five percent of the patients were women, with involvement by metastatic breast carcinoma the most common clinical pattern. The mean length of time from diagnosis of the primary neoplasm until presentation for prophylactic surgery of the hip was 4.6 years. Eighty-one percent of the impending fractures were located in an intertrochanteric or subtrochanteric location (Fig. 9–2).

The majority of these patients were treated by elective stabilization of their impending fracture with internal fixation devices such as a Zickel nail or some other form of a nail plate device (Table 9–1). Eleven percent of the patients were treated by resection of their proximal femur and reconstruction with a total hip arthroplasty due to disseminated disease and poor bone stock. Nine of the 53 patients were treated with adjunctive methyl methacrylate. The average length of hospitalization was 23.8 days, and the overall complication rate was 14% (Table 9–1). Six percent of the patients were diagnosed as having a deep vein thrombosis, which represented the most common complication. None of the patients expired in the hospital. The mean survival after surgery for pa-

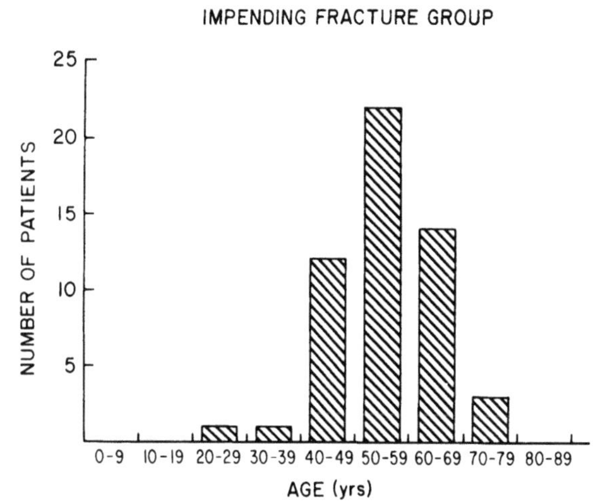

FIG. 9–1 Age distribution of impending fracture group.

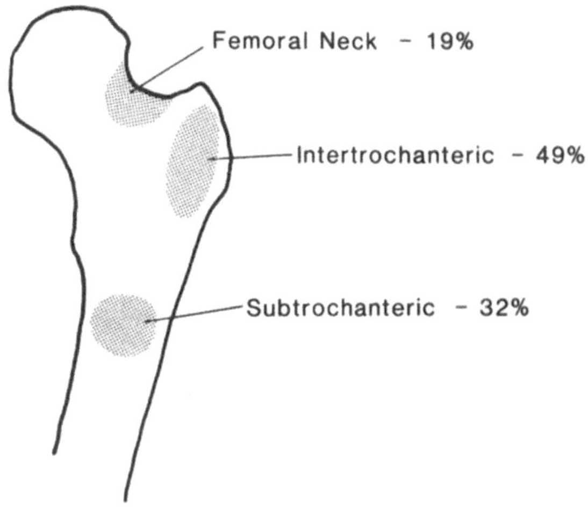

FIG. 9–2 Location of impending fractures.

tients with an impending fracture of the hip was 15.4 months.

A similar group of patients ($n = 46$) presented with a pathological fracture of the proximal one-third of the femur (Figs. 9–3 to 9–6). This was during the same time period and represented a consecutive group of patients treated from 1971 to 1979. None of these patients was able to ambulate and presented as an emergency with a pathological fracture. The average age was 55.3 years with 80% of the patients being women (Fig. 9–7). Breast carcinoma again represented the most common primary neoplasm, occurring in 59% of the patients. Nine percent of the patients presented with a pathological hip fracture and were found to have an unknown primary carcinoma at biopsy (Table 9–2). These patients underwent extensive diagnostic evaluations to attempt to locate the primary neoplasm, but these attempts were unsuccessful. Excluding these four patients, the mean length of time with a known primary neoplasm was 4.4 years. Eighty-five percent of the patients had a pathological fracture in either a femoral neck or subtrochanteric location (Fig. 9–8).

TABLE 9–1 Clinical Data for Impending Fracture Group

Location of the Primary Disease (%)		Treatment of Metastatic Foci (%)		Complications (%)	
Breast	73	Total hip arthroplasty	11	Death	0
Lung	9	Nail plate	43	Failure of stabilization	2
Prostate	4	Hemiarthroplasty	6	Deep vein thrombosis	6
Renal	8	Zickel nail	30	Deep wound infection	2
Unknown	0	Ender nail	8	Pneumonia	0
Myeloma/leukemia	2	Intramedullary nail	2	Peroneal nerve palsy	2
Gastrointestinal	0			Cerebral vascular accident	0
Cervix	2			Pyelonephritis	2
Bladder	2			Total	14

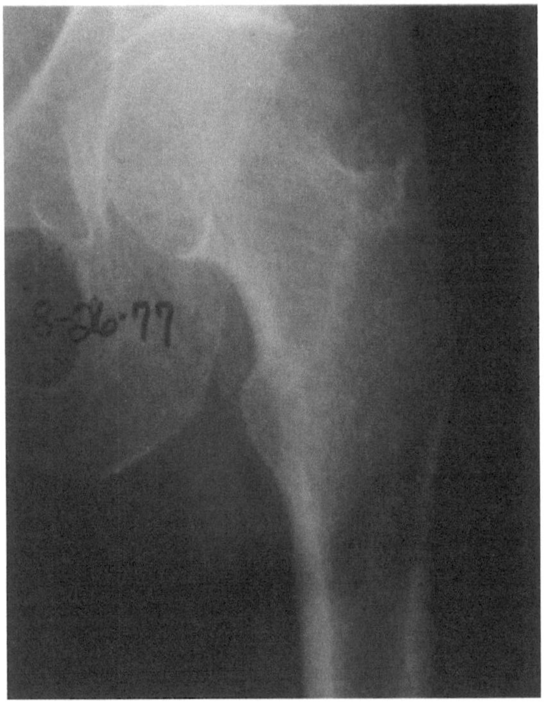

FIG. 9–3 A 58-year-old woman with breast carcinoma metastatic to the left hip subtrochanteric region.

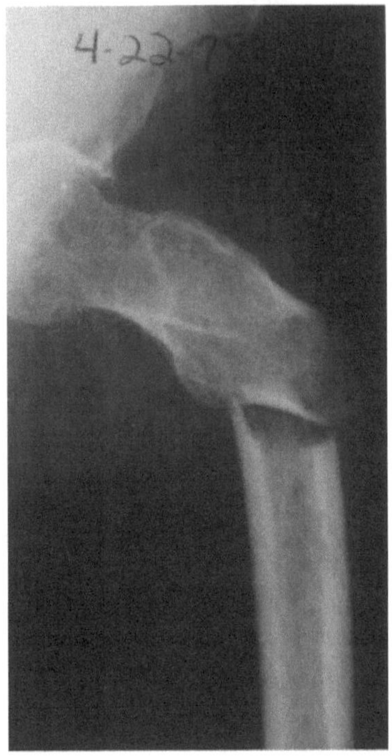

FIG. 9–5 Same patient as in Figs. 9–3 and 9–4. Three days later the patient presented with a pathological fracture. Small dark spots are artefacts.

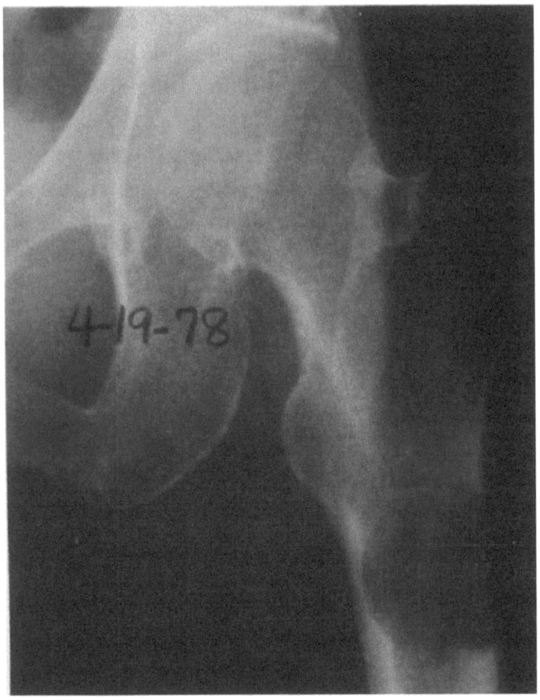

FIG. 9–4 Same patient as in Fig. 9–3. Eight months later with further progression of the destruction. Note the total loss of lateral cortex and the 50% loss of medial cortex. Small dark spots are artefacts.

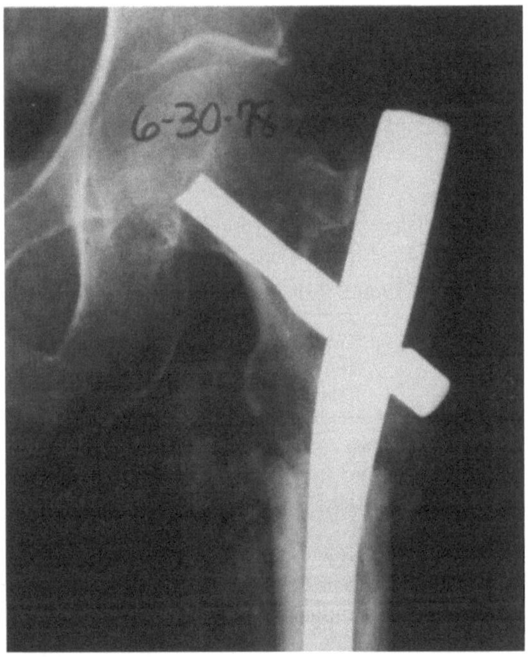

FIG. 9–6 Left hip stabilized with Zickel nail.

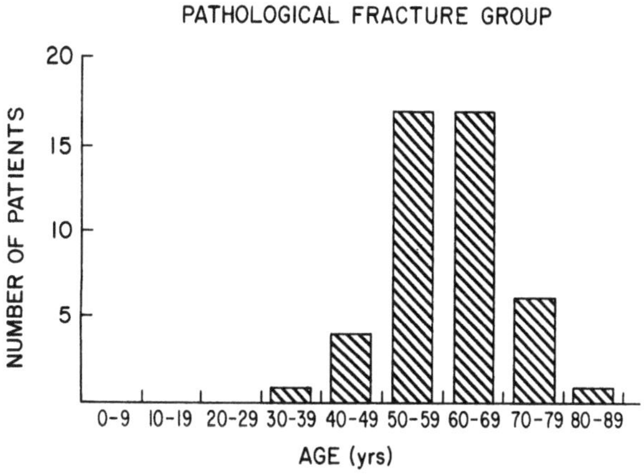

FIG. 9–7 Age distribution of pathological fracture group.

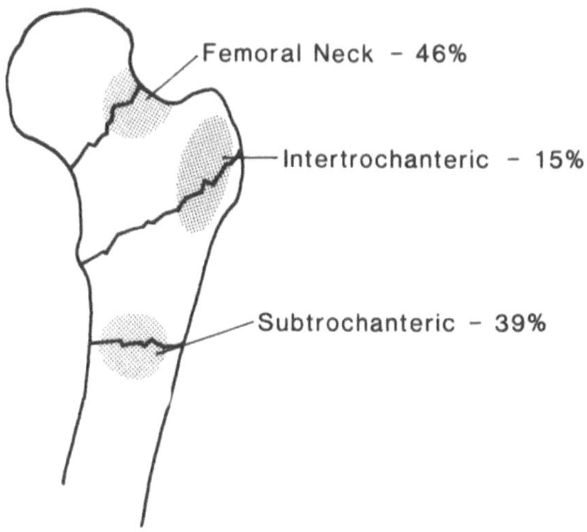

FIG. 9–8 Locations of pathological fractures.

Thirty-five percent of the patients were treated with a hemiarthroplasty because of the common occurrence of femoral neck fracture (Table 9–2). Twenty-one were, in addition, treated with methyl methacrylate to improve fixation. The methyl methacrylate was used either as a buttress to fill the cavity after curettage of the metastatic tissue or within the femoral canal to help transfer forces from the intramedullary device to the cortical bone. The average length of hospitalization for this group of patients was 26.3 days. Eleven of these patients expired in the hospital an average of 27.2 days after surgery (Table 9–2). Seven of 11 of these patients expired because of respiratory insufficiency secondary to pneumonia. Three expired because of malignant pleural effusion or malignant ascites with secondary atelectasis and respiratory insufficiency. One patient expired from a pulmonary embolus. Five patients who were treated with internal fixation for their pathological fracture had a loss of fracture fixation (Figs. 9–9 and 9–10). None of these patients was treated with adjunctive methyl methacrylate. The 21 patients who were treated with a prosthetic replacement had no major complication due to mechanical failure. The survival of this group of patients was 9.6 months.

After retrospectively reviewing these 99 patients with either an impending fracture or a pathological fracture of the proximal femur, we thought that prophylactic surgery did play an important role in their management. The surgery is performed electively when the patient is the best medical candidate for surgical intervention and anesthesia. The operative mortality rate was 0%, compared to 26% for those patients treated after a pathological fracture. Using the clinical parameters of age, sex, length of time with metastatic

TABLE 9–2 Clinical data for Pathological Fracture Group

Location of the Primary Disease (%)		Treatment of Metastatic Foci (%)		Complications (%)	
Breast	59	Total hip arthroplasty	13	Death	26
Lung	11	Nail plate	27	Failure of stabilization	11
Prostate	13	Hemiarthroplasty	35	Deep vein thrombosis	0
Renal	2	Zickel nail	13	Deep wound infection	2
Unknown	9	Ender nail	6	Pneumonia	2
Myeloma/leukemia	4	Intramedullary nail	6	Peroneal nerve palsy	0
Gastrointestinal	2			Cerebral vascular accident	2
Cervix	0			Pyelonephritis	0
Bladder	0			Total	43

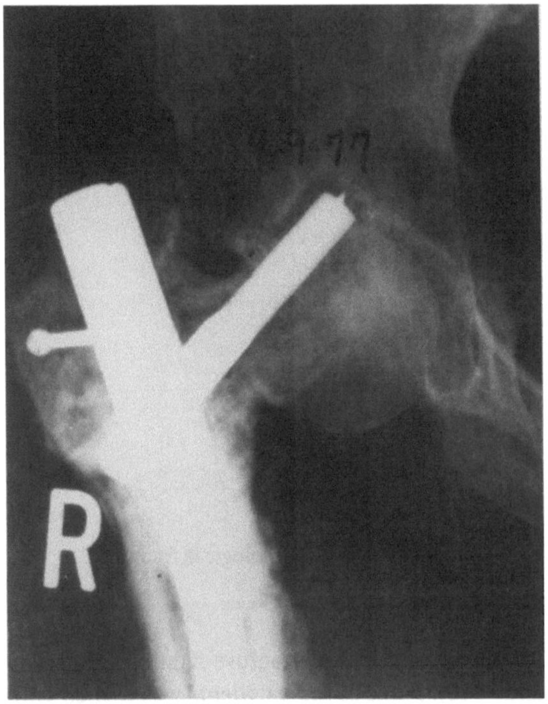

FIG. 9–9 A 57-year-old woman with breast carcinoma metastatic to the right subtrochanteric region and the femoral neck. The subtrochanteric area was well stabilized. However, the femoral neck fractured with varus deformity and loss of fixation.

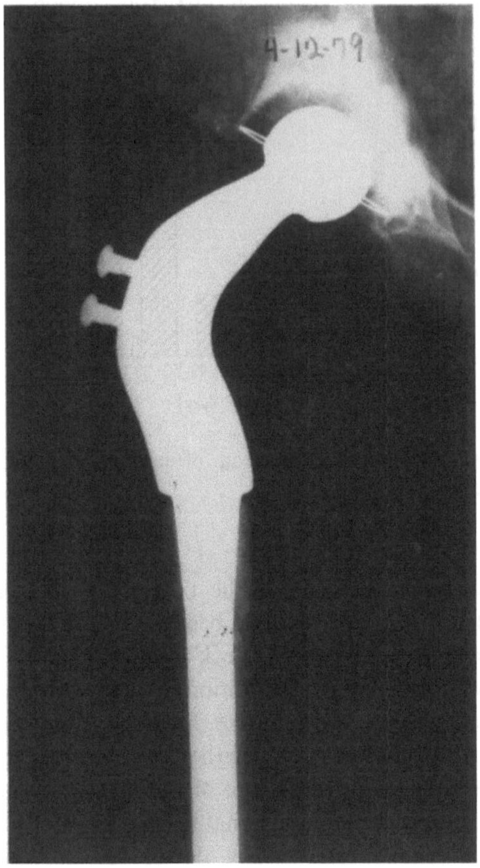

FIG. 9–10 The patient in Fig. 9–9 was treated with a prosthetic replacement.

disease, and location and type of metastatic disease, there was no statistical difference between the pathological fracture group and the impending fracture group. In conclusion, we could not attribute this major difference in mortality to clinical differences between the two groups. The next question we sought to answer more objectively was what constituted an impending fracture.

Biomechanics of the Proximal Femur and Its Relation to Pathological Fracture

Ward in 1838 made the original contribution dealing with the weight-bearing system of the proximal femur. He described the medial compressile and lateral tensile trabeculae. Koch in 1917 created a mathematical model of weight transmission across the proximal femur.[27] He concluded that the trabeculae correspond to trajectories of maximal compressile and tensile forces and postulated five normal groups of trabeculae. Other authors have included the action of muscles about the proximal femur and their effects on the forces in both compression and tension. Bone is twice as strong in compression as in tension. The ultimate tensile strength of the proximal femur is between 10,000 and 20,000 pounds per square inch (psi). Rybicki et al. determined that the tensile force during one-legged stance in the proximal femur is in the area of 6640 psi.[36] It is obvious that the forces generated during the stance phase of the gait rather closely approximate the ultimate tensile strength of the proximal femur—and this is a normal bone. In diseased bone (e.g., significantly weakened by metastatic disease, however, the ultimate tensile strength of the proximal femur is far less. Using this information, one can postulate that metastatic lesions involving the primary tensile trabeculae in the area of the lateral proximal femur would significantly weaken the bone (Figs. 9–11 and 9–12). In a retrospective analysis of 39 patients

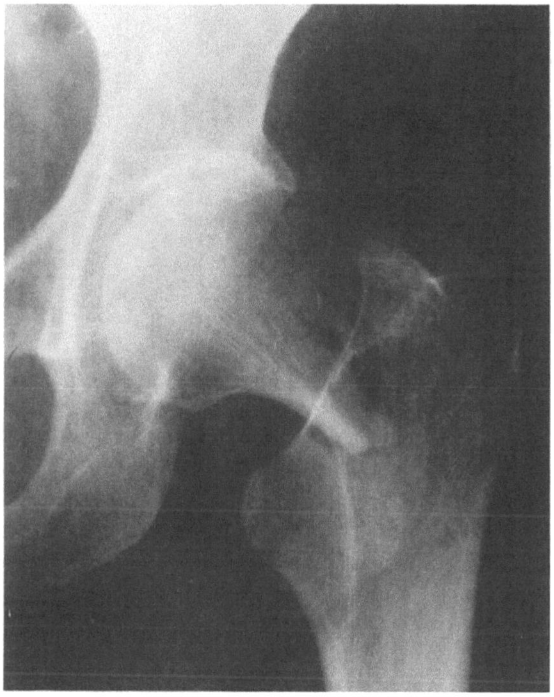

FIG. 9–11 A 76-year-old woman had metastatic breast carcinoma with a pathological hip fracture. Note the primary destruction of the tensile trabeculae.

FIG. 9–12 The patient in Fig. 9–11 was treated with a calcar replacement hip prosthesis and captured acetabulum.

with metastatic hip disease, we were able to categorize two types of radiological bone destruction: geographic and permeative. We next determined whether either type of radiological destruction involved primarily the tensile trabeculae, the compressile trabeculae, or both. We found that 11 of 12 patients with destruction of primarily the tensile trabeculae of the proximal femur went on to pathological fracture. We further found that of 12 patients with primary involvement of the compressile trabecule of the proximal femur, only one went on to pathological fracture. All five patients with involvement of both the compressive and tensile trabeculae went on to pathological fracture. When the destruction was characterized by diffuse permeative involvement of the proximal femur, which was present in 10 patients, the pathological fracture occurred in the subtrochanteric region in all patients. We concluded that this type of radiological destruction placed the patient at significant risk for fracture in the subtrochanteric area.

It is important that prior to determining an impending fracture that x-ray films be obtained in at least two planes. All too frequently we found that among patients who had a radiograph of the hip in only the anteroposterior plane only minimal destruction of the proximal femur was demonstrated. When a lateral radiograph was obtained, rather extensive destruction was found. The one plane radiograph can often be misleading in detecting the total extent of the destruction. In recent years we have used computed tomography to delineate the destruction in the proximal femur and have found it to be very accurate in presenting a three-dimensional representation of the amount of disease.

Definition of an Impending Fracture and Treatment

We currently use both clinical and radiological information to determine the presence of an impending fracture. The clinical information reveals the need for increasing analgesia; the disability for recreational, vocational, or daily living activities; the increasing pain; and the increasing dependency on accessory apparatuses for ambulation. Objective clinical data reveal the inability to initiate an independent straight leg raise, pain elicited in the groin or thigh with passive hip rotation, and measureable thigh or buttocks atrophy. The radiological criteria include osseous destruction located in areas of primary tensile trabeculae or destruction of greater than 50% of the cortex in the area of the calcar or subtrochanteric region. At least two plane radiographs must be taken to delineate this destruction. The radiological criteria, however, must be correlated with the clinical information previously stated to indicate the needs for prophylactic surgery.

Once the patient with an impending fracture is identified, treatment is varied. Knowledge of systemic data, including the source of the primary, other skeletal involvement, other organ system involvement, survival prognosis, and oncological management, is necessary prior to management decision. Therapeutic modalities for the impending pathological fracture with geographic type of destruction is based on its anatomical localization. These lesions can be categorized into subcapital, intertrochanteric, and subtrochanteric. Most of these impending fractures can be treated by nail plate fixation. We prefer a sliding hip screw similar to that used for traumatic hip fractures. Subtrochanteric geographic lesions are best treated by the Zickel device or some other form of intramedullary implant. The fixation is augmented with methyl methacrylate whenever possible. If the type of destruction is permeative, involving the proximal femur, we prefer to do a resection of the proximal femur with prosthetic reconstruction. This may necessitate hemiarthroplasty for femoral neck lesions if adequate calcar is present to seat the prosthesis. If no calcar is present, a calcar replacement prosthesis is used. We prefer resection with prosthetic reconstruction for permeative lesions because of the high incidence of failure of fixation with this type of radiological destruction.

When performing resection of the proximal femur with prosthetic reconstruction, it is important to have available as stock items in the operating room a wide range of prostheses so that intraoperative decisions can be made regarding treatment. We stock a calcar prosthesis with a 32-mm head with stem lengths ranging from 150 to 220 mm. The neck replacement lengths range from 55 to 70 mm with 5-mm increments (Fig. 9–13). The 32-mm head is adaptable for either a cemented acetabular component or an uncemented captured acetabular component (Fig. 9–12). We also stock proximal one-third of the femur replacements with 32-mm head diameters. The stem lengths range from 140 to 180 mm. The replacement lengths range from 80 to 200 mm (Fig. 9–14). The replacement lengths are in 10-mm increments. A selection of hemiarthroplasty prostheses of a solid-stem Austin Moore type with variable head diameters should also be available (Fig. 9–15). At the time of resecting the proximal femur, an intraoperative decision regarding the level of resection is made based on the adequacy of cortical bone for seating of the implant. We prefer to resect down to uninvolved cortical bone, replacing the additional length of proximal femur with a longer prosthesis to minimize the likehood of future subsidence. A prosthetic length is chosen that will provide stability of the hip joint after trial reduction of the hip. Stem length is determined by the presence of disease distally in the femoral diaphysis that requires intramedullary stabilization (Fig. 9–16). When the proximal one-third of the femur is replaced with a 32-mm head prosthesis, the acetabular component can be either cemented or captured.

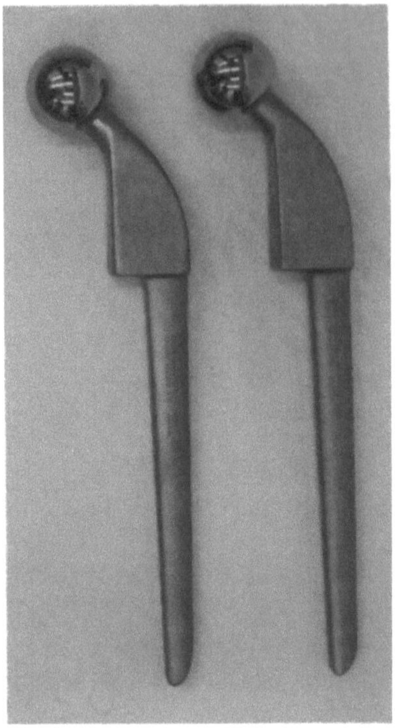

FIG. 9–13 Calcar replacement prostheses.

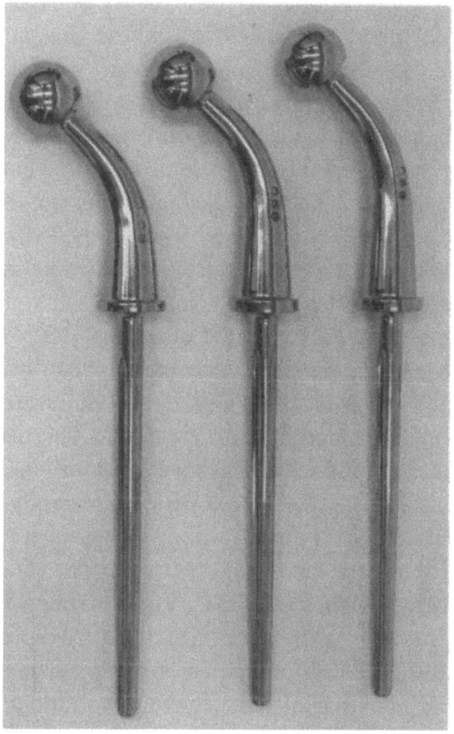

FIG. 9–14 Proximal one-third of the femur replacement prostheses.

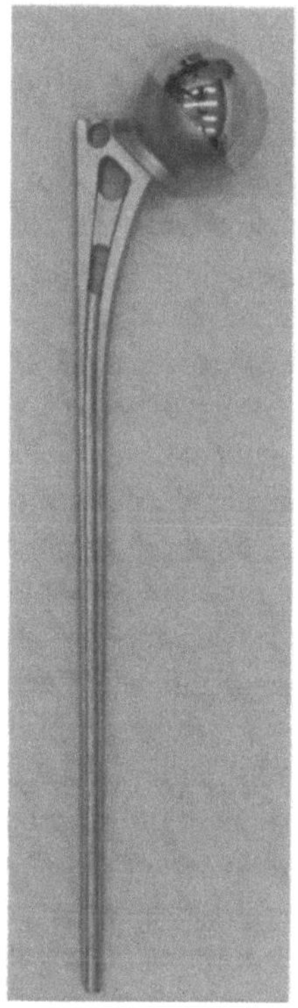

FIG. 9–16 Long-stem Austin Moore prosthesis to stabilize the femoral diaphysis.

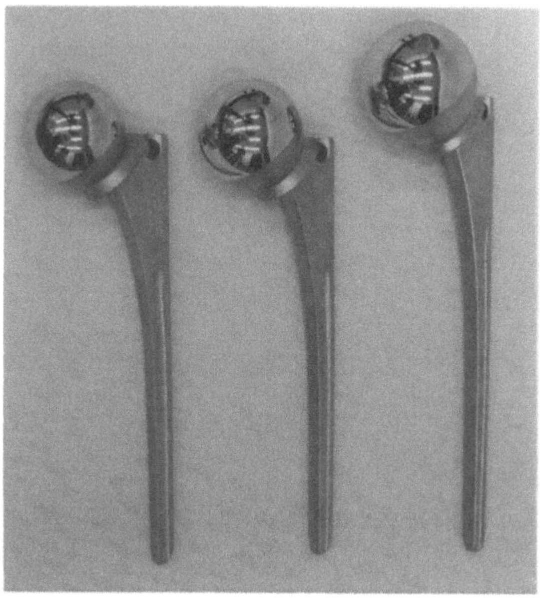

FIG. 9–15 Solid-stem Austin Moore prostheses.

Reconstruction of the soft tissues amounts to suturing the abductors to the vastus lateralis to form a lateral soft tissue buttress. Suturing the abductors to the prosthetic device has not proved successful.

Recommendations for Treatment of Pathological Fractures of the Proximal Femur

Once a pathological fracture occurs, we believe that all patients should undergo surgical treatment unless the patient is moribound and has a very limited life expectancy or cannot tolerate the anesthesia necessary for treatment of the pathological fracture. Justification for this rather aggressive management program is the fact that with surgical intervention, even if the patient cannot be made ambulatory, improved nursing care is facilitated and relief of pain is achieved.

Pathological fractures are treated in a manner similar to that for traumatic fractures in the given anatomical area using conventional techniques. The most common location of these fractures is the femoral neck, and if a patient presents with a displaced femoral neck fracture some form of arthroplasty is performed. For the most part, we treat these patients with a cemented solid-stem hemiarthroplasty with or without a captured acetabular component. If it is elected to reconstruct the hip with a hemiarthroplasty without an acetabular component, a solid-stem Austin Moore prosthesis is used with cement. If marked calcar destruction has occurred, we use either a cemented calcar replacement prosthesis or a proximal one-third of the femur replacement as previously described for impending fracture treatment. The decision to include an acetabular component is based on the coexistence of acetabular disease. Often necessary in the acetabular reconstruction is a wire mesh or Protrusio ring. In addition, we have employed bone grafts and other forms of internal fixation to help support the acetabular component.

Intertrochanteric fractures can usually be treated by internal fixation using a sliding compression nail. It is important to stabilize these fractures in the operating room, and we use the same indications for stability as for traumatic intertrochanteric fractures. These indications include lack of medial or posterior support due to comminution or tumor destruction. If the intertrochanteric fracture is unstable, we stabilize the fracture in the operating room by performing a medial displacement and valgus pinning with osteotomy of the greater trochanter. If additional medial support is necessary owing to destruction in that area, we curet out the tumor and fill the cavity created with methyl methacrylate to act as a medial buttress. If the lag screw part of the compression nail lacks firm fixation in the femoral neck and head prior to implantation, we inject methyl methacrylate into the previously reamed hole. These fractures heal well so long as they are stabilized using whatever technique is necessary.

Subtrochanteric fractures present a major problem in stabilization. As previously stated, the majority of these fractures are secondary to diffuse permeative destruction involving the proximal one-third of the femur. If the fracture is associated with adequate bone stock of the proximal femur, we treat it with a Zickel nail. Other forms of intramedullary devices can be used, e.g., a Kuntscher rod, if the fracture is far enough distal to the lesser trochanter. When performing intramedullary fixation of subtrochanteric fractures, we augment the fixation with intramedullary methyl methacrylate. The cement is injected into the medullary canal using a pressurizing cement gun so that an adequate bone cement interface can be achieved around the intramedullary device. For those subtrochanteric fractures with diffuse permeative destruction of the proximal femur, we recommend a proximal one-third of the femur replacement after tumor resection (Figs. 9–17 and 9–18). The advantage of this procedure is early mobilization and full weight-bearing.

Once surgical treatment of the metastatic focus has been accomplished, very careful postoperative monitoring is crucial. This is especially true for patients with pathological fractures. The patients are at much increased risk for respiratory insufficiency, so we monitor these patients carefully postoperatively with an indwelling intraarterial catheter for arterial blood gas determinations and chest radiographs when indicated. Vigorous chest physical therapy with intermittent positive-pressure breathing devices and other mechanical methods for mobilization of secretions are routinely used. We do not hesitate to use postoperative ventilatory

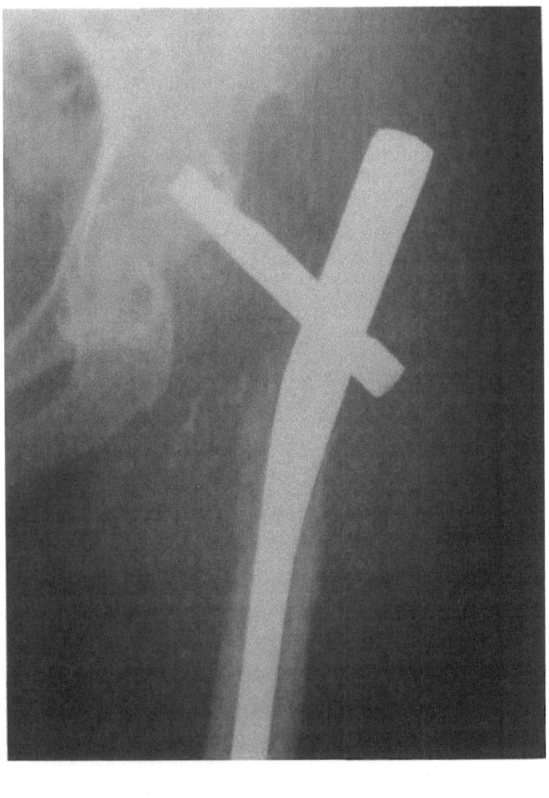

FIG. 9–17 A 54-year-old patient stabilized 2 years earlier for pathological subtrochanteric fracture. Note the progression of the disease involving the femoral neck.

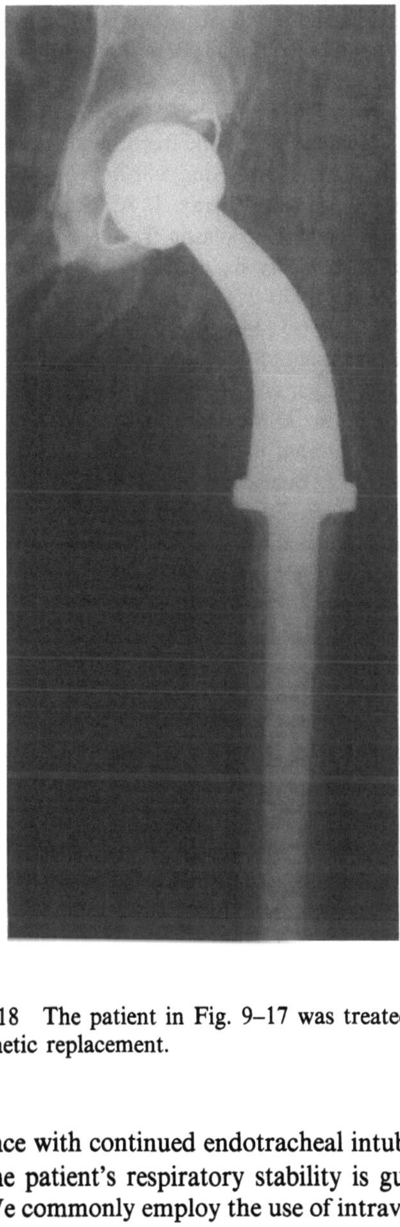

FIG. 9–18 The patient in Fig. 9–17 was treated with a prosthetic replacement.

assistance with continued endotracheal intubation until the patient's respiratory stability is guaranteed. We commonly employ the use of intravenous antibiotics as part of the surgical procedure and for the first 24 hours after the surgical procedure. Early mobilization of the patient is crucial. The patients are mobilized from the bed the day after surgery and are ambulated in a physical therapy environment as soon as they can tolerate it. Ambulatory aids are determined based on the type of surgical procedure performed and the stability of the hip. Consideration for adjunctive treatment of the metastatic disease is given about 2 weeks after surgery once primary soft tissue wound healing has occurred. We commonly use prophylactic medications, including aspirin and warfarin, for the prevention of deep vein thrombosis. The patients are commonly irradiated. Irradiation is reserved for patients with residual neoplastic disease; however, in those treated by resection with prosthetic reconstruction or by curettage of tumor with methyl methacrylate irradiation is not routinely undertaken. These patients must be carefully followed by both the orthopedic surgery service and the oncology service. We do not justify performing surgery on metastatic disease of the hip for improvement in survival but, rather, for improved quality of life. This can often be achieved, although great care must be taken in the management of these rather fragile patients.

References

1. Altman, H.: Intramedullary nailing for pathological impending and actual fractures of long bones. Bull. Hosp. Joint Dis., 13:239, 1952.
2. Beals, R. K., Lawton, G. D., Snell, W. E.: Prophylactic international fixation of the femur in metastatic breast cancer. Cancer, 28:1350, 1971.
3. Bennish, E. L., Hammond, G.: Treatment of actual and imminent pathologic fractures of the femur by intramedullary nailing. Surg. Clin. North Am., 35:865, 1955.
4. Bremner, E. L., Jelliffe, A. M.: The management of pathological fracture of the major long bones from metastatic cancer. J. Bone Joint Surg., 40B:652, 1958.
5. Carlson, D. H., Adams, R.: The use of methylmethacrylate in repair of neoplastic lesions in bones. Radiology, 112:43, 1974.
6. Clain, A.: Secondard malignant disease of bone. Br. J. Cancer, 19:15, 1965.
7. Coran, A. G., Banks, H. H., Aliapoulios, M. A., Wilson, R. E.: The management of pathologic fractures in patients with metastatic carcinoma of the breast. Surg. Gynecol. Obstet., 127:1225, 1968.
8. Devas, M. B., Dickson, J. W., Jelliffe, A. M.: Pathologic fractures: treatment by internal fixation and irradiation. Lancet, 2:484, 1956.
9. Douglas, H. O., Jr., Shukla, S. K., Mindell, E.: Treatment of pathological fractures of long bones excluding those due to breast cancer. J. Bone Joint Surg., 58A:1055, 1976.
10. Ehrenhart, J. L., Tidrick, R. T.: Intramedullary bone fixation in pathologic fractures. Surg. Gynecol. Obstet., 88:519, 1949.
11. Enis, J. E., Hall, M. F., Sarmiento, A.: Methylmethacrylate in neoplastic bone destruction. In: *The Hip: Proceedings of the Hip Society.* St. Louis, Mosby, 1973, pp. 118–138.
12. Fidler, M.: Prophylactic internal fixation of secondary neoplastic deposits in long bones. Br. Med. J., 1:341, 1973.

13. Fitts, W. T., Jr., Roberts, B., Ravdin, I. S.: Fractures in metastatic cancer. Am. J. Surg., 85:282, 1953.
14. Francis, K. C.: Prophylactic internal fixation of metastatic osseous lesions. Cancer, 13:75, 1960.
15. Gitelis, S., Sheinkop, M. B., Hammerberg, K., Brugliera, P.: The role of prophylactic surgery in the management of metastatic hip disease. Orthopedics, 5:1004, 1982.
16. Griessman, H., Schuttemeyer, W.: Wietere Erfahrungen Mit Der Marknogelung Nach Kuntscher An Ber Chirungischen Universitalsklinch Kiel. Chirurg, 17/18:316, 1947.
17. Grunert, U.: Pathologuiche Fracturen (Spontan-Fracturen). Dtsch. Z. Chir., 76:254, 1905.
18. Haberman, E. T., Sache, R., Stern, R. E., et al.: The pathology and treatment of metastatic disease of the femur. Clin. Orthop., 169:70, 1982.
19. Harrington, K. D.: The management of acetabular insufficiency secondary to metastatic malignant disease. J. Bone Joint Surg., 63A:653, 1981.
20. Harrington, K. D., Johnston, J. O., Turner, R. H., Green, D. L.: The use of methylmethacrylate as an adjunct in the internal fixation of malignant neoplastic fractures. J. Bone Joint Surg., 54A:1665, 1972.
21. Harrington, K. D., Sim, F. H., Enis, J. E., et al.: Methylmethacrylate as an adjunct to internal fixation of pathological fractures: experience with three hundred and seventy-five cases. J. Bone Joint Surg., 58A:1047, 1976.
22. Hejna, W. F., Fossier, C. H.: Surgical aspects of metastatic bone disease. Illinois Med. J., 136:704, 1969.
23. Higinbotham, N. L., Marcove, R. C.: The management of pathological fractures. J. Trauma, 5:792, 1965.
24. Jaffe, H. L.: *Tumors and Tumorous Conditions of Bones and Joints.* Philadelphia, Lea & Febiger, 1958.
25. Jensen, T. M., Dillion, W. L., Reckling, F. W.: Changing concepts in the management of pathological and impending fractures. J. Trauma, 16:496, 1976.
26. Johnston, A. D.: Pathology of metastatic tumors in bone. Clin. Orthop., 73:8, 1970.
27. Koch, J. C.: The laws of bone architecture. Am. J. Anat., 21:177, 1917.
28. Lane, J. M., Scuico, T. P., Zolan, S.: Treatment of pathological fracture of the hip by endoprosthetic replacement. J. Bone Joint Surg., 62A:954, 1980.
29. Lehman, O.: Problems of pathological fractures. Bull. Hosp. Joint Dis., 12:90, 1951.
30. Levy, R. N., Sherry, H. S., Siffert, R. S.: Surgical management of metastatic disease of bone at the hip. Clin. Orthop., 169:62, 1982.
31. Mickelson, M. R., Bonfiglio, M.: Pathological fractures in the proximal part of the femur treated by Zickel-nail fixation. J. Bone Joint Surg., 58A:1067, 1976.
32. Murray, J. A., Parrish, F. F.: Surgical management of secondary neoplastic fractures about the hip. Orthop. Clin. North Am., 5:887, 1974.
33. Parrish, F. F., Murray, J. A.: Surgical treatment for secondary neoplastic fractures: a retrospective study of ninety-six patients. J. Bone Joint Surg., 52A:665, 1970.
34. Poigenfurst, J., Marcove, R. C., Miller, T. R.: Surgical treatment of fractures through metastases in the proximal femur. J. Bone Joint Surg., 50B:743, 1968.
35. Ryan, J. R., Dowe, D. E., Salciccioli, G. G.: Prophylactic internal fixation of the femur for neoplastic lesions. J. Bone Joint Surg., 58A:1071, 1976.
36. Rybicki, E. F., Simonen, F. A., Weis, E. B.: On the mathematical analysis of stress in the human femur. J. Biomech., 5:203, 1972.
37. Schocker, J. D., Brady, L. W.: Radiation therapy for bone metastasis. Clin. Orthop., 169:38, 1982.
38. Schurman, D. J., Amstutz, H. C.: Treatment of neoplastic subtrochanteric fractures. Clin. Orthop., 97:108, 1973.
39. Sherry, H. S., Levy, R. N., Siffert, R. S.: Metastatic disease of bone in orthopedic surgery. Clin. Orthop., 169:44, 1982.
40. Sim, F. H., Daugherty, T. W., Ivins, J. C.: The adjunctive use of methylmethacrylate in fixation of pathological fractures. J. Bone Joint Surg., 56A:40, 1974.
41. Sim, F. H., Hartz, C. R., Chao, E. Y. S.: Total hip arthroplasty for tumors of the hip. In: *The Hip: Proceedings of the Fourth Open Scientific Meeting of the Hip Society.* St. Louis, Mosby, 1976, pp. 246–259.
42. Smedal, M. I., Salzman, F. A.: Treatment of metastatic bone tumors. Wis. Med. J., 47:675, 1948.
43. Tachdjian, M. O., Compere, C. L., Ravin, P. H.: Pathologic fractures of the hip. Surg. Gynecol. Obstet., 109:13, 1953.
44. Welch, C. E.: Pathologic fractures due to malignant disease. Surg. Gynecol. Obstet., 62:735, 1936.
45. Yablon, I. G., Paul, G. R.: The augmentive use of methylmethacrylate in the management of pathological fractures. Surg. Gynecol. Obstet., 143:177, 1976.
46. Zickel, R. E., Mouradian, W. H.: Intramedullary fixation of pathological fractures and lesions of the subtrochanteric region of the femur. J. Bone Joint Surg., 58A:1061, 1976.
47. Zimskind, P. D., Surver, J. M.: Metastasis to bone from carcinoma of the breast. Clin. Orthop., 11:202, 1958.

CHAPTER 10

Intertrochanteric Osteotomy for Adult Hips

RAYMOND G. TRONZO AND RICHARD F. SANTORE

Introduction

When the first edition of Volume I, *Surgery of the Hip Joint*, was published in 1973, total hip arthroplasties were in their infancy. Their potential was to replace all other forms of hip reconstruction. The chapter on intertrochanteric osteotomies was written together with Professor Müller at a time when only the European surgeons had accumulated enough experience to retain any enthusiasm for the operation. Now 14 years later, much has been learned about the performance of a total hip replacement and the comparison to osteotomities has been rekindled. Total hip replacement is not for everybody, nor is it the panacea for treating all hip disorders. Cemented systems have failed to solve the long-term problem of endurance for an artificial implant for a patient who has a life expectancy in excess of 20 years. Biologically fixed implants are now in their infancy and face an even tougher challenge in gaining credibility because of early failures of fixation, confusion of designs, and chaotic parameters regarding patient candidacy and choice of procedure. Press fit versus beaded coatings versus wire mesh versus powdered porosity versus short stems versus long stems versus curved stems versus straight stems versus titanium versus cobalt chromium versus hemispheres versus screw-in cups versus truncated cones will be the mixture for a long debate. It will surely require very mature minds with long-term objectivity before any meaningful data is produced. In the meantime, those arthritic victims 20 to 50 years of age remain in limbo. Or do they? Concerned hip surgeons met in Boston in May of 1986 to revive interest in the potentials for intertrochanteric osteotomies. The meeting was chaired by Poss and Millis. It was an excellent forum but dominated again by the European experts. Surely in the near future this operation will assume a strong footing among American surgeons who will soon accumulate their own data on an excellent operation.

The Swiss AO plates and instruments were so well designed 18 years ago and the technique of executing the osteotomy so perfected that they remain the standard today. For that reason both are being reproduced here, in the current chapter, with a few minor refinements in the chapter's original composition. There are some new observations that must be added at this point in time. Bombelli's contribution with his flexion/extension osteotomy is being recognized here as written by one of his star students, Richard Santore.

The haunting question with this procedure is whether the articular hyaline cartilage can regenerate itself after an osteotomy. It has been shown repeatedly that when an osteotomy works well, the joint space becomes widened and smoother. Does this mean that the cartilage has the capability of regenerating? It appears that, indeed, it does according to new clinical findings presented at the Boston symposium by H. Mankin. He and others working at the cellular level of investigation are finding more evidence that when the proper mechanical realignment is made, a number of favorable cellular changes take place in the cartilage environment that make regeneration possible. This scientific observation confirms what a Southern rural orthopedic surgeon once told me when we discussed the cartilage response after an osteotomy—"It happened once. It will happen again"—(the wisdom of D. Simmons). Just what exactly these changes are remain to be proven. Over the years, gleaned from clinical experience, certain guidelines have evolved.

An Update

Age remains an important parameter. Anyone beyond the age of 50 is not a good candidate for an intertrochanteric osteotomy unless there is a very good spherical head whose integrity is being threatened by a singular *large cyst,* which should be evacuated, filled with bone grafts through a slot in the neck, and then unstressed by a varus osteotomy. For patients in their early 20s, refer to the excellent work of Millis in Volume I, Chapter 14.

Range of motion is an important preoperative assessment. Müller states that flexion less than 60° is an unfavorable preoperative situation. Moscher considers a total range of motion of less than 80° will most likely end in a poor result. However, a younger patient with such a stiff hip from contractures can still be considered for a realignment osteotomy because it will help improve gait and protect the opposite hip, lumbar spine, knees, and feet from secondary damage.

The *disease state* that responds best to an osteotomy is early degenerative arthritis with a relatively round head. Congenital deformities and other mechanical deformities with secondary damage, such as in slipped ephiphysis and Perthes disease, respond better than idiopathic hip degeneration. Bilateral disease has a negative effect on the outcome of this operation. If the first hip is successful then the second hip can be expected to follow the same pattern. Rheumatoid arthritis, or inflammatory disease, and Paget's disease are contraindications to an osteotomy. Any protrusio carries a poor prognosis for an osteotomy. Any cysts in the head which appear to communicate with cysts in the acetabulum ("kissing lesions") will do poorly with an osteotomy.

Expectations can be predicted from the patient's early response. If there is little prompt relief of pain, the operation will likely fail. Conversion to a total hip should be delayed for up to a year after the osteotomy has healed well and remodeling has been maximized. Early good results seldom deteriorate before 15 to 20 years.

Capsulectomy is advocated as being beneficial to the outcome of the operation. It decreases joint pressure. It also helps in regaining motion. Tight adductors and/or a tight iliopsoas should also be released as well as a tight rectus tendon.

Today it is best to perform the osteotomy with *x-ray control.* This author uses a fracture table. Wagner uses a glass top operating table.

Preoperative planning can be much more accurate by examining the patient under anesthesia with the use of an imaging x-ray machine. This procedure can more accurately determine if and how much of a bi-plane osteotomy should be done, extension or flexion, along with the varus or valgus osteotomy. CAT or NMRs may aid in the planning. Three-D scans are the thing of the future. At this point in time there is little information to report because these techniques improve almost daily with each new generation of machine.

Overview of Individual Designs

It is more common today to combine osteotomies. Lengthening or shortening the leg should be considered. When a varus osteotomy is done the leg may be shortened enough to create an uncorrectable limp so that the leg may be lengthened later with an autogenous bone graft. When valgus osteotomy is done the leg may be made too long so that it should be shortened at the time of the initial osteotomy. Radical corrections must not be done because the resultant deformity will make conversion to a total hip arthroplasty impossible or unnecessarily difficult—which will jeopardize the results.

Varus osteotomies are the most common design used. Where there is early involvement from congenital dysplasia it can easily be combined with a Chiari osteotomy. Narrowing of the joint space medially from degeneration can be improved by a varus osteotomy. It is critical that adequate abduction is available, otherwise an adduction contracture can be bothersome. It is almost always followed initially by a Duchenne-Trendelenberg gait. It not infrequently requires prolonged physiotherapy. For this reason the Swiss no longer take out more than a 15° wedge. They also will combine it with displacement of the greater trochanter more distally in order to eliminate this awkward gait (Fig. 10–6).

A *valgus osteotomy* is done when there is improved congruency in adduction. The medial part of the femoral head is shifted up under the weight bearing part of the acetabulum. This is especially appropriate for old slipped epiphysies.

A *medial displacement osteotomy* (McMurray Osteotomy) by itself is seldom done. It is indicated when there is medial compartment arthritis, little head deformity, and no difference in congruity from varus to valgus.

Lateral displacement is combined when a valgus osteotomy is done of more than 25°. It is also done when there is a coexistent valgus knee deformity.

An *extension osteotomy* is performed when a flexion contracture or deformity exists as demonstrated by the Thomas test. It is combined with release of iliopsoas and/or rectus femoris tendons. Be reminded that it will throw the head into varus.

A *flexion osteotomy* will correct a posterior deformity such as in slipped epiphysis. It is most useful in treating avascular necrosis. Up to 40° can be cut out in order to place intact areas, or virgin bone, of the posterior section of the femoral head into the weight bearing part of the acetabulum.

Derotation is usually done simultaneously with the other forms of osteotomies to correct any residual rotation of the leg. It does nothing to the mechanics of the femoral head but will improve gait and lessen strains on the knee.

Varus Osteotomy

Pauwels had tried over thirty years ago to explain why this type of osteotomy is of benefit in the treatment of the osteoarthritic hip. He defined osteoarthritis as a disturbance of the equilibrium between the load on the joint surface and the biological resistance of the tissues such that the load exceeds the biological resistance. Pauwels, having established this definition, then attempted to diminish the load on the joint surfaces. He found that if the angle of inclination between the femoral neck and shaft is decreased in a number of different types of osteoarthritis, the surface areas of both the acetabulum and the femoral head, which come under stress, are increased; the length of the lever arm of the abductors is increased while all the muscles acting on the hip joint are relaxed (Fig. 10–1). There is considerable diminution of the joint load frequently resulting in a most surprising regeneration of the joint space.

Later it became evident that the change of direction of the acting compressive and tensile stresses lead to a remodeling of the internal architecture of the femoral head and neck (Fig. 10–2).

Indications A varus osteotomy is the method of choice in those cases in which reduction of the neck angle of inclination achieves the above goals. A varus osteotomy is indicated for: (1) the subluxating dysplastic valgus hip, (2) early osteoarthritic hip with narrowing of the joint space medially, (3) a subcapital fracture which has united in valgus

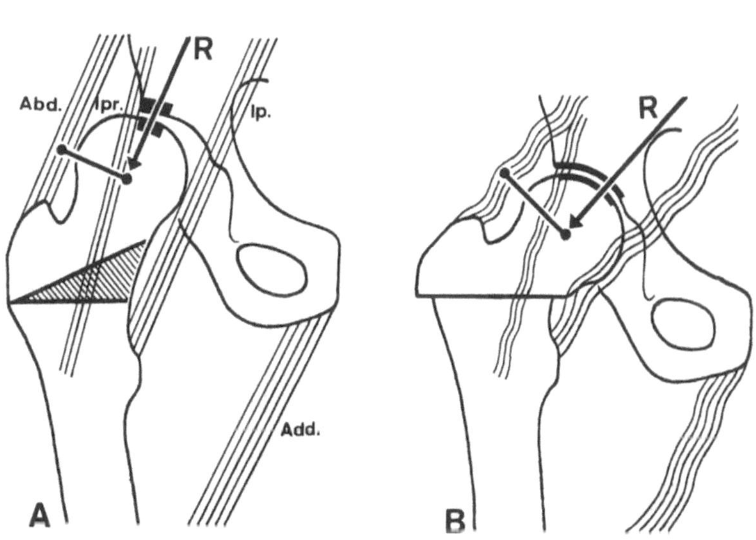

FIG. 10–1 Mode of action of a varus osteotomy in osteoarthritis of the hip. **A** In a painful osteoarthritic hip the abductors and adductors, the iliopsoas, and the rectus femoris muscles are in spasm. The areas under pressure of the femoral head and acetabulum are relatively small. The effort arm, i.e., the distance between the center of the femoral head and the abductors, is short. **B** After a varus osteotomy the tension in the muscles is reduced, the areas under pressure of the femoral head and acetabulum are considerably enlarged, and the effort arm is made longer.

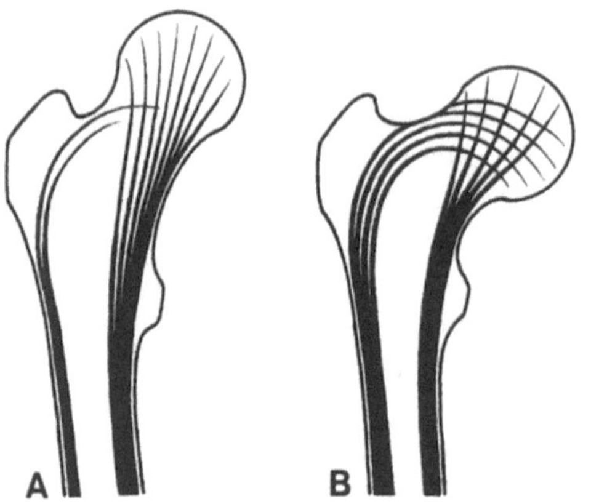

FIG. 10–2 Influence of varus osteotomy on the internal architecture of the femoral head and neck. **A** A coxa valga is subjected almost entirely to compressive stresses. Thus the internal architecture of the femoral neck shows a preponderance of compression trabeculae. **B** In contrast, in a coxa vara there are both compression and tension trabeculae. The change of a coxa valga to a coxa vara results in remodeling of the internal architecture of the femoral neck in response to the new stresses. This remodeling influences the local blood supply as well as the repair phenomena.

with early osteoarthritis, and (4) early avascular necrosis with minimal collapse of the femoral head. Before the decision is made to carry out a varus intertrochanteric osteotomy, both hip joints must be carefully examined clinically and radiologically. See Indications, Table 10–5.

Preoperative Clinical Assessment With the help of the Thomas test, the existence of any flexion contracture is evaluated. Next the maximal range of abduction and adduction is measured. This measurement is carried out by noting the excursion of the limb in relationship to a line dropped at 90° to a line joining the anterior superior iliac spines. See Figure 10–3 to appreciate the importance of realigning the hip with the knee. In neutral position this reference line passes laterally to the patella. When assessing abduction, it is best to fix the other hip joint. This is done by abducting the hip to its limit, then letting the leg hang with the knee flexed over the edge of the table. The abduction of the other hip is then carried out slowly so as not to cause discomfort to the patient.

The range of external and internal rotation is measured with the patient in the prone position. The so-called rectus phenomenon can also be elicited; it is present when flexion of the knee increases a flexion contracture of the hip.

A maximal distance between the malleoli in

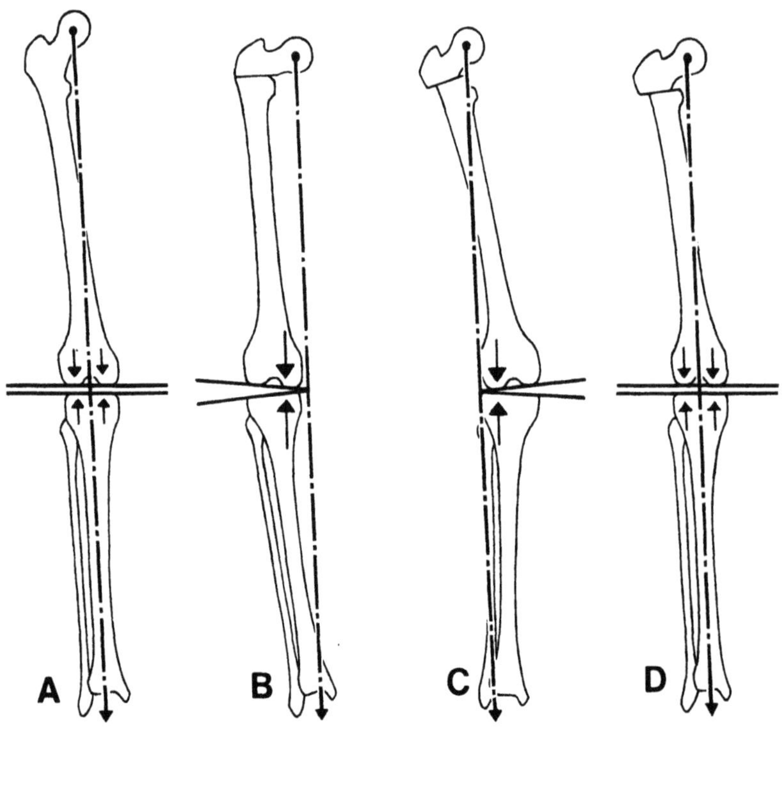

FIG. 10–3 Influence of medial displacement of the shaft on the loading of the knee joint. **A** Under normal anatomical circumstances according to Lanz both halves of the knee joint are equally loaded. **B** Simple varus osteotomy results in a varus leg with excessive loading of the medial half of the knee joint. **C** Simple medialization without a change of the neck–shaft angle results in a genu valgum where only the outer half of the knee joint comes under pressure. **D** When the femoral shaft is medialized at the time of a varus osteotomy, the preoperative angle between the mechanical and anatomical axis is reconstituted and the pressure relations of the knee joint restored to normal.

abduction and adduction is important for follow-up examinations. The *functional shortening or lengthening* of the leg is of far greater importance than the effective distance between the anterior superior iliac spine and the tip of the malleolus because the clinical difference between the legs can be evaluated.

The patient's back and knee joints must obviously be examined. Axial deviation such as genu valgum or genu varum must be taken into consideration when plans are made to carry out an intertrochanteric osteotomy.

Contraindications We have found that cases with fixed external rotation of 25° or more (measured in the prone position) are not suitable for an intertrochanteric osteotomy. Despite operative correction of the external rotation, the deformity recurs and leads to an unsatisfactory result.

Another contraindication for a varus osteotomy is flexion limited to 60° or less, even if all other factors seem to favor the procedure (Table 10–2).

Preoperative X-rays In the anteroposterior projection of the pelvis, the knee joints must touch and the patelli must face as much forward as possible. In hips with a good range of motion, we have found the standard projection taken with the knees bent over the edge of the table most useful. One must be able to see the iliac crests on the x-ray in order to establish immediately the presence of an adduction contracture. Functional x-rays in maximal abduction and adduction must also be obtained. These are done in order to judge the position of the femoral head in the acetabulum in the two extreme positions. *In taking these x-rays, the pelvis is fixed by abducting or adducting the other hip.* Of the two positions, the abduction position is of greater importance. Abduction may be painful; maximal abduction may have to be attained very slowly and with some discomfort to the patient. The patient should be sedated with a narcotic. In cases with an adduction contracture, an x-ray with the hip in maximal abduction can be taken only under general anesthesia after an adductor tenotomy. Internal rotation is usually full in cases of early osteoarthritis and particularly in dysplastic hips in young patients. In such cases, one further x-ray, namely, the Dunn projection, can be taken (see Vol. I, Chapter 8, Pizzutillo, page 184). This projection is necessary to determine the degree of anteversion of the femoral neck. If anteversion must also be corrected, then an x-ray is taken with the patient lying on his stomach in maximal abduction and internal rotation.

From the anteroposterior projections of the hip, that of Dunn, and the functional projections, the real inclination angle of the femoral neck (neck-shaft angle) and the anteversion (AT) angle are determined. In these views the best position for the femoral head in the acetabulum usually becomes apparent. In an unsatisfactory position, particularly in those cases where the portion of the weight-bearing surface cannot be increased by abduction, the varus osteotomy should not be recommended until an x-ray under anesthesia (or even until an adductor tenotomy) has been done. A significant incongruence spells doom for a varus osteotomy. The lateral projection is helpful in appraising the global concentricity of the femoral head. If it is flattened to any significant degree, the osteotomy will probably fail.

Examining the patient under an imaging machine on a glass top table will yield considerable information.

Calculation of The Angles of Correction In an osteotomy of any long bone, six possible corrections can be carried out: (1) in the frontal plane: varus/valgus; (2) in the sagittal plane: flexion/extension; (3) in the horizontal plane: internal/external rotation. The displacement does not have to be only (4) medialization or lateralization but can be also (5) a dorsal or a ventral displacement or (6) a shortening or a lengthening.

Experience has shown that in carrying out an intertrochanteric osteotomy the most important correction is in the frontal plane, namely, a varus or valgus alignment, and therefore must be most carefully calculated. A varus osteotomy should not exceed 15°. As already mentioned, the first goal of the operation is to increase the surface area of contact which is under pressure between the femoral head and the acetabulum. This occurs only when the joint surfaces are congruent. The varus angle of maximal congruity is not always discernible on the x-ray taken with the hip in maximal abduction. The experienced surgeon knows that carrying out a capsulotomy medially at the calcar and cutting through the femur in the intertrochanteric area lead to a considerable increase in the varus amount, which can never be judged preoperatively from the abduction x-ray. *It is for this reason that preoperative drawings are so important.*

The degree of correction necessary in the sagittal plane depends on the degree of flexion contracture and external rotational deformity. A flexion contracture is almost always present in advanced osteoarthritis of the hip. In such cases an *extension osteotomy* of 10 to 30° is performed. The external rotational deformity is corrected by internally rotating the distal fragment. This lessens the likelihood of recurrence of postoperative external rotation. However, it must be noted that an extension osteotomy of 30° causes simultaneous adduction of 10° to 15°, depending on whether the CCD angle measures 120° or 135°. This indirect adduction must also be considered in preoperative planning. (For the technique of the extension osteotomy, please see Fig. 10–13.) In early osteoarthritis or in the so-called coxa valga luxans (dysplastic hip), internal rotation can surpass external rotation. The Dunn projection indicates that in these cases anteversion is usually greater than 20°. In such cases, the excessive anteversion must be corrected and reduced to an angle of 20°. This is achieved by externally rotating the distal fragment.

Calculating Medial Displacement Medialization must be carefully calculated preoperatively in order to retain the physiological angle between the mechanical and anatomical axis (Fig. 10–3). This is important in preventing a possible genu varum or genu valgum, which would result in overloading of the inner or outer part of the knee joint (Fig. 10–3). Any preoperative axial deviation in the knee joint must of course be taken into consideration when plans for the surgical procedure are developed. Thus, in a genu valgum the medialization will be minimal, whereas in a genu varum medialization will be considerably greater. In an adult patient whose legs are straight preoperatively, the medialization measures approximately 12 mm. This can be represented schematically (Fig. 10–4).

The Combination of Varus Osteotomy with Another Procedure Here consideration is given to the following procedures: transposition of the greater trochanter distally, acetabuloplasty (Chiari osteotomy, see Figure 10–5), tenotomy, bone grafting of the large acetabular or femoral-head cysts, and capsulectomy.

In a case where the angle between the femoral neck and shaft is 125° or less, a varus osteotomy of 20° or 30° would result in a coxa vara with the greater trochanter lying higher than the center of rotation of the femoral head. This would produce a marked shortening and simultaneous weakening of the hip abductors, and the patient would have a permanent limp. *The transfer of the greater trochanter* distally can be easily combined with a varus osteotomy if modern up-to-date operative techniques are employed (Fig. 10–6). An *acetabuloplasty* is indicated when the ventral portion of the acetabular roof is shallow, as seen in some dysplastic hips. Although Pauwels has repeatedly demonstrated the brilliant possibilities of carrying out only a varus osteotomy in such cases we feel that, whenever the CE angle of Wiberg is less than 10°, a ventrolateral plasty of the acetabular roof should be performed, using a wide iliac-crest graft after a pelvic osteotomy (Fig. 10–5). In a patient with a positive *rectus femoris test* which remains positive after a varus intertrochanteric osteotomy, the rectus femoris must be divided proximally at its origin. Similarly in a residual flexion contracture, the *iliopsoas* must be divided; in a residual

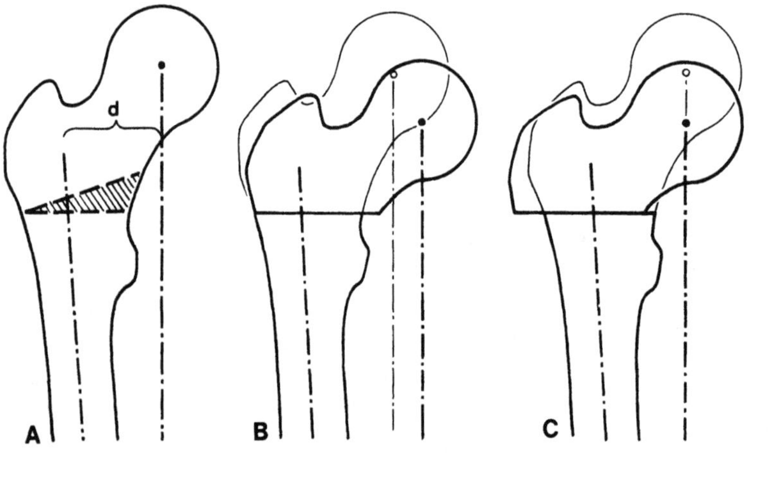

FIG. 10–4 Measure of medial displacement in a varus osteotomy. **A** Prior to surgery the distance (*d*) between the femoral–shaft axis and the center of the femoral head measures 3 to 5 cm. **B** Simple varus osteotomy lengthens this distance considerably. **C** Medialization of the shaft of 10 to 15 mm allows return to normal of the distance between the anatomical axis and the center of the femoral head. The angle between the mechanical and anatomical axis remains unchanged.

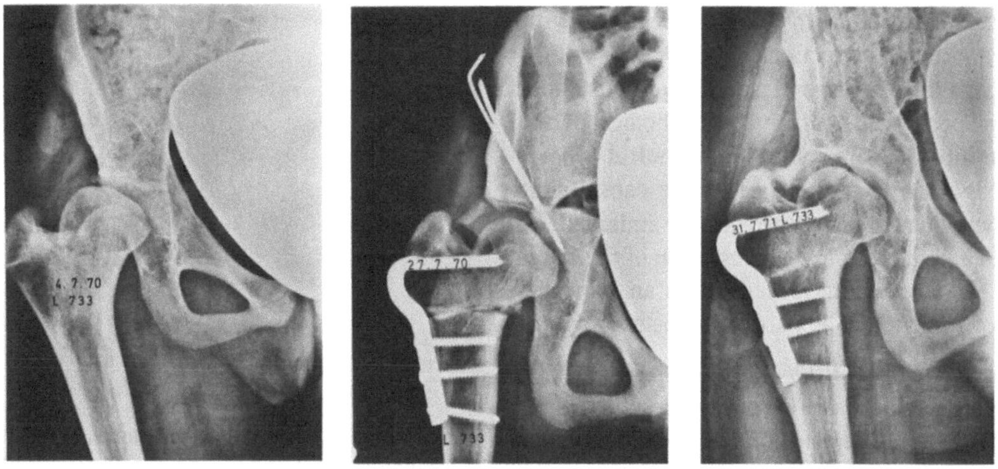

FIG. 10–5 A 13-year-old girl with subluxation of the hip due to inadequacy of the acetabular roof. A varus osteotomy above would leave the hip still uncovered for proper weight-bearing, so a Chiari osteotomy and a graft were combined with a varus osteotomy.

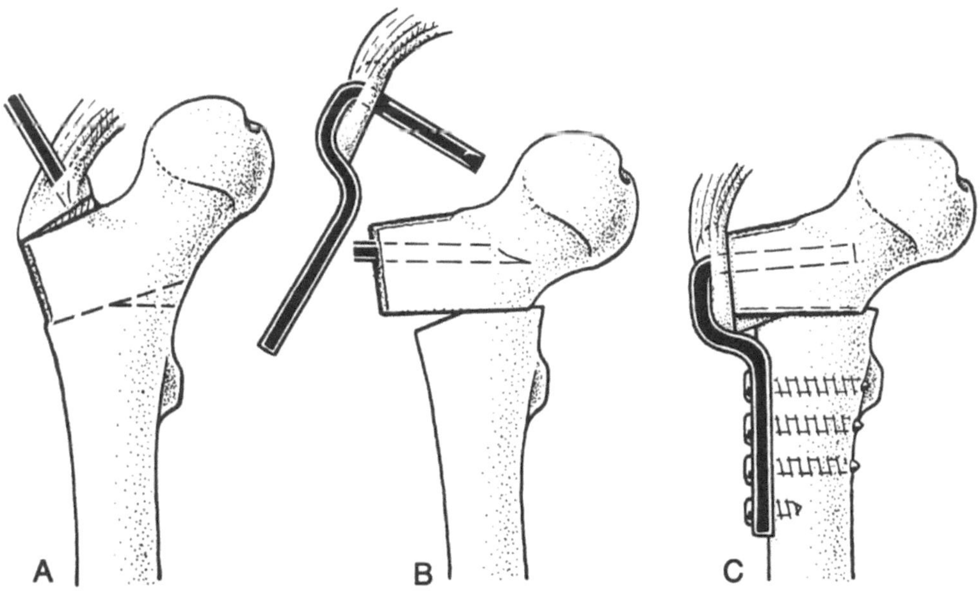

FIG. 10–6 Technique of distal transfer of the greater trochanter at the time of a varus osteotomy. **A** Before the greater trochanter is osteotomized a 3.2-mm drill bit is used to drill the greater trochanter prior to inserting a special seating chisel which allows a 1-inch deep, U-shaped cut in the greater trochanter. The seating chisel is removed and a horizontal cut is made, amputating the trochanter with the attached abductor muscles. **B** Thereafter the seating chisel is inserted in the usual fashion (see Fig. 10–15) into the femoral neck, the medial wedge is removed, and the proximal fragment is tilted into varus. A right-angled blade plate allows 20 mm of displacement. The blade of this blade plate is then passed through the previously cut U-shaped trough in the amputated greater trochanter. **C** The seating chisel is then removed, and the blade of the blade plate is inserted into the femoral neck. If the greater trochanter should break off, the abductors can be fixed to the bow of the blade plate with a tension band wire.

external rotational deformity, the small external rotators or the *adductors* are divided if they are tight and block abduction.

At the time of surgery, a *capsulotomy* is almost always performed and any loose bodies present in the hip joint are removed. A ventral *synovectomy* is done if at the time of the capsulotomy the synovium is hypertrophied or inflamed. *Do not* do a "bumpectomy" or resection of the lateral lip of the acetabulum because it is an important area of remodeling as part of the osteotomy.

Shortening Through the Varus Osteotomy The shortening which almost always results from a varus osteotomy depends on the size of the medial wedge. If the varus angle is 20° and the medial wedge is resected as suggested by Pauwels, that is, from the full width of the osteotomy surface, then the shortening will be 2.5 cm. If, however, only the medial half of the osteotomy surface is resected and the resected wedge is inserted laterally at the time of reduction of the osteotomy surfaces, the shortening is reduced to 1.5 cm. Thus, whenever shortening is undesirable, the medial wedge is excised from half of the osteotomy surface only (Fig. 10–7).

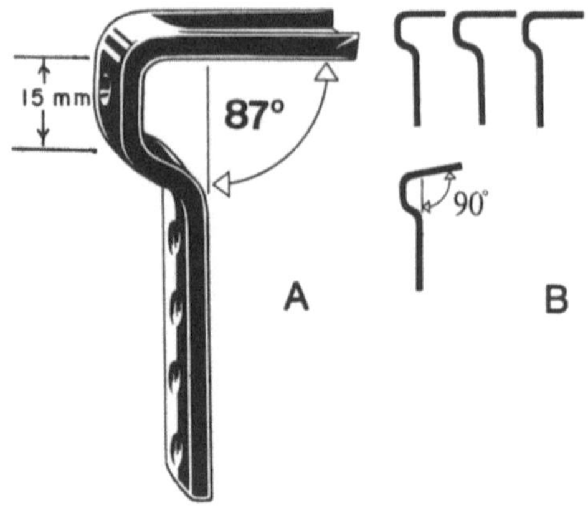

FIG. 10–8 ASIF right-angled blade plates for the intertrochanteric osteotomy. **A** The standard blade plate has three angles. The angle between the blade and the plate is 87°. **B** When the blade plate is placed under tension, this angle opens up to 90°, and medialization of 15 mm is possible. The bow is provided with a hole which allows fixation of the blade plate to the calcar with a malleolar or a cortex screw. The blade has a U-profile and measures 50 mm. A 40-mm blade can be used for varus osteotomies in old teenagers and young adults. Two size blade plates allow a medialization of 20 or 10 mm.

Internal Fixation The ASIF right-angle blade plates are rigid and the profile of the blade is U shaped (Fig. 10–8). The U shape of the blade causes the least interference with the circulation of the femoral head and lends strength which exceeds that of the strongest three-flanged nail. The fixation is so rigid that the patient is allowed free

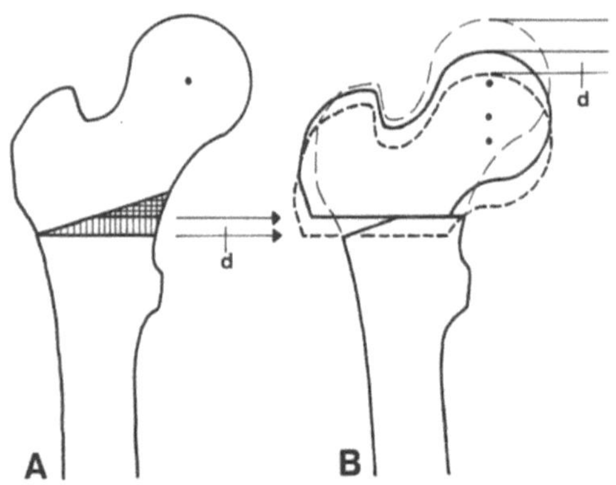

FIG. 10–7 Length gained by resection of a small medial wedge which is subsequently inserted on the lateral side. **A** The two wedges placed medially are shown. **B** The gain in length by resecting the smaller wedge equals that distance (*d*).

movement of the hip joint immediately after surgery and ambulation within a few days.

Previously a right-angled blade plate was used with a blade length of 70 to 80 mm. From experience it has been learned, however, that in an intertrochanteric osteotomy stable internal fixation is achieved by utilizing the tension-band principle. In order to accomplish this, a blade length of only 40 to 60 mm is needed. It has been found that if the blade is longer, within a few months resorption of bone takes place around the tip of the blade. This is the result of a discrepancy in the modulus of elasticity between the femoral neck and the blade of the blade plate. The *standard-angle blade plate* contains a fixed angle of 87° which opens to 90° once the blade plate is placed under tension. The 40-mm blade is to be used in young patients with hard cancellous bone. In all other cases, the 50-mm blade should be regarded as the standard length. The available blade plates allow a medialization of 10, 15, or 20 mm. A medialization of 15 mm is standard. This allows full compensation in the changes produced between the anatomical and mechanical axis of the femur in a varisation of 20 to 25°. The distance between the blade and the bow of the plate portion is 15 mm (Fig. 10–

8). This distance must be fully utilized, resulting in a bony ridge of 15 mm between the osteotomy cut and the blade portion of the blade plate. A hole in the middle of the bow permits the insertion of a screw to fix the plate to the calcar when the bone is osteoporotic.

A slit is especially fashioned in the last hole of the plate to allow for insertion of the tension device which actually impacts the cut surfaces together.

Necessary Instruments A special seating chisel (Fig. 10–9) is the most important instrument used in preparing the seat for the angled blade plate. We employ *triangular positioning plates* in calculating any angles of correction during surgery. The *chisel guide,* which is fixed to the seating chisel, is employed in judging the amount of extension of the distal fragment (Fig. 10–9). Proper handling of the seating chisel, its guide, and the triangular positioning plates has made x-ray control during the procedure easier.

The *slotted hammer* (Fig. 10–10*A*) is needed to control the rotation of the seating chisel in insertion and it also serves in extraction of the seating chisel once the seat is cut. The impactor has been modified in the last two years by adding the screw hole to the bow in the angled blade plate.

The following instruments are also necessary: long tension device with a Kardan key and an open spanner, a flat 15-mm chisel (used to enlarge the hole for the seating chisel), 6 Hohmann retractors and instruments necessary for screwing the plate to the shaft. We have found the oscillating saw almost indispensable. Four to six Steinman pins are also necessary to determine the direction of the seating chisel and for rotational control during the procedure, see Figures 10–11 and 10–12.

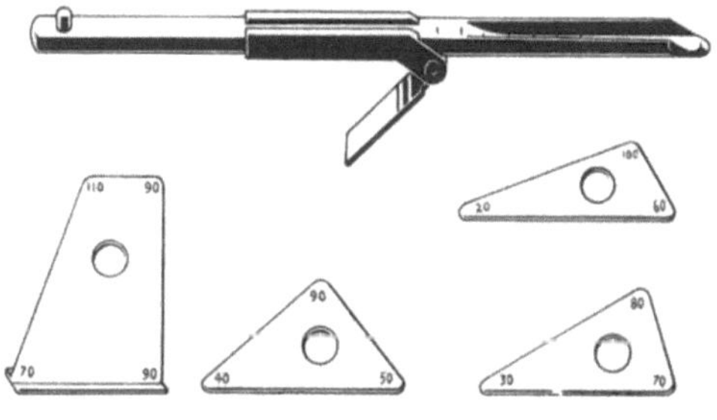

FIG. 10–9 Seating chisel with the chisel guide, which allows one to determine the sagittal plane, and the other metal positioning plates of various angles.

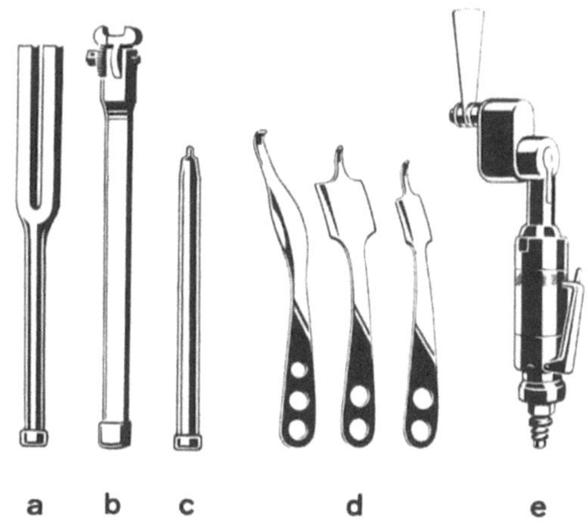

FIG. 10–10 Additional instruments for carrying out a varus osteotomy: slotted hammer (*a*), blade holder for insertion and extraction (*b*), impactor (*c*), three Hohmann retractors (*d*), oscillating saw (*e*).

The Technique of Varus Osteotomy

Incision The incision is a straight lateral one (see Figs 10–37 and 10–38). The capsule is incised anteriorly along its neck axis. It does no harm to excise the anterior part of the capsule and the hypertrophied ilio-inguinal ligament which is often responsible for adduction-flexion contractures. At this point even the iliopsoas tendon can be cut and allowed to move freely to seek its own

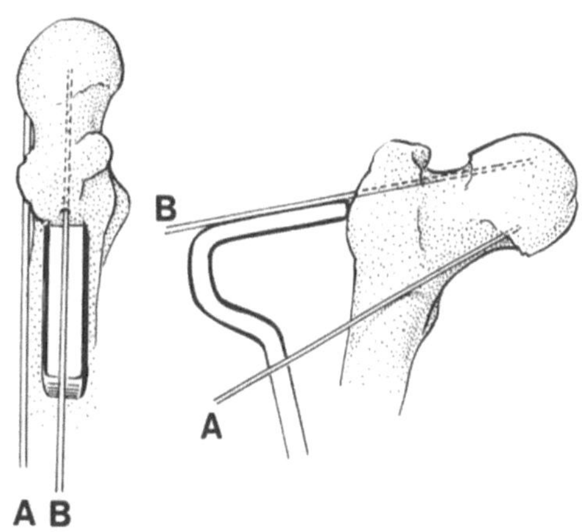

FIG. 10–11 Two medium-sized Steinmann pins are excellent guides for helping to determine the precise cut. **A** The lower pin aligns the direction of the neck so the blade is driven into the center of the neck. **B** The top pin is parallel to the lower but angled for the osteotomy cut after being positioned from the proper angle scales (Fig. 10–9).

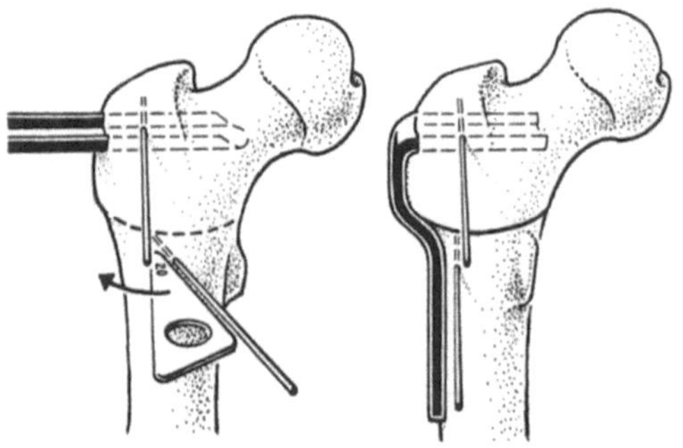

FIG. 10–12 Determination of the rotational plane. If a derotation osteotomy is to be carried out in a freely movable hip, two Kirschner wires are inserted in the frontal plane. These should subtend the angle of derotation between them.

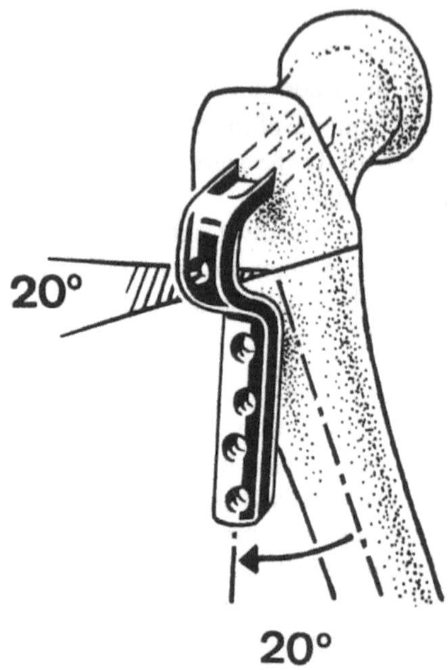

FIG. 10–13 Extension osteotomy as seen from the side. A flexion contracture is corrected by removing a wedge with a dorsal base. At the end of the procedure this wedge is inserted ventrally into the osteotomy. The reverse procedure is done for a flexion osteotomy.

level of attachment. Anterior osteophytes are not chipped off. These were formally removed but experience has shown that they do not block any motion and that they are active growth which will contribute to the regeneration process. Any hypertrophied synovium is excised.

Placement of Guide Pins and Chisel Two smooth Steinmann pins (⁹⁄₆₄") are placed to aid in judging angles (Fig. 10–11). The first pin (A) is laid on top of the femoral neck and then driven into the lip of the femoral head and no further. The second pin (B) is drilled into the tip of the greater trochanter parallel to the first pin in the sagittal plane and then parallel to the 70° template in the frontal plane. Figure 10–15 illustrates the progression of the procedure. It is best to use a fracture table or a glass top operating extension for precise control with an image x-ray machine.

Now the chisel guide is driven into the neck at a level just below the top border of the femoral neck and certainly no lower than the middle of the neck. It will follow the direction of pin B, but parallel to pin A, and is driven in on 40 or 50 mm (depending on which blade is to be used).

If rotation is to be corrected, two additional pins are placed perpendicular to the shaft above and below where the osteotomy will be made (Fig. 10–12). At the end of the osteotomy and derotation, the two pins must come to be parallel to one another unless an additional extension wedge is removed (Fig. 10–13).

Great emphasis is placed on the proper handling of the seating chisel because it ultimately determines the position of the plate. The slotted hammer is used to hold the chisel firmly in place, thus keeping it from rotating as it is driven into the femoral neck.

Determining the Site and Direction of the Bone Cuts Bone must be retained between the blade and the cut surface of the upper fragment; otherwise, compression will be inadequate and there will be subsequent loss of fixation. (See Fig. 10–14 for possible variations.) A spot is marked with an osteotome 15 mm from the bottom of the seating chisel (Fig. 10–15). The bone is cut along a line parallel to the chisel in both its frontal and sagittal planes. The leg is adducted and the bone opens up widely.

The 15° bone wedge (15° ± 75° = 90°) becomes easy. From the middle of the cut surface of the distal fragment a mark is made with an osteotome. From this point, the operator saws across into the medial portion perpendicular to the long axis of the femoral shaft. The resultant wedge will automatically measure 15° if the original cut had been planned at 75°.

Driving in the Blade Plate The upper fragment is held with a towel clip. The chisel is gently

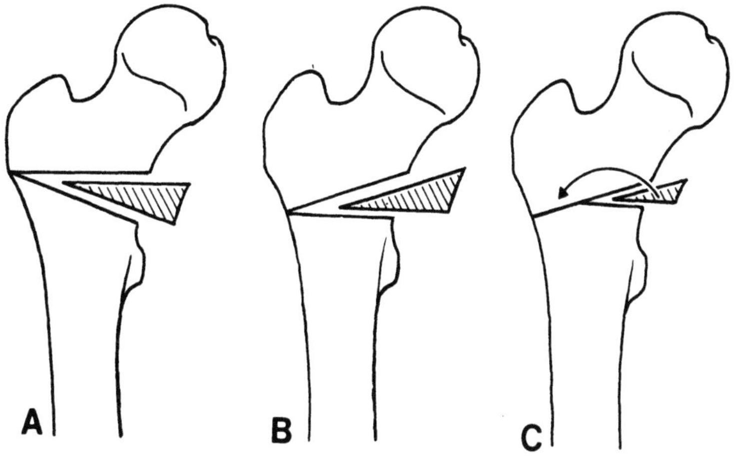

FIG. 10–14 Direction of the osteotomy cuts. **A** According to Pauwels one should begin the cut at the rough line of the greater trochanter and carry the proximal osteotomy at right angles to the shaft, with the distal cut coming to lie obliquely in the direction of the lesser trochanter. This original technique of Pauwels (**A**, **B**) hinders correction of the rotation. In addition, the lateral bone bridge is too small to use a right-angled blade plate. **C** By using an oscillating blade, precise cuts can be made as depicted. The smaller wedge of bone taken medially is turned around and placed laterally.

tapped out with the slotted hammer mallet, while its spatial relations are mentally retained. The blade plate is tapped in until its base is firmly seated against bone. If the upper fragment is unusually soft bone, a cancellous screw is inserted into the hole in the upper curved portion of the plate.

The shaft is brought over to the plate which is aligned parallel with its long axis. It is fixed into place by the special holding clamp (Verbrugge) which is nicely curved to serve as a retractor once in position. The clamp is placed as far up on the plate as possible. Any planned rotational correction is made.

Attachment of the Tension Device The distal end of the shaft is cleared so that the tension device can be easily attached. The incision is extended if necessary. A short screw is used so that only the lateral cortex is drilled. The clamp is loosened slightly and the wedge is placed into the lateral gap. Its sharp edge may have to be trimmed a bit before it will fit snugly into place. The fragments are slowly compressed together while the rotational position is constantly checked. The socket wrench is used first and the final moves are made with the open-ended wrench. If all corrections appear to be in order, the two middle screws are fixed into the shaft, the Verbrugge clamp is removed and the final screws are inserted. A short screw is used through the lateral cortex only in the last hole in order to smooth out the gradation between normal elastic bone and the rigid plated segment. Two examples are illustrated in Figures 10–16 and 10–17.

Intertrochanteric Valgus Osteotomy

The technique for the valgus or abduction osteotomy is very similar (Fig. 10–18) to that of a varus osteotomy only in reverse. Usually the same right-angled blade plate or the 90° blade plate is used. The bone wedge which has to be resected is based laterally. This wedge can also be reversed and inserted medially.

The valgus osteotomy is almost always combined with an extension osteotomy, as shown in Figure 10–13. The posterolaterally based bone wedge is then inserted in front or anteromedially.

Our example (Fig. 10–19) is that of a 55-year-old man with long-standing osteoarthritis of the hip, the result of a slipped femoral epiphysis. Five years after a valgus osteotomy of 25° and an extension osteotomy of 20°, the patient was free of pain and was able to ski and walk for hours without discomfort. The cartilage space, which had vanished preoperatively, returned to normal three years from the time of surgery. In performing such a valgus osteotomy, it is usually necessary to osteotomize the lesser trochanter in order to relax the iliopsoas (Table 10–4).

Chiari Osteotomy

The Chiari osteotomy is valuable to augment coverage of the femoral head especially in treating congenital dysplasia (Fig. 10–5). The surgical technique is covered in detail by Millis in Vol. I, Chapter 14, Fig. 14–33. One should also review an excellent paper by Graham, et al. (4).

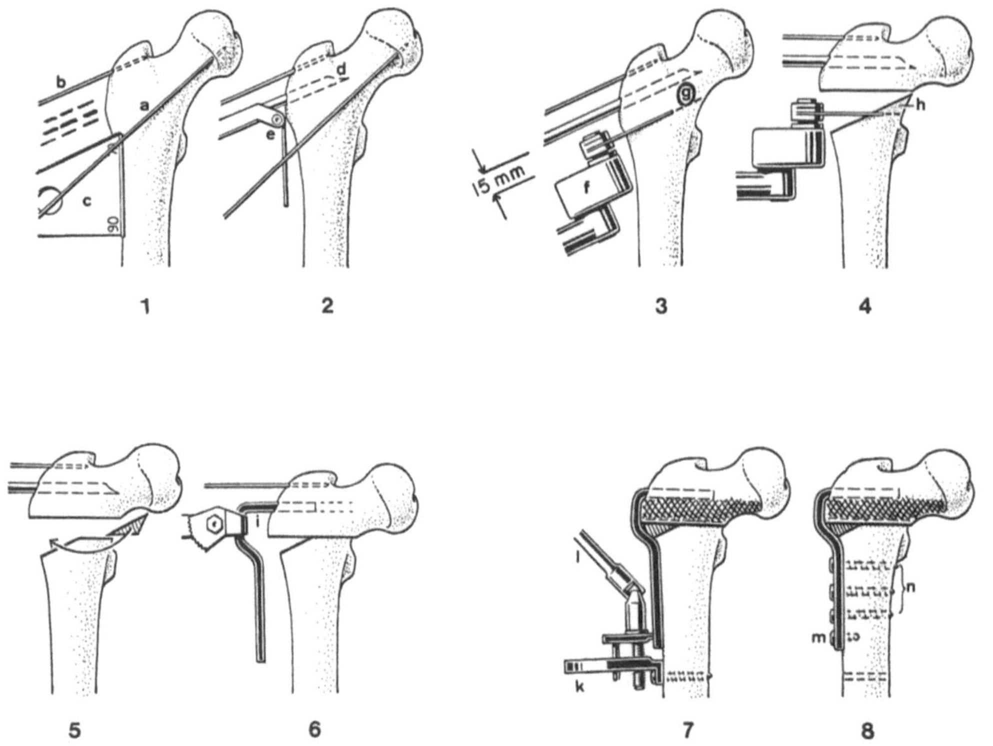

FIG. 10–15 Intertrochanteric varus osteotomy. **1** Make a lateral incision through the skin and fascia lata, extending it from the tip of the greater trochanter 20 cm distally. Reflect the vastus lateralis forward and then insert one Hohmann retractor below the calcar and one above the neck just medial to the greater trochanter. Next, do a wide anterior capsulotomy in line with the femoral neck and examine the joint. Introduce one Kirschner wire (*a*) along the front of the femoral neck and advance it into bone at the head–neck junction. This Kirschner wire (*a*) corresponds to the femoral neck axis. A second Kirschner wire (*b*) is introduced into the greater trochanter parallel with the first Kirschner wire and with the quadrangular positioning plane (*c*). This gives both the frontal planes and the femoral-neck axis of transversal plane. **2** Approximately 2 cm proximal to the point where the osteotomy is to be carried out, with an osteotome cut a hole in the cortex wide enough to receive the seating chisel (*d*). This hole should be as anterior as possible. The chisel is fitted with a removable chisel guide (*e*). The chisel is hammered into the middle of the femoral neck to a depth of 4.5 cm and parallel to the second Kirschner wire. The small flap on the chisel guide (*e*) serves to indicate the sagittal plane. **3** Introduce a wide Hohmann retractor behind to protect the soft tissues. The osteotomy is now carried out with the oscillating saw (*f*). A cut is made parallel to the seating chisel (*g*). The distance from the base of seating chisel *must* be 1.5 mm. to the osteotomy otherwise there will be inadequate bone stock to allow the plate to compress the bone together as depicted by dark areas in 7 and 8. **4** Using the seating chisel as a lever, open the osteotomy by tilting the proximal fragment into varus. It is now possible to excise a small wedge (*h*), based medially, by beginning in the middle of the osteotomy surface of the distal fragment and making the cut at right angles to the long axis of the femoral shaft. **5** Remove the small medial wedge. This small wedge is subsequently inserted laterally between the osteotomy fragments. **6** Hammer out the seating chisel. Now insert the right angle blade plate (*i*), making certain that it is inserted exactly into the channel cut for it by the chisel. **7** Reduce the osteotomy and maintain the reduction by fixing the plate to the femoral shaft with a Verbrugge clamp. Check now for rotational position of the lower extremity in extension. If the osteotomy has been correctly reduced and if no rotational deformity is present, a 3.2-mm hole is drilled and tapped 2 cm distal to the plate. Now insert the tension device (*k*), fix it to the femoral shaft, and begin tightening the screw on the tension device, first with the socket wrench with cardan joint (*l*) and subsequently with the open-end wrench. Once the osteotomy surfaces have been placed under maximal compression, flex the hip as much as possible and again check for rotation. **8** Now insert a short screw (*m*) into the last hole of the plate. This screw is short in order to smooth out the gradation between normal elastic bone and the rigid plated segment.

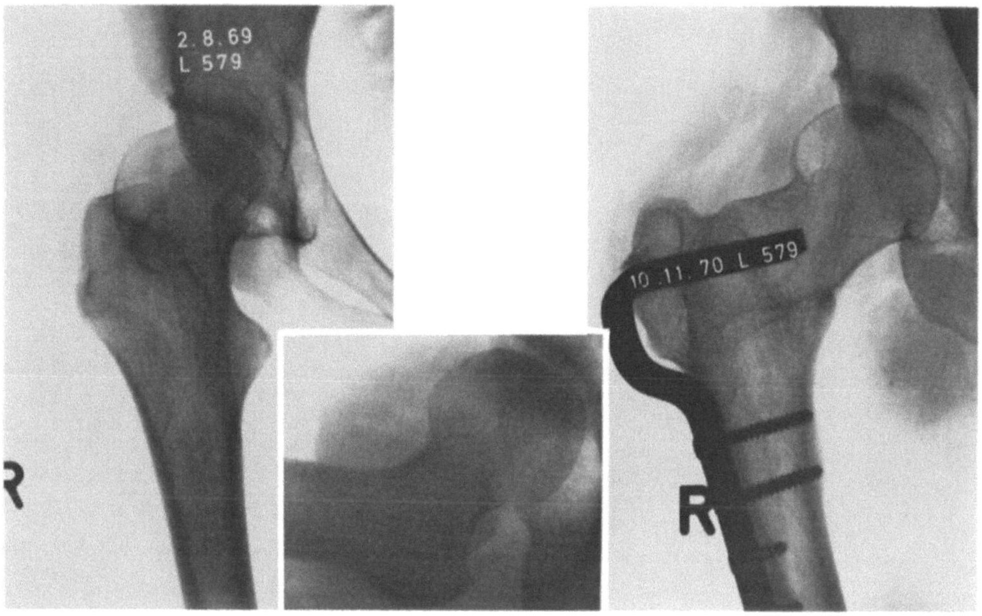

FIG. 10–16 Coxa valga luxans in a 32-year-old patient. The femoral neck is antevertel 65°. The x-ray film 1 year after varisation of 20°, derotation of 45°, and transfer of the greater trochanter distally shows that the biomechanical relations of the hip joint were restored almost to normal.

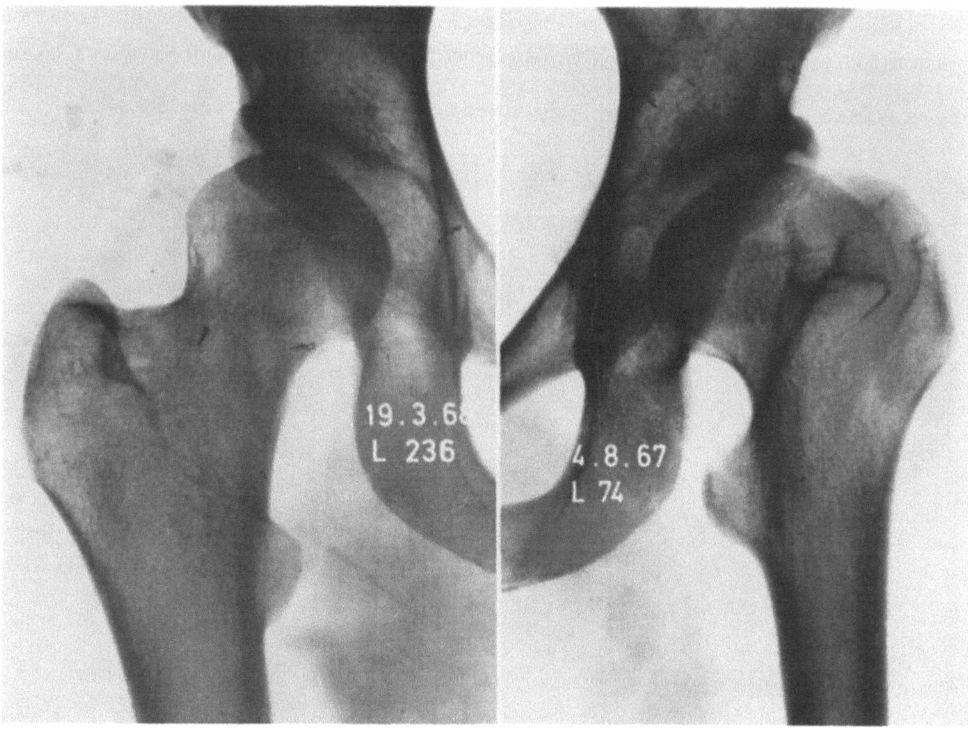

FIG. 10–17A Early bilateral osteoarthritis in a 22-year-old woman with a coxa valga luxans on the right and a subluxing femoral head on the left.

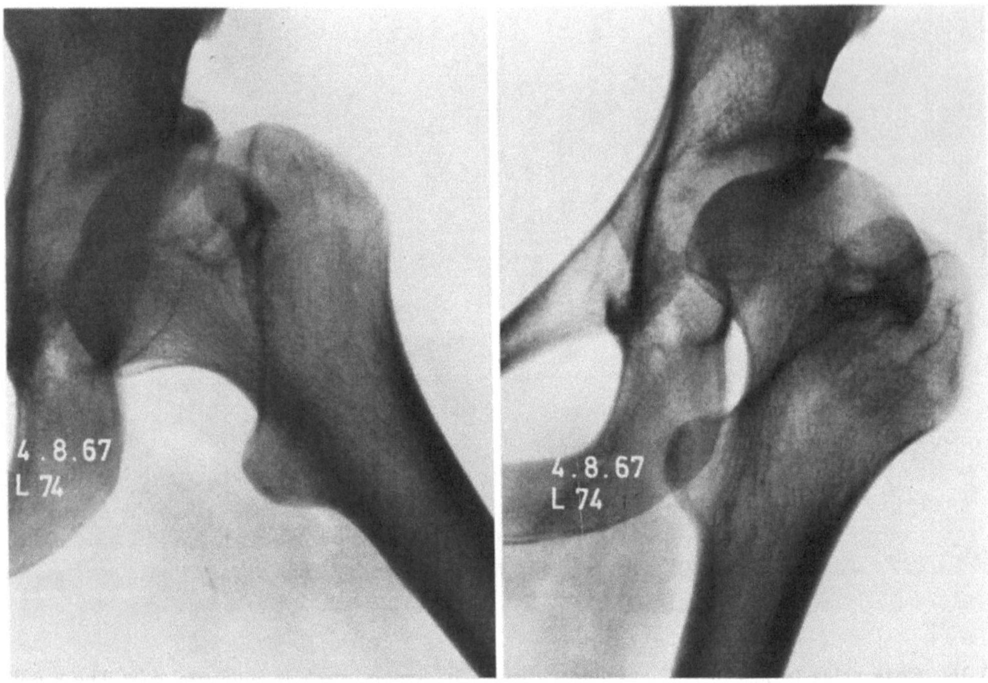

FIG. 10–17B X-ray films in maximal abduction and adduction were obtained. In abduction there is much better centralization of the femoral head in the acetabulum and better joint congruency. For this reason a varus osteotomy was chosen.

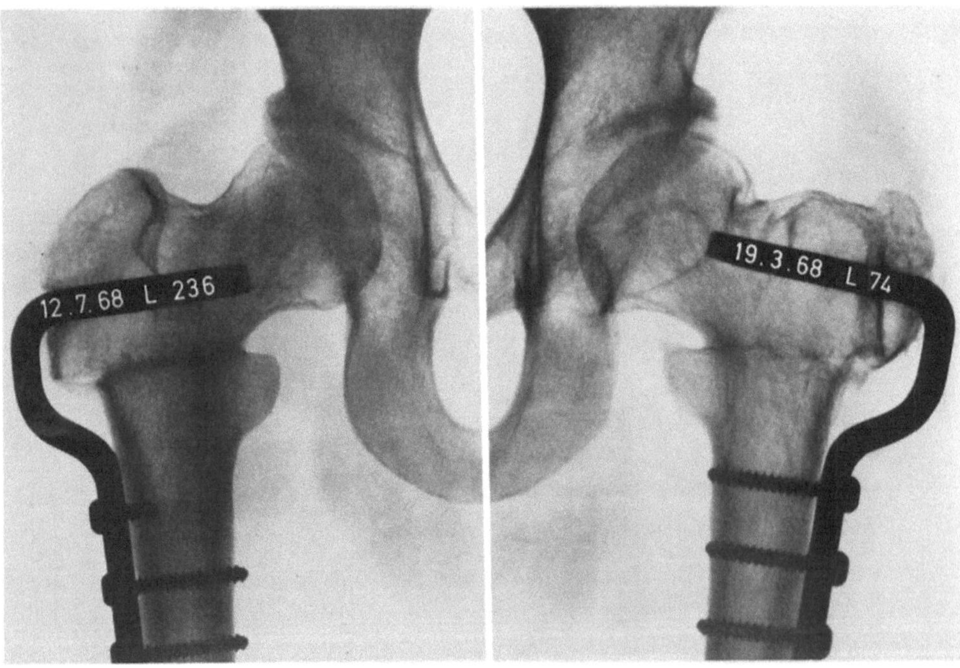

FIG. 10–17C Postoperatively it can be seen how the greater trochanter was transferred distally and fixed with the plate. On the right, an intertrochanteric osteotomy was carried out with excision of a wide medially based wedge. This allowed correction of the 3-cm shortening of the leg on the left.

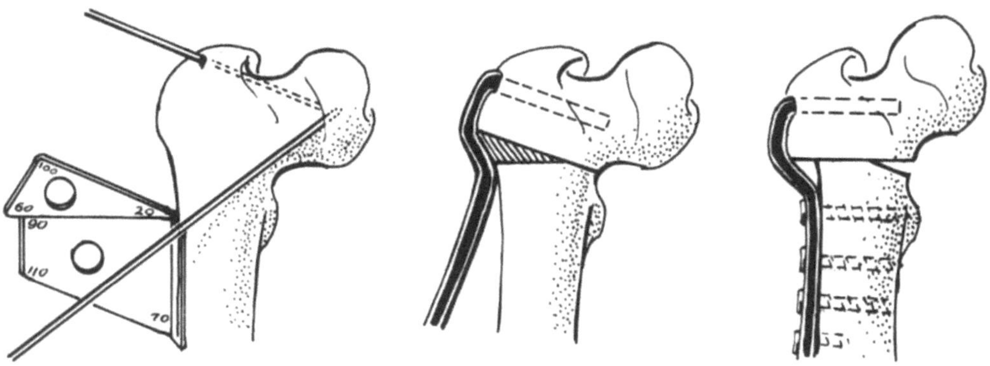

FIG. 10–18 Valgus osteotomy. The plate is driven cranially into the neck of the femur. The bone wedge which is excised is based laterally.

Postoperative Care

Prophylaxis for thrombophlebitis begins preoperatively. This consists of deep breathing exercises, and is continued postoperatively. The suction drains are removed at 24 to 48 hours from surgery. When the drains are removed, we begin with active and passive mobilization of the joints. At the end of one week, we begin ambulation with the aid of two crutches, and on the 7th to 10th postoperative day the patient is discharged. Partial weight bearing of 10 to 15 kg (determined with the aid of a scale) is allowed. In the immediate postoperative period attention is directed to mobilization of the knee joint, which must have regained at least 90° of flexion at the time of discharge (at the end of 3 to 4 weeks). In about 5 percent of cases, the knee must be manipulated under anesthesia to regain an acceptable range of motion.

Two crutches are used for four months to protect the healing and reorganization of the hip joint from any excessive stress. At the end of this period the patient goes to one crutch, and later to a cane. Active training of the hip musculature with the help of pulleys, bicycles and swimming is highly recommended.

An objective and subjective assessment of the success or failure of an osteotomy can be carried out only at the end of one year. If a widening of the joint space and the healing of the internal ar-

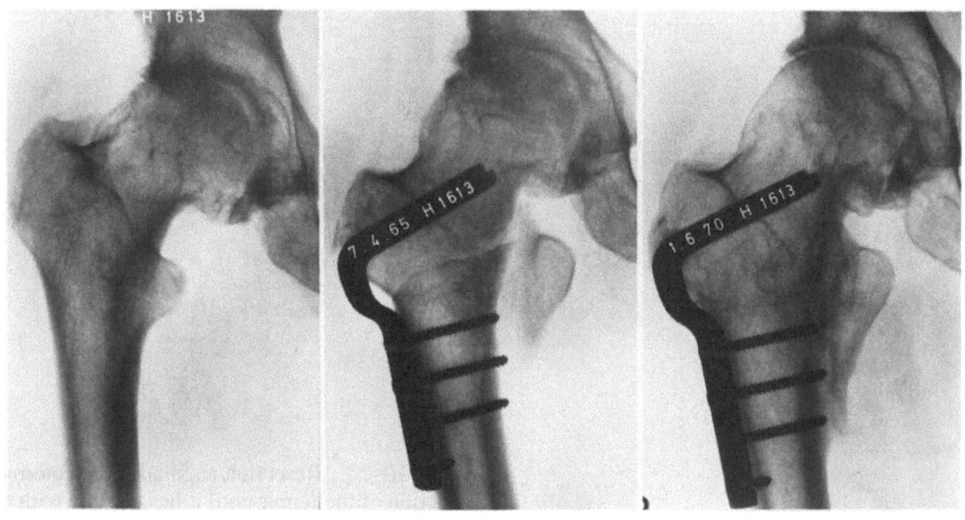

FIG. 10–19 **A** A 55-year-old patient with an osteoarthritic hip secondary to a slipped femoral epiphysis. The joint space has disappeared. **B** Three weeks after an osteotomy of 25° valgus and 30° extension. **C** Five years later the joint space is much wider, and the patient is pain-free.

chitecture of the femoral head and of the acetabulum are noted, the osteotomy can be considered a success. The absence of symptoms is usually short lived if no improvement in the x-ray picture has occurred.

Possible Complications Loss of fixation may result from inadequate bone stock between the plate and osteotomy site. At least 15 mm of bone is necessary to prevent fracturing of this segment. If the complication of a break of the lateral bridge

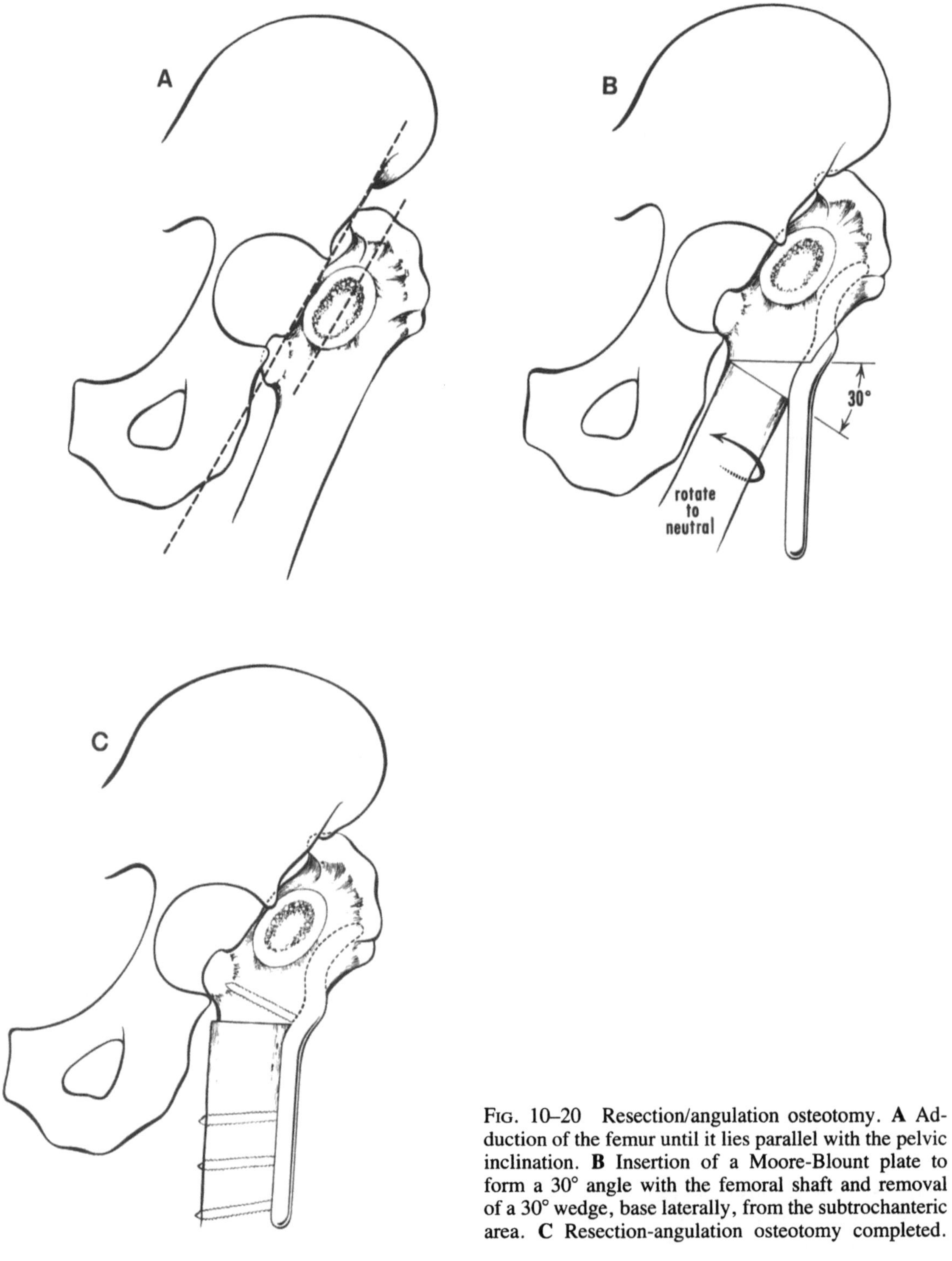

FIG. 10–20 Resection/angulation osteotomy. **A** Adduction of the femur until it lies parallel with the pelvic inclination. **B** Insertion of a Moore-Blount plate to form a 30° angle with the femoral shaft and removal of a 30° wedge, base laterally, from the subtrochanteric area. **C** Resection-angulation osteotomy completed.

arises, fixation can be secured in two ways: a new plate with a 20-mm recess can be used and its blade inserted more cranially, or a tension-band wire can be passed around the insertion of the abductors and onto the greater trochanter around the bow of the angle plate. The blade should never be inserted, pulled out and reinserted, or anchorage will be compromised. Therefore the blade must be inserted in the channel precut by the chisel with great care and precision.

In young adults, the cancellous bone of the proximal femoral metaphysis is very hard. A channel should be predrilled with a 3.2-mm drill bit before the seating chisel is driven. Otherwise the bone can be fractured all the way into the femoral neck.

Compromise of the retinacular vessels supplying the femoral neck may result if the tip of the Hohmann retractor presses against the posterior superior area of the neck.

Improper correction usually results from poor preoperative planning, but a second cause can be poor placement of the osteotomy. If the first cut is made too far up into the neck, too much varus displacement can occur as compression is applied, causing the fragments to slide along the neck. The cuts must be kept just above the lesser trochanter, thereby keeping the osteotomy well within the intertrochanteric zone.

Pseudarthrosis is a direct result of any one of the technical errors mentioned above.

Resection/Angulation Osteotomy

For completeness sake the resection/angulation osteotomy is being reproduced for it may have more than historic value in today's complicated world which is demanding more and more creative orthopedics to solve complex problems. It was one of the earliest osteotomies which was championed by Milch[5] is therefore also called a Milch osteotomy, or pelvic support osteotomy, Figure 10–20. As failures in total hip replacements mount from the shear numbers being done there is a renewed search for some alternate avenues for salvage pro-

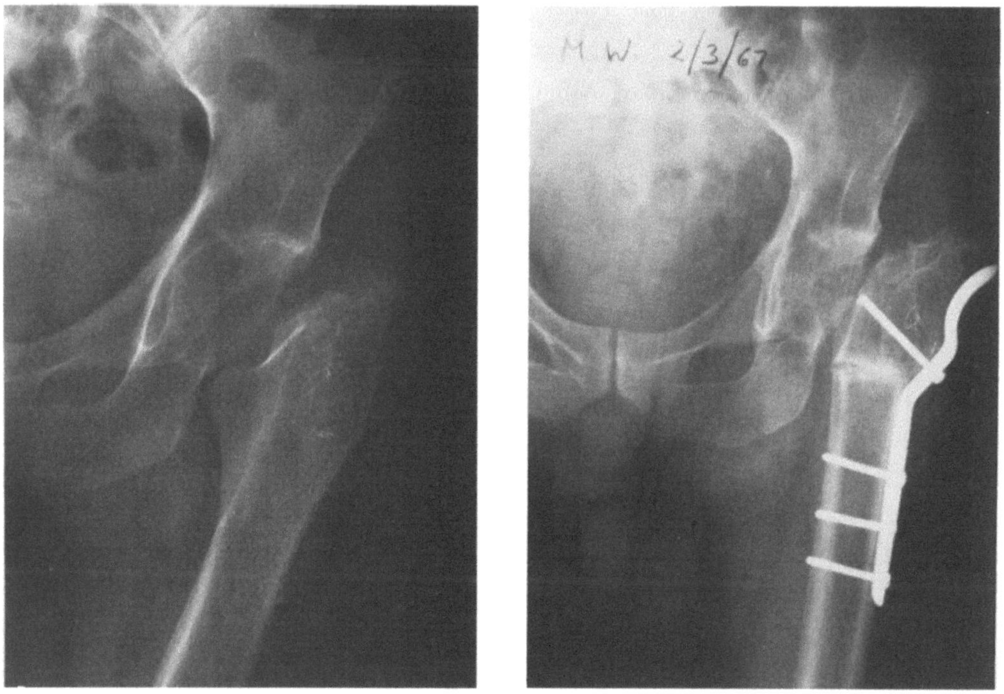

A B

FIG. 10–21 **A** Head and neck of the femur were removed. Purulent material was found in the hip joint. Antibiotic suction-irrigation treatment was carried out for 4 weeks, followed by intermittent traction for an additional 4 weeks combined with physiotherapy to mobilize the hip and strengthen the hip muscles. The wound healed without complications. **B** Three months later, abduction osteotomy was performed. The patient now walks without support of a cane, against advice, and is pain-free.

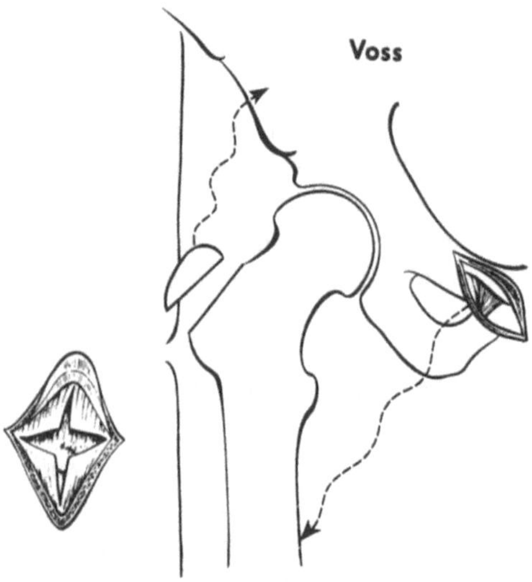

FIG. 10–22 Voss "hanging hip" operation achieved by osteotomizing greater trochanter and releasing adductor tendons at pubis.

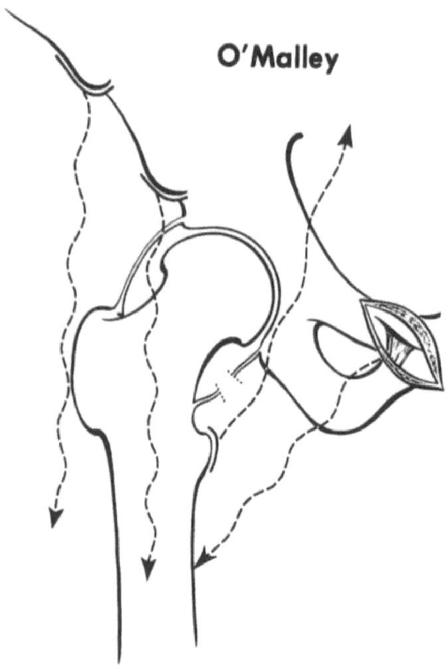

FIG. 10–23 O'Malley "hanging-hip" operation done by a capsulectomy and adductor tenotomy.

cedures. The younger hip surgeon should have access to information about this old but useful operation. It can be used as a salvage procedure to save another salvage operation such as a failed Girdlestone, Figure 10–21. "Muscle release" operations are more of the same historically. Voss and O'Malley were proponents of performing an extensive soft tissue releases which lossened the hip and decompressed the joint,[6] Figures 10–22 and 10–23. In comparison to an osteotomy it is less traumatic with an almost immediate relief of pain. Kuntscher properly labled it the "hanging hip operation."[7]

References

1. Müller, M. E.: *Die hüftnahen Femurosteotomien.* Stuttgart. Thieme Verlag, 1971.
2. Pauwels, F.: Des affections de la hanche d'origine mécanique et leur traitement par l'ostéotomie d'adduction. Rev. Orthop., 37:22, 1951.
3. Pauwels, F.: Ueber eine kausale Behandlung der Coxa valga. Z. Orthop., 79:305, 1950.
4. Graham, S., Westin, G. W., Dawson, E., and Oppenheim, J. J.: The Chiari Osteotomy., Clin. Ortho. 208:249, July, 1986.
5. Milch, H.: The "pelvic support" osteotomy. J. Bone Joint Surg., 23:581, 1941.
6. Mueller, K. H.: Muscle release operation about the hip, in Surgery of the Hip Joint, 1st Ed., (Tronzo, R. G. ed.), pp. 748–758, Lea & Febiger, 1973, Philadelphia.
7. Küntscher, G.: die Behandlung der coxarthrose nach Voss, Arch. Klin. Chir, 301:383, 1962.

Bombelli Osteotomy (Extension Osteotomy)*

Osteotomy of the proximal femur in the surgical treatment of osteoarthritis of the hip has a history which dates back to the late years of the nineteenth century in continental Europe. Even before the advent of roentgenography, osteotomies were performed by Kermission for difficult cases of late congenital dislocation. In the early mid-portions of this century, contributions were made by von Baeyer, Lorenz, Schanz, Putti, and others. Most of the scientific and clinical writing was done in the German and French literature.

Pauwels devoted intense interest to the study of the fundamental biomechanics of the hip. He made substantial clinical contributions to the treatment of fractures and pseudarthroses of the femoral neck and to the surgical management of osteoarthritis of the hip by means of osteotomy at the intertrochanteric level. One of his disciples, Renato Bombelli of Italy, has made further advances for "superolateral" osteoarthritis.

The Bombelli series was remarkable because of the high percentage of patients who benefited and the fact that follow-up was performed 11 years after the surgical procedure for each patient. Within the theoretical framework of Bombelli, the role of osteotomy in the surgical treatment of osteoarthritis is viewed as contributing principally to increasing, in the long run, the total surface area of interacting articular surfaces. In the short run, transient reduction in the forces in the hip is achieved during the postoperative period by mechanical alterations in the geometry of the proximal femur, the direct surgical modification of muscle forces, and the use of gait support with partial weight-bearing.

The technique of *valgus extension osteotomy* as practiced by Bombelli is presented in detail later in this section. Other contemporary leaders in the technology and practice of osteotomy include Müller, Schneider, Wagner, Morscher, and Maquet among others.

Osteotomies in Review

As clearly noted by Blount, from both a practical and historical point of view osteotomies can be grouped into those based on displacement of the shaft and those based on angulation of the shaft in one or more planes. Many procedures, in fact, were combinations of the two techniques and could be designed to include adjustment of leg length and control of rotational deformity as needed.

The *displacement osteotomies,* associated with the names McMurray, Lorenz, Putti, and von Baeyer, are rarely performed today and are mostly of historical interest. This type of osteotomy was used primarily in the treatment of osteoarthritis. Technically, it was performed either transversely or obliquely, at or in proximity to the level of the lesser trochanter. The distal fragment was displaced medially with the objective of stable impingement of the proximal portion of the distal fragment against the inferior rim of the acetabulum. A partial transfer of the weight-bearing function of the joint directly to the pelvis was the ultimate goal. Discomfort from this impingement was often reported, and the simultaneous performance of intraoperative obturator neurectomy

* This section of the chapter was written by Richard F. Santore.

with each displacement osteotomy was openly advocated.

For many years no internal fixation was used. The inadequate control of the fragments as well as the long period of required bed rest in plaster were serious drawbacks until the advent and adoption of internal fixation.

Medial displacement of the shaft did not, in fact, result in transfer of weight-bearing function of the hip joint directly to the pelvis, as was often argued, Medial transfer did succeed in relaxing the iliopsoas and adductor musculature with a resultant favorable reduction in these forces across the joint. With medial displacement of the shaft, an upward thrust to the medial aspect of the cut surface of the proximal fragment ensues. This results in an angulatory repositioning of the proximal fragment in the frontal or coronal plane which is identical qualitatively to that which occurs upon adduction positioning of the lower extremity or after valgus osteotomy. In those cases which would benefit from biomechanical and anatomical consequences of valgus repositioning, as we now understand them, the effects would be favorable. However, in cases in which varus osteotomy would be indicated on a morphological basis, the long-term results would be predictably less favorable.

A review of the literature is not as helpful as it might be hoped, as detailed descriptions of the radiological morphologies pre- and postoperatively for each case are rarely reported.

The shape of the femoral head, whether spherical, elliptical, or severely deformed by osteophytes and/or collapsed, the neck shaft angle, the presence and magnitude of acetabular dysplasia, and the type and magnitude of femoral head subluxation or coverage deficiency all play important roles in the preoperative planning. *Should conversion to total hip arthroplasty be required in the future, the substantial deformity of the proximal femoral anatomy created by the combination of valgus and medial displacement makes the conversion much more difficult.*

The mechanical effects of medial displacement on the knee must be carefully considered as well. Valgus of the proximal fragment results in lateralization of the weight-bearing axis at the knee, even without lateralization of the shaft. The combination of valgus and medialization of the shaft further exaggerates the adverse affects on an otherwise normal knee and predisposes to a valgus knee deformity. Therefore deliberate lateralization of the shaft is now performed to compensate for this adverse biomechanical effect at the knee. In the infrequent circumstance of coexistent ipsilateral medial compartment osteoarthritis of the knee, the valgus effect on the knee is advantageous. Therefore lateral displacement of the shaft may be electively omitted if formal correction of the knee deformity is not contemplated. However, if the osteoarthritic process at the knee level is of sufficient magnitude to warrant consideration of a surgical procedure in the near future, both joints may more appropriately be addressed independently. This leads to a decision to laterally displace the shaft in the intertrochanteric osteotomy for the hip and to proceed at a later date with tibial osteotomy or arthroplasty of the knee. Varus osteotomy, on the other hand, results in medial displacement of the weight-bearing axis at the knee level. Medial displacement of the shaft at the time of intertrochanteric osteotomy serves to offset this effect at the knee level.

In addition to its role in the treatment of osteoarthritis, the *angulation osteotomies* were used in the management of deformities, fractures, and nonunions. The osteotomy of Schanz was performed in the subtrochanteric region with its apex medially and a resultant valgus or adduction effect on the femoral head. As with displacement osteotomies, significant deformity in the architecture of the proximal femur resulted.

Patient Selection

From the clinical perspective, ideal candidates are those who are highly motivated and who understand the cost/benefit ratio of osteotomy in a realistic sense (Tables 10–1 and 10–2). Age in and of itself is not a contraindication to the procedure. Physical age, not chronological age, should be the determining criterion. Motion of 60° or more in the flexion arc correlates with better long-term results. Patients should have 15° or more of abduction prior to varus osteotomy and 15° or more or adduction prior to valgus osteotomy.

TABLE 10–1 Clinical Indications for Osteotomy

Cooperative patient
Physiologically young
Adduction 15° (for valgus osteotomy)
Abduction 15° (for varus osteotomy)
Motion in flexion arc of 60° or more

TABLE 10–2 Contraindications for Osteotomy

Absolute contraindications	
	Neuropathic arthropathy
	Active infection
	Osteopenic bone
	Inflammatory or rheumatoid arthritis
Relative contraindications	
	Stiff joint (motion in flexion arc < 30°)
	Contralateral arthrodesis
	Advanced physiological age
	History of prior osteotomy

Absolute contraindications to osteotomy included neuropathic arthropathy, evidence of active infection, osteopenia, and evidence of inflammatory or rheumatoid arthritis. Relative contraindications include stiffness of the joint with motion in the flexion arc of less than 60°, a contralateral arthrodesis or contralateral stiff hip, and a history of failed osteotomy.

Although successful osteotomy can be performed in the presence of moderately advanced morphological changes, restoration of normal or near-normal motion in a hip which was stiff preoperatively cannot be expected. Particularly with regard to this criterion, patients may be disappointed if they gauge their results against the early results after total hip replacement surgery. In the 11 year follow-up study the average preoperative motion in the flexion arc was 51°. At follow-up it was only 63°. In terms of pain relief and the longevity of the result, even patients with preoperative flexion of 30° or less had long-term results comparable to those with relatively mobile hips. However, displeasure with the limitations inherent in hypomobility of the hip was the single most frequent objection raised by patients when asked to assess their results objectively.

When osteotomy is performed in the presence of significant preoperative stiffness, i.e., flexion of less than 30°, arthrodesis may result. When the stiff arthritic hip is unilateral and the patient is young, postoperative, spontaneous arthrodesis is not an unacceptable outcome so long as the patient is prepared for this possible outcome.

Theoretical Considerations

To this day the rationale for the osteotomy procedure remains controversial and a clear explanation for the effectiveness of osteotomy in relieving pain remains elusive. In general, satisfactory, even good or excellent, relief of pain accompanies many of the various osteotomy procedures, at least for a finite period of time. The paucity of long-term follow-up studies in the literature makes quantification of the success rates of the various procedures difficult to verify. The author and Professor Bombelli have concluded a long-term follow-up study of a consecutive series of osteotomies performed by Bombelli in 1971. It was ascertained that 82% of patients had little or negligible pain after a minimum of 11 years from the time of surgery. In this study 92% of the consecutive series of 50 patients were retrieved for long-term follow-up (Table 10–3).

Theories concerning the relative importance of rotating new articular cartilage into the weight-bearing region, increasing the thickness of the articulation, altering the biomechanics of the hip joint toward a more favorable balance, decreasing the vascular pressure within the femoral head, or increasing the overall surface area of the weight-bearing region are theoretical explanations for the good results. Although there is likely some validity to each of these concepts, none as yet has satisfied the demands of reproducible scientific documentation. Nevertheless, there is a body of information in the literature which supports the thesis that intertrochanteric osteotomy of the proximal femur effectively relieves pain in the adult arthritic hip. Certain criteria have evolved for the indications for (Table 10–1) and against (Table 10–2) intertrochanteric osteotomy.

TABLE 10–3 Clinical Results in 50 Consecutive Cases

Parameter	No. of Patients	Harris Score at Follow-up
Total patients (hips)	50	95
Deceased	2	85
Lost to follow-up	2	69
Eliminated	1	45
Patients reviewed	45	
Results		
Excellent	19	
Good	15	
Fair	7	
Poor	4	
Total	45	

The Harris hip score is widely used to quantify the status of the hip: 44 points for absence of pain, 51 points for various aspects of function, and 5 points for motion.

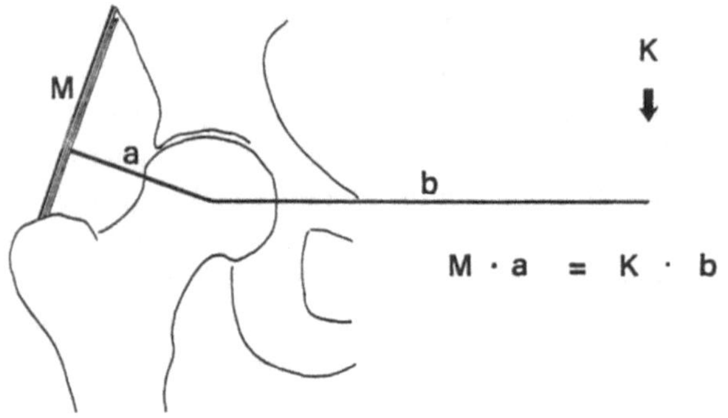

FIG. 10–24 Lever arm balance of forces acting at the center of rotation of the femoral head. *M*, abductor force; *a*, lever arm of the abductors, from the center of rotation of the femoral head to a point perpendicular to the line of action of the abductors. *K*, body weight minus the weight of the supporting limb. *b*, lever arm of the body weight.

As popularized by Pauwels, biomechanical analysis of the hip is facilitated by considering the hip joint as a fulcrum above which stable balance of lever arm forces occur in single limb stance (Fig. 10–24). In order to result in a level pelvis in a single limb stance, the abductor forces (M)—acting through lever arm a, which transverses the distance from the center of rotation (CR) of the femoral head to a point perpendicular to the angle of insertion of the combined abductors—must be in equilibrium with the force of the body weight (K) minus the weight of the supporting limb, acting through lever arm b, which spans the distance from the center of rotation of the femoral head to the line of center of gravity of the body. Overall balance of forces is expressed in the equation $M \times a = K \times b$. Factors which affect the magnitudes of the variables of this equation affect the overall size of the net lever arm forces. A theory of the mechanical etiology of osteoarthritis has emerged from the work of Bombelli based on the concept of the vertical nature of the primary acting forces in the hip and the role of anatomical variations in the inclination of the acetabular weight-bearing surface.

The abductor force (M) is factored into vertical

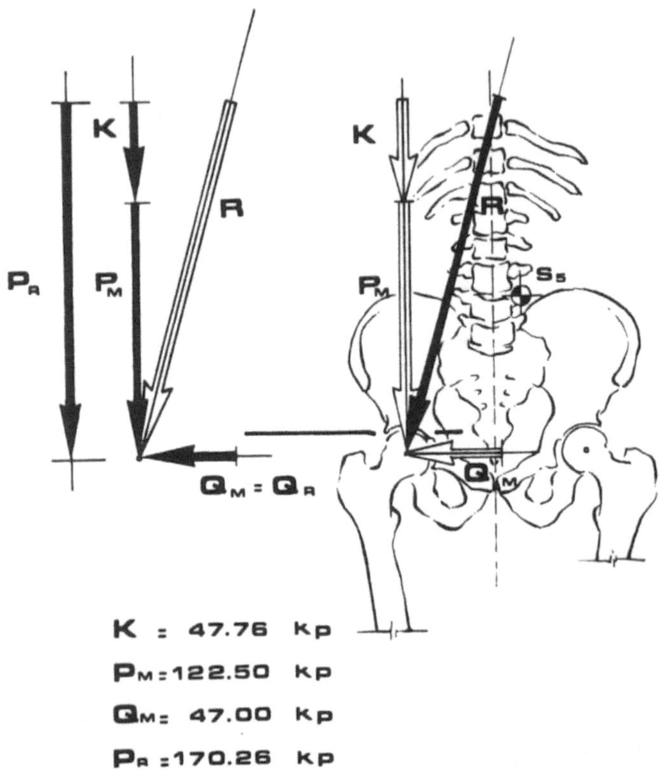

FIG. 10–25 Derivation of force *R*. It is the resultant of the vertical forces P_M and K and the horizontal force Q_M. For reason of simplicity: $P_M + K = P_R$ and $Q_M = Q_R$.

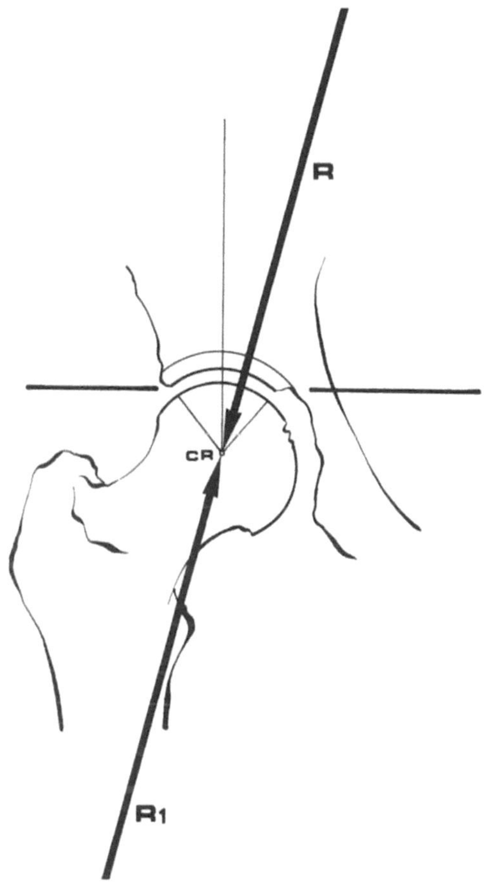

FIG. 10–26 Force R is countcracted by an equal and opposite force R_1, which represents the counterthrust from the ground.

and horizontal component vectors to complement the vertical nature of the gravity force of the body weight (K).

Direct addition of the gravity force of the body weight (K) and the vertical component of the abductors permit retrograde trigonometric computation of the resultant force (R) (Fig. 10–25). Force R is the resultant force of the lever arm forces and proves to be identical in magnitude and direction to that computed by Pauwels using different methodology.

An equilibrium state is then considered in which a counterforce (R_1) is postulated to be equal in magnitude and opposite in direction to the resultant force R (Fig. 10–26). Vectors of the theoretical counter-force are factored perpendicular and parallel to the plane of inclination of the acetabular weight-bearing surface (Fig. 10–27). The ground rules of this theoretical equilibrium state thus make the component vectors equisitely sensitive to variations in the inclination of the acetabular weight-bearing surface (Fig. 10–28). Superolateral

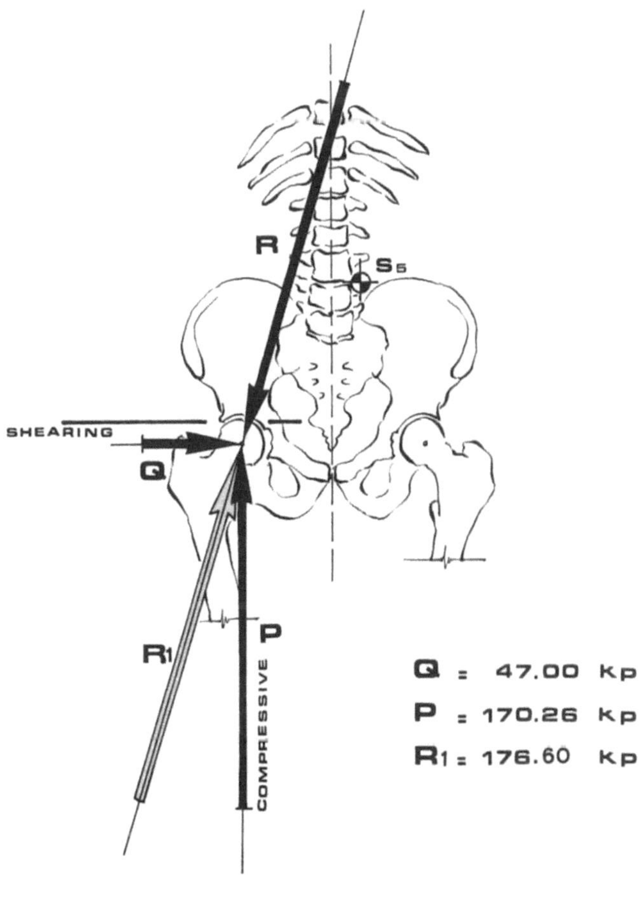

FIG. 10–27 The two effects of force R_1. The concave WBS of the acetabulum in a normal hip has a horizontal direction. The oblique force R_1, pushing the femoral head against a horizontal WBS, may be resolved into a shearing force (Q) and a compressive force (P).

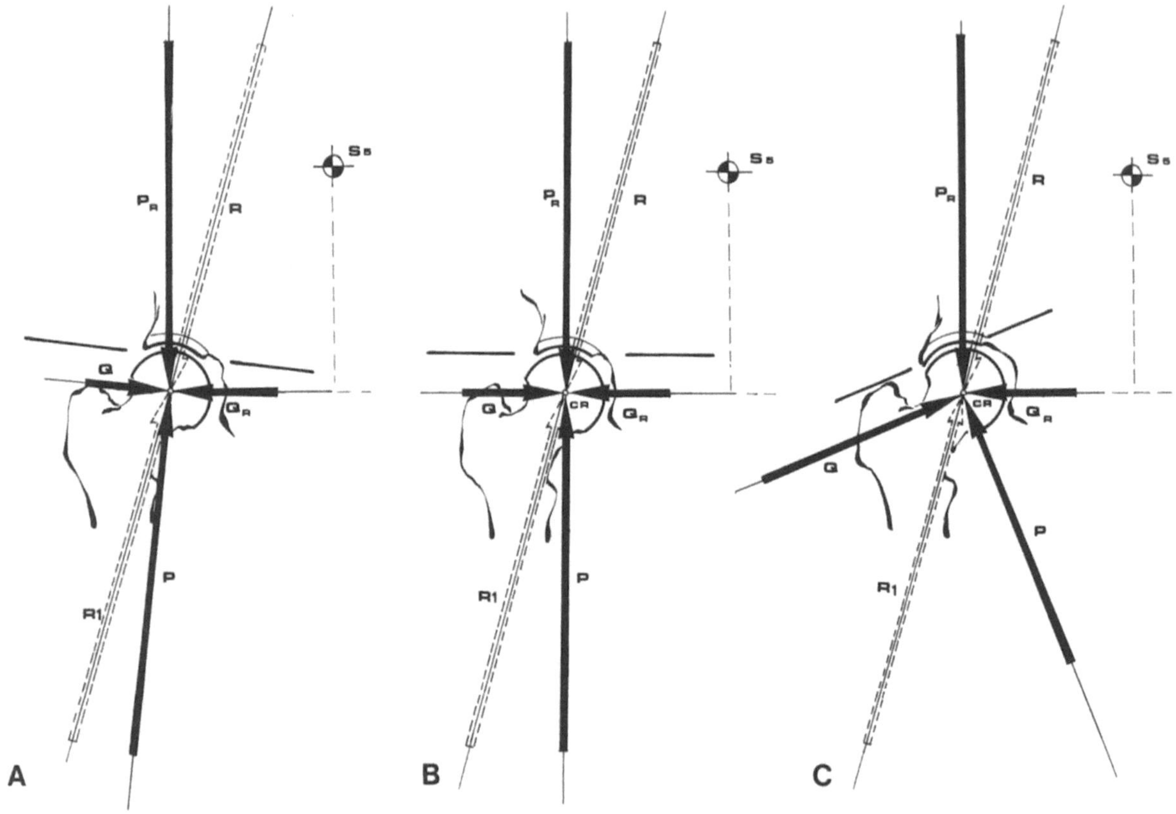

FIG. 10–28 In cases of an oblique weight-bearing surface (WBS) the normal mechanics of the hip are deranged. **A** When the WBS has a craniolateral inclination, force Q, parallel to it, points caudally and medially and decreases in magnitude, and force P, perpendicular to the WBS, points craniomedially and increases in magnitude. **B** Only when the WBS has a horizontal direction are normal mechanics in the hip achieved, i.e., forces P_R and P are equal and opposite in direction, as well as the horizontal forces Q_R and Q. **C** When the WBS has a craniomedial inclination, force Q points craniomedially and increases in magnitude, and force P points craniolaterally and reduces in magnitude. In both **A** and **C** the equilibrium between P_R and P and Q_R and Q is lost.

and superomedial variations in the inclination of the acetabular weight-bearing surface result in alterations in both the magnitudes and directions of the component vectors of the counter resultant force. Variations in the magnitudes and directions of these vectors have been shown by Bombelli to correspond with certain types of mechanical osteoarthritis.

Biomechanical Aspects

From the biomechanical perspective varus and valgus osteotomies favorably influence the net magnitude of the lever arm forces by manipulating the lengths of the principal lever arms and, in the case of the varus osteotomy, by a direct effect on the length, tension, and angle of insertion of the abductors.

Varus osteotomy (Fig. 10–29) results in an elevation of the greater trochanter relative to the center of rotation of the femoral head. Simultaneously, the length of the abductor lever arm (a) increases, the angle of insertion of the abductors (M) becomes more horizontal, and the length–tension relation of the abductors decreases. All three factors contribute to weakening of the abductors and a decrease in the net lever arm forces acting on the hip. This is so effective that Trendelenburg gait invariably is seen for 6 months to 2 years postoperatively. In some cases the effect is permanent, and trochanteric advancement is necessary to restore a normal gait pattern.

After valgus osteotomy, point-to-point contact

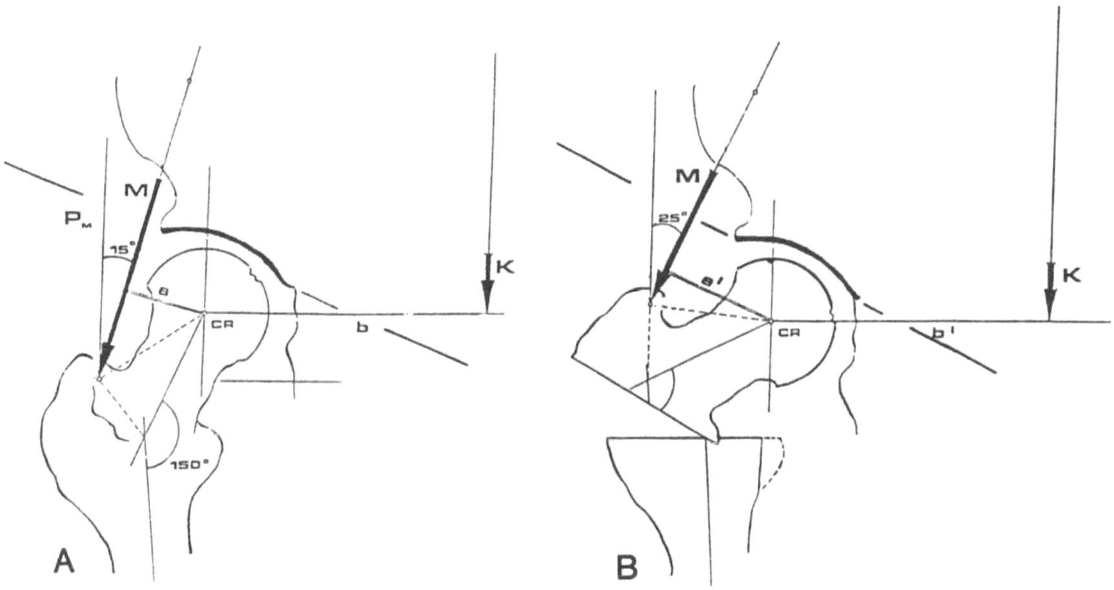

FIG. 10–29 **A** Lever arm forces in coxa valga subluxans. Note the laterally inclined acetabulum, the valgus neck shaft angle, and the vertical inclination of the abductors. **B** After varus osteotomy the biochemical consequences include a more horizontal angle of insertion of the abductors, proximal displacement of the greater trochanter, increase in the length of the abductor lever arm (*a'* greater than *a*). All contribute to a reduction in the magnitude of forces at the hip joint.

is provoked between the inferomedial osteophyte of the femoral head (capital drop) and the osteophyte along the medial acetabular wall (curtain osteophyte) (Fig. 10–30). This action, it is reasoned, transiently transposes the center of rotation of the femoral head to the point of contact of the osteophytes, resulting in an increase in lever arm *a* and a decrease in lever arm b; this in turn results in a decrease in the abductor force due to a lever arm effect. However, valgus osteotomy also results in a direct effect on the abductors consisting in an increase in the length–tension relation of the muscle itself and a more vertical line of insertion of the abductors to the greater trochanter. These direct effects on the abductor muscles, considered in isolation, increase the forces in the hip joint attributable to the abductors. Thus in valgus osteotomies a relaxing osteotomy is performed on the greater trochanter to offset the direct effects on the abductors imposed by the angulatory repositioning in the frontal plane. Therapeutically, valgus and varus osteotomies result in decreased loads, facilitating healing and reconstitution of fibrocartilaginous and osseous tissues during the postoperative period.

Factors which contribute to a reduction in load applied to the hip and a decrease in unit load at the articular surface include the biomechanical consequences of varus and valgus repositioning as noted above, a reduction in the muscular tension across the hip joint achieved by transection of the iliopsoas tendon in all cases, and the relaxing osteotomy of the greater trochanter in valgus cases.

Additional factors include the direct weight-bearing function of the osteophytes. In certain cases roof osteophytes and/or capital drop osteophytes contribute significantly to an increase in the size of the weight-bearing surface of the hip joint. Finally, a prolonged period of crutch-supported gait further protects the hip from the full forces of normal ambulation.

Osteophytes

Exploitation of the remodeling potential of osteophytes is one of the key building blocks on which the logic of valgus osteotomy has been constructed (Table 10–4). The major osteophytes recognizable in the arthritic hip are represented in Figure 10–31 based on the original work of Bombelli. Note the osteophytes in the superior cervical and in-

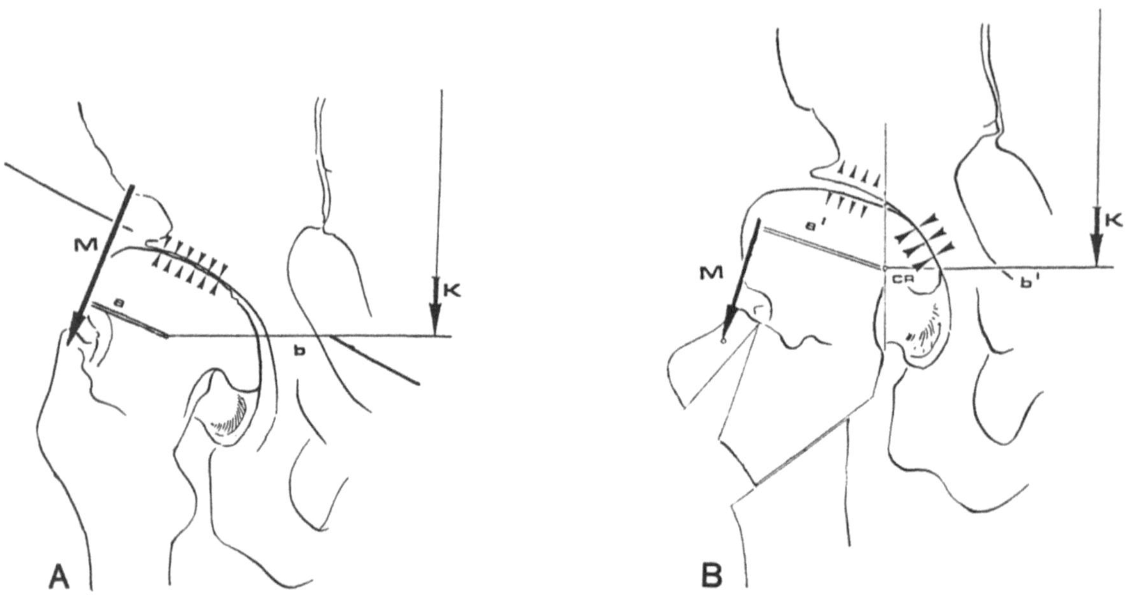

FIG. 10–30 **A** Dysplastic hip with mushroom-cap deformity of the femoral head, large capital drop osteophyte of the inferomedial aspect of the femoral head, and obliteration of the superolateral joint space. **B** After valgus osteotomy note the fulcrum effect of osteophyte impingement medially, with opening up of the superolateral joint space; the relaxing, opening-pocket partial osteotomy of the greater trochanter; and the transient medial displacement of the center of rotation which results in lengthening of the abductor lever arm (*a*, *a′*) and shortening of the lever arm of the body weight (*b*, *b′*). The opening-pocket greater trochanteric osteotomy directly relaxes the abductors, which would otherwise have been put on stretch by the valgus angulatory change. An overall reduction in forces results.

feromedial (capital drop) regions on the femoral head. The development of these osteophytes in conjunction with superior collapse of the femoral head is responsible for the characteristic "mushroom-head" appearance of the femoral head seen in cases of *late congenital dislocation* of the hip or acetabular dysplasia. An osteophyte is seen

TABLE 10–4 Indications for Valgus or Valgus-Extension Osteotomy

Osteoarthritis superimposed on dysplastic hip
Acetabular dysplasia with mushroom cap elliptical deformity of the femoral head, well developed capital drop and osteophytes, early roof osteophyte
Osteoarthritis in false acetabulum of congenitally dislocated hip
Coxa vara
Osteonecrosis with collapse of femoral head and osteophyte proliferation
Vertical subcapital fracture in a young patient
Anteromedial acetabular dysplasia with equitorial osteoarthritis or coxa profunda

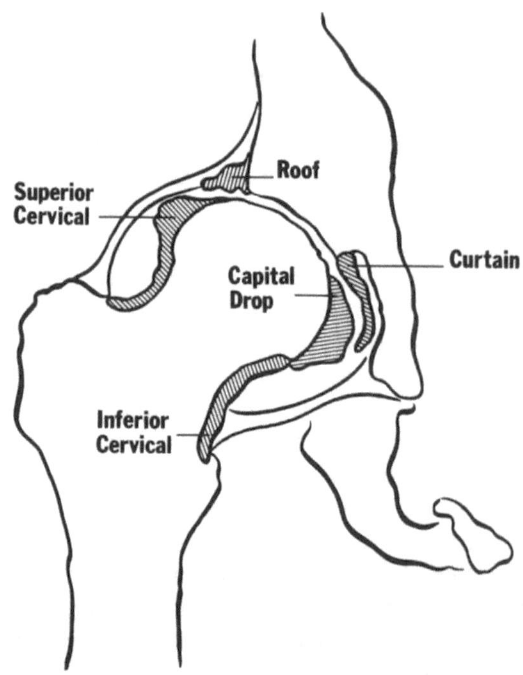

FIG. 10–31 Major osteophytes recognizable in the arthritic hip.

along the medial acetabular wall and is referred to as the "curtain" osteophyte. At the lateral superior margin of the acetabulum a "roof" osteophyte is seen projecting laterally.

In the frontal plane the valgus realignment was believed by Bombelli to result in direct traction on the superior aspect of the hip joint capsule, which has a stimulating effect on the roof osteophyte. It was further reasoned that a temporary fulcrum develops at the point of contact between the capital drop and curtain osteophytes, which contributes to a reduction in load at the superior aspect of the head (Fig. 10–32).

In a *dysplastic hip,* particularly one in which the head is poorly covered laterally, the performance of a valgus osteotomy might seem inappropriate, even illogical. It can be reasoned, certainly, that the head is being projected into a position away from, and not toward, the acetabulum in a manner which would tend to diminish, not enhance, congruency and coverage.

In fact, in younger patients a prominent postoperative roof osteophyte seldom develops, and simultaneous or subsequent pelvic osteotomy may be required to provide adequate long-term coverage for the femoral head. In older patients, however, a roof osteophyte forms consistently after valgus osteotomy, particularly in those cases in which a roof osteophyte is thought to participate in the weight-bearing function of the acetabular weight-bearing surface in a manner analogous to that of the bone graft placed at the lateral margin of the acetabulum in the shelf procedure. Additionally, in valgus osteotomies the capital drop osteophyte, which at times is quite large, is brought up into a functional weight-bearing position. In long-term postoperative radiographs, incorporation of the capital drop osteophyte into the femoral head can be seen.

Figure 10–33 demonstrates a case of osteoarthritis secondary to acetabular dysplasia with a mushroom-head deformity of the femoral head,

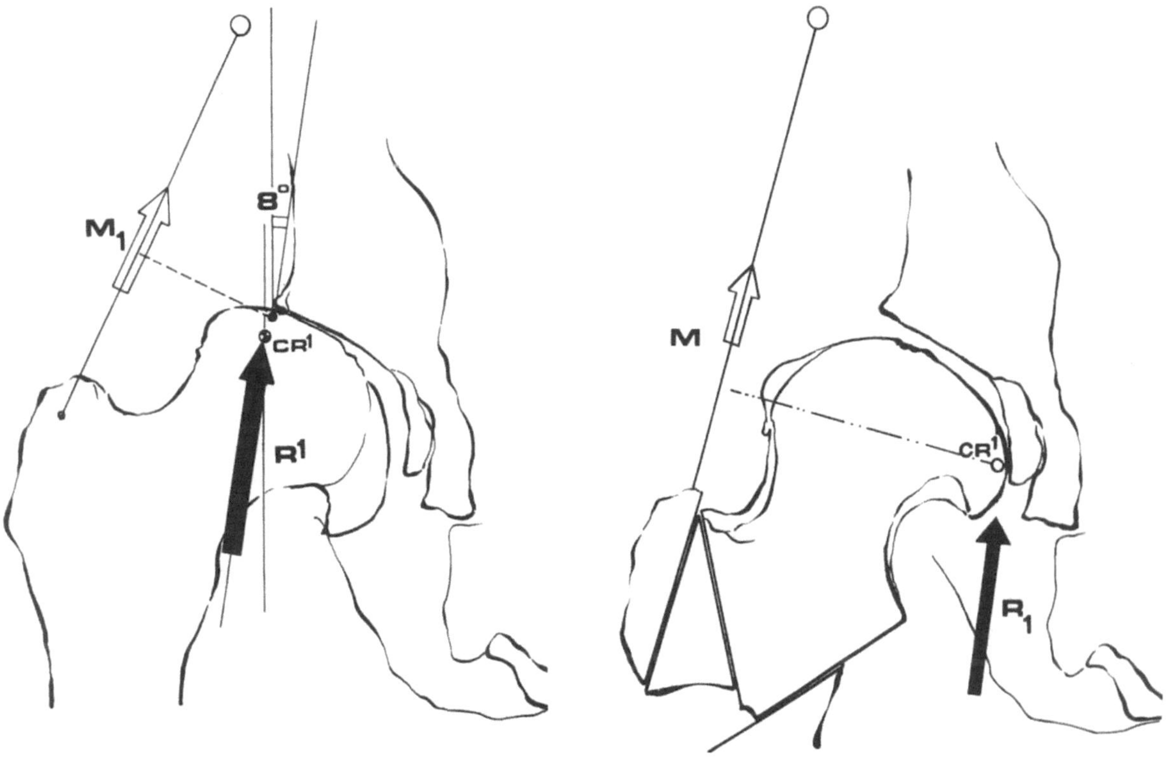

FIG. 10–32 By doing a valgus-extension osteotomy the capital drop on the femoral head comes into contact with the curtain osteophyte in the acetabulum. The contact area acts as a nonpainful fulcrum for the head and holds the joint surfaces apart. The space obtained becomes filled with synovial fluid, which acts as a buffer. The part of the head which previously had become deformed owing to excessive pressure has been relieved of this pressure and in some cases regains its normal shape.

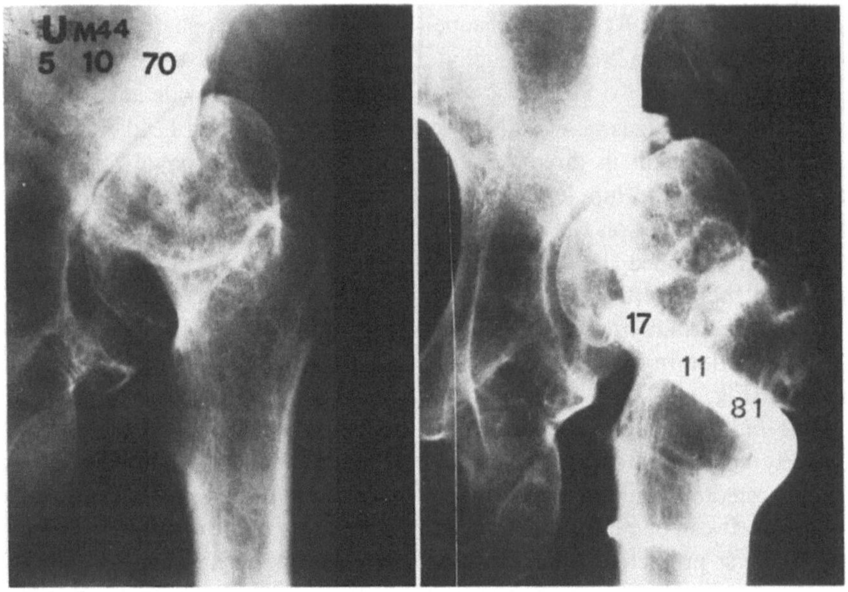

A B

FIG. 10–33 **A** Osteoarthritis secondary to acetabular dysplasia. **B** Successful treatment by a valgus/extension osteotomy.

proximal subluxation, and joint space narrowing. Eleven years later good joint space is seen with moderate enlargement of the roof osteophyte, though the head remains uncovered superolaterally.

Role of Extension

After hundreds of osteotomies, Bombelli recognized an almost universal tendency for the femoral head to be uncovered anteriorly as well as laterally, particularly in cases of acetabular dysplasia. By incorporating a correction in the sagittal plane over and above that needed to offset any preexisting flexion contracture, a significant increase in acetabular coverage of the anterior aspect of the femoral head was achieved. This evolved as an integral part of the osteotomy procedure, in both varus and valgus angulatory correction cases. The rationale is illustrated and explained in Figure 10–34.

Varus Osteotomy

In the frontal plane the proximal fragment can be manipulated to result in a valgus or varus change in the neck shaft angle relative to its preoperative value.

A virtual sine qua non among the criteria for a *varus osteotomy* is the presence of a spherical femoral head and a congruent, well-preserved joint space (Table 10–5). Abduction of the extremity generally results in a radiographically appreciable increase in femoral head coverage. The femoral head need not be perfectly spherical but must be smooth, congruent, and without evidence of collapse; in short, the athritic damage to such a joint will be minimal. If left alone and given medication with advice to "Let's wait until we are forced into surgery," the joint will steadily progress to a grossly distorted hip as seen in Figure 10–34.

A case with excellent indications for a varus osteotomy is seen in Figure 10–35. It is a case of *early* degenerative joint destruction. The head is seen to be slightly elliptical though smooth and regular. The joint space is congruent. A valgus neck shaft angle is apparent. Anterolateral dysplasia of the acetabulum is present with evidence of sclerosis on the acetabular side and cysts of small magnitude on both acetabular and femoral sides. Seven years after a varus osteotomy the joint space is seen to be well preserved and congruent. The patient was comfortable and active, and coverage of the head is improved. The cysts have resolved, but moderate sclerosis is still present.

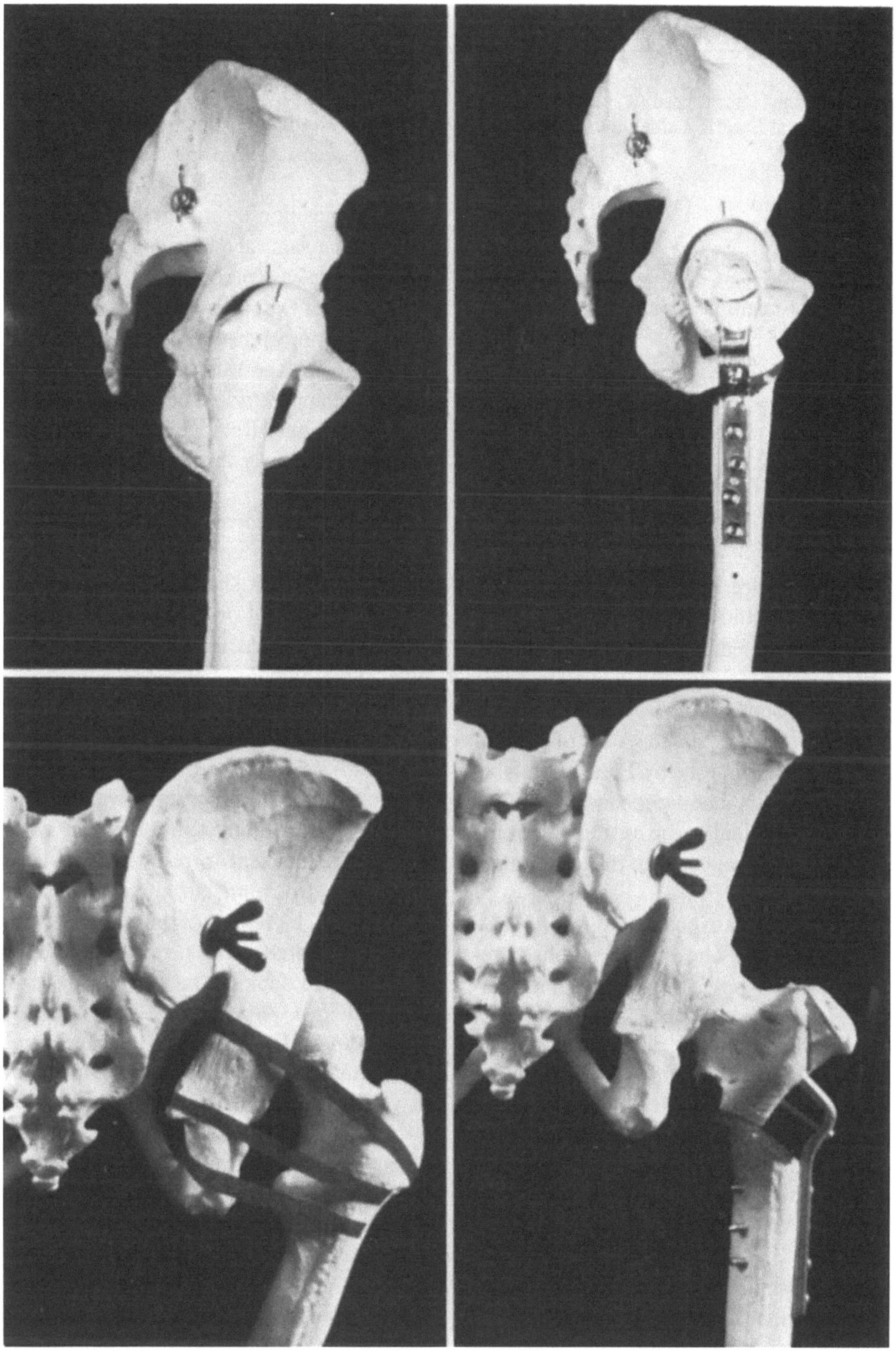

A

B

FIG. 10–34 Importance of extension component in osteotomy for superolateral types b, c, and d OA. **A** Lateral view, showing how the femoral head moves forward, upward, and laterally out of the acetabulum. This movement reduces the WBS of the joint and provokes pain. To reduce the pain, by increasing the WBS, the patient twists his pelvis toward the slipping femoral head. The pelvis fruitlessly chases the escaping head. The increasing contraction of the muscles (iliopsoas and rectus femoris) necessary to incline the pelvis leads in time to a permanent contraction of their fibers. For this reason the flexion of the hip joint becomes permanent. The extension component of the osteotomy centers the head in the acetabulum, and detaching the muscles eliminates the effect of their contraction. **B** Posterior view. Extension component of the osteotomy allows the head to be centered again in the acetabulum. The internal rotation of the shaft performed during the operation corrects the external rotation of the limb.

Table 10–5 Varus Osteotomy

Contraindication	
	Deformation of the femoral head (a spherical or congruent femoral head is a sine qua non for varus osteotomy)
Indications	
	Coxa valga subluxans
	Coxa valga
	Concentric osteoarthritis
	Osteoarthritis superimposed on malunited subcapital fracture in a valgus position
	Osteonecrosis in the absence of femoral head deformity (see section on osteonecrosis)

Valgus-Extension Osteotomy: Surgical Technique of Bombelli

Wide surgical exposure is strongly advocated to ensure precise visual and manual control of bony fragments, correct placement of the osteotomy cut and internal fixation device, and adequate room for use of the AO compression device. Initial exposure is depicted in Figure 10–36. A set of colored illustrations on this technique by Poss is available from the Upjohn Co.[31] The tensor fascia lata has been divided longitudinally and retracted anteriorly to expose the interval between the tensor muscle and the abductors.

The interval is further exposed, and wound towels are sewn into place. The vastus lateralis is reflected anteriorly to expose the proximal and midportions of the femur. The exposed femur and capsule of the hip joint are depicted in Figure 10–37. The vastus lateralis is lifted away from the femoral shaft in an L-shaped fashion by cutting away the inferior border of the muscle and then vertically from the greater trochanter. Anterior subluxation of the femoral head is encountered in this case of osteoarthritis secondary to acetabular dyplasia.

The skeletal situation is represented in Figure 10–38 as viewed from the lateral perspective. Flexion of the hip is performed until the head is covered anteriorly as confirmed by palpation or visual inspection (Fig. 10–39).

In the example shown, flexion of approximately 30° results in markedly improved coverage in the sagittal plane. Osteotomy is subsequently performed in the flexed position and the distal fragment, i.e., thigh and leg, then extended to a neutral position on the operating table. Because of this "extended" position of the distal fragment relative to the proximal fragment, which remains fixed in its newly established position in the acetabulum, the maneuver acquired the term "extension" (Fig. 10–40).

The acquisition of improved femoral head coverage in the sagittal plane can be appreciated by reviewing the case presented in Figure 10–41. This component of the overall procedure has particular importance in valgus cases, as substantial gains in coverage in the sagittal plane can offset, to a degree, the apparent loss of coverage in the frontal or coronal plane. Remodeling of the capital drop is often particularly impressive in a review of the axial radiographs.

One effect of correction on the sagittal plane is that extension confers an obligatory varus change in the neck shaft angle, the magnitude of which is dependent on both the magnitude of the extension performed and the preexisting neck shaft angle. This angular, geometric interdependency has been quantified and reported by Bombelli.[3]

Let us assume that a correction of approximately 15° is considered desirable in the frontal plane on the basis of preoperative tracings of the anteroposterior radiographs. In other words, 15° of valgus is sufficient to result in impingement of the capital drop and curtain osteophytes and a concomitant increase in the superolateral joint space. If the preexisting neck shaft angle is 130°, as in the case depicted here, an extension of 30° will result in a postoperative neck shaft angle of 126°. In practical terms, 5° of excess valgus in the frontal plane is necessary to end up with the net valgus determined to be optimal on the basis of the tracings. Thus a 20° valgus correction intraoperatively will result in a net valgus of 15° when a simultaneous extension correction of 30° is performed. Similar calculation, with reverse compensation, must be done in various osteotomy cases.

After establishing the magnitude of extension required, a relaxing opening-pocket osteotomy of the greater trochanter is performed, leaving the superior cortex and posterior soft tissues intact (Fig. 10–42).

The seating chisel is positioned in the neck and head at an angle synchronous with the fact that a 130° AO blade plate will be used and a 20° valgus correction is to be obtained.

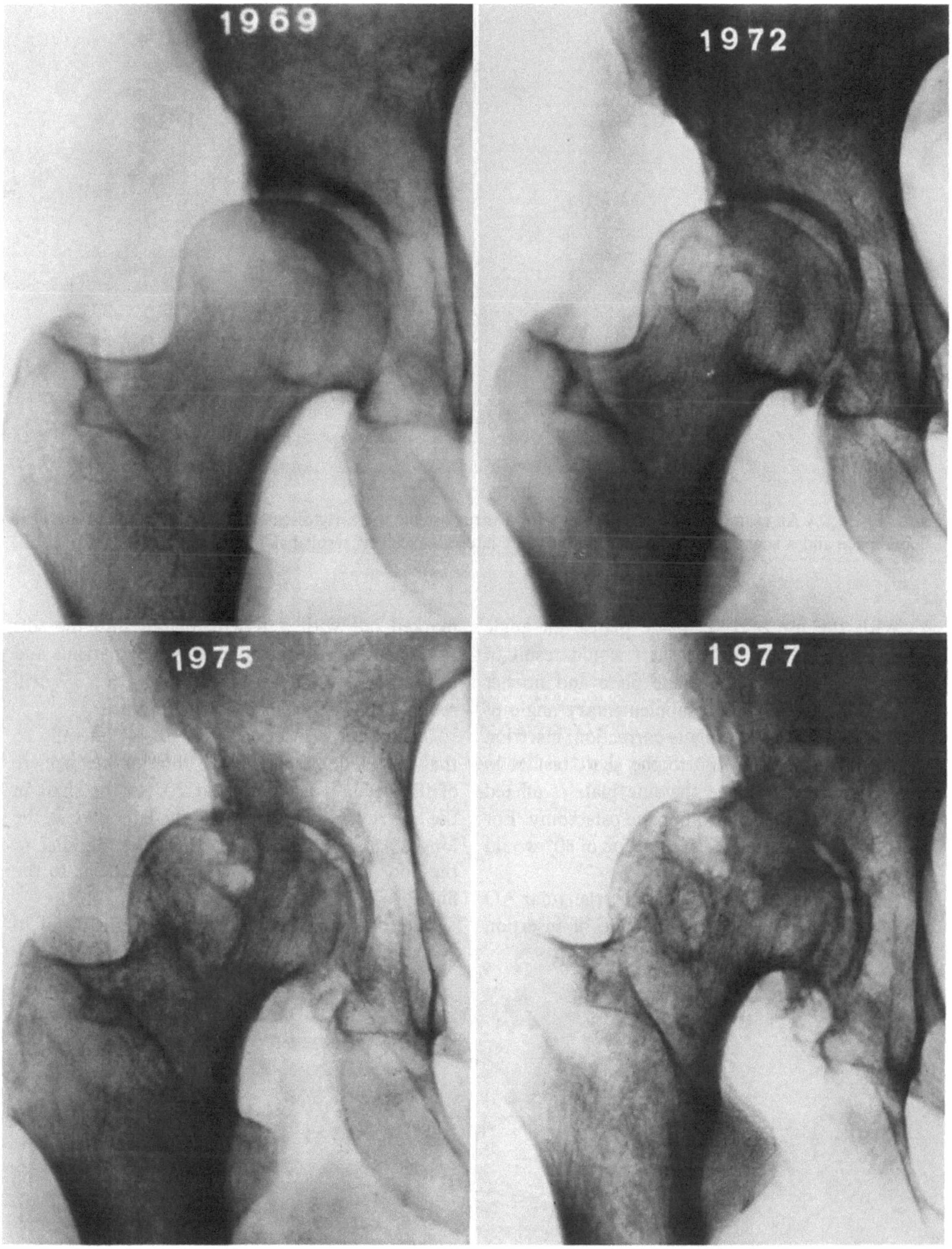

FIG. 10–35 (Top) A case of early degenerative destruction that would benefit from varus osteotomy. (Bottom) Cysts continued to enlarge and the head is grossly distorted from being so neglected.

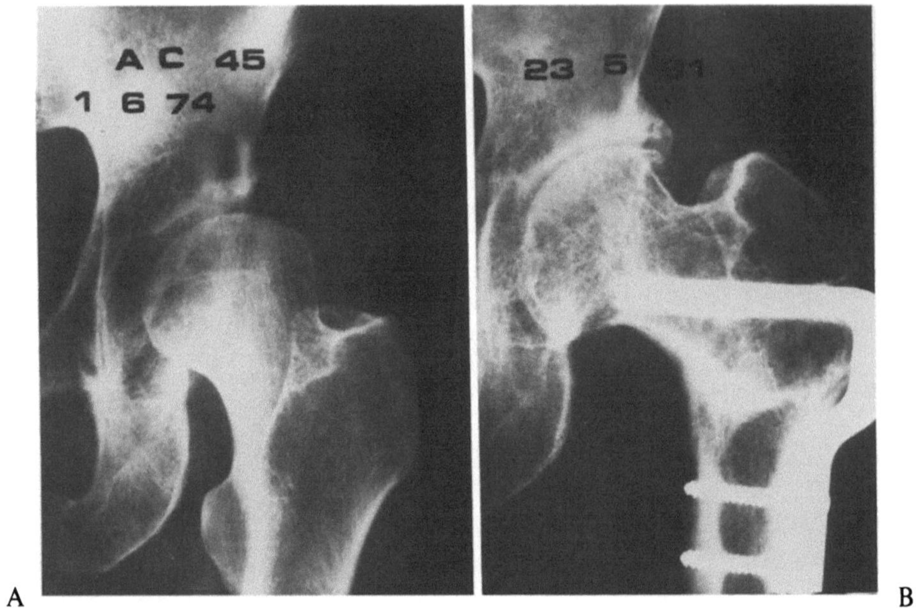

FIG. 10–36 **A** An example of an excellent case for a varus osteotomy; early disease, a spherical head, a congruent joint space and a slightly varus neck. **B** Seven years later an excellent result has been maintained.

With the use of 130° blade plates, an angle of insertion of 50σ to the shaft would result in neutral insertion of the blade plate and no net correction, as 50° is the supplementary angle of 180°. For a 20° frontal plane correction, insertion of the blade plate at 70° to the shaft results in the 20° correction once the side plate is affixed to the shaft of the femur after the osteotomy. For a 30° correction, an angle of insertion of 80° would be needed, etc.

As depicted in Figure 10–43, the triangular AO angle guides are used and the line of insertion marked out with a K-wire placed into the soft tissues anterior to the bone. In young patients and those with dense bone, predrilling with a 3.2 drill reduces the risk of inadvertent fracture.

The chisel is inserted (Fig. 10–44) laterally so that the blade resides in the inferior hemisphere of the head. It is inserted at 70° to the shaft in the anterior projection. From the lateral view, the long axis of the chisel is maintained parallel to the floor and the short axis perpendicular to the floor.

The osteotomy is performed 1.5 cm distal to

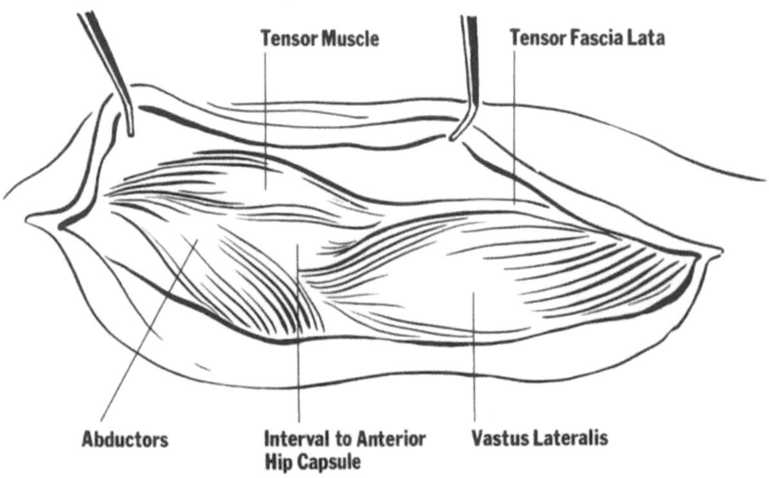

FIG. 10–37 Initial exposure for the valgus-extension osteotomy using a straight lateral inversion.

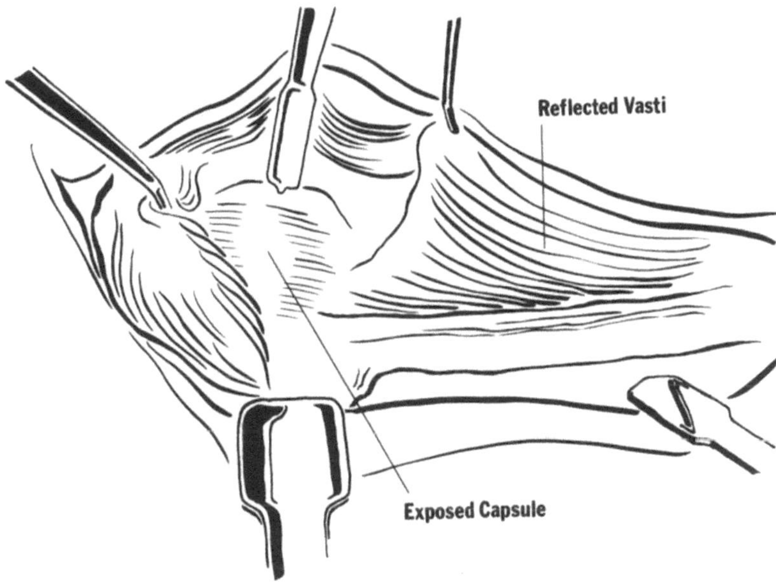

FIG. 10–38 The femur and the capsule of the hip joint are exposed. Note that a wide capsulectomy is to be performed.

the site of chisel insertion. It is important to leave adequate bone between the osteotomy site and the locus of the blade plate in order to avoid fracture at the time of interfragmentary compression (Figs. 10–45 and 10–46).

The osteotomy is done perpendicular to the long axis of the femur. Depending on the leg lengths preoperatively, a wedge may then be removed from the proximal aspect of the distal fragment. The wedge is designed to be a simultaneous closing wedge laterally and posteriorly to accommodate the dual objectives of valgus and extension and to increase the surface area of bony contact (Fig. 10–47). If rotatory correction is desired, wedges

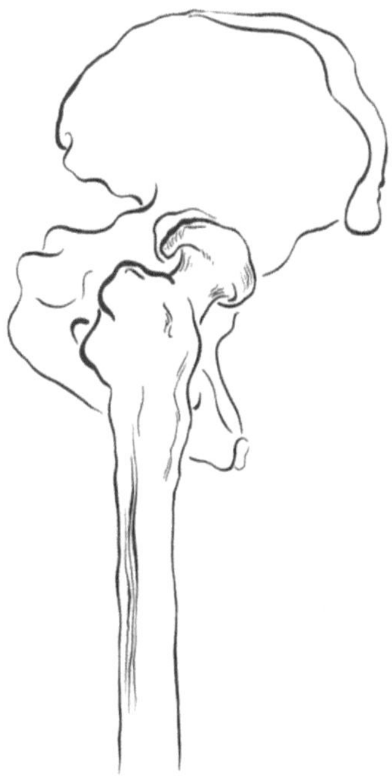

FIG. 10–39 Skeletal representation from the lateral perspective. Head is subluxating anteriorly.

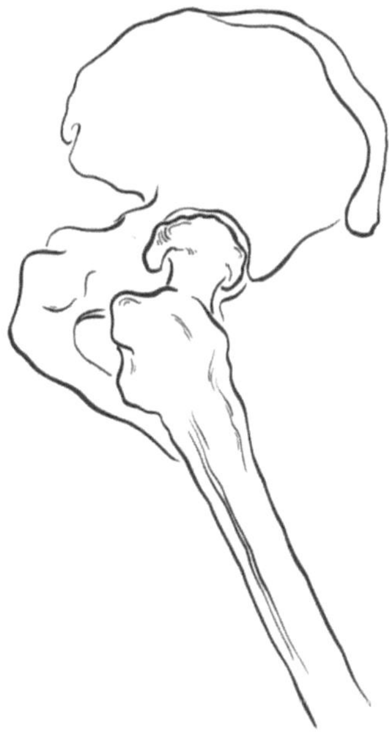

FIG. 10–40 Valgus-extension osteotomy: The hip is flexed until the head is covered anteriorly which can be seen once the thickened capsule has been excised.

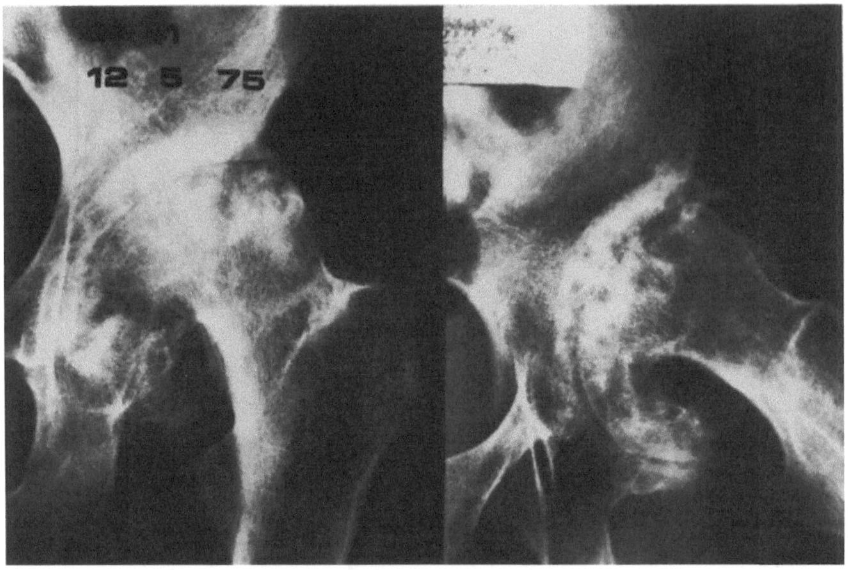

A

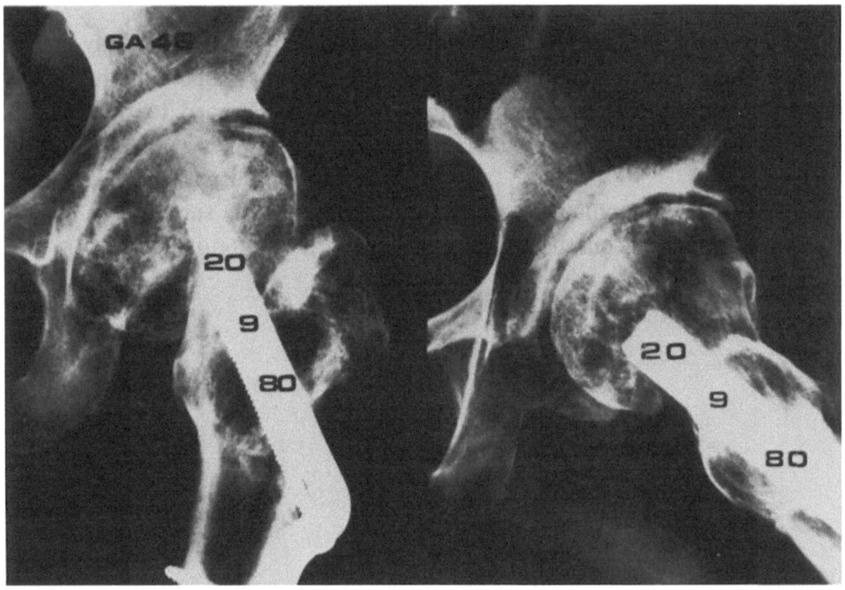

B

FIG. 10–41 **A** Preoperative x-ray of an ideal candidate for a valgus/extension osteotomy to correct an old congenital dysplasia. **B** Postoperative x-ray of same patient illustrating a healthier looking joint which is widened and smoother in contour.

should be removed after osteotomy and rotatory correction.

The blade plate is then carefully inserted into the tract of the chisel. The blade selected is deliberately longer than measured, permitting lateralization of the shaft fragment in order to avoid a valgus effect at the knee level which might otherwise result. For the purpose of engineering strength, the blade plates have an offset L-shape which tends to result in medial displacement of the distal fragment. This effect, desirable in varus osteotomies, has a potentially deleterious effect in valgus cases. An example of a medially displaced shaft due in part to blade plate design is seen in Figure 10–48. Current technique with lateralization of the shaft is seen in Figure 10–49. The iliopsoas tendon is released prior to the internal fixation (Fig. 10–50).

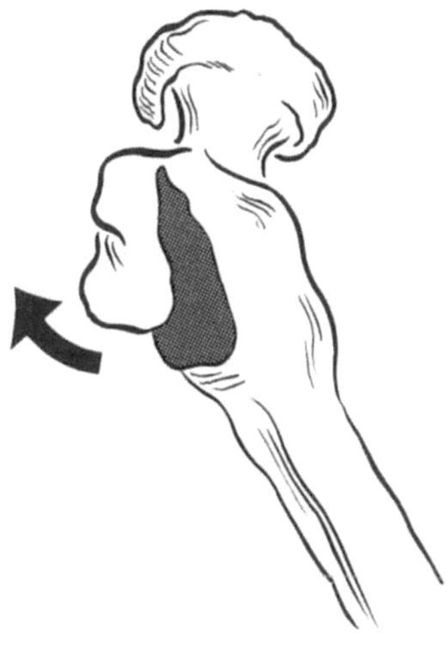

FIG. 10–42 A relaxing osteotomy of the greater trochanter is performed with care to protect the superior cortical hinge. Arrow shows the direction of the displacing the trochanter like a green stick fracture.

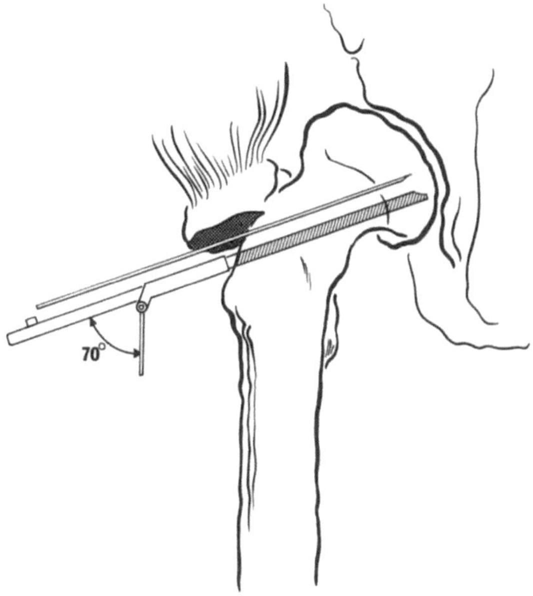

FIG. 10–44 The chisel is inserted laterally, following the final position of the guide pin.

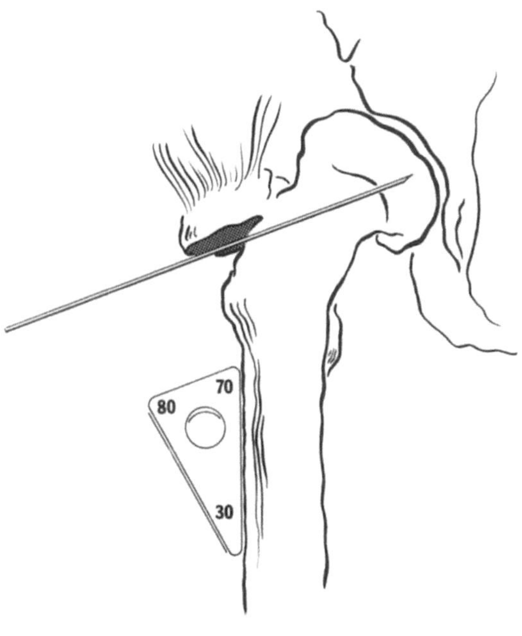

FIG. 10–43 AO angle guides are used and the line of insertion marked with a k-wire placed along the anterior femoral neck. The pin placement should be checked with an imaging x-ray.

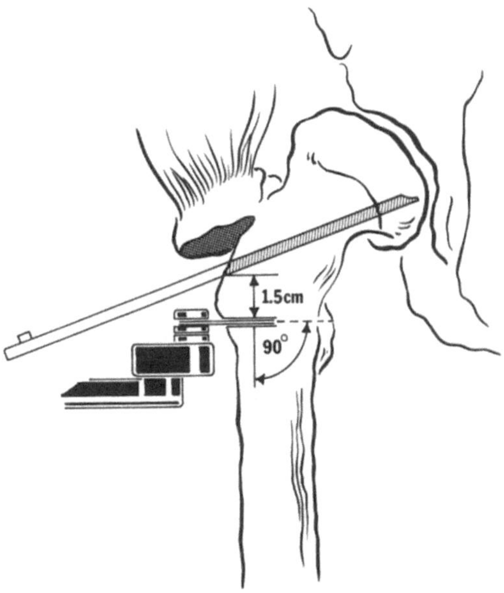

FIG. 10–45 Osteotomy is performed 1.5 cm distal to the site of chisel insertion. *The 1.5 cm space is critical for it accommodates the shoulder of the bone plate.*

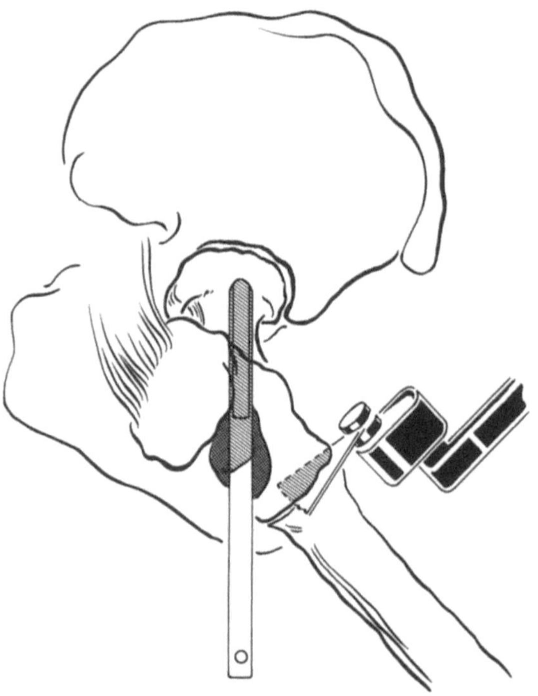

FIG. 10–46 Adequate bone is left between the osteotomy site and the blade plate as the osteotomy is completed.

The AO Compression device is used to secure compression of the fragments. Prior to full compression, the proximal screw is inserted into the proximal fragment to secure the position of the blade in the head and neck (Fig. 10–51). The distal screw is placed only through the lateral cortex to provide a transition from the rigid plate segment to the normal elastic properties of the femur.

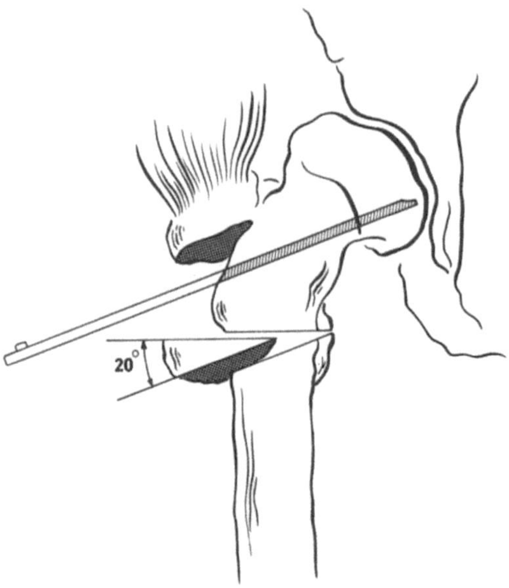

FIG. 10–47 A wedge is removed from the upper edge of the distal fragment by doing a second osteotomy.

Hemostasis is carefully controlled. The previously removed wedge is placed into the opening wedge pocket of the greater trochanter. Four or six medium suction drains are placed in the wound at various levels. The vastus lateralis is closed over

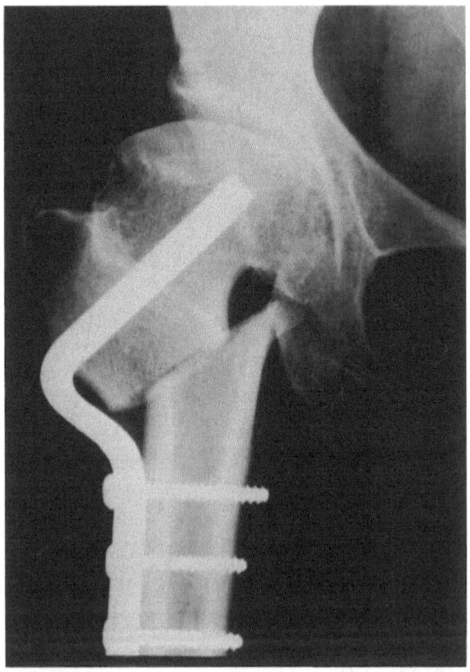

FIG. 10–48 Medially displaced shaft after wedge has been properly resected.

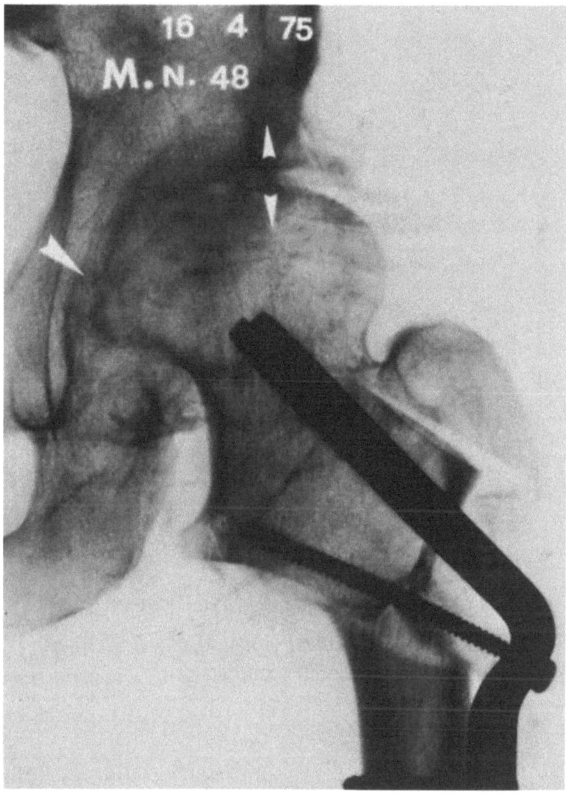

FIG. 10–49 Lateralization of the shaft should be no more than one third of the width of the shaft.

the plate. The remainder of closure is routine. The final appearance of the osteotomy prior to closure is shown in Figure 10–52.

Role of Osteotomy in Osteonecrosis

A middle-aged man engaged in heavy work for a living who has developed arthritis secondary to osteonecrosis with collapse of the femoral head is a potential candidate for an osteotomy (Fig. 10–53). The surgical management of cases such as this one represents one of the more difficult challenges in contemporary orthopedic therapy. Therapeutic options are limited. By virtue of age and activity level, the patient is not a suitable candidate for conventional total hip replacement. Ar-

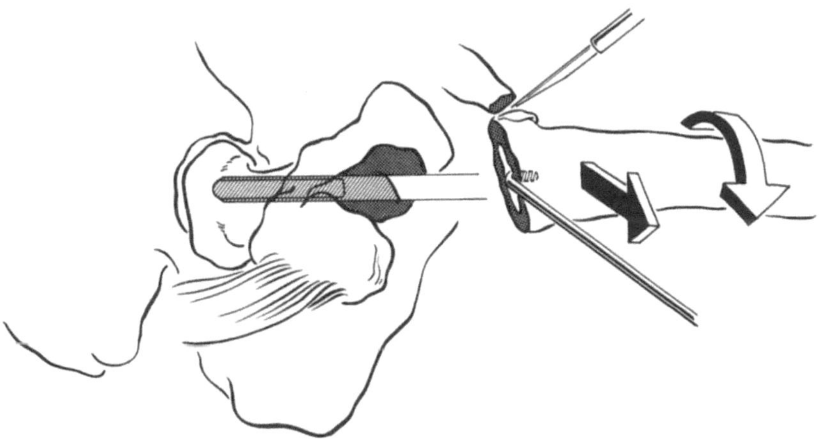

FIG. 10–50 Iliopsoas tendon is released as the shaft is pulled laterally and externally rotated.

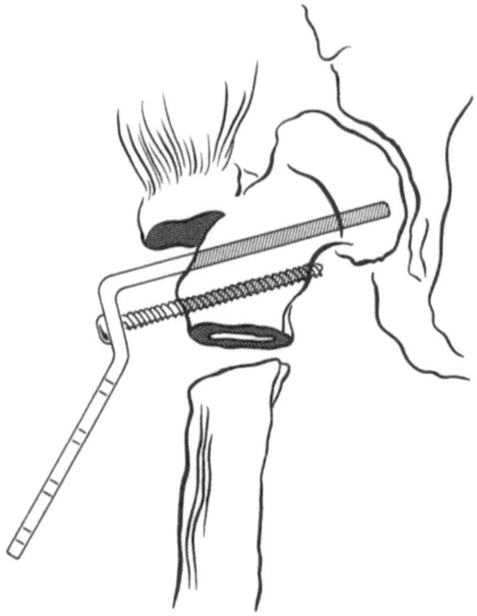

FIG. 10–51 Proximal screw is inserted into the proximal fragment for additional fixation.

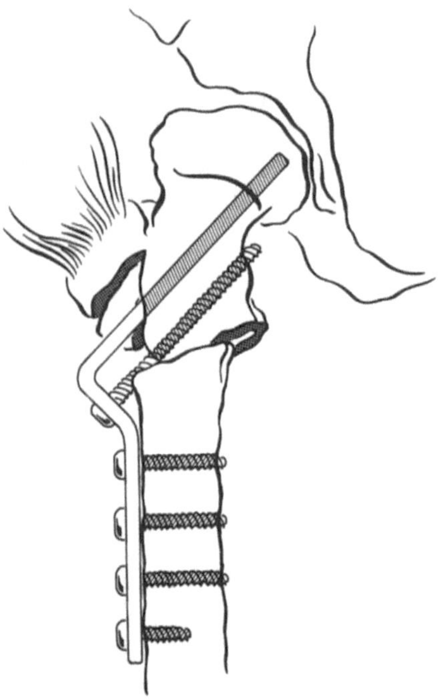

FIG. 10–52 Completed osteotomy. See Figure 10–49 for matching x ray of finished operation.

throdesis is potentially problematic in a condition which so often proves to be bilateral. As outlined before, the fact that femoral head deformity has occurred rules out the possibility of varus osteotomy or a rotational osteotomy of the Sugioka type.

In June 1976 a valgus osteotomy was performed by Bombelli with lateralization of the shaft resulting in immediate relief from pain. X-ray films from January 1978 (Fig. 10–53) and June 1982 (Fig. 10–54) are shown in which preservation of the joint space is well seen, as is partial remodeling of the femoral head. Photographs of the patient in June 1982 show the patient performing deep knee bends and wide abduction (Fig. 10–55). The patient was engaged in unrestricted work-related and recreational activities. In the difficult area of osteonecrosis of the femoral head, certainly all results cannot be expected to turn out so favorably. Once collapse of the femoral head has occurred, the paucity of viable alternatives helps to justify valgus intertrochanteric osteotomy.

The management of osteonecrosis in its earliest stages prior to collapse of the femoral head is an order of magnitude more difficult. Firstly, it is impossible to reliably predict those cases which will evolve into near-complete necrosis of the femoral head and those in which the necrotic area will be confined to a more limited geographic dimension.

Flexion osteotomy, varus osteotomy, combinations of these, core-drilling, or simple observation have all been advocated. The decision is complicated enormously by the fact that osteonecrosis is often bilateral and occurs at the time of prime economic productivity. The economic consequences of several years of diminished work capacity or complete disability can be catastrophic for both patient and family. The pressure to "do something" mounts quickly.

None of the available options are completely satisfactory. An endoprosthesis (uncemented or cemented, uni- or bipolar) or total hip replacement in a middle-aged active individual may prove to be the first act in a tragic drama which ultimately leads to multiple revisions and infection, girdlestone, or both. Thus osteotomy is not an "easy out." Though exact statistics are not yet available, results with osteotomy are less reliable than those documented for osteoarthritis. On the other hand, an osteotomy is less drastic than replacement arthroplasty for the younger patient.

Early varus osteotomy may well be followed

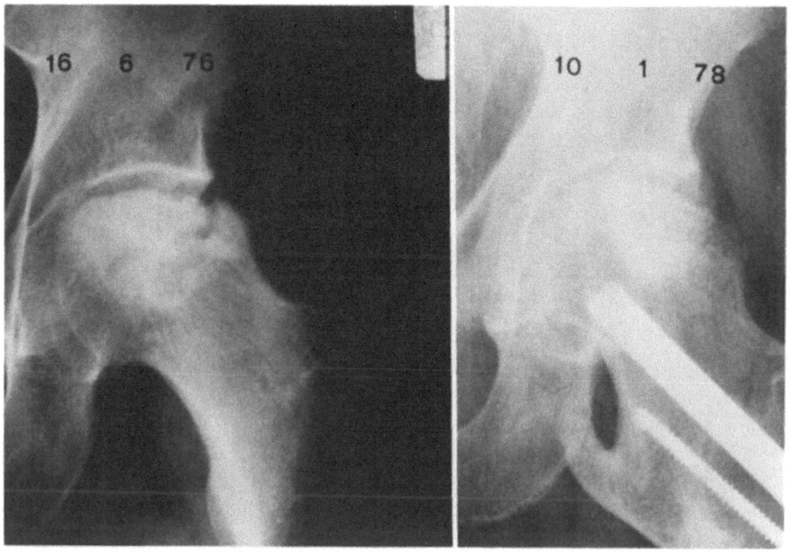

FIG. 10–53 **A** Osteonecrosis with collapse of the femoral head. **B** Seven months later after osteotomy.

by pannecrosis and collapse of the femoral head with failure due to recurrent arthritis. Varus osteotomy is a viable option in cases in which no significant collapse has occurred and the necrotic segment appears stable and limited (Fig. 10–56). European hip experts (Wagner, Morsher) are enthusiastic about biplane osteotomies in flexion and extension. Wagner[30] claimed that 85% of his patients had pain relief at a 5-year follow-up. His average realignment was 45° of flexion with 20° of valgus. The technique is demanding.

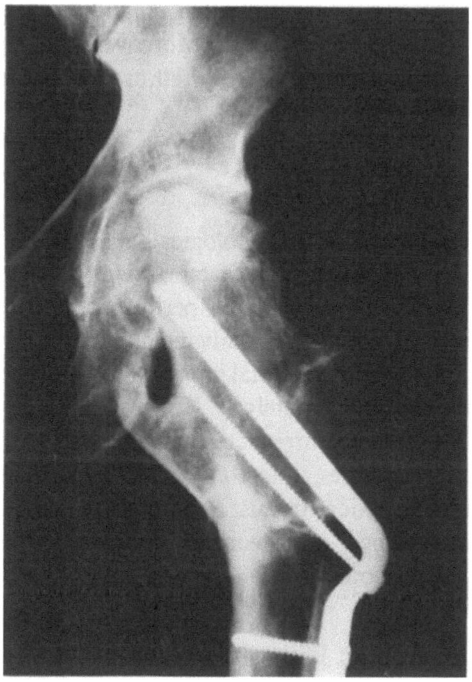

FIG. 10–54 Same patient as in Fig. 10–53, 6 years after osteotomy.

Ideally, one would want to wait for collapse, of the femoral head and development of a medial head osteophyte before proceeding with a valgus osteotomy. However, significant time may be required for this morphological evolution. Also, at the time of surgery the hip may be extremely stiff and the ability to gain motion from the osteotomy procedures is limited. Arthrodesis, in general, is untenable because of the high incidence of simultaneous or subsequent bilateral involvement.

Though conversion of a failed osteotomy to total hip replacement is possible, particularly if shaft displacement has been properly executed, it is significantly more difficult than a virgin total hip replacement. One must always view osteotomy for osteonecrosis as a possible first step in an eventual total hip replacement. Though many case histories highlight the potential advantages of osteotomy, it is by no means either a universally applicable or successful maneuver for the osteonecrotic hip, a condition difficult to successfully treat by any means.

Postoperative Management

Breathing exercises and calf exercises begin immediately after operation. Low-dose coumadin or aspirin is administered. Trunk and extremity exercises commence in bed on the first postoperative

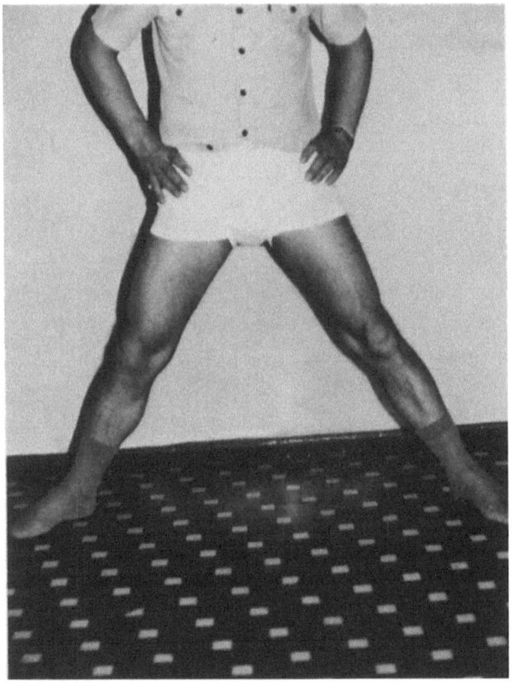

A

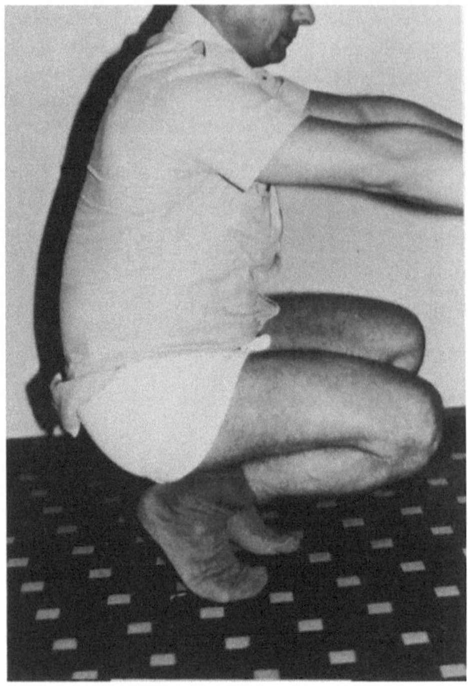

B

FIG. 10–55 A Same patient as in Fig. 10–53, 6 years after osteotomy; no pain and excellent function. B Same patient as figure 10–53. Note excellent flexion.

day and progress daily. The four to six postoperative closed suction drains are removed after 48 hours. Partial weight-bearing ambulation with a walker is normally begun by the fourth or fifth postoperative day and is progressed to partial weight-bearing ambulation with two Canadian crutches as tolerated. No passive or active assisted exercises are permitted. After independent transfers, ambulation, and stair training have been completed, patients are discharged on a program of daily active range-of-motion exercises in all planes. After 5 to 6 months patients convert to the use of one crutch for as long as it is needed.

The results of one long-term follow-up study included information about the duration of crutch support. The average time for the use of two crutches was 6.6 months. A cane or one crutch was then used for an average of 4.6 months. Thus after osteotomy gait support was required for an average of more than 11 months.

Analysis of Results of Bombelli Osteotomy

Study of the long-term results has helped to confirm the efficacy of osteotomy and to clarify the indications, both clinical and morphological. As seen in Table 10–3 after 11 years there were 19 excellent, 15 good, 7 fair, and 4 poor results among the 45 patients available for study. Seventy-five percent of patients had either a good or excellent result at the 11-year mark. Moreover, 49% of patients had a Harris score of 90 or above after 11 years.

Age

Physiological, not chronological, age is the principle consideration. Other factors being equal, osteotomy can be successfully performed in patients over the age of 60. With advancing age, the threshold for conventional total hip replacement becomes lower and appropriately so. However, in those who wish to resume unrestricted occupational or recreational activities, osteotomy offers a particularly attractive option. It must be emphasized, however, that evidence of osteopenia mitigates strongly against osteotomy.

Radiographic Patterns

Particularly suitable for osteotomy are cases in which the neck shaft angle is valgus, the femoral

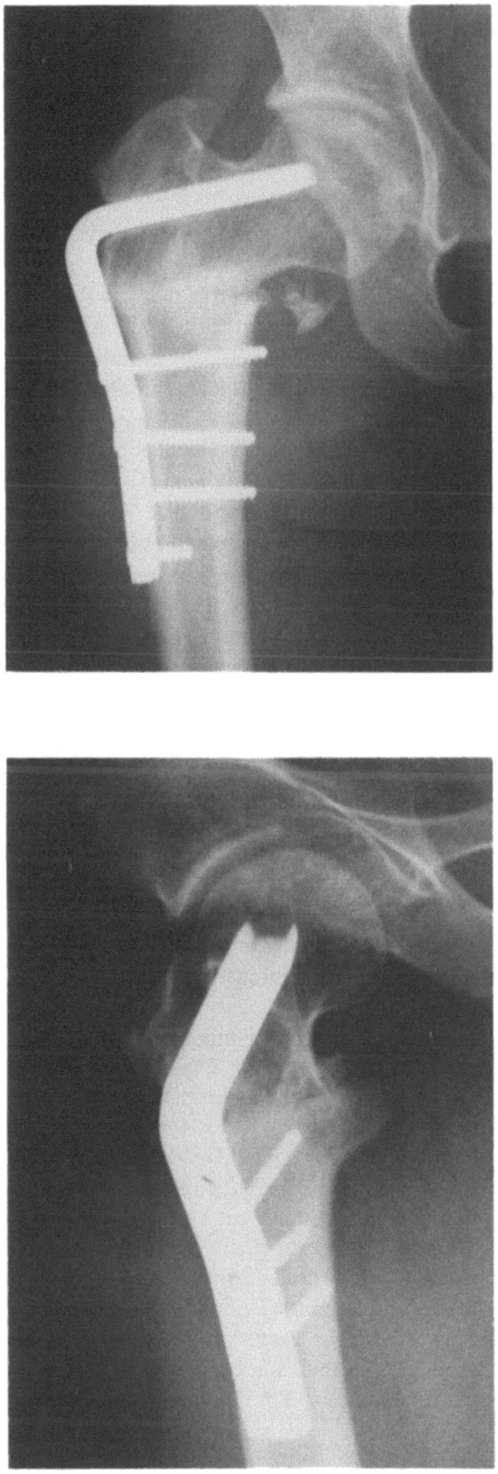

FIG. 10–56 An example of femoral head necrosis treated with a flexion/varus osteotomy. The patient was a 23-year-old female, who had sustained an undisplaced femoral neck fracture at age 11. These x-rays are 18 months later with almost complete relief of pain and early filling in of defect. Initial head sphericity was well retained. (Courtesy R. G. Tronzo.)

head spherical, and the acetabulum dysplastic superolaterally. Bombelli reported a case in which there was excellent head coverage, joint space, and resolution of sclerosis 8 years 4 months after varus osteotomy. A similar excellent result is seen in the case shown in Fig. 10–32. In our long-term follow-up study, more than 90% of patients with this morphological pattern had excellent results after 11 years.

The next most favorable subgroup is that with the combination of a mushroom-cap femoral head deformity, a large capital drop osteotphye, an early roof osteophyte, and lateral acetabular dysplasia. Seventy-five percent of patients in this subgroup had good or excellent results after 11 years.

Clinical Perspective

Osteotomy is not a procedure which, resurrected in an updated form, will or should challenge the appropriate role of conventional total hip arthroplasty in the elderly population. However, in well-selected young patients with suitable radiographic and clinical features, it represents an extremely attractive alternative to arthroplasty and complements the surgical options available to the reconstructive orthopedic surgeon. It is particularly useful as a salvage procedure for arthritis secondary to acetabular dysplasia or congenital dislocation of the hip. Relief from pain has been excellent in a high percentage of patients followed for many years. The freedom to engage in unrestricted activities after the recovery period and the substantial gain in time before the need for conversion to total hip replacement can be gratifying to surgeon and patient alike.

With regard to younger arthritic patients, the resurgence of interest in cup arthroplasty, arthrodesis, and osteotomy as true conservative procedures is justified. Younger patients with relatively small loss of motion tend to gain more motion after an osteotomy. Those with less motion either retain the same or lose a little.

References

1. Adam, A. and Spence, A. J.: Intertrochanteric osteotomy for osteoarthritis of the hip: a review of fifty-eight operations. J. Bone Joint Surg., 40-B:219–226, 1958.
2. Blount, W. P.: Proximal osteotomies of the femur. In Instructional course lectures. AAOS, 9:1–29, J. W. Edwards, Ann Arbor, 1952.

3. Bombelli, R.: Osteoarthritis of the hip, pathogenesis and consequent therapy. Springer Verlag, Berlin, 1976.
4. Burrows, H. J., Murley, A. H. and Shephard, E.: Displacement oseotomy for osteoarthritis of the hip: results more than twenty years later. J. Bone Joint Surg., 37-B:158, 1955.
5. Campbell, J. P. and Jackson, J. P.: The treatment of osteoarthritis of the hip by osteotomy. In proceedings of the British Orthopaedic Assoc. J. Bone Joint Surg., 37-B:167–8, 1955.
6. Chandler, H. P., Reneck, T., Wixson, R. L. and McCarthy, J. C.: Total hip replacement in patients younger than thirty years. J. Bone Joint Surg., 63-A:1426–34.
7. Detenbeck, L. C., Coventry, M. B. and Kelly, P. J.: Intertrochanteric osteotomy for degenerative arthritis of the hip., Clin. Ortho. Rel. Res., No. 86, July-Aug., 1972.
8. Ferguson, A. B., Jr.: The pathological changes in degenerative arthritis of the hip and treatment by rotational osteotomy. J. Bone Joint Surg., 46-A:1337–52, 1964.
9. Gudmundsson, G.: Intertrochanteric displacement osteotomy for painful osteoarthritis of the hip. Acta Orthop. Scand., 41:91, 1970.
10. Harris, W. H.: Role of intertrochanteric osteotomy in the treatment of arthritis of the hip. Surg. Cl. N.A., 49:4, 1969.
11. Harris, N. H. and Kirwan, E.: the results of osteotomy for early primary osteoarthritis of the hip. J. Bone Joint Surg., 46-B:477, 1964.
12. Kirmission, E.: De l'ostéotomie sous-troch-anterienne appliqué à certains cas de luxation congenitale de la hanche., Rev. d'Orthip., 5:137–46, 1894.
13. Lorenz, A.: Über die Behandlung der irreponiblen angeborënen Hüftluxation und der Schenkelhals-pseudarthrosen mittels Gabelung (Bifurkation des oberen Femurendes). Wiener Klinische Wochenschrift, 32:997, 1919.
14. Malkin, S.: Femoral osteotomy in the treatment of osteoarthritis of the hip. Br. Med. J., 1:304–5, 1936.
15. Maquet, P.: A biomechanical approach to the surgical treatment of osteoarthritis of the hip. Rev. Med. Liege, 24:146–169, 1969.
16. McMurray, T. P.: Osteoarthritis of the hip joint. Br. J. Surg., 22:716, 1935.
17. Müller, M. E.: Intertrochanteric osteotomy in the treatment of the arthritic hip joint. In Surgery of the Hip Joint, Lea & Febiger, Chapter 22, Philadelphia, 1973.
18. Müller, M. E.: Die hüftnahen Femurosteotomien, Stuttgart. Thieme Verlag, 1971.
19. Ottolenghi, C. E., Napolitano, M. F., Frigerio, E. and deNapolitano, N. B.: Effects of intertrochanteric osteotomy on the hip joint. Clin. Orthop., 39:157, 1965.
20. Pauwels, F.: The place of osteotomy in the operative management of osteoarthritis of the hip. Triangle, 8(6):196–210, 1968.
21. Pauwels, F.: Neue Richtlinien für die operative Behandlung der Koxarthrose, F. Enke Verlag, 1935.
22. Pauwels, F.: Basis and results of etiological therapy of osteoarthritis of the hip joint. In Neuviéme congrés de la société internationale de chirurgie orthopèdeque et de traumatologie (Vienne, September 1–7, 1963), Vol. 2, Vienna, Verlag der Wiener Medizinischen Akademie, pp. E31-E50; T51-T84, 1965.
23. Putti, V.: L'ostéotomie intertrochanterienne dans le traitement des pseudarthroses du col du femur. Presse méd., 101:1841, 1937.
24. Schanz, A.: Zur Behandlung der veralteten angeborenene Hüftverrenkung. Múnchener medizinische Wochenschrift, 69:930, 1922.
25. Schanz, A.: Über die nach Schenkelhalsbrüchen zurückbleibenden Gehstörungen. Duetsche medizinische Wochenschrift, 51:730, 1925.
26. Von Baeyer, H.: Operative Behandlung von nicht reponierbaren angeborenen Hüftverenkungen. Münchener medizinische Wochenschrift, 65:1218, 1918.
27. Pauwels, F.: Atlas of biomechanics of the healthy and diseased hip. Berlin, Springer Verlag, 1975.
28. Osbourne, G. V. and Fahrni, W. H.: Oblique displacement osteotomy for osteoarthritis of the hip. J. Bone Joint Surg. 32-B:148–160, 1950.
29. Bombelli, R.: Oseoarthritis of the hip, second edition, Heidelberg, Springer Verlag, 1983.
30. Wagner, H.: Intertrochanteric osteotomy for treatment of femoral head necrosis. Symposium on upper femoral osteotomies, Boston, 1956.
31. Poss, R.: Valgus/extension osteotomy for primary protrusio acetabuli and coxa vara. Strategies in Orthopedic Surgery. Vol. 5, No. 2, May 1986.

CHAPTER 11

Hip Arthrodesis

B. G. WEBER

Until 20 years ago, hip arthrodesis (HA), intertrochanteric osteotomies, and arthroplasties (Smith-Petersen) were standard procedures for the treatment of osteoarthritis of the hip joint. The use of arthroplasty got a tremendous boost during the early 1960s owing to Charnley's total hip replacement (THR), which has since become "the hip operation" throughout the world. With the good results obtained with THR, osteotomies, HA, and other arthroplasties have lost their attraction, and HA is today an almost forgotten operation. At the recent 1984 Perkins Memorial Symposium in London, for example, only 10 of the 180 attending orthopedic surgeons had done an HA themselves. This observation is typical for today's training of orthopedic surgeons.

The interest in other surgical treatments of the painful hip seems to have increased again, because THR lack long-term durability. The author has been asked many times recently to bring HA back into the orthopedic mind. The conclusions at all three recent meetings were the same:

1. THR is not the operation of choice for young patients.
2. Osteotomies of the proximal femur and of the pelvis do have a place in young patients with an osteoarthritic hip.
3. HA offers the most reliable results but is least accepted by the patients because its reputation is poor.

It is the task of this chapter to reshape the reputation of HA because THR is, by far, not able to fulfill all the needs in hip surgery.

History of HA

The first HAs were described by Albert (1882), Heusner (1884), Lampugnani (1885), Daraignez (1891), Dollinger (1891), Lagrange (1892), and von Winiwater (1895). Albee is supposed to have done the first HA in the United States in 1908. All these HAs were of the *intraarticular* type, requiring prolonged plaster fixation and bed rest.

The first *extraarticular* HAs for tuberculosis were done by Wilson (1927, 1933) and Albee (1929) using iliofemoral bone grafts. For the same purpose, the ischiofemoral graft was recommended by Trumble (1931–32), used in a modified technique by Maragliano (1969), and used with a subtrochanteric osteotomy by Brittain (1952). The nailing of a denuded hip joint to obtain fusion has been stressed by Watson-Jones (1938), Burns (1939), Van Ness (1939).

The value of the HA for certain conditions is generally accepted. However, three major difficulties call its reputation into disfavor: (1) too high a rate of nonunion; (2) the necessity of plaster fixation and bed rest; and (3) frequent disability from immobilization.

Various ideas have been proposed to prevent nonunion. Davis (1954) used a pedicle iliofemoral bone graft to preserve circulation. Apley and Denham (1955), after nailing the denuded hip joint, completed their operation with a subtrochanteric osteotomy, the lever arm of the leg then no longer transmitting disturbing mobility to the HA itself. Cattaneo (1959) tried double grafting: an iliofemoral and transarticular tibial graft.

Other techniques attempted to stabilize the fusion in order to obviate the need for external immobilization. Charnley (1953, 1955) increased bony contact and stability by creating a central dislocation, which was then fixed by a compression screw parallel to the femoral neck. Alvik (1962, 1963) stabilized the denuded hip joint with a long Smith-Petersen nail and a powerful plate and screws. Küntscher (1953), May and Manuck (1962), Dwyer and Cass (1961), Dwyer (1964), and Onji et al. (1965) used a Küntscher nail, running down from the iliac crest to the femoral shaft. Müller (1967) innovated a method of hip fusion utilizing compression with double plates. To increase the contact of bone, he described a transverse osteotomy of the pelvis similar to the Chiari procedure. Teinturier (1966) exerted compression between the fragments with an ASIF system but added a pedicle iliofemoral graft of the greater trochanter. Gertsch (1966), Dreyer and Pingel (1969), and Wiedmer (1969) published the technique and results of hip fusion with the so-called cobra-head compression plate, which was developed by Schneider as a refinement of Müller's double-plated fusion combined with a pelvic osteotomy.

The history of HA ends with a distinct tendency to use some form of internal fixation in order to avoid plaster fixation, which frequently causes unnecessary stiffness of at least one knee (on the fused side). A successful HA must (1) have a wide contact area of raw bone, (2) have sufficiently strong stabilization of the bony components, and (3) permit almost immediate ambulation.

Since the early 1960s there have been thousands of publications on THR. Discussion is still open on the problem of anchorage and materials. In contrast, there have been only a small number of reports on HAs over the last 12 to 15 years: Carter and Wickstrom (1971), Hauge (1973), Weber (1973), Liechti (1974), Gore (1975), Ramadier and Lecestre (1976), Fulkerson (1977), Liechti (1978, 1983), and Sponsell et al. (1984).

All authors agree that HA has a place in hip surgery. There were no descriptions in the literature of hip fusion after THR, which could be desirable after failed arthroplasty. On the other hand, the conversion of HA to a THR is well known to every surgeon doing THRs: Brewster et al. (1975), Hardinge et al. (1977), Lubahn et al. (1980), and Courpied et al. (1981).

Sponsell et al. (1984) reviewed the history of 53 patients who had had a HA longer than 20 years and were younger than 35 years at the time of the operation. They expressed what the younger orthopedic surgeons should know: "Until improved technology allows a more durable THR, particularly in patients who are less than 35 years old, the results of this study indicate that arthrodesis may be far superior to arthroplasty on young patients."

However, as early as 1963 Alvik summarized his ideas on Arthrodesis and arthroplasty of the hip joint:

> From 1943 till 1960, 360 hip joints with osteoarthritis, severe posttraumatic conditions, and congenital dislocations (adults) were operated upon, the procedure being arthrodesis or some type of other arthroplasty. Osteoarthritis has been the main indication for surgery. The result after arthrodesis is far superior to arthroplasty. . . . The treatment of choice of severe disabling bilateral hip lesions is arthrodesis on the one side and arthroplasty on the other. . . . Persistent low back pain after hip arthrodesis is not common providing the ancylotic hip has a functional good position giving the spine a good alignment. . . . An osteochondrotic lumbar spine is no contraindication for hip arthrodesis providing a good alignment of the spine follows after the fusion. . . .

It is the task of this chapter to direct attention to one of the several alternatives to THR: HA. It will become evident that there are still clear-cut indications for the "forgotten hip operation."

HA in Relation to Other Hip Surgery

Material 1961 to 1971

Since the introduction of THR at the Department of Orthopedic Surgery of the Kantonsspital St. Gallen in 1961, the number of hip osteotomies and especially of HAs has dramatically decreased (see Graph 11–1). From 1961 to 1983, there were 745 HAs performed, though only a few during the latter of those years. In 1983, there were 187 THRs, 24 osteotomies, and 5 HAs done for the treatment of osteoarthritis of the hip in adults. Three publications were based on our HA experience:

Weber (1973): 111 patients from 1967 to 1969 with a follow-up of 111

Liechti (1974) and its translation into English (Liechti, 1978): 583 patients from 1961 to 1971 with a follow-up of 300

Liechti (1983): A redo study with an expanded number of patients from 1961 to 1980, i.e., 672 with a follow-up of 400

General Experience with HA

The outcome of these three studies are identical, the only difference being the number of operations, i.e., patients being included. The general experience with HA can be summarized as follows:

1. Patients with HA are mostly pleased and satisfied (85%) with the result over 10 and 20 years (and probably longer).
2. A good HA on one side with no serious involvement of the other lower limb joints allows an almost normal life with regard to walking, sports, and working.
3. Low back problems are no contraindication to a HA; on the contrary, low back pain may be improved with a HA in a good position.
4. There is no age limit for HA. Elderly patients with a painful, almost stiff hip are accustomed to stiffness and do not suffer from stiffness after HA. They are, however, delighted because of permanent relief of pain after HA.
5. A HA is best in the presence of a normal hip on the other side, but it is also compatible with a good result of an osteotomy or a THR.
6. Absolute contraindications of HA are a stiff ipsilateral knee, a stiff contralateral hip, and severe low back problem.
7. HA does not cause severe difficulty with sexual mechanics.
8. The HA operation is far more difficult to perform than THR.

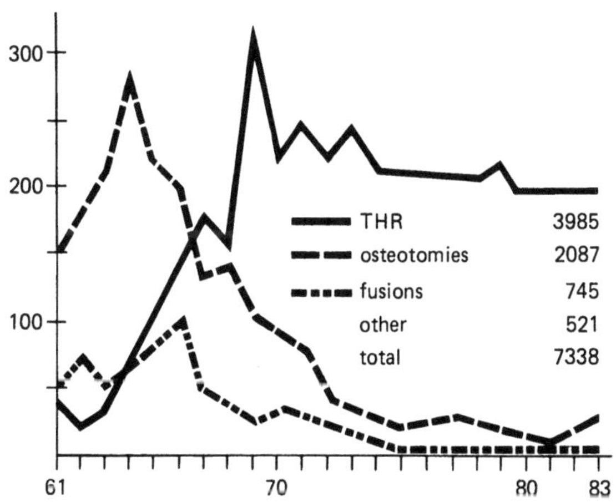

GRAPH 11–1 Hip surgery at St. Gallen, 1961–1983.

HA from 1972 to 1981 (Unpublished Results)

In view of the reborn interest for HA, the 82 patients' histories with hip fusions of the years 1972 to 1981 had been reviewed in 1983 by myself and Nittner, registrar at our department. The questions are: What are the indications, i.e., is there still a place for HA today? What were the results? Which techniques were used for HA?

Available Data The case histories and x-ray films of all 82 patients were examined.

Patients with HA	82
Dead at time of study	14
Lost to follow-up	14
Personal follow-up	54

General Data The general data look much the same as the data of our former studies.

Women	28
Men	54
Age 28–78	45 years
Bilateral disease	18
Body weight	73 kg
Body height	170 cm

There is no upper age limit for HA, i.e., for an old patient with an almost stiff and painful hip. Bilateral disease is no contraindication to HA if the opposite hip has few symptoms or has been successfully treated with osteotomy or THR. The body size of the HA patients were average. Very tall patients and obese patients have poorer results than small and light patients.

Primary osteoarthritis or idiopathic necrosis	40	75%
Secondary osteoarthritis: CDH, Perthes', epiphysiolysis	21	
Posttraumatic osteoarthritis	14	17%
Septic hip	6	8%
Tuberculosis	1	

Degenerative hip disease is by far still the most frequent indication for HA. It is, however, the number of HAs which have decreased in favor of THR. A review of the individual cases is revealing: today HA is restricted to patients who cannot expect a good and long-lasting result from an osteotomy or THR, or in whom a THR would be contraindicated. Such contraindications are: (1) an age younger than 60 years; (2) physically very active patients, i.e., farmers, heavy laborers; (3) local conditions poor for anchoring the THR components; and (4) infection.

Operations Prior to HA Some patients had had previous surgery.

Osteotomy	12	
Fracture nailing	12	
Slipped epiphysis fixation	2	33%
Infection drainage after hematogenous coxitis	1	
No surgery	55	67%

The decision for HA was made in one-third of the cases after failure of a previous treatment and in two-thirds according to the indications listed above.

Reoperations after HA The 41% rate of reoperations after HA was high. Not counting those with removal of metal, every third patient underwent a second operation.

For nonunion	14	17%	
Alignment–osteotomy	6	6%	28%
For fracture of the femur	4	5%	
Metal removal	11		13%
Total	34		41%

The rate of *nonunions* (all have been reoperated with rigid plating, some with additional graft) was higher in the present series than previously. In the first series of 111 HAs, only eight nonunions had occurred that required surgery (7%). The explanation for this is that today HA is used mainly for problem cases, whereas in previous series it was used for "easy" cases. Another point is that because of the small number of fusions the young orthopedic surgeon lacks training with this operation, which results in poor technique and nonunion.

Alignment osteotomies are necessary in cases of HA with an unfavorable position of the leg—a position other than 20° of hip flexion, 0° to 5° adduction, and 0° to 15° of external rotation. To attain that position, an intertrochanteric osteotomy with rigid plate fixation may be indicated. In case of genu valgum—not an infrequent occurrence after HA—a supracondylar varus osteotomy with plate fixation is indicated.

In young patients *metal removal* makes sense in order to reduce the risk of fatigue fracture of the femur at the lower end of an HA plate. Fatigue fractures (stress concentrating fractures) at the lower plate end have been successfully treated by another laterally applied plate, bridging the fracture.

Results of 54 HAs from 1972 to 1981

As mentioned, among the earlier series of 82 HAs, 54 patients were available for follow-up 3 to 12 years after fusion. Of these, 53 patients did not ask for "more" surgery in relation to their HAs at the time of follow-up; one patient suffered pain from a nonunion.

Subjective Rating of the Results It is almost unbelievable that patients with HAs are practically without exception satisfied by the result.

Very satisfied	47	(87%)
Satisfied	6	(11%)
Not satisfied	1	(2%)

This fact was also true in our previous series, which had almost the same rate, thereby qualifying HA against other procedures very positively.

Walking Capacity The results of the HAs in terms of walking ability are as follows:

Unlimited	34	(63%)
More than 1 km	19	(35%)
Less than 1 km	1	(2%)

The patient's walking capacity does not depend on the HA but on the other hip, the knee joints, the feet, and occasionally on the problem of low back pain. All our patients with limited walking capacity were afflicted with one or more such additional pathological findings.

Use of a Cane The use of a cane is an indication not of the HA result but of additional problems which require "manual" assistance for walking.

No cane	39	(72%)
One cane	12	(12.5%)
Two canes	3	(5.5%)

Limited walking capacity and the use of a cane are not determined by the HA. Patients with HA and sound or symptom-free other joints and low back are able to perform sports activities such as hiking, skiing (alpine or cross country), swimming, and tennis.

Pain after HA No sound HA caused pain.

None	32	(60%)
Moderate	18	(33%)
Strong	4	(7%)

Pain from other sources, however, limited the physical activity and often required the use of a cane.

Pain Localization

Opposite hip	10	(18%)
Ipsilateral knee	6	(11%)
Contralateral knee	2	(4%)
Low back	4	(7%)

Most frequently it is the opposite hip that impairs the patient's well-being and physical activity. With bilateral degenerative hip disease, the opposite hip may not yet be treated, or after treatment the patient may not be free of symptoms. The same may be true for the knee joints and the back problem. HA must therefore always be considered with regard to the whole patient.

Opposite Hip Joint Of the 54 patients, 44 had no pain from the opposite hip joint, 10 patients suffered pain, and 3 of them asked for surgery in the near future: one for a loose THR and two for THR.

Mild osteoarthritis	3	10	(18%)
Moderate osteoarthritis	4		
Severe osteoarthritis	2		
THR with pain	1		
THR without pain	7	44	(82%)
Normal hip	37		

Low Back Pain The experience with low back pain and HA is remarkable but fits exactly with the statement of Alvik (1963). Low back pain may be improved after HA when a severe limping hyperlordosis—scoliosis of the lumbar spine, leg length—discrepancy is corrected with the HA.

No back pain preop.	37
No back pain postop.	33
= Back pain after HA	4
Back pain preop.	17
Back pain postop.	6
= Improved	11
No back pain preop.	37
No back pain postop.	44

As in our previous series, there are fewer patients with low back problems after HA than before HA. Low back pain, however, may be persistent and not tolerated such that the HA must be reduced to a THR. We had five cases in 20 years, but only two patients were subjectively pleased despite a radiologically good THR in all five instances. In three patients the back problem did not improve. The regained joint mobility of about 40° was rather disappointing for all five patients and did not improve their physical capacity as they had expected.

Techniques for HA

It must be emphasized that HA is a difficult surgical procedure. However, the patient's risk is small in the hands of an expert. Our standard methods and some possible techniques for extraordinary problems are described below. The technique must be selected according to the particular case.

Anesthesia, Position Mostly peridural and occasionally general anesthesia with intubation is utilized. Four or five bottles of blood must be available. The patient lies on his or her back on a common operating table. Beginning at the navel distally, the abdomen, pelvic area, and both legs are disinfected and covered with plastic drapes. This is the best method to obtain the right position for an HA.

Exposure The lateral approach (Fig. 11–1) is used for all types of HA. An incision is made over the greater trochanter more or less upward and downward, splitting the fascia and freeing the capsule between the tensor fasciae latae and the gluteus medius. The gluteus minimus and gluteus

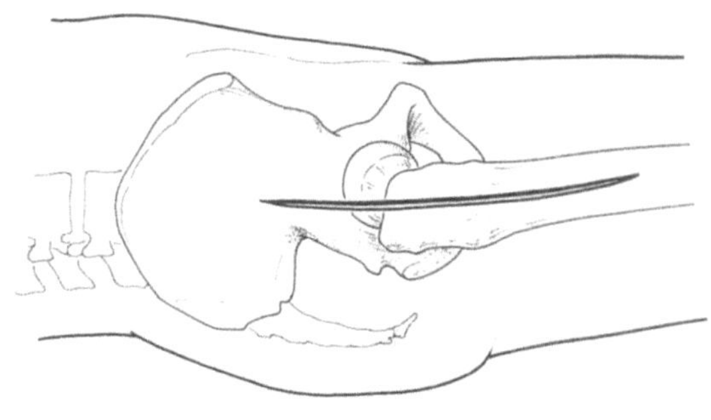

FIG. 11–1 Skin incision. Patient is supine on an ordinary operating table, both legs draped, both iliac crests and spines exposed for axial assessment. A straight incision is made, more or less extending over the greater trochanter, depending on the technique of fusion to be used.

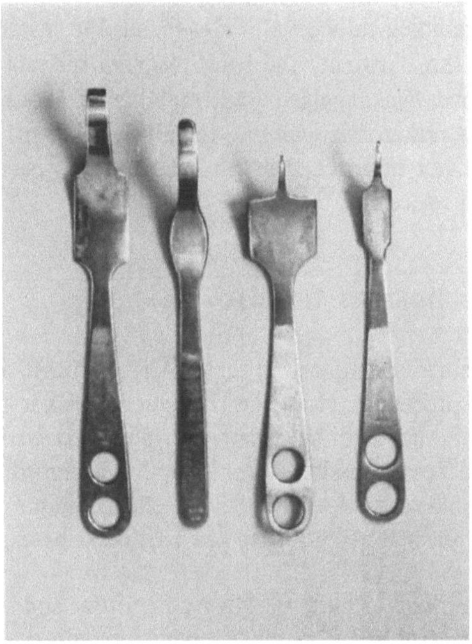

FIG. 11–2 Hohmann retractors. These four retractors from the ASIF instrumentarium are essential for hip fusions.

medius are detached from the greater trochanter and along the capsule to the acetabulum. The laterosuperior aspect of the acetabular roof and the adjacent ilium are denuded. The proximal vastus lateralis is dissected and detached along the linea aspera after ligating the perforating vessels. Hohmann retractors are inserted (Fig. 11–2). A large Hohmann retractor over the eminentia iliopectinea between the pelvis and iliacus muscle protects the pelvic contents. A smaller retractor through the sciatic notch meets the large retractor. A further Hohmann retractor with its apex set in the ala iliaca keeps the pelvitrochanteric musculature off the acetabular roof. A fourth retractor keeps off the vastus fibularis ventral to the femur (Fig. 11–3).

Pelvic Osteotomy

Technique The capsule is partially resected cranially. The top of the femoral head is removed with a large flat osteotome. The acetabular roof is now visible. A transverse pelvic osteotomy is done 1 cm above, crossing the roof. The osteotomy is performed in small steps with osteotomes and the oscillating saw. It must be horizontal or, better, angled slightly downward 5° to 10°. The plane of bone contact between the femoral head and the ilium is perpendicular to the load axis, providing optimal stability and sound union. A disc of pelvic bone is removed step by step until the internal cortex, still protected by the two main Hohmann retractors, becomes visible. To facilitate removal of the bony slice, a spreader is used to open the osteotomy gap (Fig. 11–4). The medial cortex is divided step by step with a small chisel. Done this way, the pelvic osteotomy is free of any risk. After the slice is completely removed, the osteotomy surfaces of acetabular roof and femoral head fall together. To improve bony contact, medial displacement of the femoral head is sometimes necessary. With a suitable lever (we use a so-called coachwork lever) the desired medial displacement is obtained. The distal pelvic fragment is rotated at the symphysis (Fig. 11–4). The limb is now placed in its final position (see below). The osteotomy surfaces should be exactly parallel. If not, a small resection of the femoral head may be needed to make them so. The osteotomy planes must be more concave than convex to provide optimal stability and to prevent rocking. Such mechanical stability of the pelvic osteotomy, i.e., of the ilium and the femoral head, makes additional bone grafting unnecessary. The fixation of the femoral head and ilium is variable, depending on the type of HA (see below). The remaining steps in the procedure follow the usual routine.

Wound Closure The operative field is washed with Ringer's solution. Two deep vacuum drains and two subcutaneous drains keep the operative field dry. Most important is a reliable suture of the pelvitrochanteric muscles to the vastus lateralis muscle, which is fastened to the tendon of the gluteus maximus (Fig. 11–5). Closure of fascia and skin is done in layers. The drains are removed after 48 hours and the stitches after 14 days.

Various HA Techniques

The choice of one or the other technique for HA is not a question of the preference of the surgeon. The decision must be made according to the given anatomical situation.

To master the problems of HA, a single operative technique is not enough—though the cobrahead plate technique (type III) is the technique of choice in three of four cases. However, it is the one of four cases which presents the real chal-

FIG. 11–3 Exposure of the hip joint. **A** The detached muscles are reflected. Two Hohmann retractors "embrace" the osteotomy level; one large Hohmann retractor exposes the adjacent ilium. **B** and **C** The two Hohmann retractors, inserted with bony contact, meet in the sciatic notch and protect the pelvic contents and the sciatic nerve.

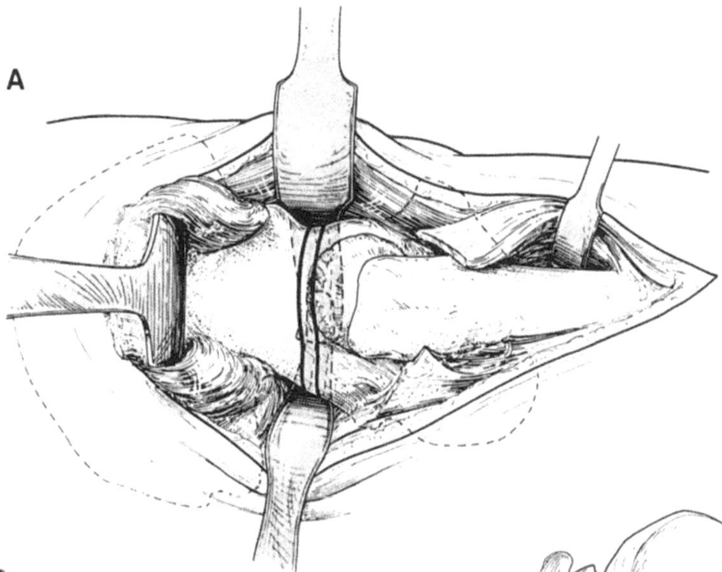

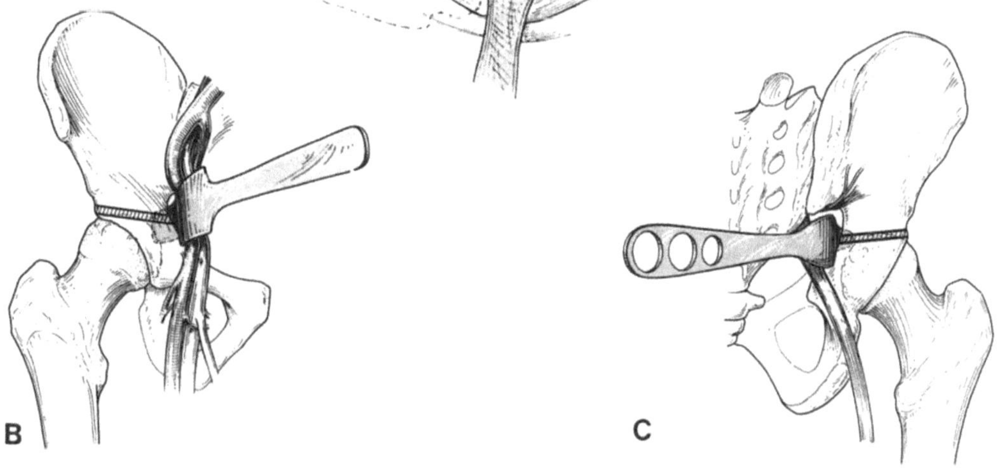

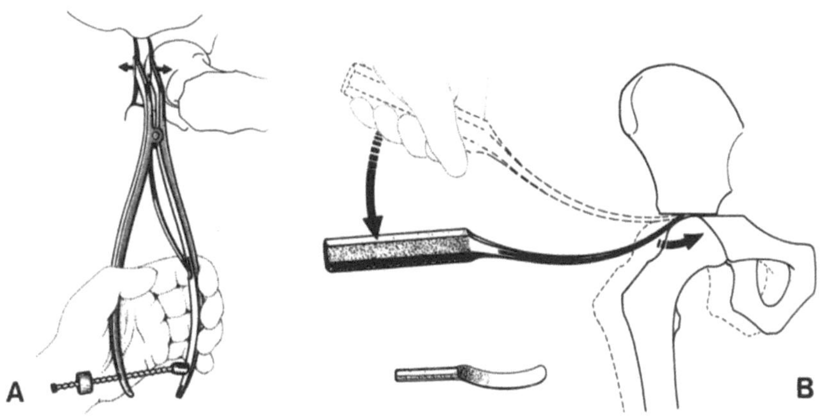

FIG. 11–4 Instruments helpful for pelvic osteotomy. **A** The spreader (seen from the side of the patient) is inserted and expanded in the osteotomy; it prevents the femoral head from approximating the ilium during removal of the bony slice from the joint. **B** The heavy lever (seen from the front of the patient) is inserted into the completed osteotomy, making medial displacement easy, though the pelvis–symphysis may be "hard."

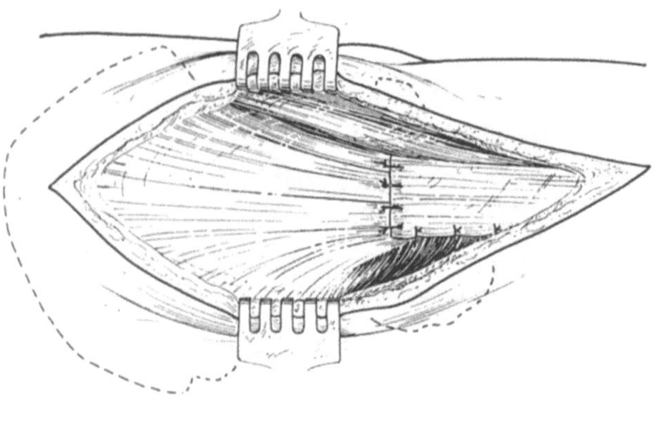

FIG. 11–5 Closure of the deep wound. The reflected muscles fall back. They are sewed up in their natural relation to each other.

lenge of HA. For this case the surgeon must be especially skilled and experienced, but where is this experience to come from at a time when HA is unknown to the majority of the younger teachers in orthopedic surgery?

Standardized HA techniques (types I, II, and III) are described in the following sections, and clinical examples are given for the atypical fusion (type IV).

HA Type I

Technique The greater trochanter is osteotomized, and the femoral neck and acetabular roof are smoothed with a curved osteotome. A pelvic osteotomy, as described, is performed to contact the two denuded osteotomy planes of the femoral head and the ilium (Fig. 11–6). The greater trochanter is prepared as a free graft, fitting onto the osteotomy as an iliofemoral bridge. This graft is then fixed to the ilium with a lag screw securing the medial displacement in the osteotomy and maintaining the valgus position of the femoral neck.

For type I HA, the vastus lateralis muscle is not detached, although it must be split. Between two slim Hohmann retractors, the femur is exposed at the intertrochanteric region. A transverse osteotomy with the oscillating saw is performed to permit free mobility of the distal fragment, preventing stress transmission at the iliofemoral junction.

Postoperative Treatment A below-knee plaster is applied to both legs. A cross bar connecting the two legs in slight abduction maintains neutral rotation. A generous slot over the fibula should be cut to prevent peroneal nerve palsy. The patient, with relative fixation, is kept in bed for 2 weeks. The plaster boots are removed under general anesthesia, and a hip spica, including the operated side, is applied. The hip joint is adjusted to increase abduction by 10°. The ideal functional neutral position is established spontaneously within the spica by loss of 10° of abduction. Over the next few days the patient, with the hip spica ending above the ankle, starts ambulating with crutches. Four weeks after the operation the hip spica is

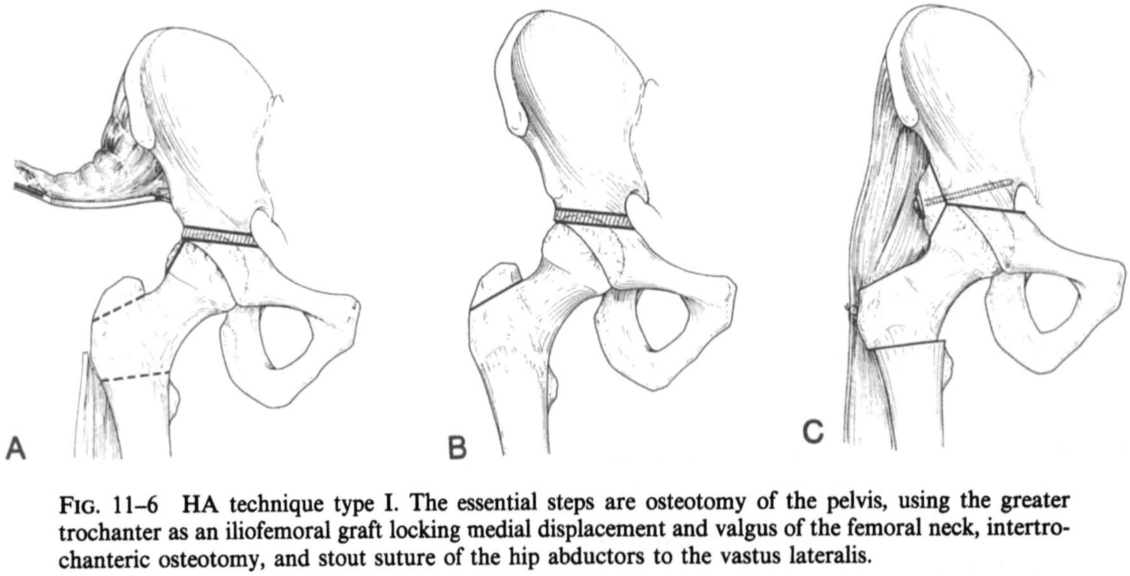

FIG. 11–6 HA technique type I. The essential steps are osteotomy of the pelvis, using the greater trochanter as an iliofemoral graft locking medial displacement and valgus of the femoral neck, intertrochanteric osteotomy, and stout suture of the hip abductors to the vastus lateralis.

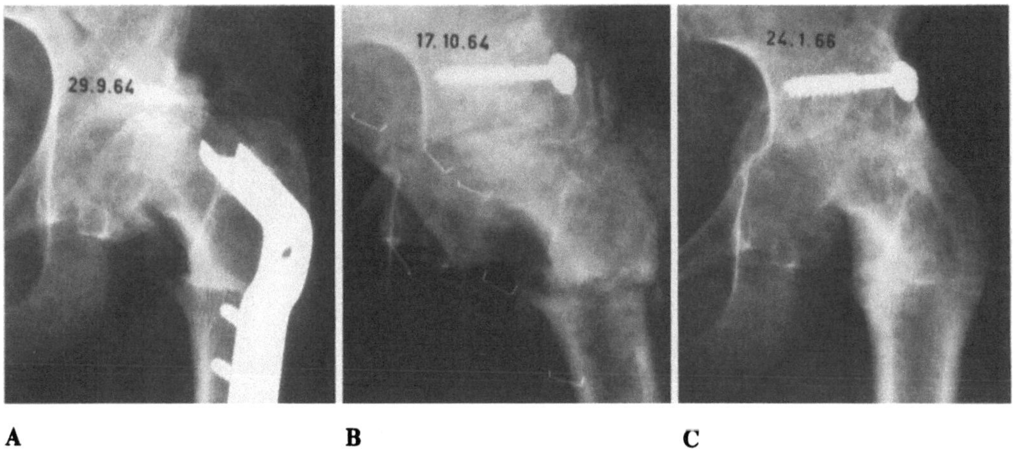

FIG. 11–7 HA type I: example. The patient is a 56-year-old woman. **A** Painful hip 4 years after unsuccessful osteotomy. **B** Two weeks after HA in a plaster spica. Note the 10° abduction. **C** Sixteen months after HA: pain-free fusion.

shortened to above the knee joint, permitting knee exercises. Discharge from the hospital occurs at this point. Fourteen weeks after surgery, the plaster is removed and x-ray films should show early union.

The patient uses crutches another 6 weeks. They are discarded after another x-ray check is made to be certain of the bony union 5 months after surgery (Fig. 11–7).

Indications Type I arthrodesis is the best procedure for a young, healthy patient who can easily tolerate plaster fixation. The specific benefit of the technique is that final positioning of the leg is postponed a few days. This can be accomplished at a more convenient time after the wound has healed and the possibility of postoperative complications has passed. Another advantage is that fatigue fracture of the femur is not to be expected.

In addition to plaster fixation, there is another disadvantage: The femoral head–neck fragment tends to tilt into varus with shortening of the leg despite the fact that the greater trochanter should prevent this. Therefore for the same indication, we prefer the next procedure.

HA Type II

Technique In contrast to the previous description, osteotomy of the pelvis (Fig. 11–8) is done

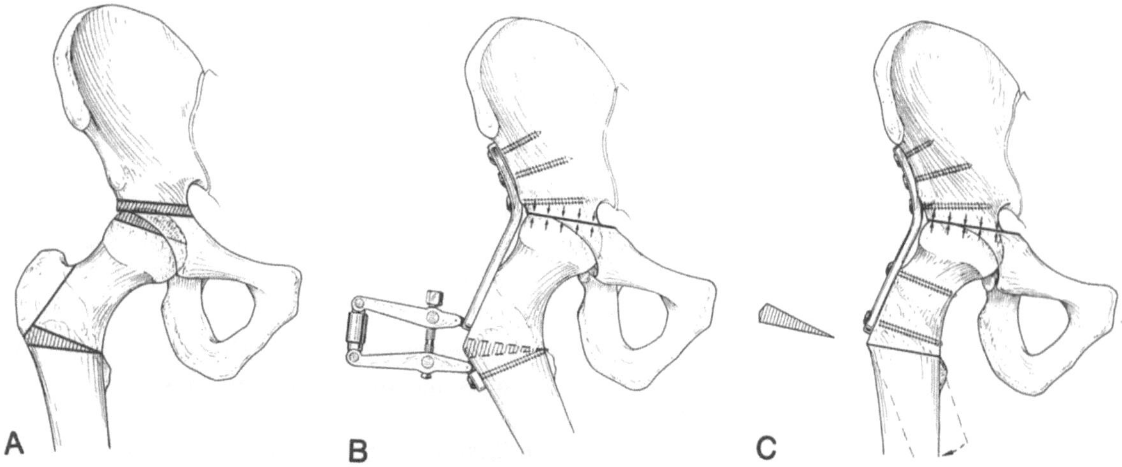

FIG. 11–8 HA technique type II. The essential steps: Osteotomy of the pelvis in valgus of the femoral neck with strong adduction of the leg; compression-impact of the osteotomy with a compression plate; intertrochanteric wedge osteotomy to correct the deformity.

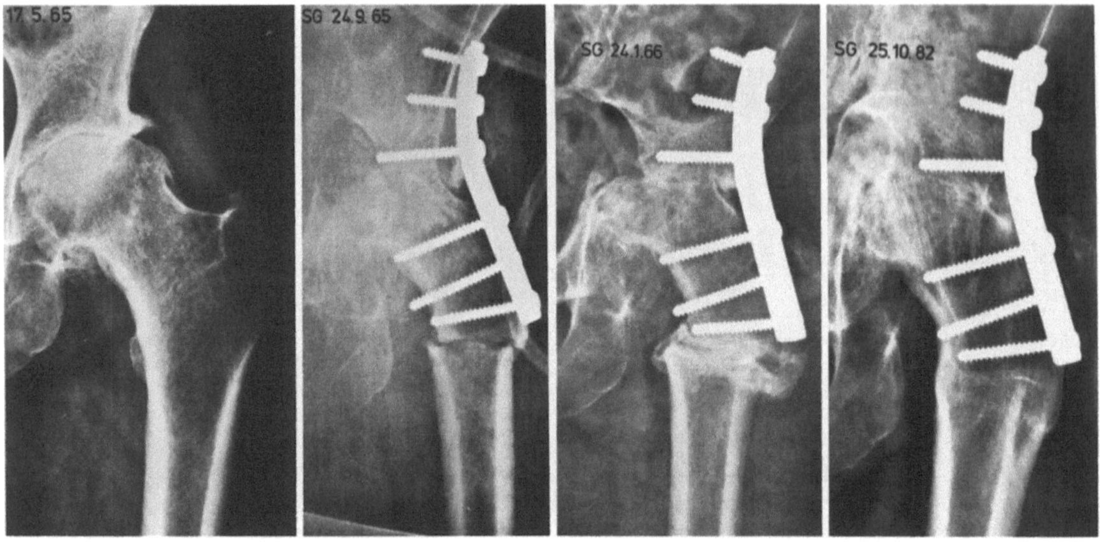

A B C D

Fig. 11–9 HA type II: example. The patient is a 50-year-old woman. **A** Unilateral painful hip joint. **B** Postoperative x-ray film. **C** Four months after HA: hip spica is discarded. **D** Seventeen years after HA: ideal HA.

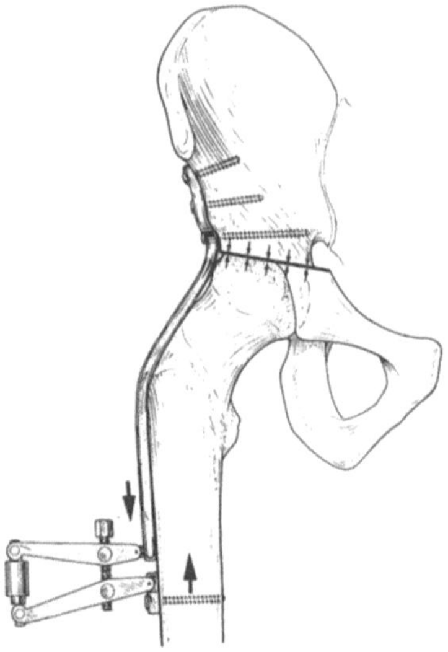

Fig. 11–10 HA technique type III. A cobra-head plate is fastened to the ilium and used as a compression plate.

with the leg in adduction so that the femoral neck is in valgus position. After the intertrochanteric osteotomy is done, the leg is brought out of adduction; consequently, some gain in leg length is achieved. The problem consists in maintaining the valgus position of the femoral neck. The following steps help: The greater trochanter is osteotomized, and the femoral neck and acetabular roof are smoothed to fit a strong, prebent ASIF plate. The plate is fastened against the ilium and runs parallel with the femoral neck. With the leg still in adduction and the neck in valgus, the ASIF compression instrument with its joint is screwed "around the corner" to the subtrochanteric cortex. Compression is applied, the femoral head and ilium are impacted, the plate is fastened to the neck, and the compression instrument is removed. To correct adduction deformity of the leg, an intertrochanteric wedge osteotomy is added. Leg length is increased 1 to 3 cm (Fig. 11–9).

Postoperative Treatment The postoperative treatment is the same as for type I HA.

Indications The indications are similar to those for type I. This procedure is preferable in cases which require leg lengthening, i.e., coxa vara, or idiopathic or posttraumatic femoral head necrosis.

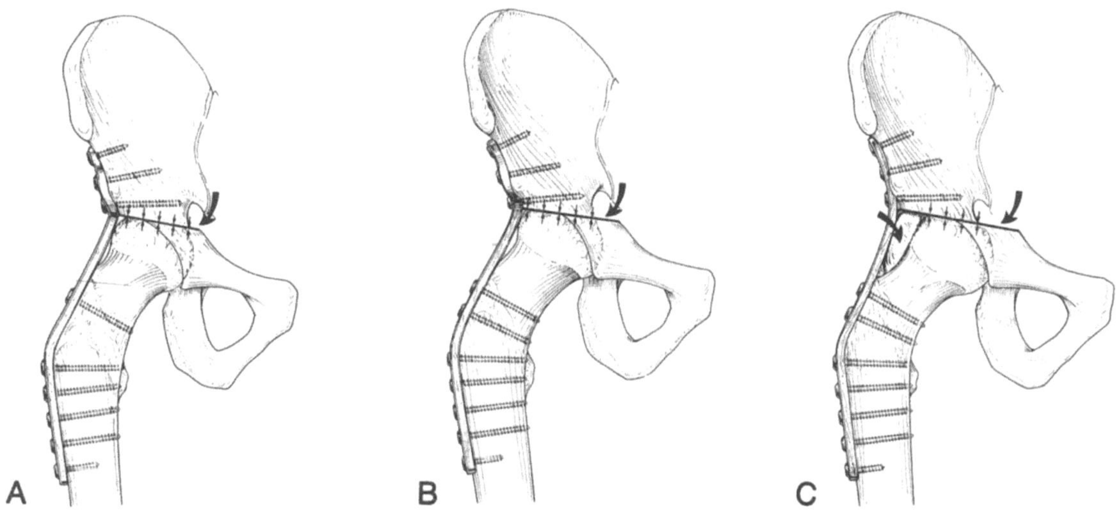

FIG. 11–11 Amount of medial displacement. The amount of medial displacement depends on the individual anatomy. **A** In a case of protrusio, no medial displacement is necessary. **B** In a case of dysplasia, moderate medial displacement is necessary. **C** In a case of a long femoral neck, the osteotomized greater trochanter fills the gap between the femoral neck and plate.

HA Type III

Technique Osteotomy of the pelvis (Fig. 11–10) is performed with the leg held in neutral position. This is checked with the landmarks of the two iliac spines and the lateral aspect of the knee joint, including an angle of 90°. With both legs draped, the feet with medial contact must be level. A sterilized goniometer may also be used. The knee joint should be in the frontal plane or in not more than 10° external rotation. The hip should be flexed not more than 20°. With the leg held in such a position, the planes of the osteotomized head and pelvis should be absolutely parallel.

The greater trochanter is osteotomized at this time. Three variations are given by the actual anatomical relation between femoral head and socket (Fig. 11–11): (1) no medial displacement; (2) moderate medial displacement; and (3) considerable medial displacement in the pelvic osteotomy. The amount of displacement depends on the coverage of the head prior to the operation. A protrusion does not need displacement, whereas subluxation–luxation requires corresponding displacement to provide adequate bony contact.

After adequate displacement is accomplished, the femur is fixed to the ilium temporarily with a stout Steinmann pin. Then a cobra plate is bent by means of the ASIF bending press or with bending irons to fit the lateral surfaces of the ilium and femoral cortex. It is important that the shaft of the plate is bent into 10° of adduction compared with the femur held in an ideal position (Fig. 11–12). The head of the cobra is fastened to the ilium above the osteotomy with six screws. The leg is moved into 10° adduction. The femoral shaft and plate should be parallel now. The compression instrument is fastened, and the hip joint is impacted. By tightening the compression instrument, the curved plate becomes somewhat stretched. Automatically the 10° of adduction is corrected and the leg, stabilized in the hip joint, falls into the desired position to the pelvis. The plate is finally fastened to the femur (Figs. 11–13 and 11–14).

With considerable medial displacement in cases with a long femoral neck, the gap between plate and neck must be filled with the osteotomized greater trochanter. The graft is fitted prior to tightening the spanner instrument, being squeezed and blocked during the compression process (Fig. 11–15).

Postoperative Treatment Bed rest is prescribed for 5 days. Ambulation is allowed thereafter on crutches, with partial weight-bearing of about 15 kg at the start (can be measured with a bathroom

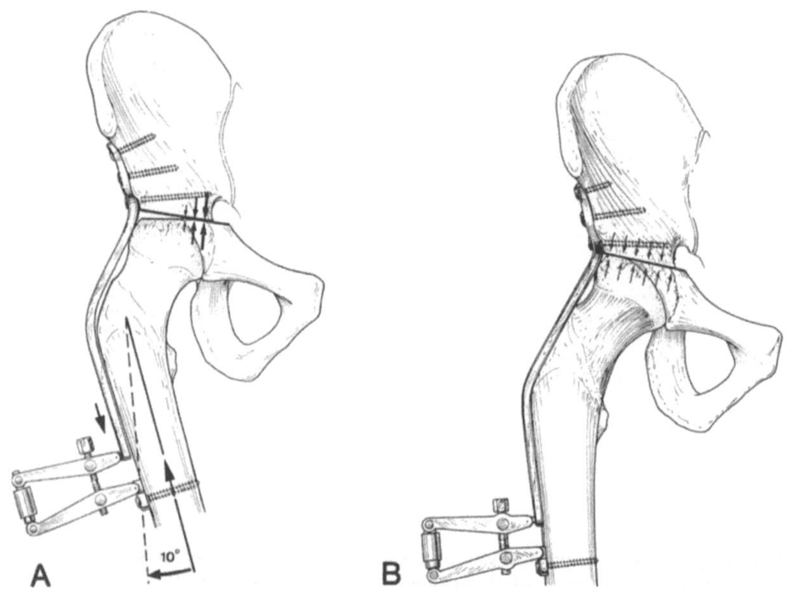

FIG. 11–12 "Overbending" of the cobra-head plate. **A** The shaft of the cobra-head plate must show 10° of adduction prior to the application of axial compression with the tension device. **B** With tensioning, the plate is "stretched," adduction disappears, and the gap between the head of the femur and the ilium collapses under the compression force.

scale). Progressive full weight-bearing is permitted within 3 months. Active knee exercises are encouraged from the first day. No external fixation is needed. A further x-ray study 3 months after surgery shows bony union as a rule.

Indications This procedure is indicated for all patients who cannot sustain bed rest and plaster fixation, i.e., especially elderly and frail patients.

Atypical HA Type IV

Technique Atypical techniques are used in children, adolescents, and adults with unusual anatomy of the hip joint. Typical are infected hip joints and anatomical defects needing "improvisation" HA (Figs. 11–16 to 11–19).

Postoperative Treatment The postoperative treatment varies according to the individual technique. Plaster–spica fixation is the rule.

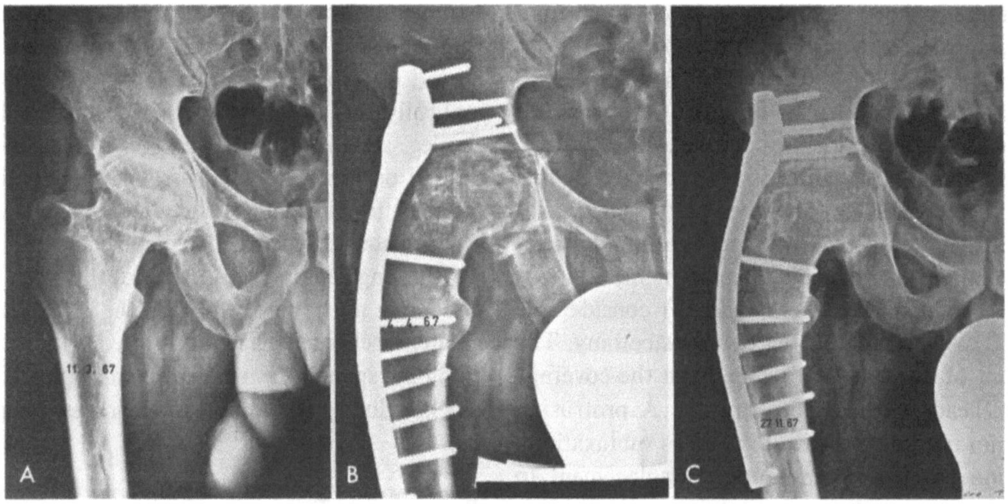

FIG. 11–13 HA type III: example. the patient is a 31-year-old man with rheumatoid arthritis. **A** Immediately before operation. Note the deep acetabulum; very little medial displacement is required at the pelvic osteotomy site. **B** Three weeks after surgery. **C** Eight months after surgery.

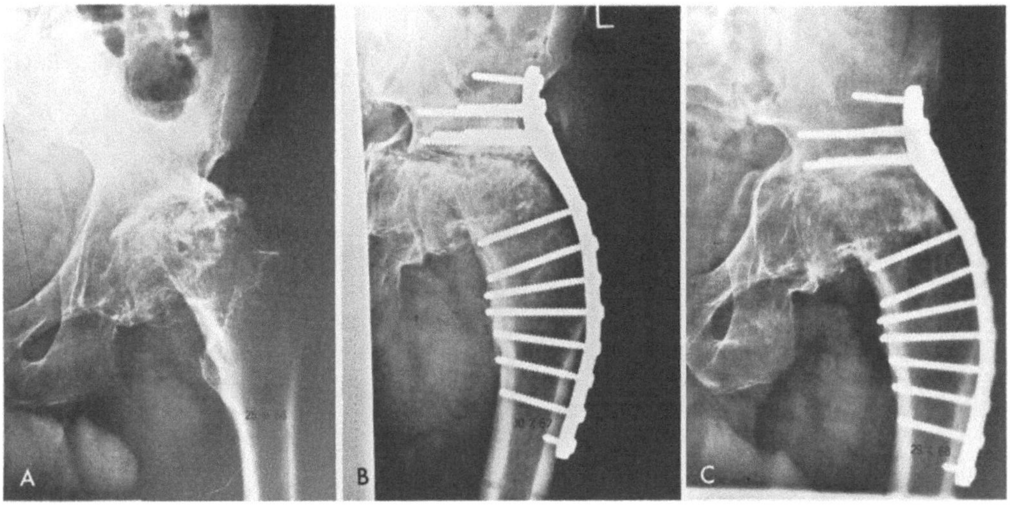

FIG. 11–14 HA type III: example. The patient is a 53-year-old man with a slipped epiphysis. Note the large, shallow acetabulum; some medial displacement is required at the pelvic osteotomy site. **A** Seven months before operation. **B** One month after operation. **C** Ten months after fusion.

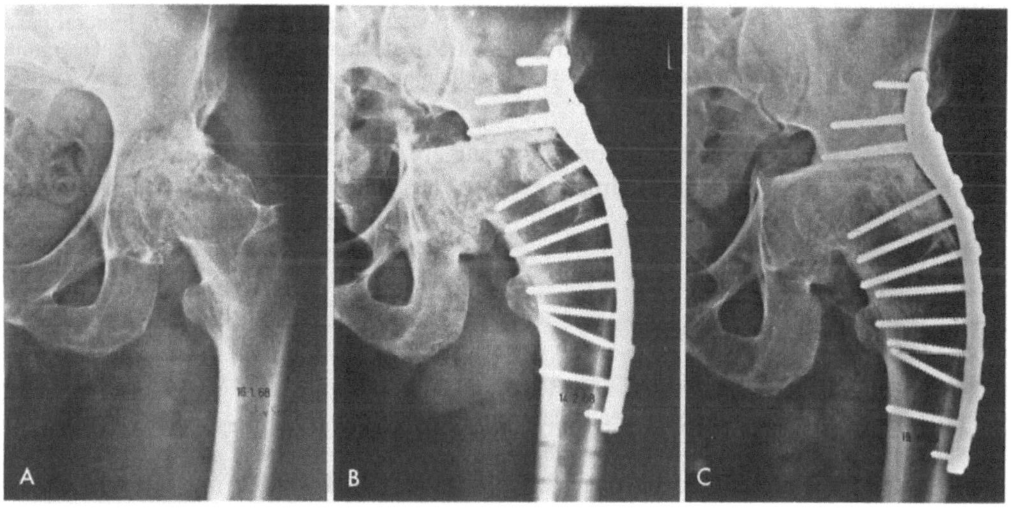

FIG. 11–15 HA type III: example. The patient is a 56-year-old man with hereditary primary disease. Note the large shallow acetabulum, the femoral head subluxated by an osteophyte of the socket floor. Much medial displacement is required at the pelvic osteotomy site. **A** Immediately before operation. **B** One month after operation. Note the greater trochanter as a free graft between the plate and the neck. **C** Twenty-two months after fusion.

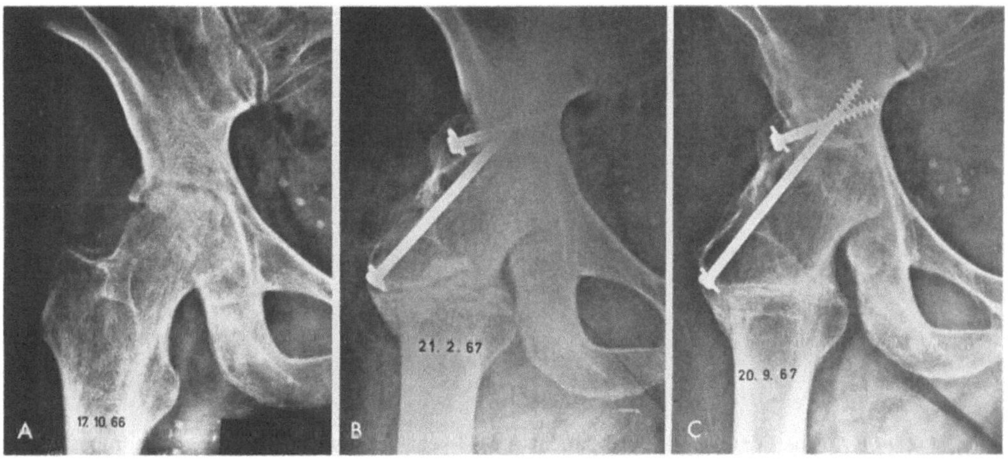

FIG. 11–16 HA type IV: example. The patient is a 39-year-old woman with acute septic arthritis, hematogenous type. **A** Immediately before surgery. **B** Fourteen weeks later. **C** Eleven months after surgery.

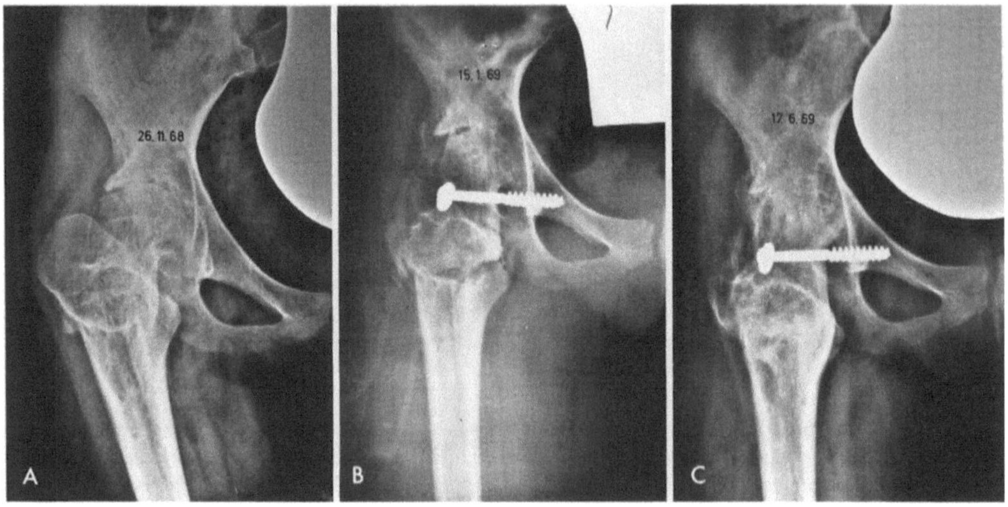

FIG. 11–17 HA type IV: example. The patient is a 16-year-old girl with a necrotic femoral head after a slipped epiphysis and subtrochanteric correction osteotomy. **A** Painful hip. **B** Operation day: femoropubic screw fixation in valgus, with lengthening. **C** Five months after surgery.

Indications Atypical HAs are performed on children and adolescents, and in unusual situations on adults.

Data Concerning HA Techniques

Fusion Techniques In our first and last series of HA, the type III technique with cobra-head plate fixation was performed in three of four cases. All these patients were out of bed and on their feet within 3 to 5 days, left the hospital 2 weeks after surgery, and used two crutches for 2 to 3 months. At that time, the HA, i.e., the osteotomy plane between the femoral head and the ilium, and the pelvic osteotomy itself had fused.

n. 119 (1967–69)			*n.* 82 (1972–81)		
Type I	3	10% (Types I–II)	Type I	—	
Type II	8		Type II	15	20%
Type III	92	75%	Type III	58	70%
Type IV	16	15%	Type IV	9	10%

Type III HA, with marked medial displacement, creates a deformity of the lesser pelvis. This

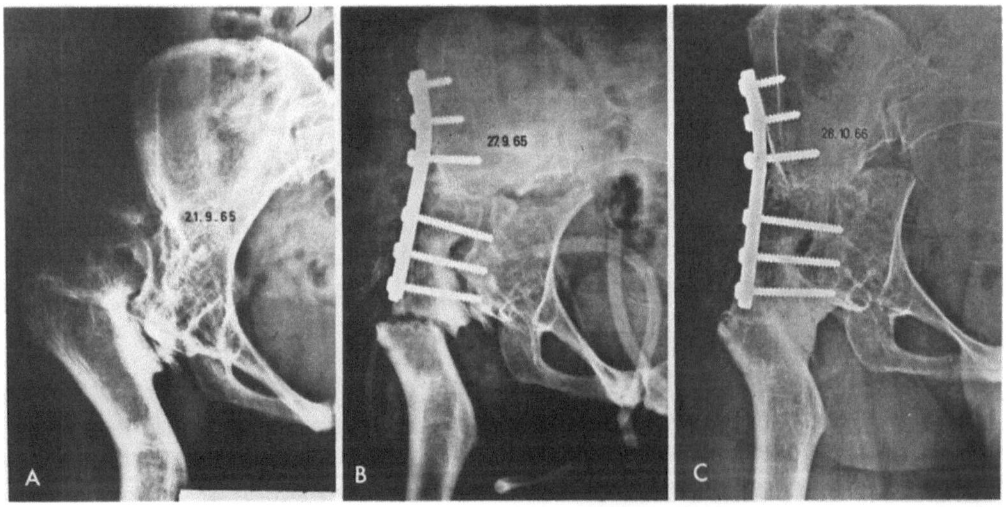

FIG. 11–18 HA type IV: example. The patient is a 43-year-old woman with congenital hip dysplasia after high diaphyseal osteotomy. **A** Painful hip. **B** Operation day. **C** Thirteen months after surgery.

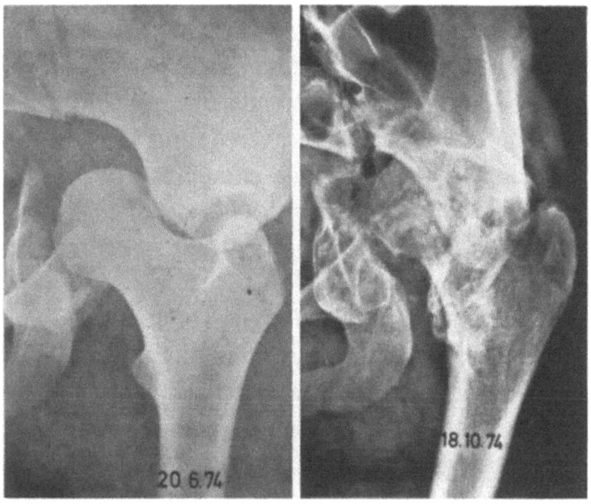

A B

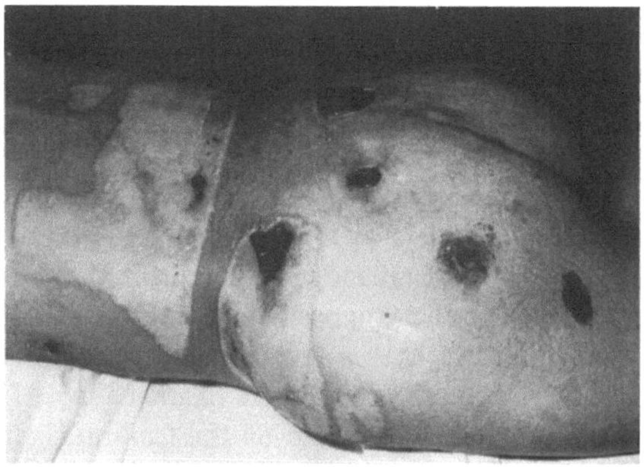

C

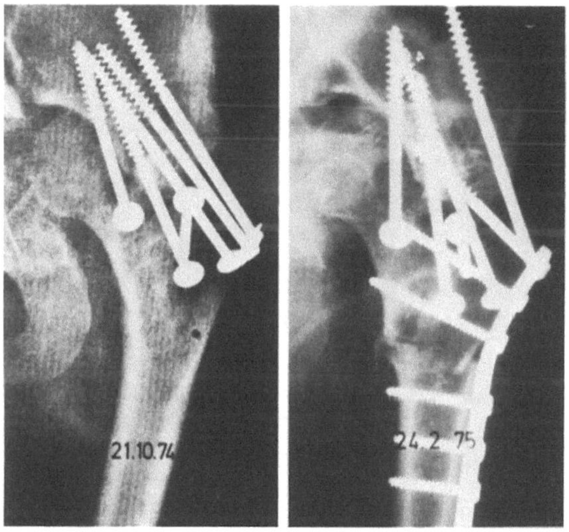

D E

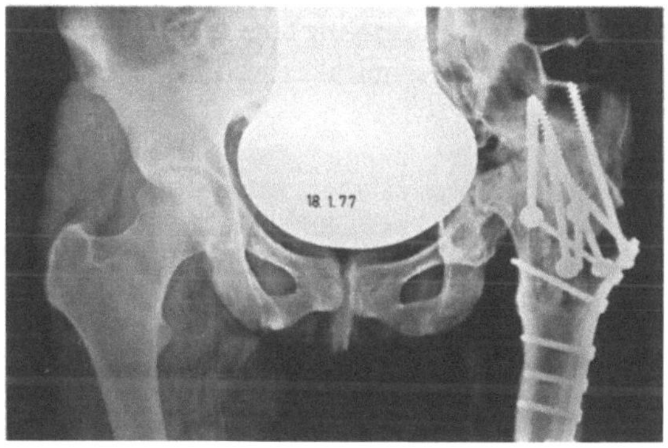

F

FIG. 11–19 HA type IV: example. The patient is a 20-year-old woman with a neglected central dislocation fracture. **A** The fracture. **B** Four months after injury, on admittance. **C** Poor general condition and poor skin condition are due to immobilization in a bilateral plaster spica. **D** First step: southern approach: fixation in situ. **E** Second step, 4 weeks later: alignment osteotomy. **F** Two years three months after admission.

may, but does not always, require cesarean delivery in women. In one of four cases, however, the anatomy of the diseased hip is altered in such a way that a cobra-head plate does not fit the lateral aspect of the hip joint. A different technique therefore is necessary, usually requiring a plaster spica for a period of 3 to 4 months.

Major Problems of HA

Reoperation of HA A *nonunion* rate of 17% contrasts with the 10% rate in our first series. There were proportionally more "problem" cases, resulting in a higher nonunion rate in the second series. Thirteen reoperations went on to union; one reoperation was unsuccessful.

n. 82 (1972–81)

For nonunion	14	17%	28%
Alignment osteotomy	5	6%	
Fracture fixation	4	5%	

The essential feature of HA nonunion is that the two fragments are well vascularized. What they need to unite is rigid fixation. Only in the minority of cases are one or both fragments badly vascularized, e.g., in cases with femoral head necrosis or tuberculosis. Necrotic tissue then must be removed, and an autogenous cancellous bone plasty is advisable. In all such cases, however, rigid fixation with compression is mandatory (Figs. 11–20 and 11–21).

Malposition of the HA or the leg, i.e., a genu valgum, should always be corrected by osteotomy. Rigid fixation at the osteotomy site allows functional after-treatment with immediate ambulation (Figs. 11–22 and 11–23).

Leg length discrepancy may require a shortening osteotomy of the opposite femur (Fig. 11–24).

Fatigue fracture is a rare complication but is characteristic of HA with plate fixation type III. These fractures are situated on the femoral shaft at the level where the metallic implant ends. Such fatigue fractures must be explained as follows: The plate absorbs mechanical stresses, bypassing stresses from the underlying bone. The bone, under such alterated mechanical conditions, is changed anatomically. The flow of stress from plate to bare bone is angulated. Such angulation of stresses dictates that bone must undergo a permanent increased turnover and permanent remodeling. Such remodeling is aimed at overcoming the unequal elasticity in the two bone compartments. At the end of the plate there may be insufficient stress protection built up by nature, and stress fracture may develop.

The treatment of a fatigue fracture is simple and reliable. In the four cases of the last series, the fracture was simply stabilized with another compression plate without grafting. Within 3 months at the most, despite immediate ambulation, a stress fracture heals far more surely than a fresh fracture would do. Such sound healing must be attributed to the hypervascularity that

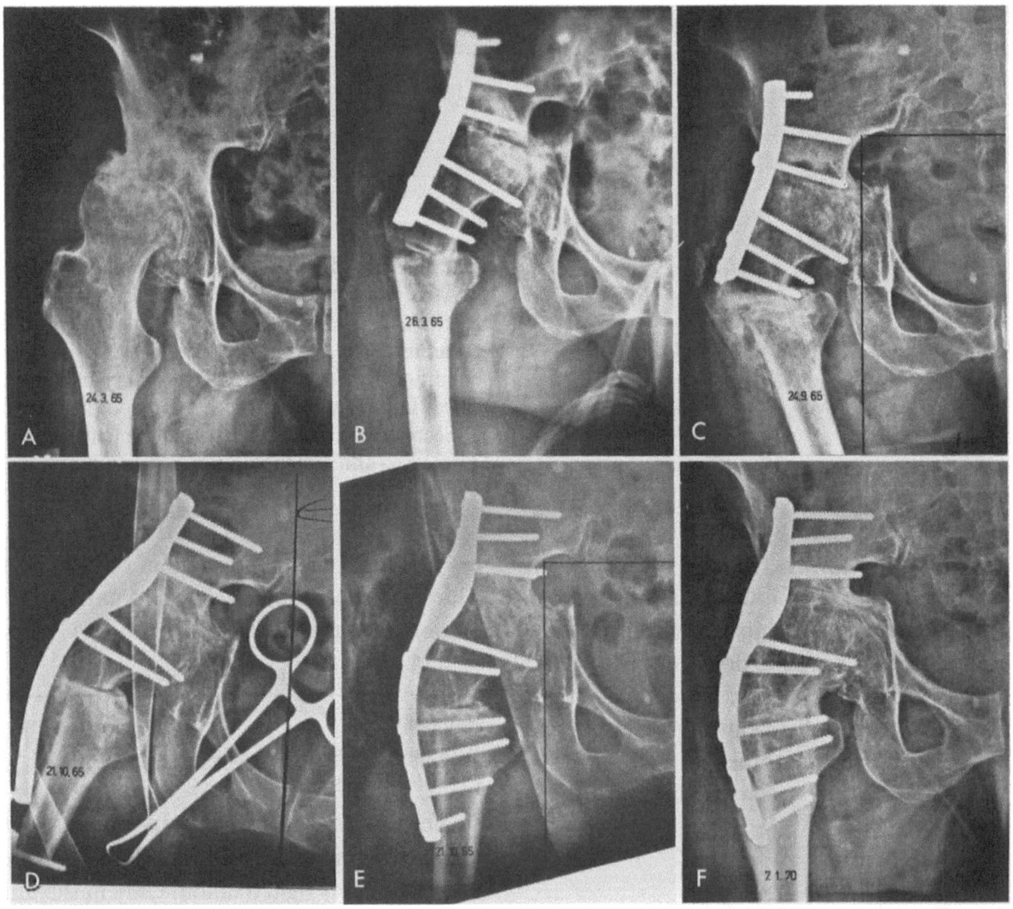

FIG. 11–20 Nonunion: intertrochanteric. The patient is a 56-year-old woman with congenital hip dysplasia. **A** Hip to be fused. **B** Operation day. **C** Nonunion of intertrochanteric osteotomy, adduction deformity, short leg. **D** Operation day: osteotomy of callus, compression plate. **E** Result of correction. **F** Late result 4 years 8 months after first operation.

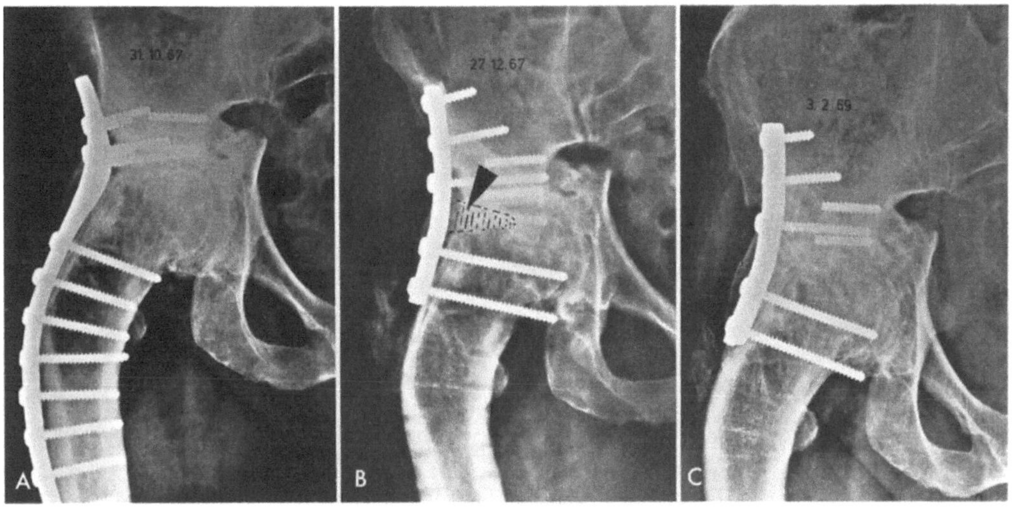

FIG. 11–21 Nonunion: iliofemoral. The patient is a 54-year-old man with congenital hip dysplasia. **A** Nonunion 1 year 8 months after surgery. Note the broken screws. **B** Small iliac bone graft squeezed into the gap under the new compression plate; he had 6 weeks bed rest, then ambulation. **C** Late result 13 months after operation for nonunion.

is not present with a normal fracture. From a biological point of view, fatigue fractures could be called "creeping" nonunions (Fig. 11–25).

Other Complications of HA

Neither in the first series of 111 HAs nor in the last series of 82 HAs did a patient die as a consequence of the hip operation. Serious thromboembolism has not occurred, all patients being systematically anticoagulated with low-dose heparin and dihydroergotamine.

Deep infection has not been seen, but septic hips were cleared of infection with or due to HA. The one tuberculous and six septic hips were the only ones that had been operated under prophylactic antibiotic treatment. All cases are operated under clean air conditions, however, explaining the

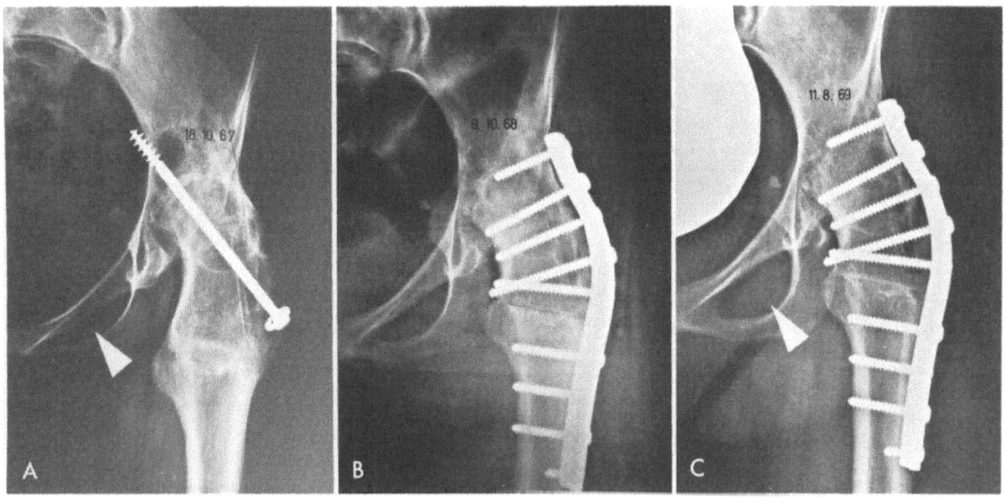

FIG. 11–22 Malposition. The patient is an 18-year-old girl with unspecific arthritis. **A** Three years after fusion. Note the flexion deformity ("narrow" foramen obturatum). **B** Day of intertrochanteric correction osteotomy with compression. **C** Ten months later. Note the normal position (foramen obturatum is "open").

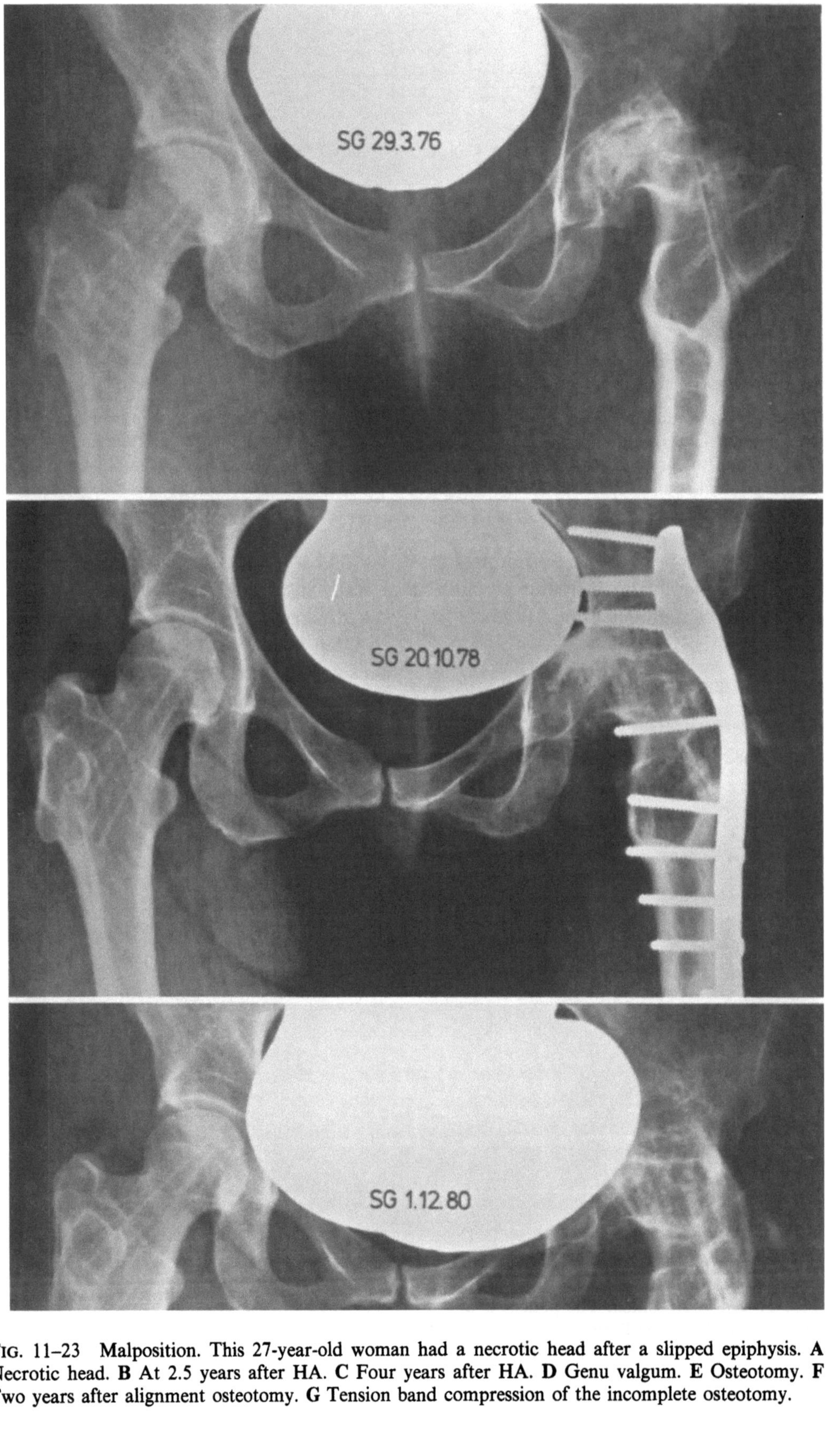

A
B
C

FIG. 11–23 Malposition. This 27-year-old woman had a necrotic head after a slipped epiphysis. **A** Necrotic head. **B** At 2.5 years after HA. **C** Four years after HA. **D** Genu valgum. **E** Osteotomy. **F** Two years after alignment osteotomy. **G** Tension band compression of the incomplete osteotomy.

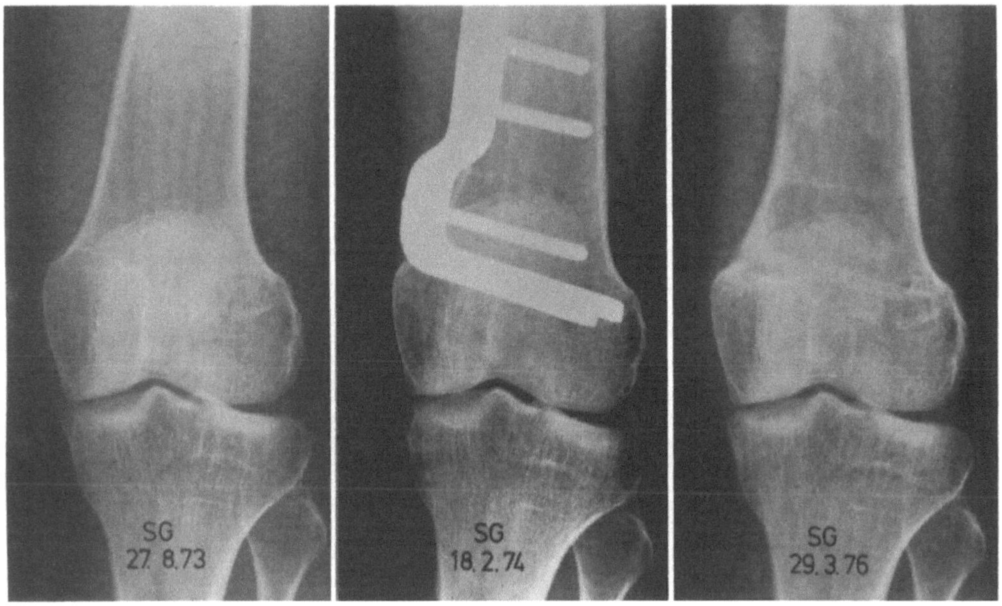

D E F

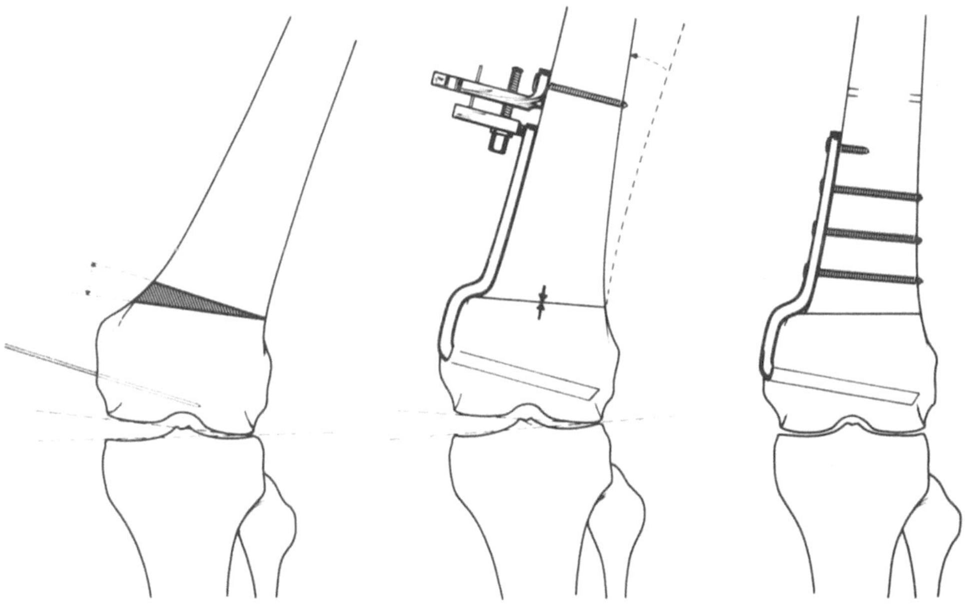

FIG. 11–23 *Continued* G

lack of wound infection. Secondary hematoma requiring surgical revision has occurred twice.

Damage to nerves and vessels is not expected if the described protection during the exposure is established. In both of our series (193 patients total), neither the sciatic nerve, the femoral nerve, nor the large pelvic vessels suffered. In another series in between, however, one case of permanent peroneal nerve palsy and one of massive hemorrhage were seen. Only ligation of the iliac interna artery could stop the hemorrhage.

Subluxations of the symphysis have been observed several times which were more or less evident on the x-ray films depending on the amount of medial displacement in the osteotomy of the pelvis. This subluxation, as an occasional finding, does not produce symptoms. It is only a curiosity of the technique (Fig. 11–26).

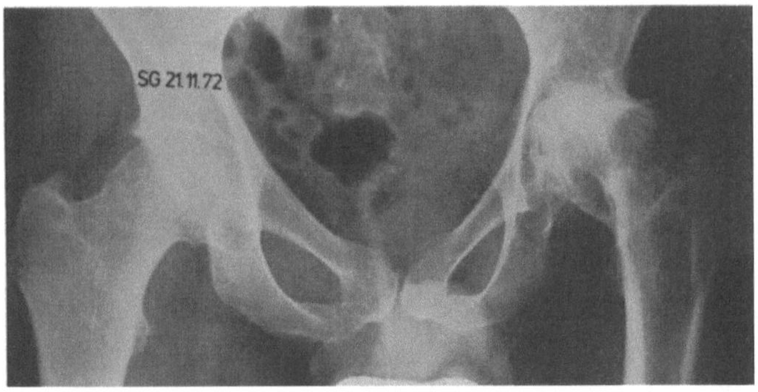

A

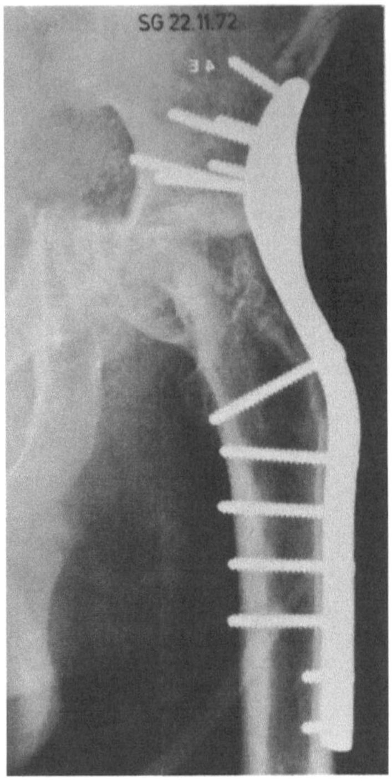

B

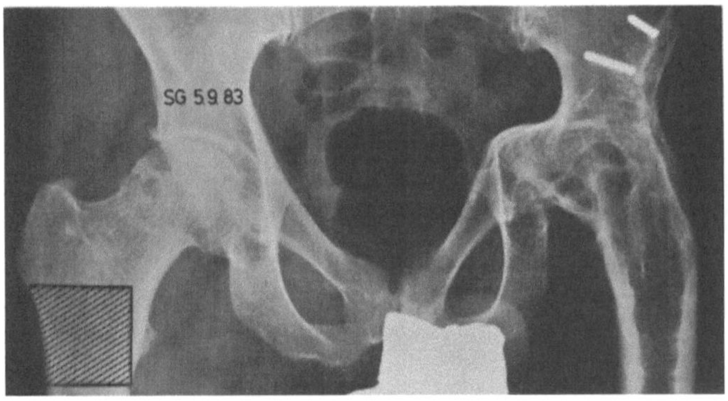

C

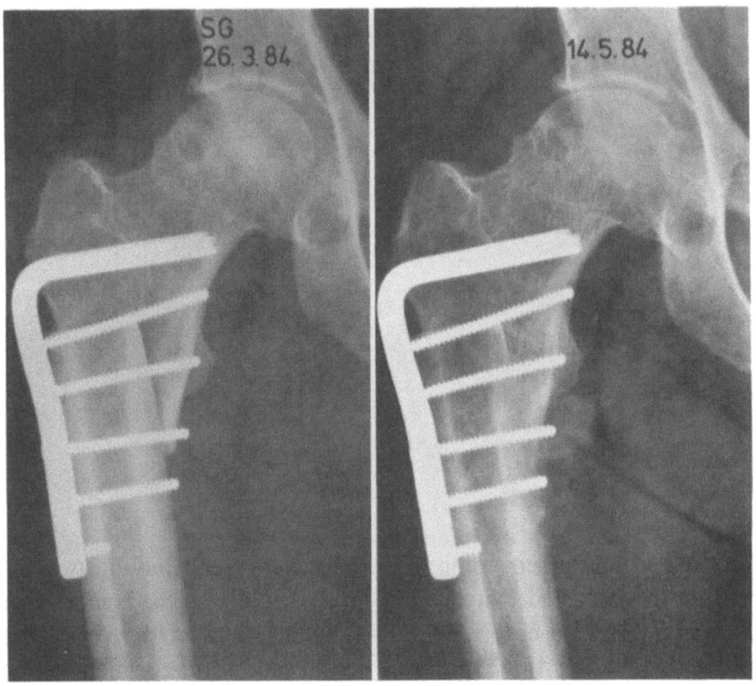

D

FIG. 11–24 Leg length discrepancy. This 52-year-old man had a slipped epiphysis. **A** Hip to be fused. **B** At operation day. **C** Eleven years after HA. Shortening was 4.5 cm. The resection is outlined on the sound femur. **D** Osteotomy and 2 months later.

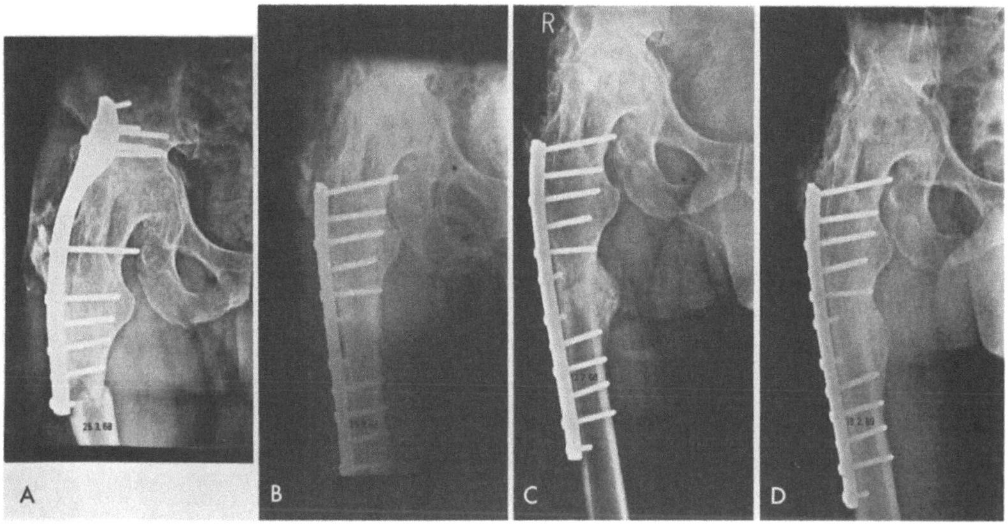

FIG. 11–25 Fatigue fracture. This 68-year-old man had congenital hip dysplasia. **A** Fatigue fracture 2 years after fusion. **B** Same day: bridging the fracture with compression plate. **C** Four months later. **D** Eleven months after fracture: sound healing.

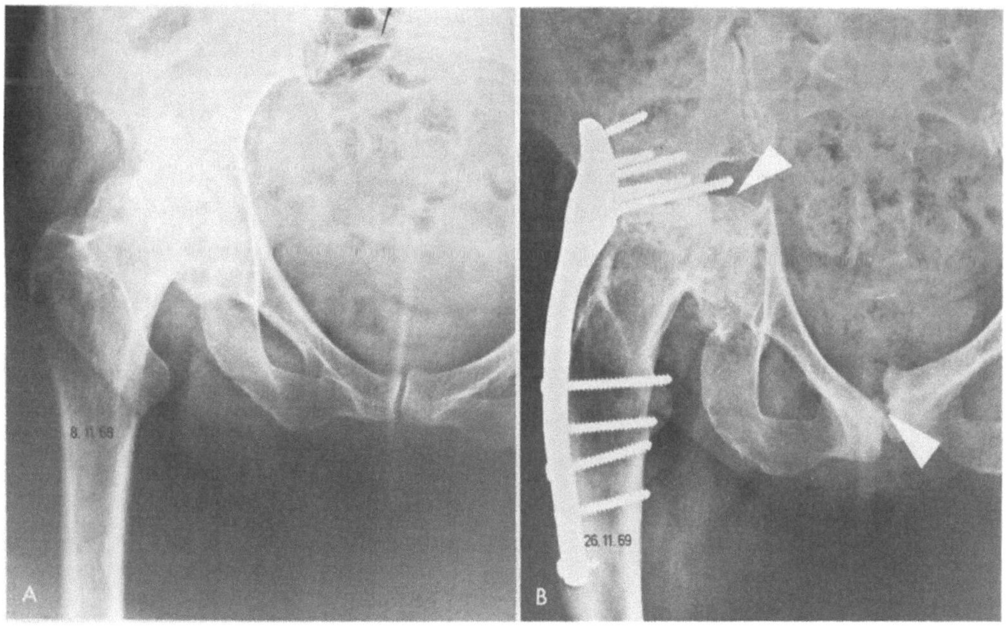

FIG. 11–26 Symptom-free dislocation of the symphysis. This 54-year-old woman had primary osteoarthritis. **A** Normal symphysis. **B** Considerable displacement of pelvic osteotomy: subluxation of symphysis with no symptoms.

HA and THR

HA on One Side, THR on the Other Side

HA is very compatible with THR on the opposite side (Fig. 11–27). Eight of 54 patients—seven with a pain-free THR, one with a THR having become loose and waiting for revision arthroplasty—had HA on one hip and THR on the other.

THR after HA

It is technically not a problem to convert an HA into a THR. We have had five such patients over

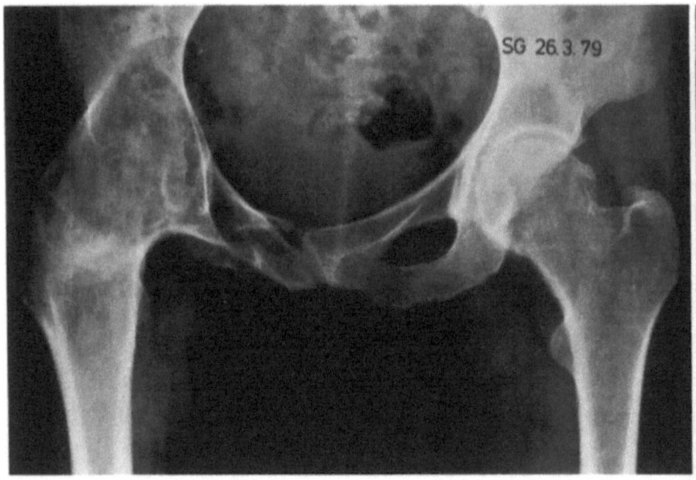

A

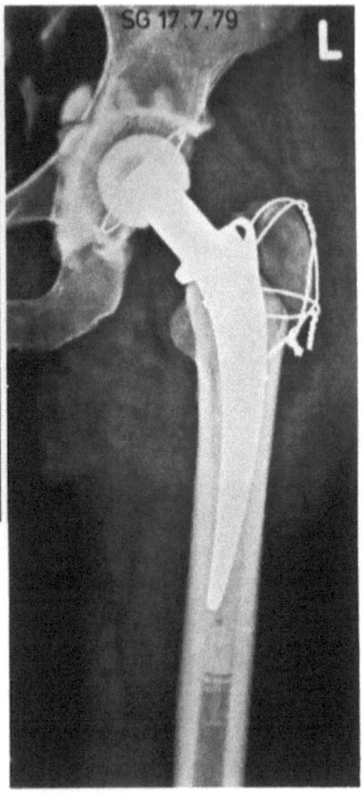

B

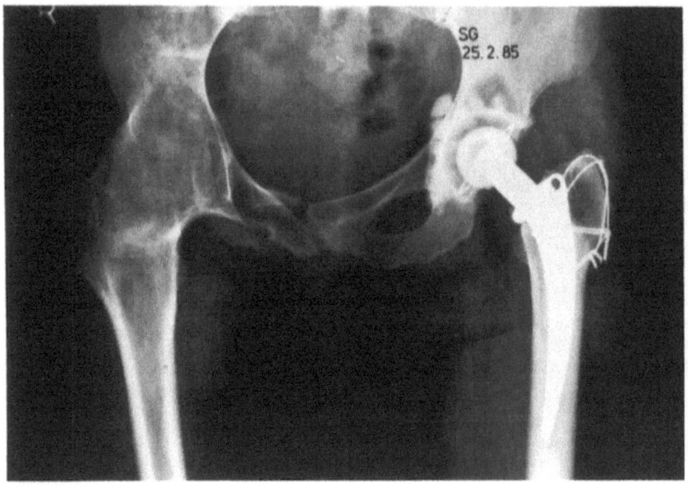

C

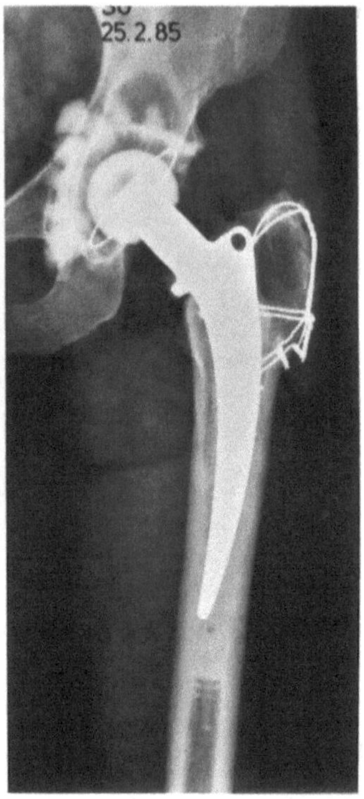

D

FIG. 11–27 HA and contralateral THR in a 55-year-old woman. **A** Fusion after septic coxitis at age 14. She had had no complaints, except the opposite hip had been painful for 4 years. **B** THR. **C** At 5.5 years after THR. **D** THR: no loosening, no wear.

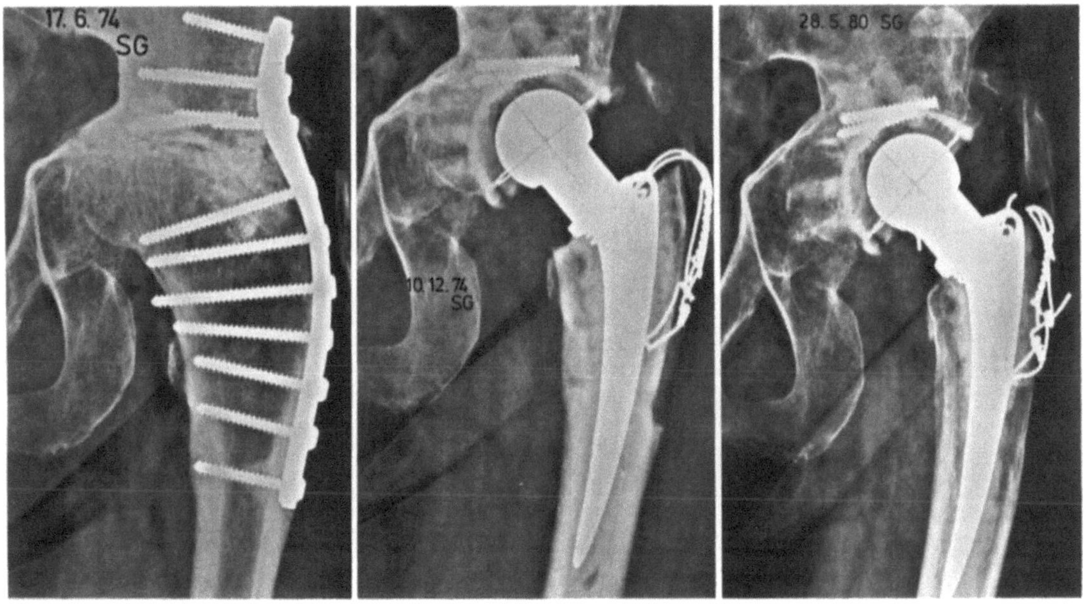

A B C

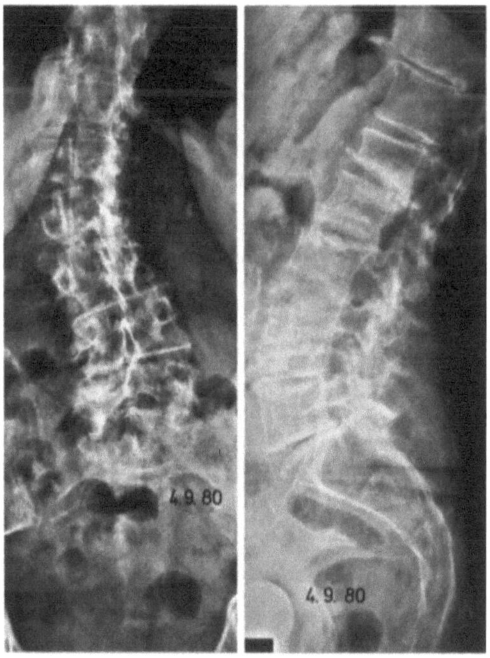

D

FIG. 11–28 THR after HA in a 67-year-old woman. **A** HA 9 years before. **B** THR, 3 weeks after surgery. **C** At 5.5 years later: Good result, but the back problem is unchanged. **D** Back pain.

the last 15 years asking for conversion. Three patients complained of low back problems; two patients, both men, no longer accepted the stiffness of the hip. Of these patients, only the latter were pleased by their regaining some hip motion (maximum 60° flexion). The low back pain patients had no relief of their pain despite regaining some hip motion (Fig. 11–28).

HA after THR

HA after removal of the THR was tried twice. Both fusions failed to unite (Fig. 11–29). Spontaneous ankylosis after THR due to ectopic bone formation may be astonishingly well accepted by the patient. Such observations influenced the decision for "cross-plating" an almost stiff hip, which became pain-free after HA (Fig. 11–30).

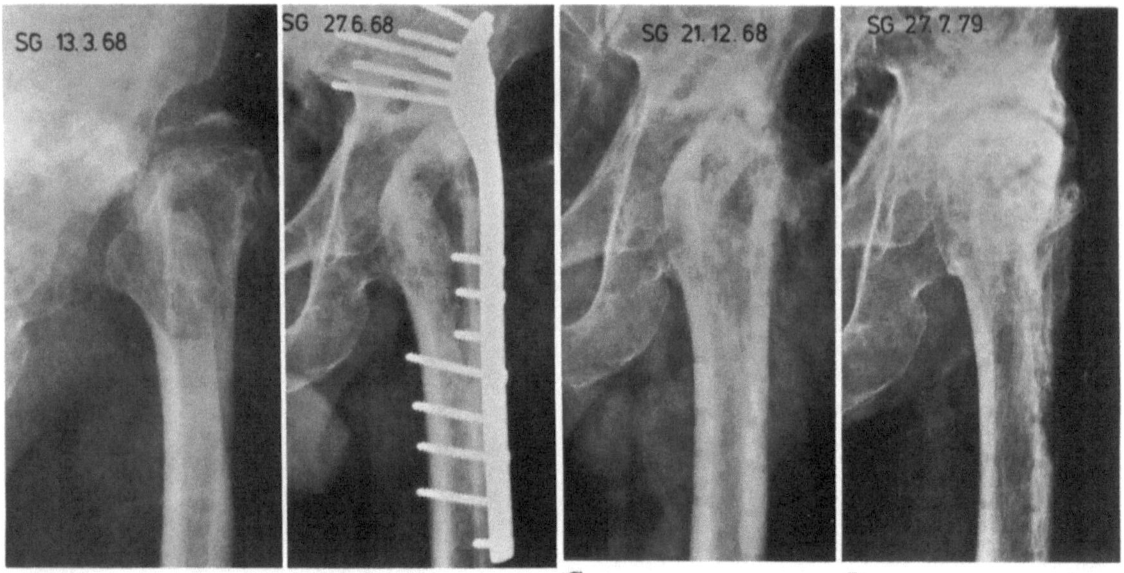

A B C D

FIG. 11–29 HA after THR and Girdlestone-type excision in a 78-year-old man. **A** Five months after excision of septic TH: unstable hip. **B** Six weeks after attempted HA. **C** Seven months after surgery: hip stable but not fused, plate already removed. **D** Six years after surgery: stable hip, no pain. Flexion 40°. Walks with a cane.

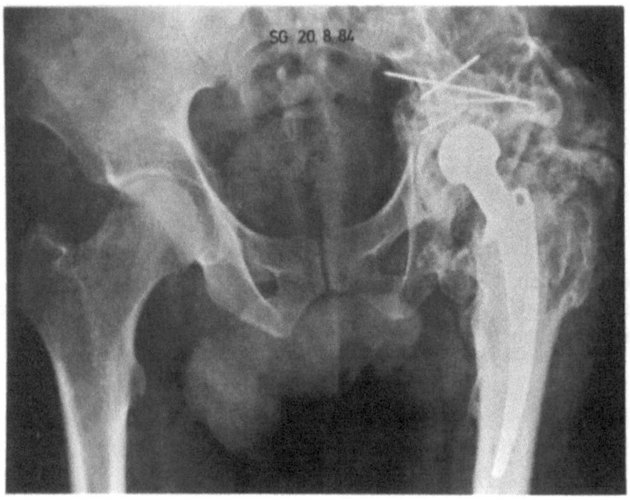

A

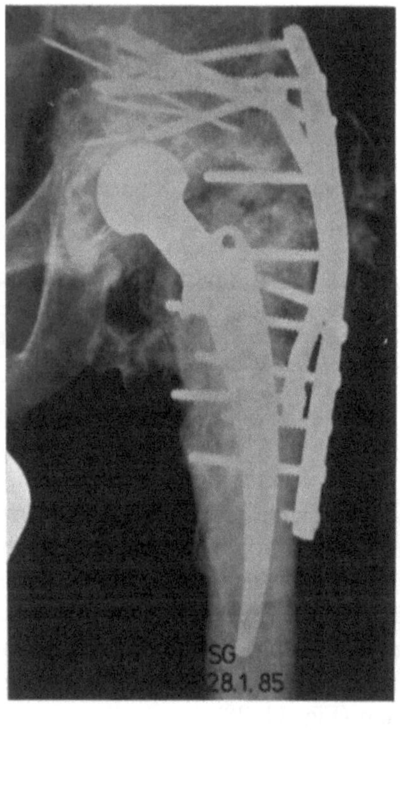

B

FIG. 11–30 HA after THR and ectopic bone formation. This 41-year-old man had had a central dislocation hip fracture 11 years before with THR 8 months later. **A** Ten years after THR: painful and stiff hip, adduction deformity. **B** Four months after "HA" with double-plating. Total relief of pain.

Conclusions and Summary

Discussion

During the years 1961 to 1983 a total of 745 HAs were performed at the Department of Orthopedic Surgery at the Cantonal Hospital, St. Gallen, Switzerland. This represents 10% of all procedures to cure osteoarthritic hip joints. HA and osteotomy have gradually decreased in favor of THR. Our actual techniques for HA, with exceptions, allow immediate or early ambulation. This is beneficial to elderly and infirm patients who would not be able to tolerate bed rest and plaster fixation. The high rate of union, the positive judgment of the result by the patients themselves, and the reliability of the procedure for the patient's future reestablishes HA as a favorable procedure for conditions otherwise poorly suited for other methods of treatment. Deleterious complications are extremely rare, and local complications can be cured easily.

The main message of our former studies (111 HAs, 400 HAs) and of the last study of 54 follow-ups consists in the fact that 80 to 90% of the patients are very satisfied with HA. The same high rate of satisfaction was found by Sponsell et al. in 1984 (53 HAs) and Callaghan et al. in 1985 (28 HAs). In 13% (Sponsell et al.), 21% (Callaghan et al.), and 0.7% of 745 HAs of our own, respectively, was the stiff hip remobilized with THR.

In contrast to such favorable findings, the reputation of HA is poor in the opinion of today's orthopedic surgeons. This must be explained by a lack of personal experience with the procedure. The situation with osteotomy of the proximal femur and of the hip socket is somewhat similar. HA and osteotomy might not be popular in the contemporary orthopedic surgical repertoire because these procedures are much more difficult to perform than THR. This reflects, at least at our department, the fact that THR is performed by everyone, whereas an osteotomy is performed only by the senior physicians. HA, however, is mostly reserved for those most experienced in hip surgery—for the chief or his partners. The "staging" according to the difficulty of the various procedures is linked with the time of training in orthopedic surgery: With 6 years of basic training, there is not enough time to perceive all the problems involved with osteotomy and HA.

It becomes more and more evident and accepted that the durability of THR is not long-lasting enough for patients with a life expectancy of more than 20 years. Osteotomy and HA therefore need to be looked at again by orthopedic surgeons. Schlegel said: "It is very easy to replace a hip. This can be done by everybody—unfortunately. But a surgeon, who is not familiar with five other reconstructive hip operations, should refrain from THR."

Such other hip operations are shelf arthroplasty; Chiari-Salter's innominate osteotomy; Wagner's periarticular osteotomy; Le Coeur, Hopf, and Steels's triple osteotomy; Pauwel's varus or valgus osteotomy; McMurray's displacement osteotomy; Bombelli's valgus osteotomy; Krucza's reconstruction osteotomy; Jaros's arthroplasty; Schanz's, Girdlestone's, Milch-Bachelor's osteotomy; Sugioca's osteotomy.

Final Remarks

The orthopedic surgeons of today are confronted with an increasing number of disasters after THR. The orthopedic surgeons of tomorrow should counteract this tendency by offering their patients more often than is currently done the well-proved alternative procedures of treatment for degenerative hip disease, HA being the most reliable.

Bibliography

Albee, F. H.: Arthritis deformans of the hip; a preliminary report of a new operation. JAMA, 1:1977, 1908.

Albee, F. H.: Extra-articular arthrodesis of the hip for tuberculosis: with a report of 31 cases. Ann. Surg., 89:404, 1929.

Albert, E.: Einige Fälle von künstlicher Ankylosenbildung an paralytischen Gliedmassen. Wien. Med. Presse, 23:725, 1882.

Alvik, I.: Arthrodesis and arthroplasty of the hip joint. Acta Orthop. Scand., 33:253, 1963.

Alvik, I.: Arthrodesis of the hip: a method allowing weight-bearing and walking postoperatively. Acta Orthop. Scand., 32:451, 1962.

Apley, A. G., Denham, R. A.: Osteotomy as aid to arthrodesis of the hip. J. Bone Joint Surg., 37B:185, 1955.

Aufranc, O. E.: The technique and illustrative cases of vitallium mold arthroplasty. In: *Die Therapie der Koxarthrose* (Rütt, A., ed.) Stuttgart, Thieme, 1969.

Bombelli, R.: *Osteoarthritis of the Hip.* New York, Springer, 1976.

Brewster, R. C., Coventry, M. B., Johnson, E. W., Jr.: Conversion of the arthrodesed hip to a total hip arthroplasty. J. Bone Joint Surg., 57A:27, 1975.

Brittain, H. A.: *Architecture Principles in Arthrodesis.* Edinburgh, Livingstone, 1952.

Buchholz, H. W.: Das künstliche Hüftgelenk. Mater. Med. Nord., 21:613, 1969.

Burns, B. H.: Fixation of the osteo-arthritic hip by nailing. Lancet, 236:978, 1939.

Callaghan, J. J., Brand, R. A., Pedersen, D. R.: Long-term follow-up of hip arthrodesis. Presented at the A.A.O.S. Meeting, Las Vegas, Jan. 26, 1985.

Carter, P. J., Wickstrom, J.: Arthrodesis of the hip: an assessment of the results in one hundred patients. South. Med. J., 64:451, 1971.

Cattaneo, R.: L'artrodesi dell'anca (con particolare riguardo alla fissazione con innesoto osseo). Arch. Ortop., 72:801, 1959.

Charnley, J.: Arthroplasty of the hip—a new operation. Lancet, 2:1129, 1961.

Charnley, J.: *Compression Arthrodesis.* Edinburgh, Livingstone, 1953.

Charnley, J.: Stabilisation of the hip by central dislocation. J. Bone Joint Surg., 37B:514, 1955.

Charnley, J.: Personal communication, 1967, 1970.

Committee on Hip Osteotomies: Fehlschläge der intertrochanteren Osteotomie bei Coxarthrose. Swiss. Orthop. Soc., 1970.

Courpied, J. P., Kerboul, M., Beller, G., Postel, M.: Arthroplastie totale sur hanche ankylosée. Rev. Chir. Orthop., 67:289, 1981.

Courpied, J. P., Postel, M.: Les indications actuelles de l'arthrodèse de la hanche chez l'adulte. Int. Orthop., 7:159, 1983.

Dahl, H.: Personal communication, 1967.

Daraignez, B. J. E.: De l'Arthrodèse. Thesis, Bordeaux, 1891.

David, J. B.: The muscle-pedicle bone graft in hip fusion. J. Bone Joint Surg., 36A:790, 1954.

Dollinger, J.: Arthrodesen bei der Kinderlähmung. Zentralbl. Chir., 18:689, 1891.

Dreyer, J., Pingel, P.: Unsere Erfahrungen bei der Hüftarthrodese mit Beckenosteotomie und Kreuzplatte. Arch. Orthop. Unfallchir., 66:310, 1969.

Dwyer, A. F.: Experience of a new method of hip arthrodesis. Aust. N.Z. J. Surg., 34:105, 1964.

Dwyer, A. F., Cass, C. A.: Internal fixation in hip arthrodesis. Med. J. Aust., 48:977, 1961.

Fulkerson, J. P.: Arthrodesis for disabling hip pain in children and adolescents. Clin. Orthop., 128:296, 1977.

Gertsch, R.: Die Arthrodese des Hüftgelenkes mit Kreuzplatte und Beckenosteotomie. Helv. Chir. Acta, 33:216, 1966.

Gore, D. R., Murray, M. P., Sepic, S. B., Gardner, G. M.: Walking patterns of men with unilateral surgical hip fusion. J. Bone Joint Surg., 57A:759, 1975.

Hardinge, K., Williams, D., Etienne, A., et al.: Conversion of fused hips to low friction arthroplasty. J. Bone Joint Surg., 59B:385, 1977.

Hauge, M. F.: The knee in patients with hip joint ankylosis: clinical survey and bio-mechanical aspects. Acta Orthop. Scand., 44:485, 1973.

Heusner, P.: Ueber Hüftresektion wegen angeborener Luxation. Zentralbl. Chir., 11:751, 1884.

Küntscher, G.: Die Technik der "geschlossenen" Hüftarthrodese. Chirurg., 24:404, 1953.

Lagrange, R.: Résection orthopédique de la hanche pour luxation pathologique. Bull. Soc. Chir. Paris, 2:132, 1892.

Lampugnani, C.: La decapitazione del femore nella lussazione congenita dell'anca; studio pratico di ortopedia chirurgica antisettica. G. Accad. Med. Torino, 33:538, 1885.

Liechti, R.: *Die Arthrodese des Hüftgelenkes und ihre Problematik.* Berlin, Springer, 1974.

Liechti, R.: *Hip Arthrodesis and Associated Problems.* New York, Springer, 1978.

Liechti, R.: Hip arthrodesis. In: *Surgery of the Musculoskeletal System* (Vol. 3; McCollister Evarts, C., ed.) New York, Churchill Livingstone, 1983, pp. 99–144.

Lubahn, J. D., Evarts, C. M., Feltner, J. B.: Conversion of ankylosed hips to total hip arthroplasty. Clin. Orthop., 153:146, 1980.

Maragliano, D.: Esiti definitive della remineralizzazione chirurgica nelle coxiti tuberculari. Arch. Ortop., 35:31, 1969.

Maragliano, D.: Nuovi punti di appoggio chirurgico nelle lussazione vere da coxite. Chir. Organi Mov., 5:225, 1921.

May, V. R., Jr., Mauck, W.: Intra-articular hip fusion with the intramedullary nail. Clin. Orthop., 25:113, 1962.

McKee, G. K.: Case presentations and results of total replacement prosthesis. In: *Die Therapie der Koxarthrose* (Rütt, A., ed.) Stuttgart, Thieme, 1969.

Müller, M. E.: *Hip Surgery.* AO Bulletin, 1967.

Müller, M. E.: Ostéosynthèse externe de compression pour arthrodèses et ostéotomies. Rev. Chir. Orthop., 39:531, 1953.

Müller, M. E., Allgöwer, M., Willenegger, H.: *Manual of Internal Fixation of Fractures: ASIF-Technique.* Berlin, Springer, 1970.

Onji, Y., Kurata, Y., Kido, H.: A new method of hip fusion using an intramedullary nail: preliminary report. J. Bone Joint Surg., 47B:690, 1965.

Ramadier, J. O., Lecestre, P.: Les indications de l'arthrodèse de la hanche. Rev. Chir. Orthop., 62:662, 1976.

Schlegel, K. F.: Hüftarthrodese: Und was ist nach ein paar Jahren? Med. Trib., 7:22, 1985.

Schneider, R.: Quoted by Wiedmer (1969).

Sponsell, P. D., McBeath, A. A., Perpich, M.: Hip arthrodesis in young patients. J. Bone Joint Surg., 66A:853, 1984.

Stewart, M. J., Coker, T. P.: Arthrodesis of the hip. Clin. Orthop., 62:136, 1969.

Teinturier, P.: Arthrodèse de la hanche: lambeau pédiculé trochantérien avec vissage ischiofémoral. Rev. Chir. Orthop., 52:645, 1966.

Trumble, H. C.: A method of fixation of the hip joint by means of an extraarticular bone graft. Aust. N.Z. J. Surg., 1:413, 1931–32.

Van Ness, C. P.: L'arthrodèse de la hanche pour arthrite déformante. Rev. Orthop., 26:771, 1939.

Von Winiwater, A.: *Lehrbuch der chirurgischen Operationen und der chirurgischen Verbände.* Stuttgart, Enke, 1895.

Watson-Jones, R.: Arthrodesis of the osteoarthritic hip. JAMA, 110:278, 1938.

Watson-Jones, R., Robinson, W. C.: Arthrodesis of the osteoarthritic hip joint. J. Bone Joint Surg., 38B:353, 1956.

Weber, B. G.: Die Rotations-Totalendoprothese des Hüftgelenkes. Z. Orthop., 107:304, 1970.

Weber, B. G.: Unsere Erfahrungen mit der intertrochanteren Osteotomie nach McMurray bei der Behandlung der Schmerzhaften Koxarthrose. Z. Orthop., 92:175, 1959.

Weber, B. G.: Hip arthrodesis. In: Tronzo, R. G.: *Surgery of the Hip Joint.* Philadelphia, Lea and Febiger, 1973, p. 759.

Wiedmer, U.: *Ergebnisse der Hüftarthrodese mit Kreuzplatte und Beckenosteotomie.* AO Bulletin, 1969.

Wilson, J. C.: Extraarticular fusion of tuberculous hip joint. Calif. West. Med., 27:774, 1927.

Wilson, J. C.: Operative fixation of tuberculous hips in children; end result study of 33 patients from the orthopaedic department of the Children's hospital. J. Bone Joint Surg., 15:22, 1933.

Zwicky, F.: The morphological method and vector associations. In: *La Méthode dans les Sciences Modernes.* Paris, Editions Science et Industrie, 1958.

Zwicky, F.: *Entdecken, Erfinden, Forschen im morphologischen Weltbild.* Munich, Droemer Knaur, 1966.

CHAPTER 12

Girdlestone Pseudarthrosis

MARVIN E. STEINBERG AND DAVID R. STEINBERG

The Girdlestone pseudarthrosis is a resection or excisional arthroplasty of the head and neck of the femur and the protruding margins of the acetabulum (Fig. 12–1). Perhaps the earliest descriptions of this procedure were those of Schmalz in 1817 and White in 1821, both of whom used it for the treatment of tuberculosis of the hip in children. In 1827 John Rhea Barton reported on a pseudarthrosis after simple osteotomy of the proximal femur followed by early motion for the treatment of a hip ankylosed in poor position. Fock, in 1861, reported on the use of femoral head and neck resection in the treatment of severe osteoarthritis of the hip.[1,15]

In 1921 Sir Robert Jones described resection of the femoral head with attachment of the greater trochanter to the stump of the femoral neck as a treatment for ankylosis of the hip joint.[24] Girdlestone in 1943 reported in detail on the procedure which has come to bear his name and which he used since 1921 for the treatment of both tuberculosis and pyogenic arthritis of the hip.[7,9,15,25] This procedure seemed to work so well that its use was extended to the treatment of patients with unilateral osteoarthritis of the hip.[25] In 1945 Girdlestone described a series of 25 cases performed between 1924 and 1940.[8] This procedure remained popular for quite some time, especially in Great Britain, where 93 cases were reported in 1950 by Taylor,[24] and 400 procedures performed over a 30-year span were reviewed by Scott in 1963.[21]

With the development of the cup arthroplasty, the femoral endoprosthesis, and particularly the total hip replacement, the Girdlestone pseudarthrosis fell into relative disuse as a primary treatment for noninfectious conditions involving the hip. At the present time, it is perhaps most useful as a salvage procedure for infected hip arthroplasties.

Indications

Prior to the advent of total hip replacement arthroplasty, the Girdlestone pseudarthrosis was used quite commonly in Great Britain and on the Continent as a primary arthroplasty for a variety of conditions, as well as for the treatment of tuberculosis and sepsis of the hip. With the excellent and predictable results now obtainable following total hip replacement, its use as a primary arthroplasty has diminished greatly. Although there are still special circumstances in which it may prove of value as a primary procedure, today it is relied on most often as a salvage method for the failed total hip replacement or any other arthroplasty, especially when complicated by infection. The surgeon should be familiar with this operation as it is often a valuable alternative when other procedures cannot or should not be done.

In order to assess the indications for this procedure properly, its advantages and disadvantages must be kept clearly in mind. The advantages are that it provides good motion, elimination of pain, durable results, and eradication of infection; it also allows future conversion to total hip replacement in most instances. The disadvantages are that a prolonged period of traction and later partial weight-bearing are required for optimum results; instability and shortening are unavoidable, thereby

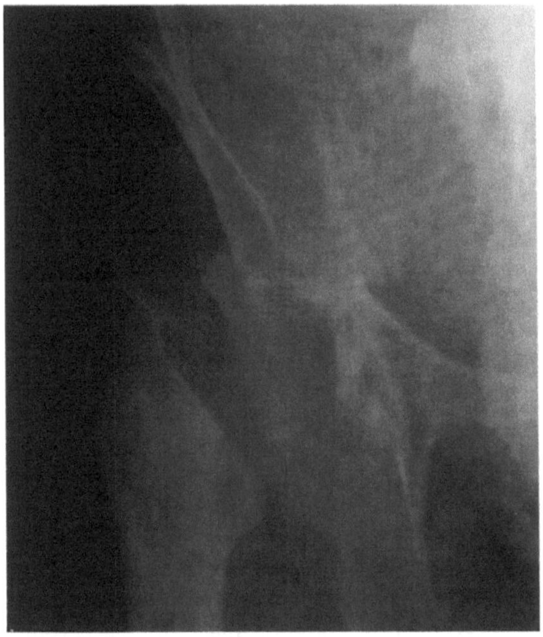

FIG. 12–1 R.P. X-ray film of a properly performed Girdlestone pseudarthrosis, with optimum postoperative management.

necessitating the use of a lift and external walking supports; and conversion to total hip replacement may be difficult.[2,5,6,11,13–19,22]

Use as a Primary Arthroplasty

Although the incidence of tuberculosis and septic arthritis of the hip have diminished considerably over the years, we are still occasionally called on to treat these conditions. The surgical treatment of acute sepsis generally involves incision, débridement, and drainage. In the chronic state, when some degree of osteomyelitis is generally present as well, more radical measures may be required. Under such circumstances, the Girdlestone pseudarthrosis may be indicated. It can usually be counted on to eradicate the infection and restore reasonable function to the afflicted joint. Under many circumstances, it is preferable to an arthrodesis. Although the pseudarthrosis is generally the definitive procedure when dealing with chronic septic arthritis, conversion to a total hip replacement might be considered at some later date if it is certain that the infection has been completely eliminated.[6,10,26]

At times one is called on to restore motion to a hip joint which has been spontaneously ankylosed because of arthritis, trauma, infection or a surgical arthrodesis. This may be because the joint itself has fused in an unacceptable position or because of knee or back pain secondary to the increased stresses placed on these regions. Although this can be accomplished by converting the fusion to a total hip arthroplasty, there are circumstances under which this may be either technically impossible or contraindicated. Such situations include cases in which there is marked deformity of the proximal femur, there is possible residual infection, the patient is young, or there are flaccid hip muscles secondary to poliomyelitis.[2,23]

Occasionally a severely debilitated patient develops contractures and deformities about the hip without true ankylosis. Proper nursing care and a more comfortable existence necessitate correction of these deformities. The Girdlestone pseudarthrosis, together with whatever soft tissue releases are required, may provide a satisfactory solution to this problem. There are also instances where a displaced or nonunited fracture of the femoral neck occurs in a patient who is not a candidate for open reduction and internal fixation, prosthetic replacement, bone grafting, or osteotomy. Here the Girdlestone procedure may be the treatment of choice.[6]

Rarely one encounters a situation in which an arthroplasty of the hip is required in a patient with severe deformities of the pelvis and the proximal femur which make it difficult or impossible to perform a total hip replacement or endoprosthetic replacement. This may be related to severe arthritic changes, ankylosing spondylitis, trauma, or congenital malformations. In these instances, when symptoms are sufficiently severe, a pseudarthrosis should be considered.[23] A pseudarthrosis may also be the procedure of choice in a variety of miscellaneous conditions, such as the Charcot joint, severe spastic disorders, and tumorous conditions about the hip (Fig. 12–2).

Salvage for Failure of Previous Joint Surgery

Perhaps the most important role for the Girdlestone pseudarthrosis today is for salvage of the infected arthroplasty or endoprosthesis. It may also be required for treatment of an established, infected nonunion of a transcervical fracture. Re-

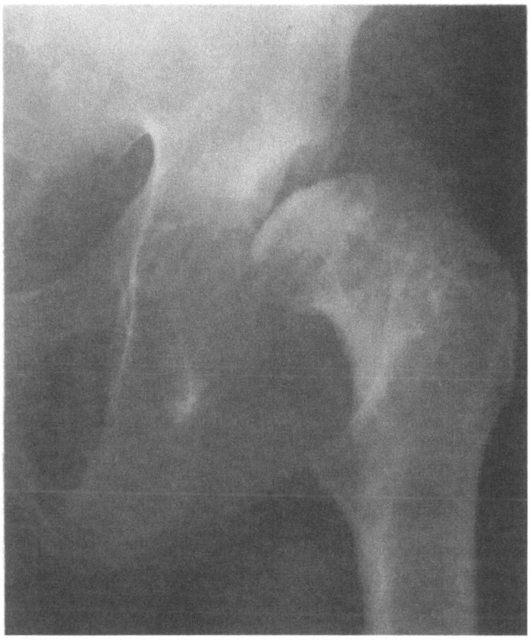

A

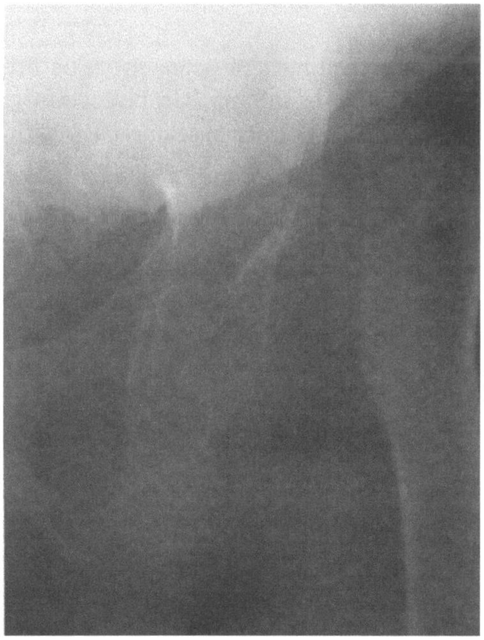

B

FIG. 12–2 F.S., a patient with acromegaly and marked destruction of the superior acetabulum. **A** Preoperative x-ray film. **B** Postoperative x-ray film.

moval of all foreign material and wide débridement of the involved bone and soft tissues is generally required to eradicate the infection. Under optimum circumstances, a total hip replacement might be performed at the same operative procedure. The incidence of recurrent infection, however, is considerably higher when a primary replacement is performed than when this replacement takes place at a later date. The minimum interval is usually considered to be 6 weeks, although many believe that more time should elapse prior to the replacement. If it is determined at the time of surgery that a total hip replacement will definitely take place in the near future, the initial procedure should be limited, with efforts made to preserve at least a part of the femoral neck and the acetabular margins (Fig. 12–3).

If it is thought unlikely that a total hip will be reimplanted in the future, the Girdlestone pseudarthrosis should be looked on as the definitive procedure. In such instances, the procedure is performed in such a way as to give the best functional results. This requires complete resection of the femoral neck at the intertrochanteric line, as well as removal of the prominent margins of the acetabulum (Figs. 12–4 and 12–5). Although this makes it more difficult to insert a total hip at a later date, it should also ensure a better result with the Girdlestone itself and make it less likely that such an additional procedure will be required. Frequently, it cannot be determined with certainty at the time of surgery whether conversion to a total hip will be required later. In these instances, we generally prefer to be less radical with excision of the superior acetabular margin but do not alter our technique as it concerns osteotomy at the intertrochanteric line.

In the majority of cases in which the Girdlestone pseudarthrosis has been used for the salvage of a septic arthroplasty or prosthesis, we allow at least 6 months, preferably a full year, to elapse prior to considering reimplantation of a total hip. It generally takes that long for the tissues to mature to the point that optimum results are obtained. If at the end of this time both patient and surgeon are dissatisfied with the result, conversion to a total hip can be undertaken once it has been determined that residual infection is no longer present.[3,5,11,16,20]

The Girdlestone pseudarthrosis may also be indicated for salvage of the failed total hip or other replacement arthroplasty without sepsis. This is especially true in the case of the multiply-operated hip. The loss of acetabular or femoral bone stock may be so great that the successful reimplantation of a total hip or other prosthesis is virtually impossible, even with bone grafts. Unfortunately, this

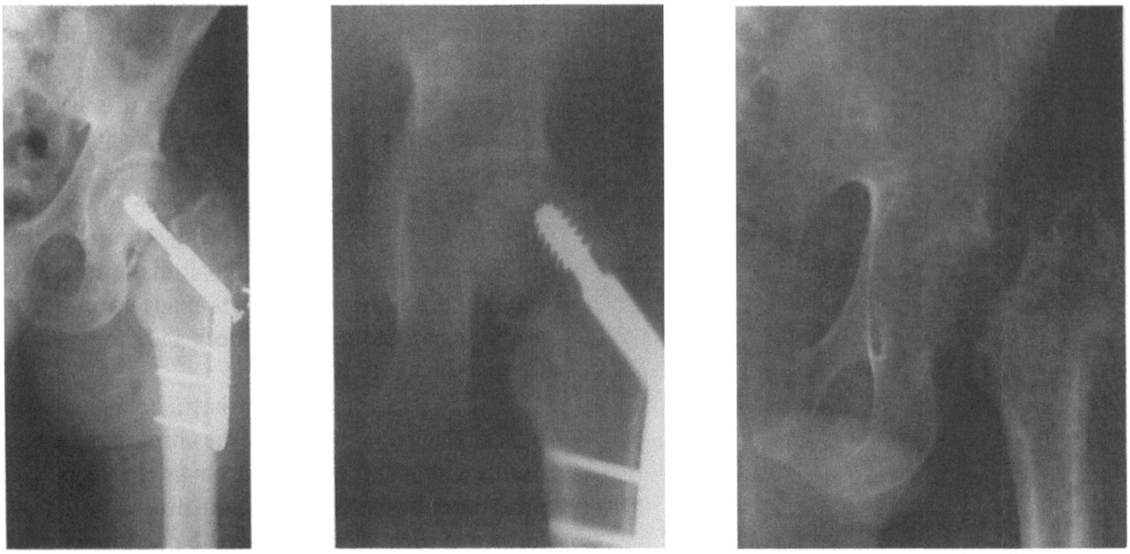

A B C

FIG. 12–3 T.W., a 23-year-old man with infected nonunion of a transcervical fracture. **A** Preoperative x-ray film. **B** Preoperative laminogram showing erosion of the femoral head around a compression screw. **C** Postoperative x-ray film following a modified Girdlestone procedure. Conversion to total hip replacement at a later date is anticipated.

situation is being encountered with increasing frequency[12] (Fig. 12–6).

Surgical Technique

The surgical technique varies considerably depending on whether the procedure is used as a primary arthroplasty or as a salvage procedure and whether infection is present.

For the treatment of acute pyogenic arthritis or tuberculosis of the hip, Girdlestone originally described a lateral transverse approach with excision of the abductor muscles and greater trochanter, as well as the head and neck of the femur. At times a medial approach with release of the adductors was also needed for adequate drainage. When used to treat sepsis in the presence of a hip ankylosed in satisfactory position, wide resection of the soft tissues alone was performed with-

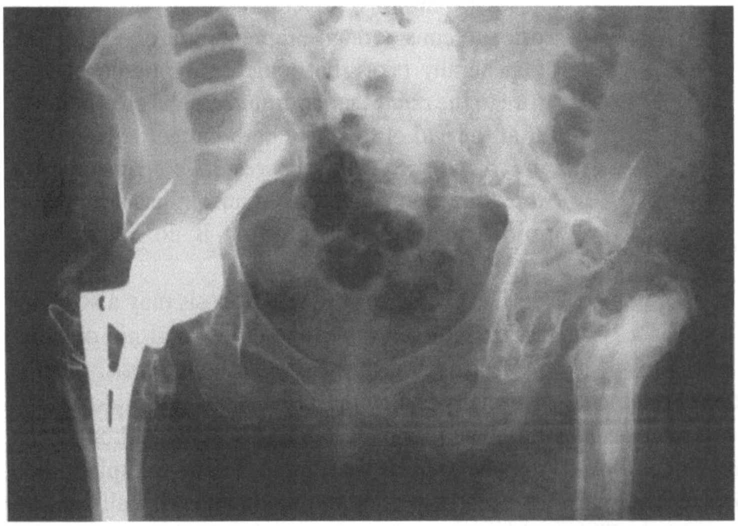

FIG. 12–4 A.P. Postoperative x-ray film of 74-year-old woman 3 years after removal of an infected noncemented prosthesis on the left. Note the presence of a well-functioning Tronzo prosthesis on the right 11 years after insertion.

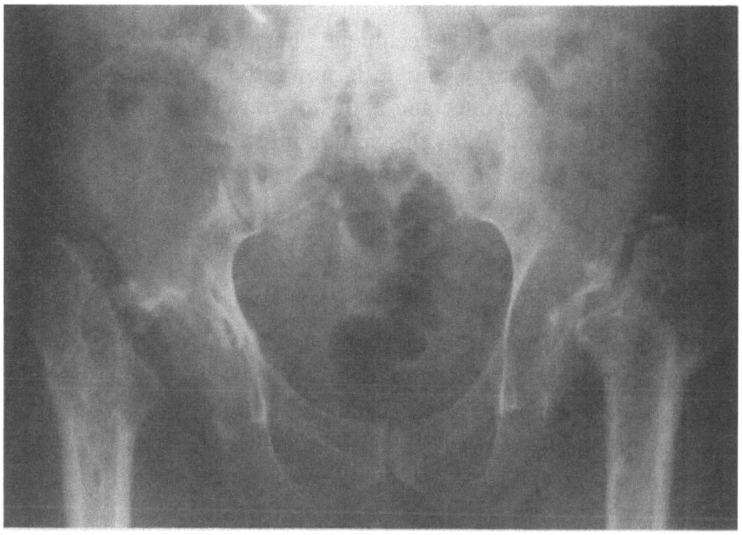

FIG. 12–5 R.P. Bilateral Girdlestone procedures following an infected Austin Moore prosthesis on the left and an infected total hip replacement on the right.

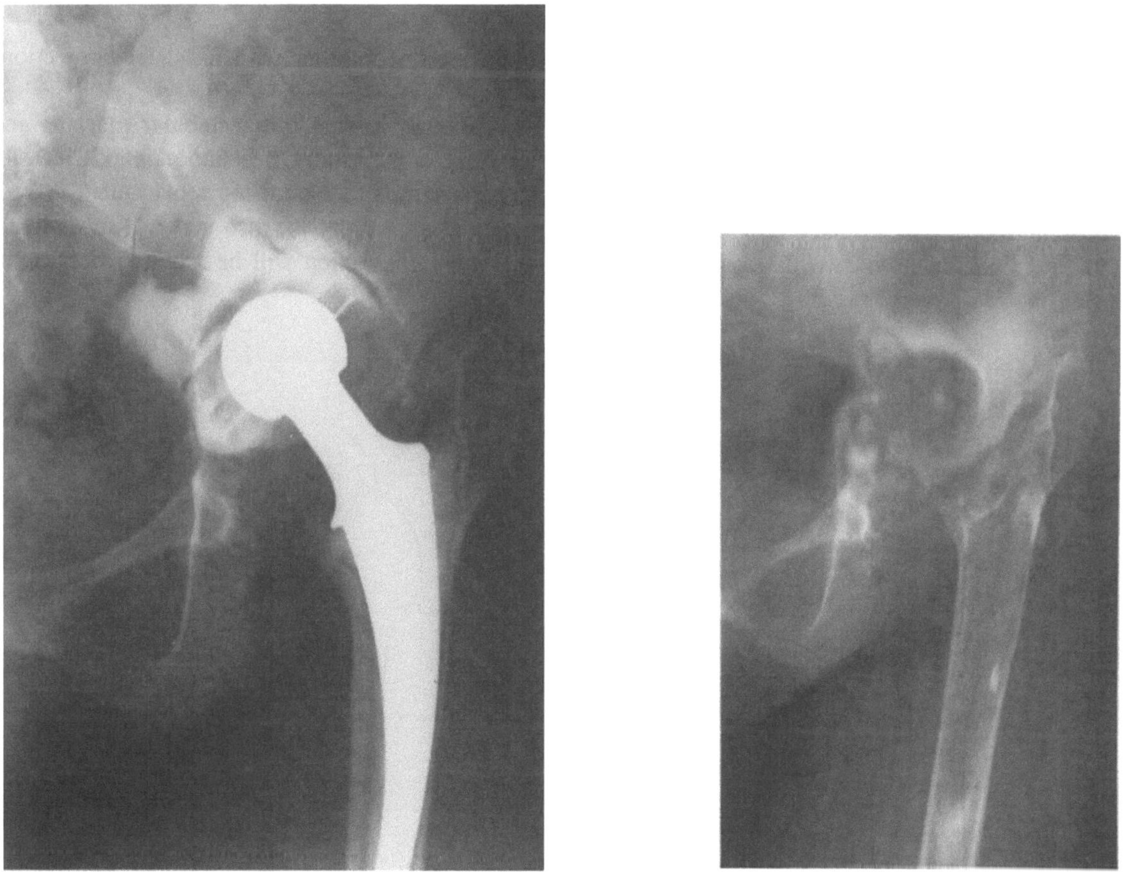

A B

FIG. 12–6 H.M. Marked loosening of femoral and acetabular components without sepsis in patient who had undergone two previous arthroplasties. **A** Preoperative x-ray film. **B** Postoperative x-ray film. An absence of bone stock, particularly in the acetabulum, led to a Girdlestone procedure rather than total hip replacement.

out removing the head and neck, thereby preserving the ankylosis.[7] The technique has been modified over the years, and it is now advised that the greater trochanter and abductor muscles should *not* be sacrificed, as this results in greater disability than when the procedure described below is used.[5,13,17,22-24]

Primary Arthroplasty (Classic Girdlestone)

An anterior iliofemoral or a posterolateral approach are preferred, although others can be used. Once adequate exposure of the acetabular margins and the femoral head and neck has been achieved, the neck is osteotomized, preferably using power instruments, in a line joining the lesser and greater trochanters. It is essential that a smooth, straight surface be left without any bony projections. The greater the surface area the better. Ideally, the bed is composed of healthy cancellous bone, and the femoral canal is not violated if it can be avoided. (When this procedure is used to revise a failed arthroplasty, this is not possible.) Any sharp margins projecting from the acetabular rim, especially superiorly and posteriorly, should be excised, either with power instruments, osteotomes, or rongeurs (Fig. 12–7). Cartilage remaining in the acetabulum is curetted or reamed down to bleeding bone. The primary goal at this point is quite simple: to leave two flat, parallel surfaces

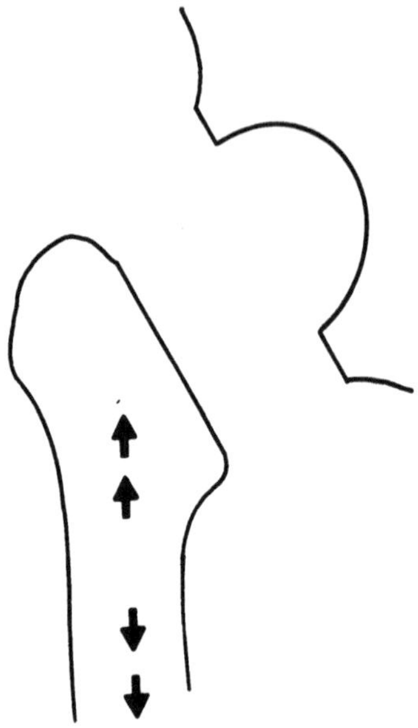

FIG. 12–8 Smooth, parallel surfaces should remain after bone resection. Skeletal traction is used to prevent proximal migration of the femur.

opposing one another with no sharp projections of bone (Figs. 12–8 to 12–10).

Although leaving the acetabular margins and a portion of the femoral neck indeed makes it easier to convert this to a total hip replacement arthroplasty at a later date, it also makes it more likely that such conversion will be required because of

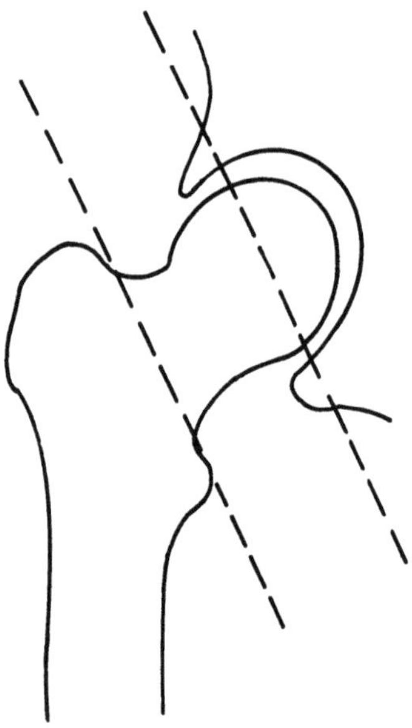

FIG. 12–7 Optimal lines of bone resection in the Girdlestone pseudarthrosis.

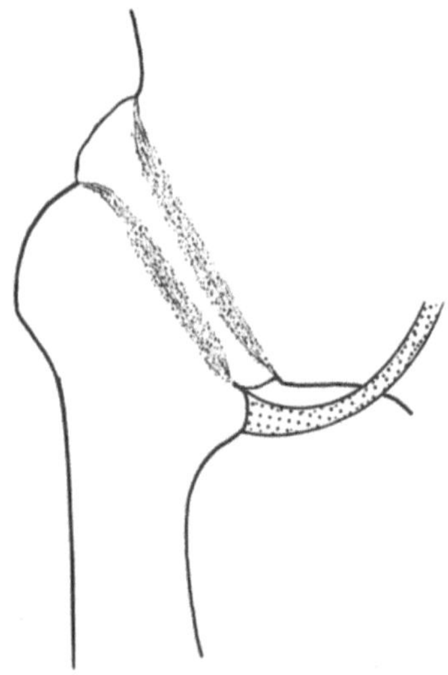

FIG. 12–9 The end-result should be two broad, smooth surfaces lying directly opposite one another and covered by durable fibrous tissue. A strong capsule and the iliopsoas tendon help prevent excessive proximal migration.

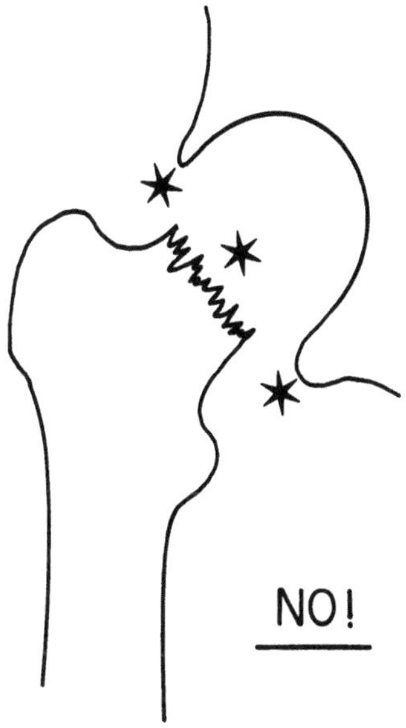

FIG. 12–10 Retention of the femoral neck and prominent acetabular margins frequently leads to poor results.

pain. The surgeon must therefore decide which approach to take in each case. If it seems certain that a conversion will be done later, sufficient bone stock is left behind. If such a conversion is unlikely, we recommend that the entire neck as well as the most prominent portion of the acetabular margin be removed. This generally leads to a good result with the Girdlestone, yet allows sufficient bone stock for later total hip implantation should this prove necessary. An allograft can always be screwed onto the acetabular roof if more bony containment is needed at the time of the revision to a total hip replacement.

Care is taken not to sacrifice unnecessarily the iliopsoas, the capsule, or other soft tissues. Although lateral transplantation of the lesser trochanter has been reported to decrease the tendency toward external rotation, this is neither completely effective nor usually required.[13] Some surgeons have combined the Girdlestone pseudarthrosis with various types of osteotomy of the proximal femur to increase the postoperative stability. Our own experience and a review of the literature suggest that this is unnecessary and probably contraindicated in the majority of cases.[2,10,14,15,17,19,26] We therefore do not describe the combined procedure. In those few cases in which additional stability is desired, an osteotomy at some later date might be considered.

The wound is closed in routine fashion. At the time of the procedure, a threaded Steinmann pin is inserted through the tibial tubercle to provide for postoperative traction in neutral rotation and slight abduction.

Revision of a Failed Arthroplasty, Ankylosis, or Treatment of Infection (Salvage Girdlestone)

The basic technique, as described above, is modified as needed for the treatment of sepsis, ankylosis, or salvage of a failed arthroplasty. When used to restore motion to a noninfected, ankylosed hip, no attempt is made to remove the remnants of the head which lie within the acetabulum. This bone actually serves a useful purpose in obliterating the dead space of the acetabulum and providing a broad, smooth, sloping surface on the lateral pelvic wall. If a good deal of the femoral neck has been preserved, it is resected by making two parallel cuts, one at the margin of the acetabulum and one at the intertrochanteric line. When little neck remains, a single cut may suffice.

When used in the treatment of a failed arthroplasty, especially with the presence of a femoral endoprosthesis, the posterior or posterolateral approach is preferred. This makes it easier to remove the femoral component and débride the medullary canal. This can usually be done without removing the greater trochanter. If the trochanter must be removed, it should be carefully reattached at the conclusion of the procedure; therefore it is best to be generous about cutting a large piece of trochanteric bone for ease in reattaching it.

In the presence of infection, a generous débridement is required to remove infected and devitalized bone and soft tissue as well as all foreign material. Abscess pouches should be sought in and around the inferior neck region. Using modern equipment, this can generally be done without the need for making a window in the femoral shaft (Fig. 12–11). When this is not possible without fear of damaging the femur, such a window should be made in the anterior upper third of the shaft. In the case of gross sepsis this may be preferred; moreover, it provides better drainage of the medullary canal (Fig. 12–12). Trochanteric reattachment is accomplished with heavy, absorbable sutures. Although a number of authors have advocated the use of ingress and egress tubes, others have found that they have not been beneficial and, in many instances, have led to a secondary infection with organisms more viru-

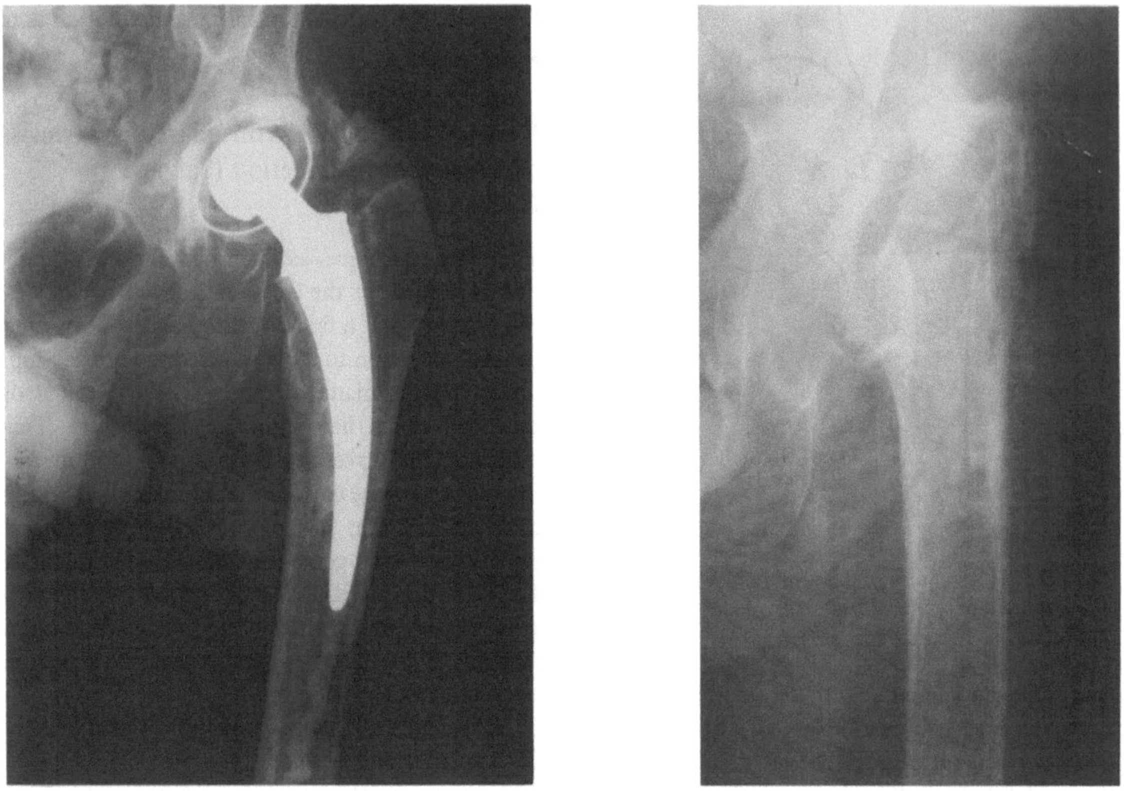

A B

FIG. 12–11 C.S. Infected and loosened total hip with extension of cement far down the medullary canal. **A** Preoperative x-ray film. **B** Postoperative x-ray film. Note that all the cement has been removed. Despite adequate traction, excessive proximal migration has occurred.

lent than those present initially.[4] The posterolateral approach is useful in that it provides dependent drainage. We prefer to close the wound very loosely with heavy wire sutures and leave three or four large Penrose drains in place.[3,5,11,16,17,19,20,21]

Postoperative Management

Proper postoperative management is perhaps just as important as meticulous attention to operative details. An adequate period of postoperative traction followed by a prolonged period of protected weight-bearing is necessary for optimum results. When done as a primary procedure, skeletal traction is employed for 4 to 6 weeks. The amount of weight generally varies from 15 to 30 pounds. The position of the limb is checked with portable x-ray films postoperatively to be sure that the proximal femur is held as far distally as possible. During this time the patient is encouraged to lie with the limb held in neutral rotation and to resist the natural tendency for external rotation. When this cannot be done actively, it can be controlled either by positioning the traction or by use of a soft boot with an adjustable horizontal cross-member designed specifically to limit external rotation of the limb.

Traction is followed by 4 to 6 months of minimal weight-bearing using crutches and an ischial weight-bearing caliper brace with the foot actually suspended a slight distance above the floor. This requires a lift on the opposite shoe. Some believe, however, that the added inconvenience of this type of brace is not warranted and rely on a more conventional ischial weight-bearing brace with the shoe touching the floor. At 6 months from surgery, the patient is gradually weaned from dependence on the brace, and later a simple cane replaces crutches. Range-of-motion and muscle-strengthening exercises are instituted during the early postoperative period and continued for quite some

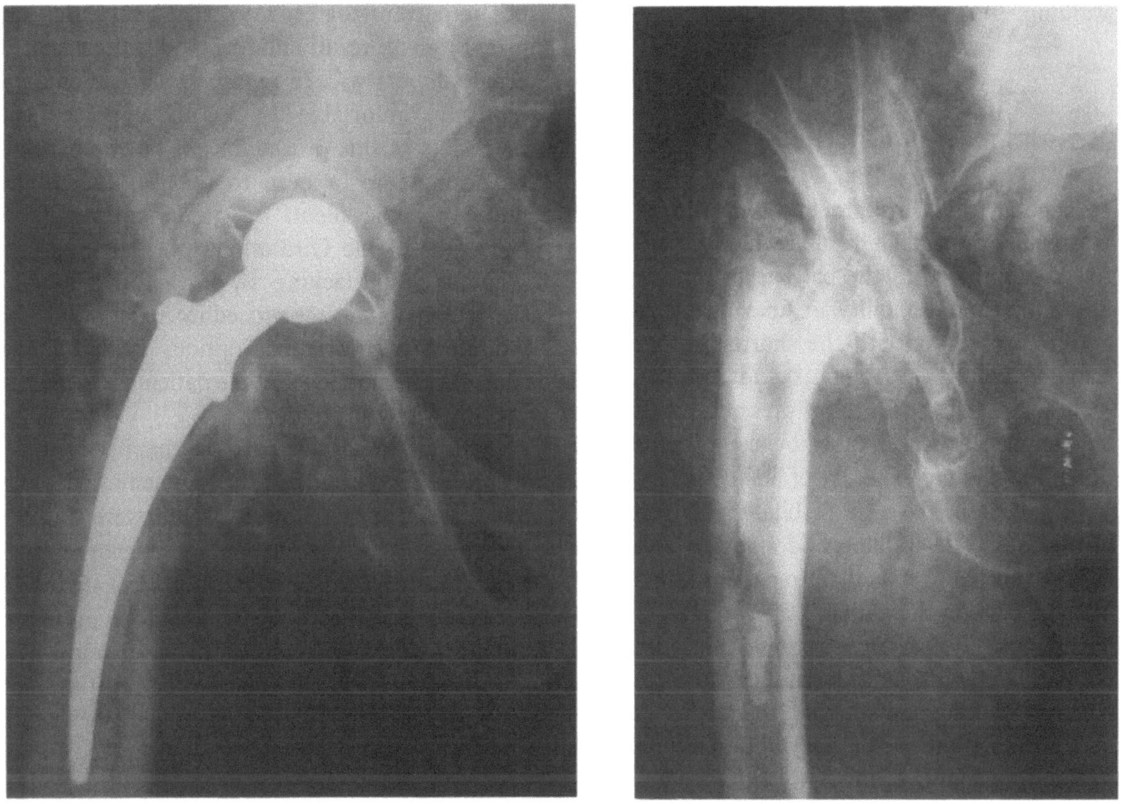

A B

FIG. 12–12 J.W. Chronically infected total hip with marked loosening of both components and intrapelvic protrusion of the acetabulum. **A** Preoperative x-ray film. **B** X-ray film 4 years after surgery. Infection was eradicated and satisfactory function achieved despite retained cement in the medullary canal and a prominent femoral neck. Note the lateral femoral window.

time. Gait training is especially important and should be started as soon as the traction has been discontinued.

In cases of revision surgery where a considerable amount of scarring is already present, it is possible to decrease the period of traction (to 3 to 4 weeks), and bracing (to 3 to 4 months) without detracting too much from the eventual result.

The objectives in the use of traction and bracing are basically threefold. If the cut surfaces of bone are held apart from one another, an adequate layer of fibrous tissue is more likely to form over both, thereby providing better articulating surfaces and a more ideal pseudarthrosis. If the bone ends are allowed to come into contact with one another, the formation of fibrous tissue may be impeded and areas of exposed bone may be left, giving rise to pain and poor function. Shortening is a natural consequence of this procedure with the mean loss of length being approximately 1.5 inches. It is diminished if the limb is held as far distally as possible during the maturation and contracture of the soft tissues about the joint. This also allows better stabilization of the joint, which, by the nature of the procedure performed, is inherently unstable.

If the patient has been properly informed of the advantages and disadvantages of this procedure, he will at this point be ready to accept the shortening and instability which are virtually unavoidable in exchange for a satisfactory range of pain-free motion. A shoe lift will be required as well as the use of a cane virtually all of the time. Occasionally, with the more stable hips the patient can walk short distances without the use of external supports, but he will have a pronounced abductor lurch. In some cases, patients feel more comfortable using two canes or crutches. Rarely, especially in the case of elderly patients, the use of a walker is required. The patient is able to sit comfortably for prolonged periods and should achieve a functional degree of standing and walking.[22-24]

Results

In general, the Girdlestone pseudarthrosis gives reasonably predictable results which generally do not deteriorate with the passage of time.[13,17,20,21] Shortening and instability are unavoidable features of this procedure, with the shortening generally ranging from 1 to 2 inches and averaging 1.5 inches. An abductor lurch is present, but this can be diminished considerably by use of a cane or other walking aid. The use of a shoe lift is necessary, except in the case of bilateral Girdlestone procedures. The walking and standing tolerance vary somewhat from patient to patient and depend in large part on the patient's age, weight, general health, and the presence of other musculoskeletal pathology. Prolonged sitting is comfortable, whereas walking and standing tolerances are limited, although they are usually within a functional range. Telescoping of the limb and a tendency toward external rotation are not uncommon. At times the degree of function is surprisingly good, as was demonstrated dramatically by a young roofer in his thirties who was able to return to his work without significant impairment, even though it required climbing ladders and walking on roofs.

There is divergent opinion as to whether the results of this procedure when used to salvage a failed arthroplasty equal those obtained when it is used as a primary operation. Generally they do not, especially if infection is present.

A matter of some concern is the disparity in results reported by different authors. The older literature as well as our own personal experience indicate that satisfactory results are obtained in approximately 80% of patients.[6,10,11,13,17-19,21,24,26] Some authors, however, report a lower incidence of satisfactory results.[3,20] We believe that this apparent disparity is based on a number of factors. "Satisfactory" is, of course, a very subjective term and is based on the opinions of both the patient and the examiner. It depends on what the procedure is being compared to and what is expected. If both the patient and the surgeon understand the advantages and disadvantages of this operation and are clear about its inherent limitations, the degree of acceptance increases considerably. Thus it is important to recognize that shortening and instability will result and a shoe elevation and external support will be required, a trade-off for a relatively comfortable hip. It is also important that the results of this procedure not be compared to the normal hip or even to the well-functioning total hip replacement. By such rigid standards, the results of the Girdlestone pseudarthrosis are of course found lacking. If, on the other hand, it is considered a salvage procedure and a reasonable option when most other options are no longer available, the surgeon and the patient are generally satisfied with the results.

Of prime importance are the manner in which the operation is done and the regimen of postoperative care that is followed. These were outlined in detail earlier in this chapter and are not repeated here. Unless meticulous attention is paid to both of these areas, the results will not be optimum. Attempts to retain remnants of the femoral neck or protruding acetabular margins and cutting short the postoperative traction or bracing frequently impair the results.[5,10,14,19,24,26]

Summary and Conclusions

Excisional arthroplasty of the femoral head and neck, although commonly referred to as the Girdlestone arthroplasty or Girdlestone pseudarthrosis, was actually in use in England and on the Continent prior to its popularization by Girdlestone. Before the advent of total hip replacement arthroplasty, it was considered a basic procedure for the treatment of both sepsis of the hip and a variety of nonseptic arthropathies. With the establishment of total hip replacement arthroplasty, its use has been quite limited. In selected circumstances it still holds a useful place as a primary arthroplasty. This is generally, however, when there is a contraindication to the performance of total hip replacement, other types of arthroplasty, or fusion. In cases of active sepsis, it is often the procedure of choice. Its major role today, however, is as a salvage procedure for the infected hip arthroplasty or prosthesis, or infected nonunion. In such instances it may be the definitive procedure, or it may be an intermediate stage designed to eliminate infection and provide a satisfactory temporary functional result until an exchange hip replacement can be performed at a later date. Occasionally, it is required as salvage for the noninfected failed total hip in which insufficient bone stock remains for the performance of another total hip replacement.

The procedure itself is not complicated. It is, however, essential that the operation be performed properly so as to provide two smooth, parallel articulating surfaces. Attention to postoperative details is also essential and includes traction for 3 to 6 weeks followed by protected weight-bearing, generally with the use of crutches and an ischial weight-bearing brace or caliper, for 3 to 6 months.

The advantages of this procedure are that it may be called on when other types of arthroplasties are contraindicated; it gives a good range of motion; it eliminates pain; the results are durable; and if necessary it can be converted at some later date to a total hip replacement. The disadvantages are that it requires a protracted period of postoperative traction and partial weight-bearing; it results in shortening, necessitating the use of a lift; it leaves the patient with definite instability, resulting in an abductor lurch and the need for at least a single cane; and the duration of standing and walking is more limited than in total hip replacement.

If the procedure and postoperative care are done properly, and if both the surgeon and the patient know what to expect, the results are generally considered satisfactory. In short, this procedure is seldom our first choice as a primary arthroplasty but may be very useful when other procedures are not possible or are contraindicated. Its primary role today is that of a salvage procedure for the failed hip arthroplasty, especially when infection is present. In this capacity it plays a very useful role.

References

1. Barton, J. R.: On the treatment of ankylosis by the formation of artificial joints—a new operation. North Am. Med. Surg. J., 3:279, 1827.
2. Batchelor, J. S.: Excision of the femoral head and neck in cases of ankylosis and osteoarthritis of the hip. Proc. R. Soc. Med., 38:689, 1944–45.
3. Bittar, E. A., Petty, W.: Girdlestone arthroplasty for infected total hip arthroplasty. Clin. Orthop., 170:83, 1982.
4. Canner, G. C., Steinberg, M. E., Heppenstall, R. B., Balderston, R.: The infected total hip prosthesis. J. Bone Joint Surg., 66A:1393, 1984.
5. Clegg, J.: The results of pseudarthrosis after removal of an infected total hip prosthesis. J. Bone Joint Surg., 59B;298, 1977.
6. Collis, D. K., Johnston, R. C.: Complete femoral head and neck resection. J Bone Joint Surg., 53A:396, 1971.
7. Girdlestone, G. R.: Acute pyogenic arthritis of the hip: operation giving free access and effective drainage. Lancet, 1:419, 1943.
8. Girdlestone, G. R.: Pseudarthrosis: discussion on the treatment of unilateral osteoarthritis of the hip joint. Proc. R. Soc. Med., 38:363, 1945.
9. Girdlestone, G. R.: Acute pyogenic arthritis of the hip: an operation giving free access and effective drainage. Clin. Orthop., 170:3, 1982 (reprinted).
10. Gruca, A.: The treatment of quiescent tuberculosis of the hip joint by excision and "dynamic" osteotomy. J. Bone Joint Surg., 32B—174, 1950.
11. Hansen, S. T., Taylor, T. K. F.: Resection of the head and neck of the femur in the management of hip-joint infections: an analysis of forty-two cases. J. Bone Joint Surg., 53A:396, 1971.
12. Harris, W. H., White, R. E.: Resection arthroplasty for nonseptic failure of total hip arthroplasty. Clin. Orthop., 171:62, 1982.
13. Haw, C. S., Gray, D. H.: Excision arthroplasty of the hip. J. Bone Joint Surg., 58B:44, 1976.
14. Milch, H.: The resection-angulation operation for hip joint disabilities. J. Bone Joint Surg., 37A:699, 1955.
15. Muller, K. H.: Resection of the femoral head and neck and resection-angulation osteotomy. In: *Surgery of the Hip Joint* (Tronzo, R. G., ed.). Philadelphia, Lea & Febiger, 1973, pp. 644–656.
16. Muller, M. E.: Preservation of septic total hip replacement versus Girdlestone operation. In: *The Hip: Proceedings of the Second Open Scientific Meeting of the Hip Society.* St. Louis, Mosby, 1974, p. 308.
17. Murray, W. R., Lucas, D. B., Inman, V. T.: Femoral head and neck resection. J. Bone Joint Surg., 46A:1184, 1964.
18. Nelson, C. L.: Femoral head and neck excision arthroplasty. Orthop. Clin. North Am., 2:127, 1971.
19. Parr, P. L., Croft, C., Enneking, W. F., et al.: Resection of the head and neck of the femur with and without angulation osteotomy: a followup study of thirty-eight patients. J. Bone Joint Surg., 53A:935, 1971.
20. Petty, W., Goldsmith, S.: Resection arthroplasty following infected total hip arthroplasty. J. Bone Joint Surg., 62A:889, 1980.
21. Scott, J. C.: Pseudarthrosis of the hip. Clin. Orthop., 31:31, 1963.
22. Somerville, E. W.: Girdlestone pseudarthrosis of the hip. In: *Operative Surgery, Orthopaedics Part I* (Rob, C., and Smith, R., eds.). Philadelphia, Lippincott, 1969.

23. Taylor, R. G.: Girdlestone's pseudarthrosis of the hip joint in patients suffering from rheumatoid arthritis and ankylosing spondylitis. In: Proceedings of the Ninth Congress of SICOT, September 1963, pp. 152–157.
24. Taylor, R. G.: Pseudarthrosis of the hip joint. J. Bone Joint Surg., 32B:161, 1950.
25. Trueta, J.: *Gathorne Robert Girdlestone.* Oxford, Oxford University Press, 1971.
26. Tuli, S. M., Mukherjee, S. K.: Excision arthroplasty for tuberculosis and pyogenic arthritis of the hip. J. Bone Joint Surg., 63B:29, 1981.

Index

G

MIX
Papier aus verantwortungsvollen Quellen
Paper from responsible sources
FSC® C105338

If you have any concerns about our products,
you can contact us on
ProductSafety@springernature.com

In case Publisher is established outside the EU,
the EU authorized representative is:
Springer Nature Customer Service Center GmbH
Europaplatz 3, 69115 Heidelberg, Germany

Printed by Libri Plureos GmbH
in Hamburg, Germany